AF788861

Veterinary Virology

Veterinary Virology

Edited by **Mel Roth**

SYRAWOOD
PUBLISHING HOUSE
New York

Published by Syrawood Publishing House,
750 Third Avenue, 9th Floor,
New York, NY 10017, USA
www.syrawoodpublishinghouse.com

Veterinary Virology
Edited by Mel Roth

© 2016 Syrawood Publishing House

International Standard Book Number: 978-1-68286-318-3 (Hardback)

This book contains information obtained from authentic and highly regarded sources. Copyright for all individual chapters remain with the respective authors as indicated. All chapters are published with permission under the Creative Commons Attribution License or equivalent. A wide variety of references are listed. Permission and sources are indicated; for detailed attributions, please refer to the permissions page and list of contributors. Reasonable efforts have been made to publish reliable data and information, but the authors, editors and publisher cannot assume any responsibility for the validity of all materials or the consequences of their use.

The publisher's policy is to use permanent paper from mills that operate a sustainable forestry policy. Furthermore, the publisher ensures that the text paper and cover boards used have met acceptable environmental accreditation standards.

Trademark Notice: Registered trademark of products or corporate names are used only for explanation and identification without intent to infringe.

Printed in China.

Contents

Preface

Virology mainly focuses on the study of viruses which have a significant impact on living organisms. This book on veterinary virology provides comprehensive insights into various diseases which affect animals, like rhabdovirus, pestivirus, foot and mouth disease virus, etc. Suitable for the students and researchers of veterinary medicine and veterinary pathology, it will be a useful tool in comprehending various viral infections and their treatment. The book will also provide innovative topics for research which interested readers can take up.

This book is a comprehensive compilation of works of different researchers from varied parts of the world. It includes valuable experiences of the researchers with the sole objective of providing the readers (learners) with a proper knowledge of the concerned field. This book will be beneficial in evoking inspiration and enhancing the knowledge of the interested readers.

In the end, I would like to extend my heartiest thanks to the authors who worked with great determination on their chapters. I also appreciate the publisher's support in the course of the book. I would also like to deeply acknowledge my family who stood by me as a source of inspiration during the project.

Editor

1

Lack of a type-2 glycosyltransferase in the fish pathogen *Flavobacterium psychrophilum* determines pleiotropic changes and loss of virulence

David Pérez-Pascual[1,2*], Esther Gómez[1] and José A Guijarro[1]

Abstract

Flavobacterium psychrophilum is an important fish pathogen, responsible for Cold Water Disease, with a significant economic impact on salmonid farms worldwide. In spite of this, little is known about the bacterial physiology and pathogenesis mechanisms, maybe because it is difficult to manipulate, being considered a fastidious microorganism. Mutants obtained using a Tn*4351* transposon were screened in order to identify those with alteration in colony morphology, colony spreading and extracellular proteolytic activity, amongst other phenotypes. A *F. psychrophilum* mutant lacking gliding motility showed interruption of the FP1638 locus that encodes a putative type-2 glycosyltransferase (from here on referred to as *fpgA* gene, *Flavobacterium psychrophilum* glycosyltransferase). Additionally, the mutant also showed a decrease in the extracellular proteolytic activity as a consequence of down regulation in the *fpgA* mutant background of the *fpp2-fpp1* operon promoter, responsible for the major extracellular proteolytic activity of the bacterium. The protein glycosylation profile of the parental strain showed the presence of a 22 kDa glycosylated protein which is lost in the mutant. Complementation with the *fpgA* gene led to the recovery of the wild-type phenotype. LD_{50} experiments in the rainbow trout infection model show that the mutant was highly attenuated. The pleiotropic phenotype of the mutant demonstrated the importance of this glycosyltranferase in the physiology and virulence of the bacterium. Moreover, the fpgA mutant strain could be considered a good candidate for the design of an attenuated vaccine.

Introduction

Flavobacterium psychrophilum is a Gram-negative bacterium and it is a member of the *Cytophaga-Flavabacterium-Bacteroides* (CFB) group. This microorganism is the etiological agent of Cold Water Disease (CWD) (as well as rainbow trout fry syndrome), one of the most important infectious pathologies, causing significant economic losses in salmonids on fish farms worldwide. Outbreaks occur at temperatures below 14 °C and mainly affect fingerlings. Currently there are no efficient commercial vaccines to protect against CWD. Besides, other approaches such as the use of immunostimulants, probiotics or lytic bacteriophages do not provide sufficient infection control. Therefore, disease management is based on fish monitoring strategies and the use of antimicrobial therapy [1,2].

In spite of being considered a fastidious bacterium because it is difficult to isolate and manipulate [3], several advances have been reported during the last few years in culture [4], experimental infection techniques [5], typing [6-9], molecular diagnosis [10-15] and genomics [16]. Furthermore, genetic manipulation systems based on transposition mutagenesis [17] and disruption of the specific genes by homologous recombination have been developed [18]. However, the mechanisms of pathogenicity of this bacterium are still unknown and little data exist about the genetic basis of virulence [19,20].

Even though protein glycosylation was once considered to be a specifically eukaryotic phenomenon, nowadays it is clear that it is widespread in prokaryotes [21,22]. In fact,

* Correspondence: david.perez@jouy.inra.fr
[1]Área de Microbiología, Departamento de Biología Funcional, Facultad de Medicina, IUBA, Universidad de Oviedo, 33006 Oviedo, Spain
[2]Present address: INRA, Institut Micalis, Équipe Peptides et Communication Bactérienne, Domaine de Vilvert, bâtiment 526, 78352 Jouy-en-Josas cedex, France

several glycoproteins described in Gram-negative pathogenic bacteria have been associated with virulence [23,24]. In the case of *F. psychrophilum,* a glycosylated protein, OmpA, has been purified and characterized [25,26]. In addition, 35 genes encoding putative glycosyltransferases have been identified in the genome of strain JIP02/86 [16]. Moreover, some members of the CFB group showed glycosylated proteins [27,28]. In particular, *Bacteroides fragilis,* forming a relevant part of the human intestinal microbiota, presented, at least eight glycoproteins which are related to the competitive colonization of mammalian intestines [28,29]. All of this suggests a relevant role of glycosyltransferases in the biology of bacteria belonging to this group.

The ability of pathogenic bacteria to cause disease depends to a large extent on the expression of specific gene-encoding factors which help them to invade the host tissues, develop the infection and evade host defenses. Amongst other characteristics, bacterial motility [30-32] and extracellular proteolytic activity [33] are considered to be involved in the infection caused by different Gram-negative bacteria. With the aim of achieving a deeper insight into the pathogenesis mechanisms of *F. psychrophilum,* a set of mutants deficient in gliding motility and extracellular proteolytic activity were isolated using the Tn*4351*-mutagenesis system [19]. In this study, a mutant with a change in the FP1638 locus was further analyzed. The interrupted gene, which encodes a type-2 glycosyltransferase, was found to be involved in the glycosylation of a 22 kDa protein. The modification of protein glycosylation in the mutant strain caused, amongst other effects, high attenuation of the virulence of the bacterium.

Material and methods

Bacterial strains and growth conditions

The strains, plasmid and primers used in this study are listed in Table 1. *Escherichia coli* strains S17-1 *λpir* [34] and BW19851 [35] were used to transfer DNA into *F. psychrophilum* THC02/90. *E. coli* strains were grown at 37 °C in 2 × TY medium (10 g of tryptone per liter, 10 g of yeast extract per liter, 5 g of NaCl per liter) with 20 g of agar per liter added for solid medium. *F. psychrophilum* THC02/90 was grown at 12 °C or 18 °C in nutrient broth (NB; Pronadisa, Madrid, Spain) or NBF [36]. Nutrient agar (NA: NB containing 1.5 g of agar/L), or nutrient agar charcoal (NAC; NA supplemented with 0.05% activated charcoal), were used for solid cultures as previously described [36]. Growth in liquid culture was carried out at 250 rpm and 12 °C and determined by measuring OD_{525nm} at different times. Stock cultures were kept in NB containing 25% glycerol at −80 °C. To observe colony spreading, *F. psychrophilum* strains were grown as previously described in 1/6NA [37]. Extracellular proteolytic activity on solid medium was visualized using NBF containing 1.5 g/mL of agar and supplemented with 0.75% gelatin [19]. Azocasein assays were performed according to Secades et al., [38] where one unit of enzyme activity [32] was defined as the amount that yielded an increase in the OD_{420nm} of 0.01 in two hours at 30 °C. For selective growth of *E. coli* S17-1 *λpir,* 50 µg/mL streptomycin was used and transformants were selected with 100 µg/mL ampicillin. Selection of *F. psychrophilum*

Table 1 Bacterial strains, plasmids and primers used in this study

Plasmid, bacterial strain or primer	Description or sequence	Source or reference
Plasmids[a]		
pEP4351	*Ori* R6K dependent protein pir,; RP4 oriT; Cm^r Tc^r (Em^r); Tn*4351* vector transfer.	[39]
pCP23	ColE1 ori, (pCP1 ori), Ap^r (Tc^r), *E. coli–F. psychrophilum* shuttle plasmid	[40]
pCP23-fpgA	*FP1638* gene, derived from pCP23.	This study
pCP23-Gfpp2	pCP23-G carrying *fpp2-fpp1* promoter	[41]
Bacterial strains		
F. psychrophilum		
THC02/90	Wild-type.	[42]
$fpgA^-$	*FP1638* mutant created by Tn*4351* transposition.	This study
fpgA+	Mutant ΔFP1638 carrying pCP23-FP1638 plasmid, complemented strain.	This study
THC02/90-G	THC02/90 strain carrying pCP23-G plasmid	[41]
THC02/90 -fpp2	THC02/90 strain carrying pCP23-Gfpp2 plasmid	[41]
$fpgA^-$ -fpp2	ΔFP1638 strain carrying pCP23-Gfpp2 plasmid	[41]
E. coli		
S17-1 *λpir*	*λpir hsdR pro thi*; RP4-2 Tc::Mu Km::Tn*7*	[34]
BW19851	RP4-2*tet*::Mu-1*kan*::Tn*7* integrant; _*uidA*:: *pir_ recA1 hsdR17 creB510 endA1 zbf-5 thi*	[35]
Primers[b]		
26-F	5'ACTG**GGATCC**AGTTTTAAGCC CGCAAA 3'	This study
26-R	5' ACTG**CTGCAG**CAATGAACTT CGTCTTG 3'	This study
TN-1	5' GGACCTACCTCATAGACAA 3'	[19]
IS4351-F	5' TCAGAGTGAGAGAAAGGG 3'	[19]
promfpp2-F	5' ATCA**GGATCC**GAGCACTACAC TTTCTAGA 3'	[41]
promfpp2-R	5' GATT**GGATCC**TGTTCGGTAGT GTAGCA 3'	[41]

[a]Antibiotic resistance phenotypes: ampicillin, Ap^r; tetracycline, Tc^r; erythromycin, Emr[b]. Antibiotic resistance phenotypes and other features listed in parentheses are those expressed by *F. psychrophilum* but not by *E. coli*.
[b]Restriction sites for cloning are in bold.

transconjugants was carried out with 10 μg/mL erythromycin and 10 μg/mL tetracycline.

DNA technology

Genomic DNA extractions were performed with the Gen Elute Bacterial DNA (Sigma-Aldrich Co., St-Louis, MO, USA) extraction kit. Plasmid DNA was purified with the Gen Elute Plasmid miniprep (Sigma-Aldrich Co.) kit.

PCR amplification products were separated on 1.5% agarose gels and bands were purified with the Illustra™ GFX, PCR DNA and the Gel Band Purification Kit gel extraction system.

Identification of Tn*4351* interrupted locus and sequencing of the surrounding DNA region

The insertion of Tn*4351* into the genome of the *fpgA* mutant strain was confirmed by Southern blot analysis. Total DNA from the mutant and parental strains was isolated and digested with *Hind*III and *Xba*I restriction enzymes. After agarose gel electrophoresis, DNA fragments were transferred to a nylon membrane (Amershan Bioscience, Uppsala, Sweden) and fixed with UV irradiation. A DIG DNA labeling and detection kit (Roche, Basel, Switzerland) was used to prepare the probe and to perform hybridization. As a probe, a 6.2 kb *Sal*I fragment from pEP4351 containing Tn*4351* transposon was used [19].

To isolate and sequence the genomic DNA flanking the Tn*4351* chromosomal insertion, DNA of the mutant strain was digested with *Hind*III followed by a re-ligation process. The resulting circular molecules were used as a template to amplify by inverse PCR the sequences adjacent to the Tn*4351* insertion site using a specific pair of primers TN-1/IS4351-F (Table 1) and the Certamp long amplification kit (Biotools B&M Laboratories, Madrid, Spain).

Automated fluorescence sequencing of the PCR amplified products was performed at the Oviedo University DNA analysis facility using BigDye 3.1 Terminator chemistry on an ABI PRISM 3100 Genetic Analyzer platform (Applied Biosystems, CA, USA). Sequences were compared to databases using the Basic Local Alignment Search Tool (BLAST) from the National Center for Biotechnology Information (NCBI).

Complementation of the *fpgA* gene mutation

To complement the fpgA mutant, the DNA sequence corresponding to the encoding gene was amplified from the parental strain by PCR, using 26-F and 26-R primers and the Expand Long Template PCR System (Roche), obtaining a fragment of 1105 pb (Table 1). *Bam*HI and *Pst*I restriction sites were introduced into the sequences of 26-F and 26-R respectively, in order to clone the PCR product into the plasmid pCP23 that has promoter activity [41] (Table 1). The resulting plasmid was designated pCP23-fpgA (Table 1). Transfer of pCP23-fpgA to *F. psychrophilum* was carried out by conjugation as previously described [17] and pCP23-fpgA was recovered from the transconjugants, digested with *Bam*HI and *Pst*I and analyzed by agarose gel electrophoresis to confirm the presence of the insert.

Transcriptional fusion analysis based on *gfp* reporter gene

The previously constructed pCP23-Gfpp2 (Table 1), derived from the GFP-based reporter vector pCP23-G [41], was used for the analysis of the transcriptional activity of the *fpp2-fpp1* operon [18] in the context of wild-type and fpgA$^-$ strains. The pCP23-Gfpp2 plasmid was introduced by transformation in *E. coli* S17 *λpir* and further conjugated into *F. psychrophilum* fpgA$^-$ and wild-type strains as described by Álvarez et al. [17], originating the fpgA$^-$-fpp2 and THC02/90-fpp2 strains (Table 1). For flow cytometry analysis, 5 mL of NB supplemented with tetracycline were inoculated with 50 μL of mid-exponential-phase cultures from fpgA$^-$-fpp2 and THC02/90-fpp2 strains. The THC02/90-G strain (Table 1) was used as the fluorescence emission negative control. They were incubated at 12 °C in NB supplemented with 10 mM $CaCl_2$ in an orbital shaker at 250 rpm. Then, early-stationary phase cultures were washed once with PBS and resuspended in 500 μL of PBS prior to fluorescence emission analysis. Promoter expression quantification was assessed in a flow cytometer (Beckman Coulter Cytomics FC 500) with 488 Ar and 633 HeNe lasers. Green fluorescence was detected on FL-14 channel (505–545 nm) and 10 000 events were acquired from each sample. All cultures were analyzed in triplicate. Fluorescence emission, with and without calcium in culture media, was assessed in a Student's *t*-test. Differences were considered significant when p-value < 0.05.

LD_{50} determination

For LD_{50} experiments rainbow trout (*Oncorhynchus mykiss*) weighing between 5 and 7 g were kept in 60-liter tanks at 14 ± 1 °C in continually flowing dechlorinated water.

On arrival at the aquarium, the fish were acclimatized to experimental conditions and 5% were selected randomly and screened for any bacteria. Samples from liver, muscle, blood and spleen were taken and plated onto permissive media (TSA and NAC) and incubated at 18 °C for 72 h. If bacterial growth was observed in these samples, the whole batch of fish was discarded for further experiments. Cultures of *F. psychrophilum* parental and fpgA$^-$ strains were grown to exponential phase, harvested by centrifugation and washed twice with PBS. Cells were resuspended in PBS and serial dilutions were prepared. Groups of 10 fish were challenged by intramuscular injection of 50 μL of dilutions containing 10^3-10^9 colony forming units (CFU) for the parental strain and 10^6-10^9 CFU for the fpgA$^-$ mutant strain, and LD_{50} was calculated ten days post-infection according to the method of Reed and Muench [43]. In the control group 10 fish were injected with 50 μL of PBS. To verify the presence of *F. psychrophilum* in dead fish, samples obtained from muscle (the injection zone), brain, liver and eyes were plated onto NAC plates (supplemented with the corresponding antibiotic for mutant strain) and incubated for 72 h at 18 °C. The assay was qualitative and was performed in order to confirm that the dead fish had a massive presence of the bacterium in different organs due to the development of septicemia. After culture, PCR was routinely used for the identification of the bacterium, using specific primers [13,19]. The results are the average of two independent experiments. Animal experiments were performed in accordance with the European legislation governing animal welfare, and they were authorized and supervised by the Animal Experimentation Ethics Committee of Universidad de Oviedo.

Analysis of protein glycosylation

The wild-type, fpgA$^-$ and fpgA$^-$ carrying pCP23-fpgA plasmid (from here, fpgA$^+$) strains were grown in NB for 120 h at 12 °C, harvested by centrifugation (10 000 rpm, 10 min) and washed twice with Tris–HCl (50 mM pH 6.8). Pelleted cells were re-suspended in 1 mL of the same buffer and cells were broken by ten 12-s sonication with 1 min intervals in an ice bath. Then, the suspension was centrifuged (12 000 rpm, 20 min, 4 °C) and aliquots of the supernatant were used for protein analysis by 14% SDS-PAGE according to the Laemmli methods. Proteins were visualized by silver and Coomassie brilliant blue staining. Glycosylated proteins were detected using the Pro-Q Emerald 300 glycoprotein staining kit (Life Technologies, Carlsbad, CA, USA), according to the manufacturer's instructions. The effect of proteinase K (50 μg/mL) and trypsin (12 μg/mL) on the glycosylated proteins was assessed by incubation of the total protein extract from the wild-type strain at 60 °C for 1 h before separation by SDS-PAGE. When a mixture of both enzymes was used, the reaction with proteinase K was carried out first. Then, an additional incubation in the presence of trypsin was performed under the same conditions. Controls without the presence of proteases were carried out simultaneously in all cases.

Genetic analysis

The BLAST program was used to compare protein sequences and Simple Modular Architecture Research Tools (SMART) [44] for detecting conserved domains. MotifScan software from MyHits was used to identify the motifs present in each sequence. The carbohydrate-active enzymes (CAZy) [45] bank was used to classify the glycosyltransferase. The ProtParam program [46] was used for molecular mass computation and SignalP3.0 [47] to predict the possible location of a signal peptide cleavage site.

Results

Analysis of the Tn*4351*-disrupted sequence of *fpgA*

A set of *F. psychrophilum* mutants were obtained by Tn*4351* insertional mutagenesis as described by Álvarez et al. [17] and then in order to study the gliding-virulence relationship, a mutant strain, defective in colony spreading, was further analyzed. Southern blot analysis of this mutant revealed a single transposon insertion in its genome (data not shown). The DNA sequence surrounding the transposon insertion was obtained by inverse PCR as described by Álvarez et al. [19]. The disrupted sequence for the isogenic mutant corresponds to the FP1638 locus (Gen Bank accession no. NC_009613) of the *F. psychrophilum* genome [16], a gene of 965 bp that encodes for a 319-amino-acid protein with a predicted mass of 38 081 Da. The transposon was inserted after nucleotide 774. The protein function corresponds to a type-2 glycosyltransferase since it presents a catalytic domain between amino acids 4 and 178, characteristic of the subfamily 2 glycosyltransferases [16]. It also shows a high level of similarity with this kind of enzyme from a variety of species such as *Dyadobacter fermentans* DSM 18053 (Gen Bank accession no. YP_003 088235.1), *Methanosarcina barkeri* Fusaro strain WcaA (Gen Bank accession no. YP_303801.1) and *Pelosinus fermentas* (Gen Bank accession no. WP_0079027).

The gene appears in the same orientation as FP1637 (Gen Bank accession no. NC_009613.3) and is separated from it by 4 bp in the genome of strain JIP02/86 of *F. psychrophilum* [16]. An identical situation was defined by PCR and further sequencing for the *F. psychrophilum* THCO2/90 strain. FP1637 codifies a protein of unknown function which exhibits high sequence identity to predicted WbhW protein of *E. coli,* similar to a glycosyltransferase enzyme [16]. A sigma 70-like promoter sequence was located twenty base pairs upstream of the FP1637 start codon (Figure 1). These results indicate that FP1637 and FP1638 loci could form an operon regulated by the promoter region mentioned.

Phenotypic characterization of fpgA$^-$ strain and complementation assays

With the aim of making a deeper analysis of the fpgA$^-$ strain, different phenotypic characteristics were studied. At 12 °C, the mutant presented a slightly lower growth rate and a decreased final cell density in comparison with the parental strain (Figure 2A). When extracellular proteolytic activity was analyzed, a significant decrease was observed in relation to the parental strain (Figure 2A).

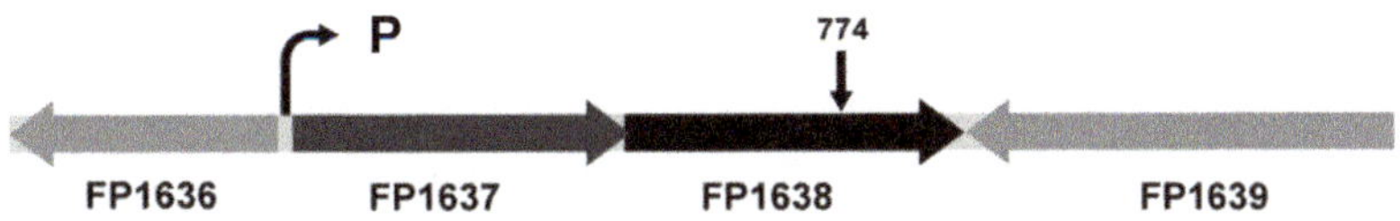

Figure 1 Genomic organization of the region surrounding the FP1638 (*fpgA*) gene in *F. psychrophilum*. The direction of transcription is indicated by arrows. The position of a putative promoter (P) involved in the regulation of both the FP1637 and FP1638 gene (separated by 4 bp) is indicated. Transposon insertion is located at position 774 of the *fpgA* locus.

In order to go further into the cause of the decrease in the extracellular proteolytic activity of the fpgA$^-$ strain, the pCP23-Gfpp2 plasmid, containing a transcriptional fusion between the *fpp2* promoter, regulating the main gene driving caseinolytic activity in the bacterium under in vitro conditions [18], and the *gfpmut3* gene, was introduced into fpgA$^-$. Strain THC02-90/G with the plasmid pCP23-G harboring a promoterless *gfpmut3* gene was utilized as a negative control and no fluorescence emission could be detected under the growth conditions tested. THC02/90-*fpp2* and *fpgA*$^-$-*fpp2* showed 117.02 ± 49.42 fluorescence relative units (fru) and 17.46 ± 3.00 fru, respectively (*p*-value 0.013). Therefore, promoter expression quantification by flow cytometry shows that, in the fpgA$^-$ background, *fpp2* promoter expression was around 85% lower than that found in the parental strain in the final-exponential phase of the growth curve.

Additionally, fpgA$^-$ showed colony spreading defects, forming non-spreading colonies with rounded edges, when grown on 1/6NA medium, whereas the parental strain presented the characteristic high spreading phenotype (Figure 2B). Complementation experiments using pCP23-

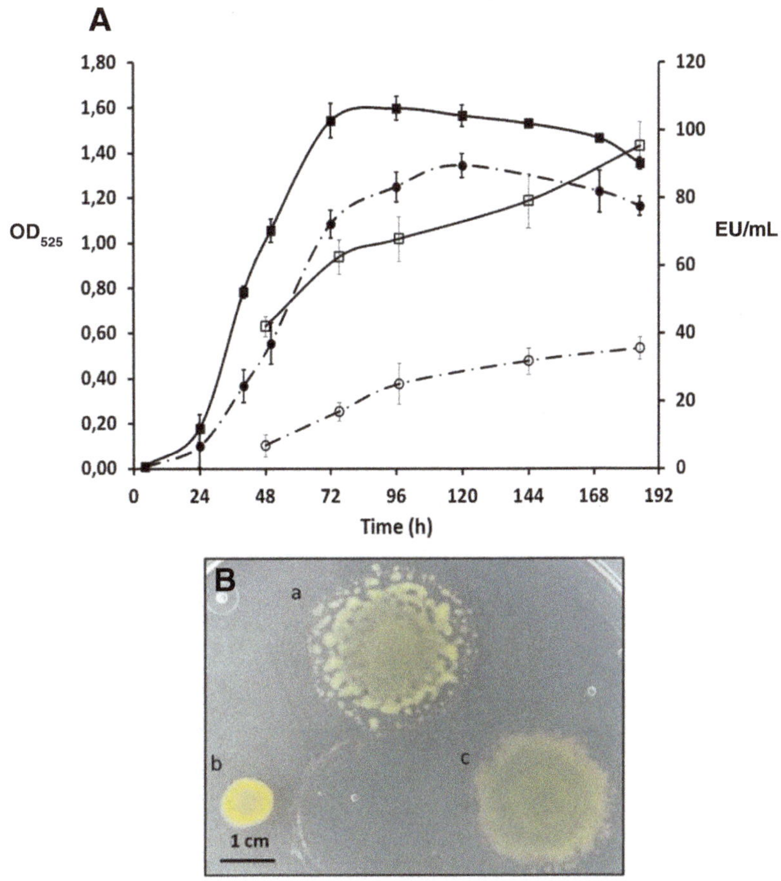

Figure 2 Growth, extracellular proteolytic activity and colony spreading of *F. psychrophilum* wild-type and fpgA$^-$ strains. (A) Growth curve at 12 °C in NBF medium, monitored by determining OD_{525}. (■) wild-type and (●) fpgA$^-$ strains. Extracellular caseinolytic activity in cell-free supernatants was determined with azocasein as described by Secades et al. [38]. (□) wild-type and (○) fpgA$^-$ strains. EU, enzyme units. **(B)** Colony spreading of *F. psychrophilum* strains grown on 1/6NA for 96 h at 20 °C according to Pérez-Pascual et al. [37]. **(a)** wild-type; **(b)** fpgA$^-$; and **(c)** fpgA$^+$ (complemented strain).

derived plasmid show that the presence of the plasmid pCP23-*fpgA* in fpgA⁻ restored both colony spreading (Figure 2B) and extracellular proteolytic activity (89.2 EU/mL at 168 h of incubation).

Protein glycosylation profile of wild-type, mutant and complemented strains

Taking account of the predicted FpgA protein function, an analysis of protein glycosylation profiles of both parental and mutant strains was carried out in order to further characterize its role. The parental strain presented a wide and diffuse glycosylated band of around 22 kDa, whereas $fpgA^-$ lacked this band, showing a new one of around 18 kDa (Figure 3A). This band could also be observed after silver staining (Figure 3B). The treatment of the extracts with different proteases show that in all proteolytic processes a new glycosylated band of about 18 kDa appeared (Figure 3C and D), suggesting a proteinaceous nature for the 22 kDa product. Different attempts were carried out in order to purify and further identify the peptide amino acid sequence of the 22 kDa glycosylated protein by mass spectrometry analysis but, unfortunately, they were unsuccessful. The complementation of the $fpgA^-$ strain with the pCP23 plasmid harboring the *fpgA* gene resulted in the recovery of the glycosylation profile of the wild-type strain, with the presence of a band of 22 kDa (Figure 3A).

LD_{50} experiments

In order to evaluate the effect of the *fpgA* mutation in the virulence of *F. psychrophilum*, LD_{50} experiments were carried out on rainbow trout. Ten days post-infection, the LD_{50} value was 2.63×10^6 CFU for the wild-type strain. Under the same conditions, $fpgA^-$ showed LD_{50} values higher than 10^9 CFU. Thus, the mutant strain for the *fpgA* locus could be considered as being highly attenuated compared to the wild-type strain. Additionally, visual examination for characteristic erosive skin lesions around the injection site showed that $fpgA^-$ infected fishes did not present any kind of tissue damage comparable to that seen in parental strain infections (data not shown). Cultures on NAC medium of samples from the different organs of dead

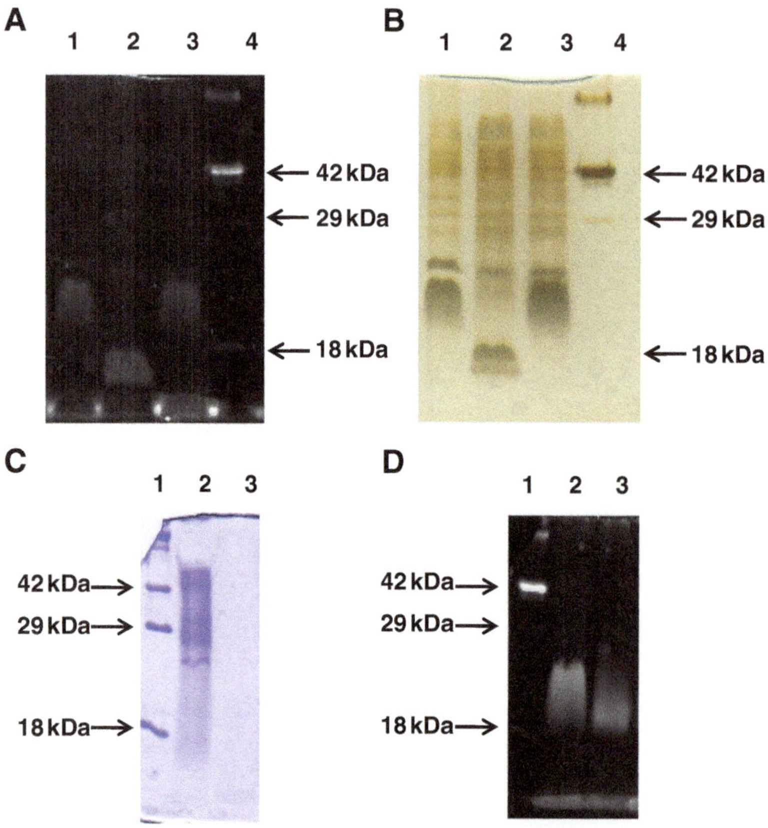

Figure 3 SDS-PAGE and gel staining of glycosylated proteins extracted from *F. psychrophilum* wild-type, $fpgA^-$, and $fpgA^+$ (complemented $fpgA^-$) strains. Total extracted proteins were separated by 14% SDS-PAGE gels that were **(A, D)** Pro-Q Emerald specific protein glycosylation; **(B)** silver; and **(C)** Coomassie blue, stained. **(A)** and **(B)**: lane 1, parental; lane 2, fpgA-; and lane 3, fpgA+. In the right of each image, the position of Candy Cane (Life Technologies, Carlasbad, Cal.) with the 42 kDa and 18 kDa glycosylated proteins is indicated (lane 4). **(C)** and **(D)**: lane 2, wild-type strain; lane 3, wild-type strain extract treated with proteinase K (similar results were obtained when trypsin and a mixture of both enzymes were used). Lane 1, Candy Cane (Life Technologies, Carlasbad, Cal.) molecular mass markers.

fish show the presence exclusively of the characteristic yellow-pigmented colonies of *F. psychrophylum*, as was expected in the case of septicemia. Routine PCR analyses show that these colonies corresponded to *F. psychrophilum* (data not shown).

Discussion

F. psychrophilum mutants obtained by Tn*4351* transposition were selected on the basis of the presence of alteration in colony spreading [19]. The fpgA$^-$ strain presented the disruption in a gene encoding a protein with a glycosyltransferase function. Its genetic context strongly suggests that the *fpgA* gene forms an operon with the FP1637 gene, due to the short distance between them (4 bp) and the presence of a promoter sequence upstream of FP1637.

Extracellular proteolytic activity and colony spreading were affected in fpgA$^-$. Complementation experiments show that the *fpgA* gene is responsible for both effects. Involvement of glycosyltransferases in bacterial motility is not limited to *F. psychrophilum*; these kind of proteins usually positioned in the outer membrane, generate polysaccharides implicated, for example, in bacterial attachment [48], an essential step for cell movement by gliding. In addition, these enzymes participate in the slime biosynthesis processes in *Myxococcus xanthus* and, consequently, are involved in the adventurous motility (A motility), where some authors proposed that the bacterium glides over a trail of polysaccharide [49,50]. In the same way, the disruption of three different glycosyltransferases in the marine bacterium *Synechococcus sp.* resulted in a non-swimming phenotype in mutant strains, indicating that these enzymes are required for motility [51].

Under the assayed conditions, most of the extracellular proteolytic activity detected from the wild-type strain is caused by the metalloproteases Fpp1 and Fpp2 whose encoding genes *fpp2-fpp1* form an operon [18]. As shown by GFP-based regulation experiments, the expression of this operon was found to be lower in the fpgA$^-$ context than that of the wild-type strain. This result suggests that the decrease of extracellular proteolytic activity detected in the *fpgA* mutant could be a consequence of down-regulation of, at least, the *fpp2-fpp1* operon. As occurring in *F. johnsoniae*, mutation in genes involved in gliding (*gld* genes) determined a change in the secretion of extracellular enzymes [52-54]. Until now, it has not been possible to establish a relationship between these two phenomena. However, it seems that a change in regulation affecting extracellular proteolytic activity occurs in parallel to the loss of the ability to move, rather than a physical interaction between the gliding machinery and the secretion systems.

The disruption of the *fpgA* gene, encoding a glycosyltransferase, caused an altered glycosylation profile in the mutant strain. While the wild-type strain presented a glycosylated element of 22 kDa, fpgA$^-$ shows an 18 kDa glycoconjugate. In any case, care must be taken when assigning a molecular mass size by SDS-PAGE in glycosylated proteins. The effect of proteolytic enzymes on the 22 kDa glycosylated band strongly suggests that it has a proteinaceous nature. The fact that a glycosylated core of 18 kDa is still present after the proteolytic treatments could be a consequence of steric impediments that might make it difficult for the proteases to gain access to the whole protein; currently, it is suggested that the addition of carbohydrates to a protein could be related to major resistance to the proteolysis process [23,55]. Taking into account that the function ascribed to FpgA corresponds to a glycosyltransferase, the results suggest that the 22 kDa protein has, at least, double glycosylation modification. One of them is probably carried out by FpgA, since the interruption of the coding locus does not involve lack of glycosylation, but a reduction of the molecular mass of the 22 kDa glycosylated protein to 18 kDa. In this sense, *B. fragilis* a member of the CFB group, presents a protein with a triple glycosylation modification [29]. Complementation experiments confirm this hypothesis since, the introduction of the *fpgA* gene into fpgA$^-$ led to the recovery of the 22 kDa glycosylated protein. It is interesting to point out that several members of the CFB group show differential glycoprotein production during their growth [28]. Thus, in *B. fragilis* 8 glycoproteins have been identified [29]; in *Elizabethkingia meningoseptica* (former *Flavobacterium meningosepticum*) [56,57] and *F. columnare*, several secreted proteins showed glycosylations [58]. These data, together with the glycosylation of the *F. psychrophilum* outer membrane protein OmpA [25,26] and the proportion of putative glycosyltransferases present in the genome of *F. psychrophilum*, strongly suggest a greater relevance of this type of enzyme in the physiology of the CFB group in relation to other bacteria, as already proposed by Fernandez-Gomez et al. [48]. The importance of the glycosylation process in the virulence of the bacterium is clear since loss of virulence in the mutant strain was definitive. The pleiotropic phenotype of the mutant strain makes the determination of the phenotypic characteristic responsible for the loss of pathogenecity, difficult. Intriguingly, in many Gram-negative pathogenic bacteria most glycoproteins were associated with pathogenesis [59]. This is the case for the glycosylation of the HWM1 adhesin of *Haemophilus influenzae* [60], the flagella in *Campylobacter jejuni* [59,61,62] and the protein-forming type IV pili in *Neisseria meningitidis* [63], amongst others. The lack of virulence seen in the fpgA$^-$ strain indicates that this strain could be a suitable candidate for the development of attenuated vaccines for the prevention of CWD. According to the pleiotropic effect generated by the mutation of the *fpgA* gene, it could not be ruled out that FpgA could be involved in a chaperon system as suggested for some glycosylated proteins in *B. fragilis* [29].

This work, together with recent data, indicates that protein glycosylation in prokaryotes and, in particular, in the CFB group could play an important role on the biology of these microorganisms, as previously suggested [28,48]. All of this could suggest that this glycosyltransferase has a regulatory role. Additionally, the avirulent mutant strain could be considered a good candidate to be used as a live vaccine in order to control the CWD.

Competing interests
The authors declare that they have no competing interests.

Authors' contributions
DP-P and EG carried out experiments. JAG conceived the experiments and drafted the manuscript. All authors read and approved the final manuscript.

Acknowledgements
The author's thanks to Dr. Beatriz Álvarez for the generously providing fpgA$^-$ mutant and to Paula Yagüe for her technical support in protein analysis. We would also like to thank Jessica Méndez, Pilar Reimundo, Roberto Navais and Desirée Cascales for their permanent help during the development of this work. Esther Gómez and David Pérez-Pascual were the recipients of respective grants from the Spanish Ministerio de Ciencia e Innovación. This project was founded by MICNN (grant AGL2009-07003).

References
1. Nematollahi A, Decostere A, Pasmans F, Haesebrouck F: ***Flavobacterium psychrophilum* infections in salmonid fish.** *J Fish Dis.* 2003,26(10):563–574.
2. Starliper CE: **Bacterial coldwater disease of fishes caused by *Flavobacterium psychrophilum*.** *J Adv Res* 2011, **2**:97–108.
3. Michel C, Antonio D, Hedrick RP: **Production of viable cultures of *Flavobacterium psychrophilum*: approach and control.** *Res Microbiol* 1999, **150**:351–358.
4. Cepeda C, Garcia-Marquez S, Santos Y: **Improved growth of *Flavobacterium psychrophilum* using a new culture medium.** *Aquaculture* 2004, **238**:75–82.
5. Garcia C, Pozet F, Michel C: **Standardization of experimental infection with *Flavobacterium psychrophilum*, the agent of rainbow trout *Oncorhynchus mykiss* fry syndrome.** *Dis Aquat Organ* 2000, **42**:191–197.
6. Izumi S, Aranishi F, Wakabayashi H: **Genotyping of *Flavobacterium psychrophilum* using PCR-RFLP analysis.** *Dis Aquat Organ* 2003, **56**:207–214.
7. Soule M, LaFrentz S, Cain K, LaPatra S, Call DR: **Polymorphisms in 16S rRNA genes of *Flavobacterium psychrophilum* correlate with elastin hydrolysis and tetracycline resistance.** *Dis Aquat Organ* 2005, **65**:209–216.
8. Arai H, Morita Y, Izumi S, Katagiri T, Kimura H: **Molecular typing by pulsed-field gel electrophoresis of *Flavobacterium psychrophilum* isolates derived from Japanese fish.** *J Fish Dis* 2007, **30**:345–355.
9. Nicolas P, Mondot S, Achaz G, Bouchenot C, Bernardet JF, Duchaud E: **Population structure of the fish-pathogenic bacterium *Flavobacterium psychrophilum*.** *Appl Environ Microbiol* 2008, **74**:3702–3709.
10. Urdaci M, Chakroun C, Faure D, Bernardet J: **Development of a polymerase chain reaction assay for identification and detection of the fish pathogen *Flavobacterium psychrophilum*.** *Res Microbiol* 1998, **149**:519–530.
11. Cepeda C, Santos Y: **Rapid and low-level toxic PCR-based method for routine identification of *Flavobacterium psychrophilum*.** *Int Microbiol* 2000, **3**:235–238.
12. Wiklund T, Madsen L, Bruun MS, Dalsgaard I: **Detection of *Flavobacterium psychrophilum* from fish tissue and water samples by PCR amplification.** *J Appl Microbiol* 2000, **88**:299–307.
13. del Cerro A, Mendoza MC, Guijarro JA: **Usefulness of a TaqMan-based polymerase chain reaction assay for the detection of the fish pathogen *Flavobacterium psychrophilum*.** *J Appl Microbiol* 2002, **93**:149–156.
14. Fujiwara-Nagata E, Eguchi M: **Development and evaluation of a loop-mediated isothermal amplification assay for rapid and simple detection of *Flavobacterium psychrophilum*.** *J Fish Dis* 2009, **32**:873–881.
15. Strepparava N, Wahli T, Segner H, Petrini O: **Detection and quantification of *Flavobacterium psychrophilum* in water and fish tissue samples by quantitative real time PCR.** *BMC Microbiol* 2014, **14**:105.
16. Duchaud E, Boussaha M, Loux V, Bernardet JF, Michel C, Kerouault B, Mondot S, Nicolas P, Bossy R, Caron C, Bessières P, Gibrat JF, Claverol S, Dumetz F, Le Hénaff M, Benmansour A: **Complete genome sequence of the fish pathogen *Flavobacterium psychrophilum*.** *Nat Biotechnol* 2007, **25**:763–769.
17. Alvarez B, Secades P, McBride MJ, Guijarro JA: **Development of genetic techniques for the psychrotrophic fish pathogen *Flavobacterium psychrophilum*.** *Appl Environ Microbiol* 2004, **70**:581–587.
18. Perez-Pascual D, Gomez E, Alvarez B, Mendez J, Reimundo P, Navais R, Duchaud E, Guijarro JA: **Comparative analysis and mutation effects of *fpp2-fpp1* tandem genes encoding proteolytic extracellular enzymes of *Flavobacterium psychrophilum*.** *Microbiology* 2011, **157**:1196–1204.
19. Alvarez B, Secades P, Prieto M, McBride MJ, Guijarro JA: **A mutation in *Flavobacterium psychrophilum tlpB* inhibits gliding motility and induces biofilm formation.** *Appl Environ Microbiol* 2006, **72**:4044–4053.
20. Alvarez B, Alvarez J, Menendez A, Guijarro JA: **A mutant in one of two *exbD* loci of a TonB system in *Flavobacterium psychrophilum* shows attenuated virulence and confers protection against cold water disease.** *Microbiology* 2008, **154**:1144–1151.
21. Schaffer C, Graninger M, Messner P: **Prokaryotic glycosylation.** *Proteomics* 2001, **1**:248–261.
22. Messner P: **Prokaryotic protein glycosylation is rapidly expanding from "curiosity" to "ubiquity".** *Chembiochem* 2009, **10**:2151–2154.
23. Benz I, Schmidt MA: **Never say never again: protein glycosylation in pathogenic bacteria.** *Mol Microbiol* 2002, **45**:267–276.
24. Schmidt MA, Riley LW, Benz I: **Sweet new world: glycoproteins in bacterial pathogens.** *Trends Microbiol* 2003, **11**:554–561.
25. Dumetz F, Lapatra SE, Duchaud E, Claverol S, Le Henaff M: **The *Flavobacterium psychrophilum* OmpA, an outer membrane glycoprotein, induces a humoral response in rainbow trout.** *J Appl Microbiol* 2007, **103**:1461–1470.
26. Merle C, Faure D, Urdaci MC, Le Henaff M: **Purification and characterization of a membrane glycoprotein from the fish pathogen *Flavobacterium psychrophilum*.** *J Appl Microbiol* 2003, **94**:1120–1127.
27. Nothaft H, Szymanski CM: **Protein glycosylation in bacteria: sweeter than ever.** *Nat Rev Microbiol* 2010, **8**:765–778.
28. Coyne MJ, Fletcher CM, Chatzidaki-Livanis M, Posch G, Schaffer C, Comstock LE: **Phylum-wide general protein O-glycosylation system of the Bacteroidetes.** *Mol Microbiol* 2013, **88**:772–783.
29. Fletcher CM, Coyne MJ, Villa OF, Chatzidaki-Livanis M, Comstock LE: **A general O-glycosylation system important to the physiology of a major human intestinal symbiont.** *Cell* 2009, **137**:321–331.
30. Gardel CL, Mekalanos JJ: **Alterations in *Vibrio cholerae* motility phenotypes correlate with changes in virulence factor expression.** *Infect Immun* 1996, **64**:2246–2255.
31. Stevens JM, Galyov EE, Stevens MP: **Actin-dependent movement of bacterial pathogens.** *Nat Rev Microbiol* 2006, **4**:91–101.
32. Wassenaar TM, Bleumink-Pluym NM, van der Zeijst BA: **Inactivation of *Campylobacter jejuni* flagellin genes by homologous recombination demonstrates that *flaA* but not *flaB* is required for invasion.** *Embo J* 1991, **10**:2055–2061.
33. Ingmer H, Brondsted L: **Proteases in bacterial pathogenesis.** *Res Microbiol* 2009, **160**:704–710.
34. Simon R, Priefer U, Puhler A: **A broad host range mobilization system for in vivo genetic engineering: transposon mutagenesis in gram negative bacteria.** *Nat Biotechnol* 1983, **1**:784–791.
35. Metcalf WW, Jiang W, Wanner BL: **Use of the rep technique for allele replacement to construct new *Escherichia coli* hosts for maintenance of R6K gamma origin plasmids at different copy numbers.** *Gene* 1994, **138**:1–7.
36. Alvarez B, Guijarro JA: **Recovery of *Flavobacterium psychrophilum* viable cells using a charcoal-based solid medium.** *Lett Appl Microbiol* 2007, **44**:569–572.
37. Perez-Pascual D, Menendez A, Fernandez L, Mendez J, Reimundo P, Navais R, Guijarro JA: **Spreading versus biomass production by colonies of the fish**

pathogen *Flavobacterium psychrophilum*: role of the nutrient concentration. *Int Microbiol* 2009, **12**:207–214.

38. Secades P, Alvarez B, Guijarro JA: **Purification and characterization of a psychrophilic, calcium-induced, growth-phase-dependent metalloprotease from the fish pathogen *Flavobacterium psychrophilum*.** *Appl Environ Microbiol* 2001, **67**:2436–2444.
39. Cooper AJ, Kalinowski AP, Shoemaker NB, Salyers AA: **Construction and characterization of a *Bacteroides thetaiotaomicron recA* mutant: transfer of Bacteroides integrated conjugative elements is RecA independent.** *J Bacteriol* 1997, **179**:6221–6227.
40. Agarwal S, Hunnicutt DW, McBride MJ: **Cloning and characterization of the *Flavobacterium johnsoniae* (*Cytophaga johnsonae*) gliding motility gene, *gldA*.** *Proc Natl Acad Sci U S A* 1997, **94**:12139–12144.
41. Gomez E, Perez-Pascual D, Fernandez L, Mendez J, Reimundo P, Navais R, Guijarro JA: **Construction and validation of a GFP-based vector for promoter expression analysis in the fish pathogen *Flavobacterium psychrophilum*.** *Gene* 2012, **497**:263–268.
42. Chakroun C, Grimont F, Urdaci MC, Bernardet JF: **Fingerprinting of *Flavobacterium psychrophilum* isolates by ribotyping and plasmid profiling.** *Dis Aquat Organ* 1998, **33**:167–177.
43. Reed LJ, Muench H: **A simple method of estimating fifty per cent endpoints.** *Am J Epidemiol* 1938, **27**:493–497.
44. SMART: *Simple Modular Architecture Research Tools*. http://smart.embl-heidelberg.de/.
45. Lombard V, Golaconda Ramulu H, Drula E, Coutinho PM, Henrissat B: **The carbohydrate-active enzymes database (CAZy) in 2013.** *Nucleic Acids Res* 2014, **42**(Database issue):D490–D495.
46. **Expasy, ProtParam tool** [http://www.expasy.ch/tools/protparam.html]
47. **SignalP 3.0 Server** [http://www.cbs.dtu.dk/services/SignalP/]
48. Fernandez-Gomez B, Richter M, Schuler M, Pinhassi J, Acinas SG, Gonzalez JM, Pedros-Alio C: **Ecology of marine Bacteroidetes: a comparative genomics approach.** *Isme J* 2013, **7**:1026–1037.
49. Wolgemuth C, Hoiczyk E, Kaiser D, Oster G: **How myxobacteria glide.** *Curr Biol* 2002, **12**:369–377.
50. Yu R, Kaiser D: **Gliding motility and polarized slime secretion.** *Mol Microbiol* 2007, **63**:454–467.
51. McCarren J, Brahamsha B: **Swimming motility mutants of marine *Synechococcus* affected in production and localization of the S-layer protein SwmA.** *J Bacteriol* 2009, **191**:1111–1114.
52. Braun TF, Khubbar MK, Saffarini DA, McBride MJ: ***Flavobacterium johnsoniae* gliding motility genes identified by mariner mutagenesis.** *J Bacteriol* 2005, **187**:6943–6952.
53. Braun TF, McBride MJ: ***Flavobacterium johnsoniae* GldJ is a lipoprotein that is required for gliding motility.** *J Bacteriol* 2005, **187**:2628–2637.
54. McBride MJ, Braun TF, Brust JL: ***Flavobacterium johnsoniae* GldH is a lipoprotein that is required for gliding motility and chitin utilization.** *J Bacteriol* 2003, **185**:6648–6657.
55. Upreti RK, Kumar M, Shankar V: **Bacterial glycoproteins: functions, biosynthesis and applications.** *Proteomics* 2003, **3**:363–379.
56. Plummer TH Jr, Tarentino AL, Hauer CR: **Novel, specific O-glycosylation of secreted *Flavobacterium meningosepticum* proteins. Asp-Ser and Asp-Thr-Thr consensus sites.** *J Biol Chem* 1995, **270**:13192–13196.
57. Reinhold BB, Hauer CR, Plummer TH, Reinhold VN: **Detailed structural analysis of a novel, specific O-linked glycan from the prokaryote *Flavobacterium meningosepticum*.** *J Biol Chem* 1995, **270**:13197–13203.
58. Vinogradov E, Perry MB, Kay WW: **The structure of the glycopeptides from the fish pathogen *Flavobacterium columnare*.** *Carbohydr Res* 2003, **338**:2653–2658.
59. Guerry P: **Campylobacter flagella: not just for motility.** *Trends Microbiol* 2007, **15**:456–461.
60. Grass S, Buscher AZ, Swords WE, Apicella MA, Barenkamp SJ, Ozchlewski N, St Geme JW 3rd: **The *Haemophilus influenzae* HMW1 adhesin is glycosylated in a process that requires HMW1C and phosphoglucomutase, an enzyme involved in lipooligosaccharide biosynthesis.** *Mol Microbiol* 2003, **48**:737–751.
61. Szymanski CM, Michael FS, Jarrell HC, Li J, Gilbert M, Larocque S, Vinogradov E, Brisson JR: **Detection of conserved N-linked glycans and phase-variable lipooligosaccharides and capsules from campylobacter cells by mass spectrometry and high resolution magic angle spinning NMR spectroscopy.** *J Biol Chem* 2003, **278**:24509–24520.
62. Young NM, Brisson JR, Kelly J, Watson DC, Tessier L, Lanthier PH, Jarrell HC, Cadotte N, St Michael F, Aberg E, Szymanski CM: **Structure of the N-linked glycan present on multiple glycoproteins in the Gram-negative bacterium, *Campylobacter jejuni*.** *J Biol Chem* 2002, **277**:42530–42539.
63. Virji M: **Post-translational modifications of meningococcal pili. Identification of common substituents: glycans and alpha-glycerophosphate–a review.** *Gene* 1997, **192**:141–147.

2

The oral and conjunctival microbiotas in cats with and without feline immunodeficiency virus infection

Scott J Weese[1*], Jamieson Nichols[2], Mohammad Jalali[1] and Annette Litster[2]

Abstract

The oral and conjunctival microbiotas likely play important roles in protection from opportunistic infections, while also being the source of potential pathogens. Yet, there has been limited investigation in cats, and the impact of comorbidities such as feline immunodeficiency virus (FIV) infection has not been reported. Oral and conjunctival swabs were collected from cats with FIV infection and FIV-uninfected controls, and subjected to 16S rRNA gene (V4) PCR and next generation sequencing. 9,249 OTUs were identified from conjunctival swabs, yet the most common 20 (0.22%) OTUs accounted for 76% of sequences. The two most abundant OTUs both belonged to *Staphylococcus*, and accounted for 37% of sequences. Cats with FIV infection had significantly lower relative abundances of Verrucomicrobia, Fibrobacteres, Spirochaetes, Bacteroidetes and Tenericutes, and a higher relative abundance of Deinococcus-Thermus. There were significant differences in both community membership ($P = 0.006$) and community structure ($P = 0.02$) between FIV-infected and FIV-uninfected cats. FIV-infected cats had significantly higher relative abundances of Fusobacteria and Actinobacteria in the oral cavity, and significantly higher relative abundances of several bacterial classes including Fusobacteria (0.022 vs 0.007, $P = 0.006$), Actinobacteria (0.017 vs 0.003, $P = 0.003$), Sphingobacteria (0.00015 vs 0.00003, $P = 0.0013$) and Flavobacteria (0.0073 vs 0.0034, $P = 0.030$). The feline conjunctival and oral microbiotas are complex polymicrobial communities but dominated by a limited number of genera. There is an apparent impact of FIV infection on various components of the microbiota, and assessment of the clinical relevance of these alterations in required.

Introduction

The body harbours vast microbial communities (microbiotas) at different body sites [1]. The microbiota interacts closely with the immune system and alterations in the immune status of the host can result in changes in the microbiota, as has been shown with the fecal, anal and oral microbiotas of humans with human immunodeficiency virus (HIV) infection [2-5]. Feline immunodeficiency virus (FIV), another lentivirus, is disseminated in the cat population worldwide [6-10]. As with HIV in humans, FIV infection can result in progressive immune dysfunction, with a corresponding increase in a variety of infectious disease risks. A variety of ocular and oral manifestations of HIV infection can occur in humans, including both infectious and non-infectious causes [11], and it is possible that alterations in the local microbiota play a role in the pathophysiology of some of these diseases. Further, the oral microbiota in humans has been shown to have an influence on various infectious diseases, including both oral (e.g. gingivitis, stomatitis, periodontitis) and extra-oral (e.g. infective endocarditis) disease, and alterations of the oral microbiota have been identified in individuals with HIV infection [2,12-14].

Understanding of the normal ocular and oral microbiotas, and changes that occur in response to FIV infection, is important for understanding the impact of FIV infection and the pathophysiology of FIV-associated opportunistic infections. The objectives of this study were to describe the conjunctival and oral bacterial microbiotas and to evaluate the impact of FIV infection.

* Correspondence: jsweese@uoguelph.ca
[1]Department of Pathobiology, University of Guelph, Guelph, Canada
Full list of author information is available at the end of the article

Materials and methods

Study population

Thirty-three cats were enrolled from a broader 5-year longitudinal controlled study investigating the clinical effects of FIV in naturally acquired infection. FIV infection status at the time of enrollment was determined by FIV antibody detection[a] and later confirmed using polymerase chain reaction (PCR) for FIV RNA[b] or virus isolation[c]. Of the enrolled cats, 19 were FIV-infected and 14 were FIV-uninfected. The cats enrolled in this study represent a convenience sample based on the timing of examination and sample collection for the larger study. FIV-infected cats were sourced from either a feline sanctuary ($n = 15$) or were privately owned ($n = 4$). FIV-uninfected cats were sourced from either the same feline sanctuary ($n = 2$) or were privately owned ($n = 12$). FIV-infected and uninfected cats were housed indoors and comingled within the sanctuary. Two of the privately owned cats, one FIV-infected and one FIV-uninfected, were allowed outdoors. None of the privately owned FIV-uninfected cats in this study were housed with FIV-infected cats. At the time of examination, all cats were re-tested for FIV antibodies.

Physical examination was performed at the time of sampling. Oral and conjunctival swab samples were collected with a sterile Dacron swab from the oral cavity or conjunctival surface, respectively. Oral health and gingival score were determined by visual inspection at the time of examination. The presence of gingivitis, stomatitis, gum recession, tooth root or furcation exposure, purulent material at the gumline, loose teeth or masses was considered evidence of dental disease. The gingival score was determined using the following scale: 0 – normal gingiva with sharp, non-inflamed edges; 1 – marginal gingivitis, minimal inflammation at free margin, no bleeding when pressure applied to the gingiva; 2 – moderate gingivitis, wider of inflammation at gingival margin, bleeding when pressure applied to gingiva; 3 – marked gingivitis, severe inflammation, bleeding can be present or absent when pressure applied to gingiva [15]. As cats were conscious during examinations, probing depths were not assessed and intraoral radiography was not performed.

The study was approved by the Purdue University Animal Care and Use Committee (protocol 1201000568).

Sequencing

DNA extraction was performed using a commercial kit[d]. The V4 region of the bacterial 16S rRNA gene was then amplified using the primers S-D-Bact-0564-a-S-15 (5′-AYTGGGYDTAAAGNG-3′) and S-D-Bact-0785-b-A-18 (5′-TACNVGGGTATCTAATCC-3′) [16]. Sequencing was performed using an Illumina MiSeq[e] and 2×250 chemistry.

Data analysis

Mothur v1.33.3 [17] was used to assemble paired end reads and perform downstream analysis. After assembly, sequence files were depleted of sequences that were not consistent with the target amplicon size (240 bp), contained any ambiguous base calls or long runs (>8 bp) of holopolymers, or did not align with the correct 16S rRNA gene region. After alignment with the Silva 16S rRNA reference database [18], chimeras were detected using UCHIME [19] and removed. Taxonomy was then assigned using the RDP taxonomy database [20] and any non-bacterial sequences that remained were removed. Sequences were then binned into operational taxon units (OTUs) at a 3% dissimilarity level.

Wilcoxon signed rank tests were used to compare relative abundances of different phylogenetic groups. Subsampling was performed to normalize sequence number for subsequent analyses [21] through random selection of a number of sequences that was chosen to optimize both sequence numbers and the number of samples that could be included. Good's coverage, diversity (inverse Simpson's index), evenness (Shannon's evenness index) and richness (Catchall) [22] were calculated and compared between groups using Wilcoxon signed rank test. Dendrograms were developed based on the Yue and Clayton measure of dissimilarity (a measure of community structure, which considers shared OTUs and their relative abundances) and traditional Jaccard index (a measure of community membership, which just considers the number of shared OTUs, not their abundance) and UniFrac [23] and analysis of molecular variance (AMOVA) were applied to compare microbial communities. Analysis of molecular variance was also used to compare communities. Principal coordinate analysis (PCoA) and indicator analysis [24] were also performed. A P value of ≤ 0.05 was considered significant for all analyses.

Results

Cats ranged in age from 5 to 12 years of age (median 7 years). There was no difference in median age of the two groups (FIV-uninfected mean 7.2y, median 8y, range 5-10y; FIV-infected mean 7.3y, median 7y, range 5-12y)

Table 1 Alpha diversity comparison (medians) of the conjunctival microbiota of FIV-infected ($n = 18$) and FIV-uninfected ($n = 11$) cats

	FIV +	FIV -	*P* value
Diversity (inverse Simpson's)	3.1	4.1	0.053
Evenness (Shannon's evenness)	0.38	0.51	0.022
Richness (Catchall)	1022	1079	0.74
Coverage (Good's coverage)	0.98	0.98	0.61

Table 2 Phyla identified in the conjunctival microbiota of FIV-infected ($n = 19$) and FIV-uninfected ($n = 13$) cats

Phylum	FIV-infected	FIV-uninfected	*P* value
Firmicutes	0.55	0.43	0.20
Proteobacteria	0.37	0.30	0.37
Actinobacteria	0.0078	0.0057	0.50
Verrucomicrobia	0.0064	0.023	0.0014
Fibrobacteres	0.0056	0.024	0.019
Spirochaetes	0.0010	0.0082	0.026
Bacteroidetes	0.0041	0.012	0.0096
Chlamydiae	0.0015	0.0015	0.54
Fusobacteria	0.00099	0.0015	0.35
Tenericutes	0.00032	0.0022	0.0005
Deinococcus-Thermus	0.00031	0.000048	0.0083
TM7	0.00017	0.00032	0.89
Acidobacteria	0.000090	0.000057	0.53
Synergistetes	0.000038	0.000059	0.34
SR1	0.000033	0.00023	0.52
Deferribacteres	0.0000067	0	0.23
Lentisphaerae	0.0000048	0.00016	0.13
Elusimicrobia	0.0000010	0.00011	0.31
Armatimonadetes	0	0.000005	0.23

($P = 0.90$). Four (31%) of the FIV-uninfected cats were neutered males and 9 (69%) were spayed females, while 12 (63%) cats in the FIV-infected group were neutered males and seven (37%) were spayed females ($P = 0.15$). Four (21%) of the FIV-infected cats were subjectively considered clinically healthy on a general physical examination, while the others had varying degrees of oral, dental, respiratory, skin or ocular disease. Six (46%) of FIV-uninfected cats were clinically normal, with the remaining cats having varying degrees of oral and skin disease. There was no difference in health status between groups ($P = 0.24$).

Conjunctival microbiota

A total of 747 559 sequences from 32 cats (19 FIV infected, 13 FIV uninfected) passed all screening tests, with sequence numbers ranging from 956 to 53 810 per sample (mean 23 361, median 21 267). A total of 9249 OTUs was identified, yet the most common 20 (0.22%) OTUs accounted for 76% of sequences. The two most abundant OTUs both belonged to *Staphylococcus*, and accounted for 37% of sequences.

Alpha and beta diversity were analysed using a subsampled population of 3422 sequences per sample. This resulted in the exclusion of samples from three cats (two FIV-uninfected, one FIV-infected) that repeatedly yielded low sequence numbers. Alpha diversity data are presented in Table 1. Cats with FIV infection had significantly lower relative abundances of Verrucomicrobia, Fibrobacteres, Spirochaetes, Bacteroidetes and Tenericutes, and a higher relative abundance of Deinococcus-Thermus (Table 2). Predominant families and genera among the FIV-infected and FIV-uninfected cats are presented in Table 3. Significant differences in the relative abundance of genera accounting for at least 0.1% of sequences are presented in Table 4.

Dendrograms based on the Yue and Clayton (community structure) and Jaccard (community membership) indices are displayed in Figures 1 and 2. There were significant differences in both community membership ($P = 0.006$) and community structure ($P = 0.02$) between FIV-infected and FIV-uninfected cats. Significant differences were also noted by AMOVA for both the Yue & Clayton ($P = 0.005$) and Jaccard ($P < 0.001$) index data. Separation of the two groups, with greater variability in membership in the FIV-infected group, was also seen with PCoA (Figure 3).

Forty significant indicator OTUs were identified (Table 5). Eleven of 22 (50%) indicator OTUs for FIV-infected cats were Proteobacteria, compared to zero of the 18 FIV-uninfected indicators ($P < 0.01$).

One OTU, *Pseudomonas*, was found in all FIV-infected cats at a relative abundance of at least 1%. *Staphylococcus* was found in 15/19 (79%) FIV-infected

Table 3 Predominant families and genera in the conjunctival microbiota of FIV-infected ($n = 19$) and FIV-uninfected ($n = 13$) cats

Family (relative abundance)		Genus (relative abundance)	
FIV +	FIV -	FIV +	FIV -
Staphylococcaceae (0.45)	Staphylococcaceae (0.27)	*Staphylococcus* (0.42)	*Staphylococcus* (0.14)
Pseudomonadaceae (0.14)	Moraxellaceae (0.20)	*Pseudomonas* (0.11)	*Acinetobacter* (0.15)
Enterobacteriaceae (0.10)	Pseudomonadaceae (0.13)	Unclassified Enterobacteriaceae (0.090)	*Pseudomonas* (0.12)
Planococcaceae (0.062)	Aerococcaceae (0.54)	*Sporosarcina* (0.052)	Unclassified Clostridiales (0.058)
Unclassified Clostridiales (0.022)	Unclassified Clostridiales (0.028)	Unclassified Pseudomonadaceae (0.038)	*Psychrobacter* (0.055)
Unclassified Bacillales (0.020)	Bacillales incertae sedis XII (0.027)	Unclassified Clostridiales (0.022)	*Aerococcus* (0.054)
Unclassified Firmicutes (0.017)	Lachnospiraceae (0.022)	Unclassified Bacillales (0.017)	Unclassified Firmicutes (0.030)

Table 4 Relative abundance of genera accounting for >0.1% of the conjunctival microbiota that were significantly different in FIV-infected (*n* = 19) and FIV-uninfected (*n* = 13) cats

Genus	FIV infected	FIV uninfected	*P* value
Staphylococcus	0.42	0.14	0.0026
Unclassified bacterium	0.051	0.19	0.0038
Unclassified Clostridiales	0.016	0.058	0.0029
Unclassified Pseudomonadaceae	0.038	0.0072	0.0096
Unclassified Firmicutes	0.011	0.030	0.0077
Unclassified Lachnospiraceae	0.010	0.036	0.0023
Fibrobacter	0.0056	0.024	0.019
5 genus incertae sedis	0.0046	0.019	0.0007
Unclassified Staphylococcaceae	0.0077	0.0010	0.0003
Unclassified Ruminococcaceae	0.0034	0.014	0.0043
Unclassified Bacteroidetes	0.0015	0.010	0.0017
Unclassified Clostridia	0.0017	0.0049	0.0018
Treponema	0.00089	0.0076	0.021
Phenylobacterium	0.0034	0.00038	0.0024

cats, while *Escherichia/Shigella* was found in 14/19 (74%) at that minimum relative abundance. In contrast, no OTUs were found at a relative abundance of at least 1% in any of the FIV-uninfected samples. *Pseudomonas* was found in 8/13 (62%) FIV-uninfected samples and was the only OTU found in at least 50% of samples at a relative abundance of 1% of greater.

Oral microbiota

There were 1 430 615 sequences from 33 samples (19 FIV-infected and 14 FIV-uninfected cats) that entered the final analysis, with sequence numbers ranging from 5587 to 94 647 per sample (mean 43 352, median 38 922, SD 24 725).

Eighteen different phyla were identified (Table 6). FIV-infected cats had significantly higher relative abundances of Fusobacteria and Actinobacteria. Similarly, FIV-infected cats had significantly higher relative abundances of several bacterial classes including Fusobacteria (0.022 vs 0.007, $P = 0.006$), Actinobacteria (0.017 vs 0.003, $P = 0.003$), Sphingobacteria (0.00015 vs 0.00003, $P = 0.0013$) and Flavobacteria (0.0073 vs 0.0034, $P = 0.030$). The eight most common classes are presented in Figure 4. The predominant genera in each group are listed in Table 7, with genera that were significantly different between the two groups in Table 8.

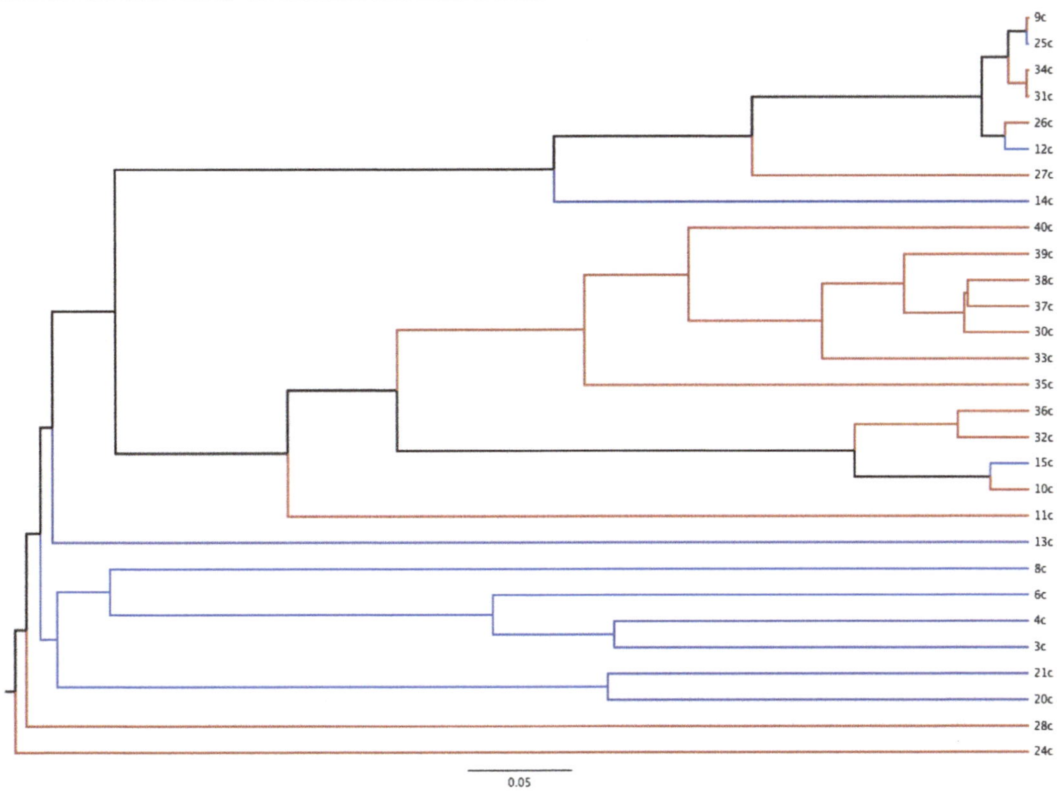

Figure 1 Bacterial community structure of the conjunctival microbiota of FIV-infected and FIV-uninfected cats. Dendrogram based on the Yue and Clayton index of dissimilarity characterizing the microbial population structure of the conjunctiva in 18 cats with FIV infection (red) and 11 uninfected (blue) cats.

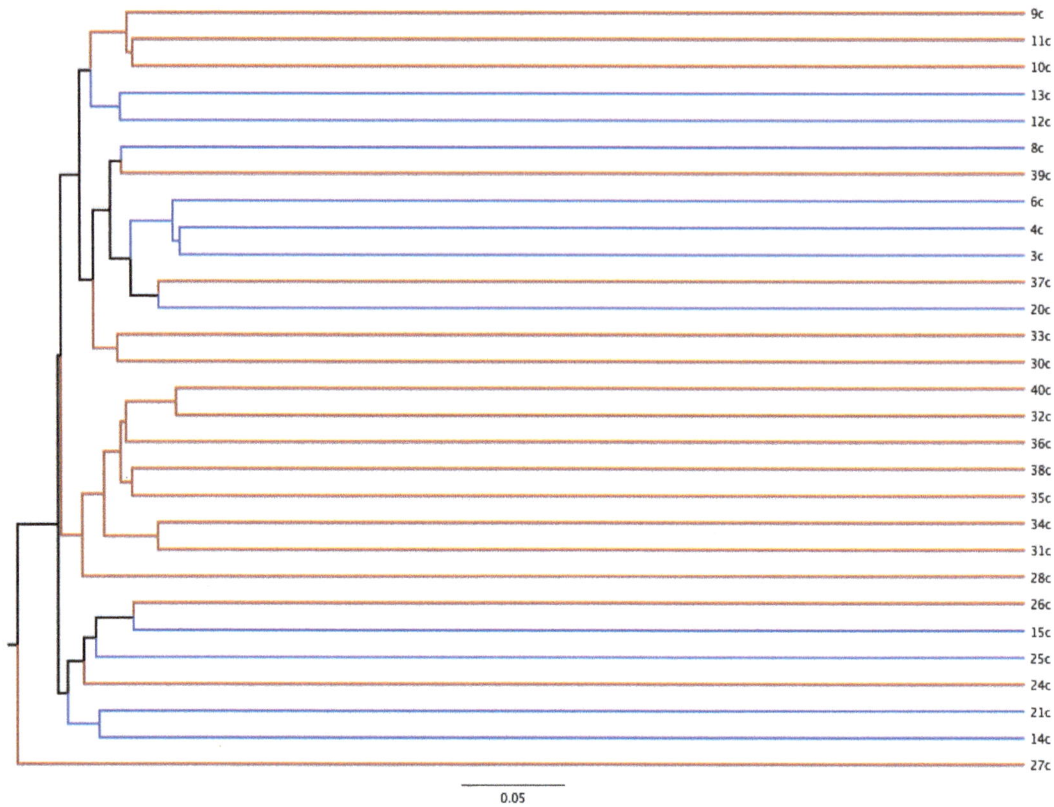

Figure 2 Bacterial community membership of the conjunctival microbiota of FIV-infected and FIV-uninfected cats. Dendrogram based on the classical Jaccard index demonstrating the community membership (operational taxon units that are present, irrespective of relative abundance) of 18 cats with FIV infection and 11 uninfected cats.

A subsample of 5587 sequences per sample was used for subsequent analysis. There were no differences in coverage ($P = 0.64$), diversity ($P = 0.44$), evenness ($P = 0.64$) or richness ($P = 0.61$) between FIV-infected and FIV-uninfected cats.

There were significant differences in microbial community structure (Yue and Clayton index, $P = 0.030$) but not community membership (Jaccard index, $P = 0.18$) by UniFrac. In contrast, there was also a significant difference between groups by AMOVA applied to a phylip-formatted distance matrix based on the Jaccard index ($P = 0.005$) but not the Yue and Clayton index ($P = 0.078$).

No OTUs were present in all cats in either the FIV-infected or FIV-uninfected groups at a minimum relative abundance of 1%. One OTU, classified as *Pseudomonas*, was present at that minimum relative abundance in 15/20 FIV-infected cats. Two OTUs, an unclassified Aerococcaceae and *Pasteurella*, were present at that abundance in 9/14 FIV-uninfected cats. Twenty indicator OTUs were identified, 16 for FIV-infected cats and four for FIV-uninfected cats (Table 9). Indicator OTUs for FIV-uninfected cats were predominantly (75%) Proteobacteria while Firmicutes were the most common indicators in FIV-uninfected cats (9/16, 56%).

Four FIV infected cats had a gingival disease score of 0, nine had a score of 1, three had a score of 2 and three had a score of 3. There were no differences in community structure ($P = 0.60$) (Figure 5) or community membership ($P = 0.99$) in FIV infected cats with and without severe gingival disease (score ≥ 2). There were also no differences between the relative abundances of any phyla or classes. Similarly, there were no differences in community structure ($P = 0.581$) and membership ($P = 0.31$) in FIV-infected cats with dental disease versus those without dental disease.

Discussion

Conjunctival microbiota

The feline conjunctiva harbours a large number of diverse phyla, albeit at a lower richness and diversity than has been described in the feline oral cavity or intestinal tract [25-27], or identified in the oral microbiota here. Yet, while the richness and diversity were lower than reported for other mucosal surfaces, the conjunctival microbiota contained an estimate of over 1000 species per sample, a count that far exceeds culture-dependent studies [28-31].

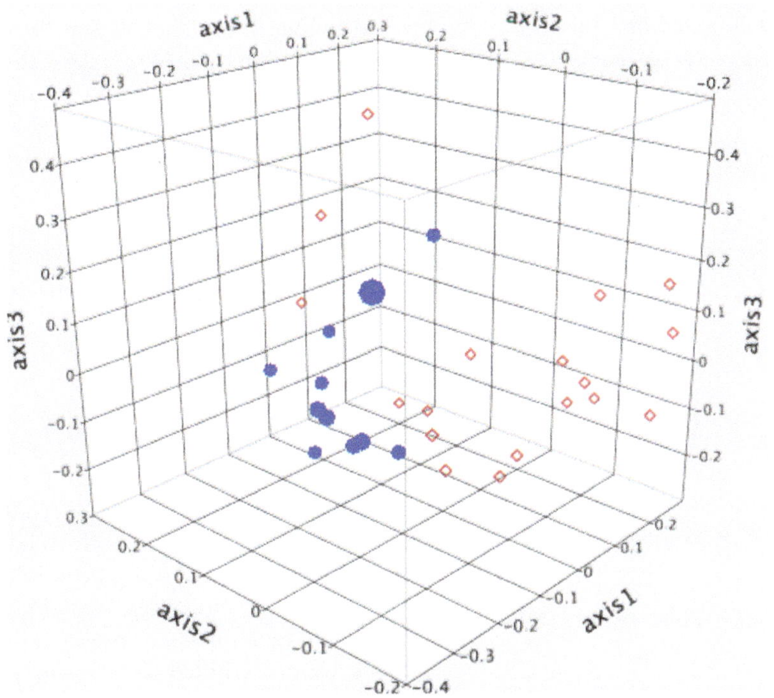

Figure 3 Principle coordinate analysis of the community membership of cats with FIV infection and uninfected controls. Three dimension principle coordinate analysis plot based on the classical Jaccard index depicting the community membership of the conjunctival microbiota of FIV-infected (n = 18, red diamonds) and FIV-uninfected (*n* = 11, blue dots) cats.

Firmicutes dominated in FIV-uninfected cats. This broad phylum, consisting of a wide range of Gram-positive bacteria, is commonly found at most body sites, albeit with different members of the phylum predominating. For example, Clostridia are dominant Firmicutes in the intestinal tract [25,26,32], while here, Bacilli were most common. This was because of the high relative abundance of Staphylococcaceae. Staphylococci are widespread commensals of mucosal surfaces and are opportunistic pathogens that can be associated with a wide range of infections, including conjunctivitis and ulcerative keratitis [29,33,34]. Their presence in the conjunctival microbiota is not surprising based on the nature of this genus and results of previous culture-dependent studies [29,31].

Proteobacteria were also common, and at a greater relative abundance (30-37%) than in many other body sites. This phylum of Gram-negative bacteria contains a variety of potential opportunistic pathogens, including *Pseudomonas* and *Acinetobacter*, two genera that were common in clinically healthy cats.

Significant differences between FIV-infected and FIV-uninfected cats in the relative abundances of numerous phyla (and corresponding lower taxonomic levels) were identified, yet these were among lower abundance phyla, the relevance of which is unclear. The difference in

Table 5 Indicator OTUs for FIV-infected (*n* = 19) and FIV-uninfected (*n* = 13) cats

FIV-infected	FIV-uninfected
Unclassified Pseudomonadaceae (3 OTUs)	5 genus incertae sedis (6 OTUs)
Staphylococcus (2 OTUs)	*Treponema* (3 OTUs)
Anaerobiospirillum (2 OTUs)	Unclassified bacterium (3 OTUs)
Elsenella	Unclassified Lachnospiraceae (2 OTUs)
Phenylobacterium	*Streptococcus*
Unclassified Aerococcaceae	*Pseudobutyrivibrio*
Pseudomonas	*Saccharofermentans*
Unclassified Bacillaceae	Unclassified Ruminococcaceae
Bifidobacterium	
Bradyrhizobium	
Akkermansia	
Cellulosimicrobium	
Thermus	
Prevotella	
Mezorhizobium	
Carnobacterium	
Unclassified Pasteurellaceae	
Succinivibrio	

Table 6 Relative abundance of phyla in the oral cavity of FIV-infected ($n = 19$) and FIV-uninfected ($n = 14$) cats

Phylum	FIV-infected	FIV-uninfected	*P* value
Acidobacteria	0.000026	0.000026	0.63
Actinobacteria	0.017	0.0035	0.0097
Bacteroidetes	0.019	0.012	0.19
Chlamydiae	0.000003	0.000028	0.65
Deferribacteres	0.000002	0.000045	0.34
Deinococcus-Thermus	0.000057	0.000039	0.15
Fibrobacteres	0.0030	0.0023	0.83
Firmicutes	0.17	0.12	0.42
Fusobacteria	0.022	0.0079	0.016
Lentisphaerae	0.00016	0.00010	0.74
Planctomycetes	0.0000014	0.0000008	0.86
Proteobacteria	0.70	0.81	0.26
Spirochaetes	0.0094	0.0064	0.86
SR1	0.0019	0.0030	0.76
Synergistetes	0.000006	0.0000009	0.69
Tenericutes	0.00041	0.00040	0.28
TM7	0.00093	0.00034	0.09
Verrucomicrobia	0.0028	0.0028	0.40

relative abundance of staphylococci was striking, with a 3-fold higher abundance in the FIV-infected group. It is unusual for one genus to comprise such a large (42%) percentage of the microbiota in any body site, and the clinical relevance of this increased relative abundance in FIV-infected cats deserves further study, given the known role of staphylococci in ocular and extra-ocular disease.

Beyond comparisons of relative abundances, there are various ecological tools that can be applied to compare communities. Here, differences in both community membership and the overall microbial community structure were noted, providing more evidence of an altered microbiota community in FIV-infected cats. Another approach is indicator analysis. This is an ecological tool that identifies OTUs that "define" a community [24]. As opposed to assessment of only relative abundance, indicator analysis evaluates both relative abundance and presence or absence in a community, to identify OTUs that are strong indicators or defining characteristics of that population by their presence. Numerous indicator OTUs were identified. Interestingly, half the indicators for FIV-infected cats were Proteobacteria, compared to none for FIV-uninfected cats. While Proteobacteria were not significantly different overall between FIV-infected and FIV-uninfected cats, the predominance of genera from this phylum as indicators in FIV-infected cats

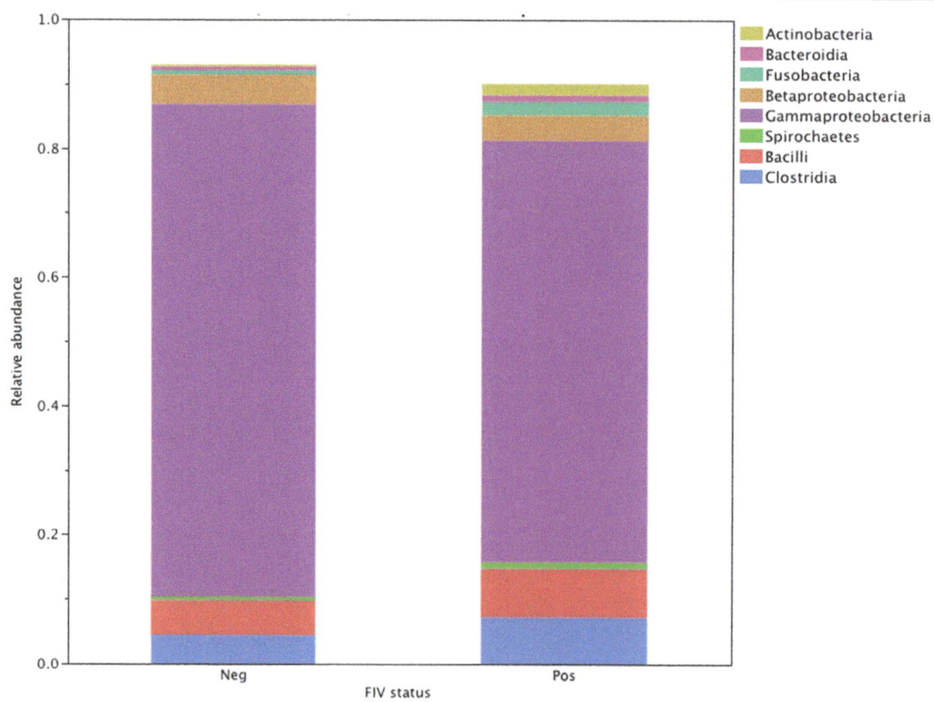

Figure 4 Predominant classes in the oral microbiota of cats with and without FIV infection. Relative abundance of the predominant classes in the oral microbiota of FIV-infected ($n = 19$) and FIV-uninfected ($n = 14$) cats. Legend: Neg = FIV-uninfected. Pos = FIV-infected. Among these predominant phyla, there were significant differences in the relative abundances for Fusobacteria (0.022 vs 0.007, $P = 0.006$) and Actinobacteria (0.017 vs 0.003, $P = 0.003$), both higher in the FIV-infected group.

Table 7 Predominant genera in the oral microbiota of FIV-infected ($n = 19$) and FIV-uninfected ($n = 14$) cats

FIV-infected		FIV-uninfected	
Genus	Relative abundance	Genus	Relative abundance
Pasteurella	0.27	*Pasteurella*	0.26
Unclassified Pasteurellaceae	0.12	Unclassified Pasteurellaceae	0.093
Pseudomonas	0.092	Unclassified Enterobacteriaceae	0.090
Mannheimia	0.060	*Acinetobacter*	0.0745
Staphylococcus	0.037	*Mannheimia*	0.061
Unclassified Clostridiales	0.030	*Pseudomonas*	0.057
Acinetobacter	0.030	*Kingella*	0.033
Unclassified bacterium	0.027	*Moraxella*	0.030
Psychrobacter	0.019	*Neisseria*	0.021
Kingella	0.018	Unclassified Clostridiales	0.020

suggests that some members of this genus can be specifically altered in response to FIV infection.

Oral microbiota

Results of this study indicate differences in the microbiota based on FIV status, although results were sometimes conflicting. There were overall differences in microbial community membership and structure in some tests (e.g. UniFrac vs AMOVA) but not others. Assessing the relevance of conflicting results is difficult. The relatively small sample size could have played a role by limiting statistical power, particularly when *P* values approached significance. Differences in the study populations beyond FIV status must also be considered. While both groups were recruited from a combination of homes and a sanctuary, the differences in distribution of those sources amongst groups could also introduce some bias.

Table 8 Relative abundances of genera that were significantly different in the oral cavity of FIV-infected ($n = 19$) versus FIV-uninfected ($n = 14$) cats

Genus	FIV-infected	FIV-uninfected	*P* value
Staphylococcus	0.037	0.003	0.004
Unclassified Actinomycetales	0.012	0.0018	0.009
Parvimonas	0.008	0.002	0.005
Streptobacillus	0.0062	0.0019	0.017
Sneathia	0.0052	0.0003	0.0011
Unclassified Flavobacteriaceae	0.0033	0.0014	0.038
Gemella	0.0038	0.00022	0.000e
Unclassified Leptotrichiaceae	0.0038	0.0009	0.0012
Peptoniphilus	0.00014	0.00067	0.022

Table 9 Indicator OTUs for FIV-infected ($n = 19$) and FIV-uninfected ($n = 13$) cats

FIV-infected	FIV-uninfected
Unclassified Pseudomonadaceae (3 OTUs)	5 genus incertae sedis (6 OTUs)
Staphylococcus (2 OTUs)	*Treponema* (3 OTUs)
Anaerobiospirillum (2 OTUs)	Unclassified bacterium (3 OTUs)
Elsenella	Unclassified Lachnospiraceae (2 OTUs)
Phenylobacterium	*Streptococcus*
Unclassified Aerococcaceae	*Pseudobutyrivibrio*
Pseudomonas	*Saccharofermentans*
Unclassified Bacillaceae	Unclassified Ruminococcaceae
Bifidobacterium	
Bradyrhizobium	
Akkermansia	
Cellulosimicrobium	
Thermus	
Prevotella	
Mezorhizobium	
Carnobacterium	
Unclassified Pasteurellaceae	
Succinivibrio	

Evaluation of specific taxonomic identifications that were different between groups can be enlightening. Two phyla, Fusobacteria and Actinobacteria, were over-represented in FIV-infected cats. The significantly higher relative abundance of Fusobacteria could be relevant given the role of members of this phylum have in oral disease in other species [35]. Increased *Fusobacterium* spp has also been identified in the anal and rectal microbiotas of people with HIV [4,5]. Of additional concern is recent evidence that *F. nucleatum* can increase re-activation of HIV in vitro, indicating a possibility that increased growth of this organism could be a risk modifier for viral replication and disease progression [36]. This has not been reported with FIV and there was no difference in the abundance of *Fusobacterium* between groups (data not presented), but the notion that an altered microbiota could influence viral activation and disease progression, independent of bacterial infection, should be further investigated in cats. Actinobacteria were also over-represented in the FIV-infected group. In humans, Actinobacteria are a component of plaque [37] and are more abundant in chronic (versus acute) tooth root infections [38], but the clinical significance in cats is currently unclear.

Phylum differences were reflected in class level differences. Additionally, Sphingobacteria and Flavobacteria, both members of the phylum Bacteroidetes, were also more common in the FIV-infected group. Both are

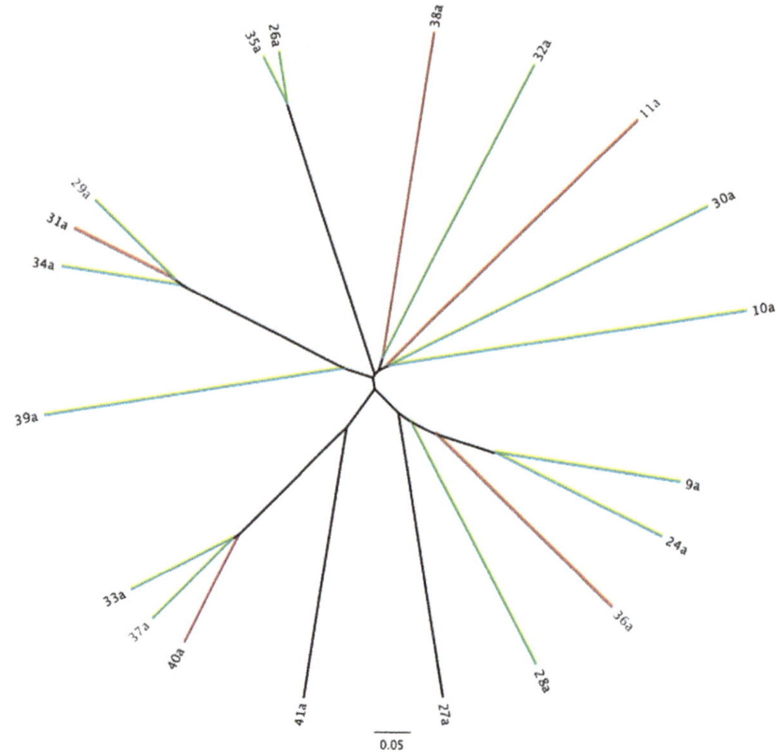

Figure 5 Oral microbial community structure in cats with FIV infection. Dendrogram based on the Yue & Clayton index of dissimilarity for the oral microbiota of 18 FIV-infected cats. Legend: Red lines indicate cats with moderate to severe gingival disease. Green lines indicate cats with mild or no gingival disease.

environmental organisms that can be found on body surfaces [39,40]. One could speculate that decreased local immune response could facilitate the survival of environmental organisms to which an individual is regularly exposed, but there is currently no supporting evidence for this. The statistically significant over-representation of various genera in FIV positive cats and the indicator species that were identified might also suggest that the oral cavity of this group is more amenable to colonization with organisms that are uncommon in healthy individuals, since these tended to be rare members of the community in FIV-uninfected cats.

The difference in staphylococci was interesting given the rather high relative abundance in the FIV-infected group (3.7%, compared to 0.3% in the FIV-uninfected group) and the range of infections that staphylococci can cause. Genus-level identification has limits because of the differences in virulence between different staphylococcal species. Speciation was not attempted because of the very limited species resolution of 16S rRNA gene sequencing for this genus. Yet, the overgrowth of this genus that consists of various important opportunistic pathogens raises concerns for infection risk in these cats.

In addition to *Staphylococcus*, other indicator OTUs for the FIV-infected group are of potential health concern, such as *Porphyromonas* (various species implicated in oral disease) [41,42], *Streptococcus* (different potential opportunistic pathogens, including oral pathogens) [43], *Parvimonas* (implicated in oral infections) [44,45] and *Gemella* (component of dental plaque that has been associated with opportunistic infections) [46,47].

The role of FIV infection in feline oral diseases such as gingivitis and stomatitis in cats is unclear, with some studies reporting an association between FIV infection and the prevalence or severity of oral infections [10], while others showing no association [48]. It has been suggested that the immune response to chronic antigenic stimulation or dysregulation of the immune response could be associated with increased disease risk [49] and both of those scenarios could involve the microbiota, as the microbiota is the primary antigenic exposure in the oral cavity and is known to closely interact with the immune system at other body sites [50,51]. Overgrowth of opportunistic pathogens residing in the oral cavity because of advanced immunocompromise is another potential cause.

There was no apparent impact of dental or gingival disease; however, this may be because of the small sample sizes of these subpopulations and the likely multifactorial nature of those diseases. Further, oral swabs provide an overview of the oral cavity but each swab is a composite swab of multiple different ecological niches that are present in the mouth. Therefore, changes in one specific location (e.g. plaque) might not be detected. The likelihood that FIV infection would predispose to oral infections also presumably relates in large part to the degree of immunosuppression. Most of the FIV-infected cats had clinical abnormalities, but the degree of immunocompromise was presumably variable and was not specifically studied. Study of cats with "feline AIDS" might provide more insight into changes associated with advanced immunocompromise.

Conclusions

The feline oral and conjunctival bacterial microbiotas are diverse microbial communities consisting of hundreds or thousands of different species, but with relatively few genera predominating. Feline immunodeficiency virus infection appears to have an impact on these microbiotas. The reasons for the apparent impact of FIV infection on these external microbial communities and the clinical relevance of altered microbiotas require further study.

Endnotes

[a]FIV/FeLV SNAP combo test, IDEXX Laboratories, Westbrook, ME, USA.

[b]IDEXX FIV realPCR test, IDEXX Laboratories, West Sacramento, CA, USA.

[c]University of Glasgow Retrovirus Research Laboratory, Glasgow, UK.

[d]E.Z.N.A. Stool DNA Kit, Omega Bio-Tek Inc., Doraville, Georgia, USA.

[e]Illumina, San Diego, USA.

Competing interests

The authors declare that they have no competing interests.

Authors' contributions

JSW and AL designed the study, based on an ongoing study designed by AL and JN. JN performed sample collection and animal data collection. MJ performed laboratory analyses. JSW performed data analysis. JSW drafted the manuscript, and all authors contributed to its revision. All authors read and approved the final manuscript.

Acknowledgements

This study was supported, in part, by a grant from the Maddie's Fund. The Purdue Maddie's Shelter Medicine Program is underwritten by a grant from Maddie's Fund, The Pet Rescue Foundation [www.maddiesfund.org], helping to fund the creation of a no-kill nation. Sequencing was performed at the University of Guelph's Advanced Analysis Centre.

Author details

[1]Department of Pathobiology, University of Guelph, Guelph, Canada.
[2]Department of Veterinary Clinical Sciences, Purdue University, 625 Harrison St., West Lafayette, IN 47907, USA.

References

1. Avila M, Ojcius DM, Yilmaz O (2009) The oral microbiota: living with a permanent guest. DNA Cell Biol 28:405–411
2. Brito LCN, Sobrinho APR, Teles RP, Socransky SS, Haffajee AD, Vieira LQ, Teles FR (2012) Microbiologic profile of endodontic infections from HIV- and HIV+ patients using multiple-displacement amplification and checkerboard DNA-DNA hybridization. Oral Dis 18:558–567
3. Lozupone CA, Li M, Campbell TB, Flores SC, Linderman D, Gebert MJ, Knight R, Fontenot AP, Palmer BE (2013) Alterations in the gut microbiota associated with HIV-1 infection. Cell Host Microbe 14:329–339
4. McHardy IH, Li X, Tong M, Ruegger P, Jacobs J, Borneman J, Anton P, Braun J (2013) HIV Infection is associated with compositional and functional shifts in the rectal mucosal microbiota. Microbiome 1:26
5. Yu G, Fadrosh D, Ma B, Ravel J, Goedert JJ (2014) Anal microbiota profiles in HIV-positive and HIV-negative MSM. AIDS 28:753–760
6. Chhetri BK, Berke O, Pearl DL, Bienzle D (2013) Comparison of the geographical distribution of feline immunodeficiency virus and feline leukemia virus infections in the United States of America (2000–2011). BMC Vet Res 9:2
7. Hosie MJ, Robertson C, Jarrett O (1989) Prevalence of feline leukaemia virus and antibodies to feline immunodeficiency virus in cats in the United Kingdom. Vet Rec 125:293–297
8. Ishida T, Washizu T, Toriyabe K, Motoyoshi S, Tomoda I, Pedersen NC (1989) Feline immunodeficiency virus infection in cats of Japan. J Am Vet Med Assoc 194:221–225
9. Nakamura Y, Nakamura Y, Ura A, Hirata M, Sakuma M, Sakata Y, Nishigaki K, Tsujimoto H, Setoguchi A, Endo Y (2010) An updated nation-wide epidemiological survey of feline immunodeficiency virus (FIV) infection in Japan. J Vet Med Sci 72:1051–1056
10. Tenorio AP, Franti CE, Madewell BR, Pedersen NC (1991) Chronic oral infections of cats and their relationship to persistent oral carriage of feline calici-, immunodeficiency, or leukemia viruses. Vet Immunol Immunopathol 29:1–14
11. Bekele S, Gelaw Y, Tessema F (2013) Ocular manifestation of HIV/AIDS and correlation with CD4+ cells count among adult HIV/AIDS patients in Jimma town, Ethiopia: a cross sectional study. BMC Ophthalmol 13:20
12. Hegde MC, Kumar A, Bhat G, Sreedharan S (2014) Oral microflora: a comparative study in HIV and normal patients. Indian J Otolaryngol Head Neck Surg 66(Suppl 1):126–132
13. Gonçalves LS, Gonçalves BML, Fontes TV (2013) Periodontal disease in HIV-infected adults in the HAART era: clinical, immunological, and microbiological aspects. Archi Oral Biol 58:1385–1396
14. Pereira VT, Pavan P, Souza RC, Souto R, Vettore MV, Torres SR, Colombo AP, de Uzeda M, Sansone C, Gonçalves LS (2014) The association between detectable plasmatic HIV viral load and different subgingival microorganisms in HIV-infected Brazilian adults: a multilevel analysis. J Periodontol 85:697–705
15. Lobprise HB (2012) Oral examination and charting. In: Lobprise HB (ed) Five minute veterinart consult clinical companion: small animal dentistry, 2nd edition. Blackwell Publishing Ltd, Ames, IA
16. Caporaso JG, Kuczynski J, Stombaugh J, Bittinger K, Bushman FD, Costello EK, Fierer N, Peña AG, Goodrich JK, Gordon JI, Huttley GA, Kelley ST, Knights D, Koenig JE, Ley RE, Lozupone CA, McDonald D, Muegge BD, Pirrung M, Reeder J, Sevinsky JR, Turnbaugh PJ, Walters WA, Widmann J, Yatsunenko T, Zaneveld J, Knight R (2010) QIIME allows analysis of high-throughput community sequencing data. Nat Methods 7:335–336
17. Schloss PD, Westcott SL, Ryabin T, Hall JR, Hartmann M, Hollister EB, Lesniewski RA, Oakley BB, Parks DH, Robinson CJ, Sahl JW, Stres B, Thallinger GG, Van Horn DJ, Weber CF (2009) Introducing mothur: open-source, platform-independent, community-supported software for describing and comparing microbial communities. Appl Environ Microbiol 75:7537–7541
18. Quast C, Pruesse E, Yilmaz P, Gerken J, Schweer T, Yarza P, Peplies J, Glöckner FO (2013) The SILVA ribosomal RNA gene database project: improved data processing and web-based tools. Nucleic Acids Res 41: D590–596
19. Edgar RC, Haas BJ, Clemente JC, Quince C, Knight R (2011) UCHIME improves sensitivity and speed of chimera detection. Bioinformatics 27:2194–2200
20. RDP [http://rdp.cme.msu.edu/index.jsp]
21. Gihring TM, Green SJ, Schadt CW (2012) Massively parallel rRNA gene sequencing exacerbates the potential for biased community diversity comparisons due to variable library sizes. Environ Microbiol 14:285–290
22. Bunge J, Woodard L, Böhning D, Foster JA, Connolly S, Allen HK (2012) Estimating population diversity with CatchAll. Bioinformatics 28:1045–1047

23. Lozupone C, Hamady M, Knight R (2006) UniFrac–an online tool for comparing microbial community diversity in a phylogenetic context. BMC Bioinformatics 7:371
24. Dufrêne M, Legendre P (1997) Species assemblages and indicator species: the need for a flexible asymmetrical approach. Ecol Monogr 67:345–366
25. Barry KA, Middelbos IS, Vester Boler BM, Dowd SE, Suchodolski JS, Henrissat B, Coutinho PM, White BA, Fahey GC Jr, Swanson KS (2012) Effects of dietary fiber on the feline gastrointestinal metagenome. J Proteome Res 11:5924–5933
26. Minamoto Y, Hooda S, Swanson KS, Suchodolski JS (2012) Feline gastrointestinal microbiota. Anim Health Res Rev 13:64–77
27. Sturgeon A, Pinder SL, Costa MC, Weese JS (2014) Characterization of the oral microbiota of healthy cats using next-generation sequencing. Vet J 201:223–229
28. Prado MR, Rocha MFG, Brito EHS, Girão MD, Monteiro AJ, Teixeira MFS, Sidrim JJ (2005) Survey of bacterial microorganisms in the conjunctival sac of clinically normal dogs and dogs with ulcerative keratitis in Fortaleza, Ceará, Brazil. Vet Ophthalmol 8:33–37
29. Shewen PE, Povey RC, Wilson MR (1980) A survey of the conjunctival flora of clinically normal cats and cats with conjunctivitis. Can Vet J 21:231–233
30. Hartmann AD, Hawley J, Werckenthin C, Lappin MR, Hartmann K (2010) Detection of bacterial and viral organisms from the conjunctiva of cats with conjunctivitis and upper respiratory tract disease. J Feline Med Surg 12:775–782
31. Espínola MB, Lilenbaum W (1996) Prevalence of bacteria in the conjunctival sac and on the eyelid margin of clinically normal cats. J Small Anim Pract 37:364–366
32. Tun HM, Brar MS, Khin N, Jun L, Hui RK, Dowd SE, Leung FC (2012) Gene-centric metagenomics analysis of feline intestinal microbiome using 454 junior pyrosequencing. J Microbiol Methods 88:368–376
33. Medhus A, Slettemeås JS, Marstein L, Larssen KW, Sunde M (2013) Methicillin-resistant *Staphylococcus aureus* with the novel *mecC* gene variant isolated from a cat suffering from chronic conjunctivitis. J Antimicrob Chemother 68:968–969
34. Lin C-T, Petersen-Jones SM (2008) Antibiotic susceptibility of bacteria isolated from cats with ulcerative keratitis in Taiwan. J Small Anim Pract 49:80–83
35. Liu P, Liu Y, Wang J, Guo Y, Zhang Y, Xiao S (2014) Detection of fusobacterium nucleatum and fadA adhesin gene in patients with orthodontic gingivitis and non-orthodontic periodontal inflammation. PLoS One 9:e85280
36. González OA, Li M, Ebersole JL, Huang CB (2010) HIV-1 reactivation induced by the periodontal pathogens *Fusobacterium nucleatum* and *Porphyromonas gingivalis* involves Toll-like receptor 2 [corrected] and 9 activation in monocytes/macrophages. Clin Vaccine Immunol 17:1417–1427
37. Xu H, Hao W, Zhou Q, Wang W, Xia Z, Liu C, Chen X, Qin M, Chen F (2014) Plaque bacterial microbiome diversity in children younger than 30 months with or without caries prior to eruption of second primary molars. PLoS One 9:e89269
38. Santos AL, Siqueira JF, Rôças IN, Jesus EC, Rosado AS, Tiedje JM (2011) Comparing the bacterial diversity of acute and chronic dental root canal infections. PLoS One 6:e28088
39. Lazarevic V, Whiteson K, Hernandez D, François P, Schrenzel J (2010) Study of inter- and intra-individual variations in the salivary microbiota. BMC Genomics 11:523
40. Hutter G, Schlagenhauf U, Valenza G, Horn M, Burgemeister S, Claus H, Vogel U (2003) Molecular analysis of bacteria in periodontitis: evaluation of clone libraries, novel phylotypes and putative pathogens. Microbiology 149:67–75
41. Booij-Vrieling HE, van der Reijden WA, Houwers DJ, de Wit WEAJ, Bosch-Tijhof CJ, Penning LC, van Winkelhoff AJ, Hazewinkel HA (2010) Comparison of periodontal pathogens between cats and their owners. Vet Microbiol 144:147–152
42. Pérez-Salcedo L, Herrera D, Esteban-Saltiveri D, León R, Jeusette I, Torre C, O'Connor A, González I, González I (2013) Isolation and identification of *Porphyromonas* spp. and other putative pathogens from cats with periodontal disease. J Vet Dent 30:208–213
43. Han YW, Wang X (2013) Mobile microbiome: oral bacteria in extra-oral infections and inflammation. J Dental Res 92:485–491
44. Topcuoglu N, Bozdoğan E, Kulekci G (2013) Presence of oral bacterial species in primary endodontic infections of primary teeth. J Clin Pediatr Dent 38:155–160
45. Uemura H, Hayakawa K, Shimada K, Tojo M, Nagamatsu M, Miyoshi-Akiyama T, Tamura S, Mesaki K, Yamamoto K, Yanagawa Y, Sugihara J, Kutsuna S, Takeshita N, Shoda N, Hagiwara A, Kirikae T, Ohmagari N (2014) *Parvimonas micra* as a causative organism of spondylodiscitis: a report of two cases and a literature review. Int J Infect Dis 23:53–55
46. Diaz PI, Chalmers NI, Rickard AH, Kong C, Milburn CL, Palmer RJ, Kolenbrander PE (2006) Molecular characterization of subject-specific oral microflora during initial colonization of enamel. Appl Environ Microbiol 72:2837–2848
47. Lo WB, Patel M, Solanki GA, Walsh AR (2013) Cerebrospinal fluid shunt infection due to *Gemella haemolysans*. J Neurosurg Pediatr 11:205–209
48. Belgard S, Truyen U, Thibault J-C, Sauter-Louis C, Hartmann K (2010) Relevance of feline calicivirus, feline immunodeficiency virus, feline leukemia virus, feline herpesvirus and Bartonella henselae in cats with chronic gingivostomatitis. Berl Munch Tierarztl Wochenschr 123:369–376
49. Sellon RK, Hartmann K (2012) Feline immunodeficiency virus infection. In: Greene CE (ed) Infectious diseases of the dog and cat, 4th edition. Saunders Elsevier, St. Louis, Missouri, pp 138–149
50. Wu S, Jiang Z-Y, Sun Y-F, Yu B, Chen J, Dai C-Q, Wu XL, Tang XL, Chen XY (2013) Microbiota regulates the TLR7 signaling pathway against respiratory tract influenza A virus infection. Curr Microbiol 67:414–422
51. McDermott AJ, Huffnagle GB (2013) The microbiome and regulation of mucosal immunity. Immunology 142:24–31
52. Maddie's Fund. [www.maddiesfund.org].

The potential spread of severe footrot in Norway if no elimination programme had been initiated: a simulation model

Gry M Grøneng[1*], Synnøve Vatn[2], Anja Bråthen Kristoffersen[1], Ola Nafstad[2] and Petter Hopp[1]

Abstract

When severe footrot was detected in Norway in 2008, a surveillance programme was initiated and followed by an elimination programme. By 2013 the disease had spread to two of 19 counties and a total of 119 (1%) sheep flocks had been diagnosed with severe footrot. A simulation model was developed to estimate the potential spread of severe footrot in Norway and to estimate the relative importance of the different spreading routes. The model parameters were based on the rate of spread of the first 38 diagnosed cases and the management and climatic factors particular for Norway. The model showed that by 2013, severe footrot would have spread to six counties and infected 16% of the sheep flocks if no elimination programme had been initiated. If this is compared with the 1% of flocks that were diagnosed in Norway by 2013, there seems to be a large effect of the implemented footrot elimination programme. By 2035, it was estimated that severe footrot would have spread to 16 counties and 64% of the sheep flocks. Such an extensive spread would probably impose a large negative impact on the sheep industry and welfare of the sheep. The most effective way to curb the spread of severe footrot was by decreasing the within county infection rate. This could be achieved by decreasing the contact between flocks or by decreasing the environmental load of *D. nodosus*, for example by footbathing sheep, culling diseased sheep or eliminating severe footrot in the flock.

Introduction

Footrot is well known in sheep-producing countries worldwide. The clinical signs range from mild inflammation of the interdigital skin to under-running and separation of the hoof horn from the sensitive tissues [1]. Footrot is a painful disease and causes lameness, poor welfare and affects ewe and lamb productivity [2,3]. *Dichelobacter nodosus* (*D. nodosus*), a Gram negative anaerobic bacterium, is the causative agent of footrot in small ruminants [1]. *D. nodosus* is divided into benign and virulent strains that can be differentiated in the laboratory by a gelatin gel test [4]. Clinical signs are often more severe when sheep are infected with the virulent *D. nodosus* strain than with the benign strain.

Severe footrot is a notifiable disease in Norway, and in 2008 the disease was diagnosed in the county of Rogaland in the south west of Norway [5]. This was the first detection of the disease in Norway since 1948 [6]. The term severe footrot has been used in Norway to include both flocks with diagnosed virulent strains of *D. nodosus* and flocks with severe clinical signs of footrot together with a positive PCR result but no bacterial isolates. A regional surveillance programme was initiated by the sheep industry in 2008, and in 2009, this was followed by a co-operative national elimination programme called the Healthy Feet Project (Animalia - Norwegian Meat and Poultry Research Centre). Between 2008 and 2011, clinical inspections were made of sheep in > 4500 sheep flocks. This includes close to 100% of the flocks in Rogaland. In addition, many of these flocks were inspected twice and some three or four times. By 2008, the disease had been detected in 1.5% of the flocks in Rogaland. The disease spread particularly rapidly in the municipality of Rennesøy, where 11.2% of the flocks were diagnosed with severe footrot in 2008 (Table 1). By 2012, severe footrot had only been detected in the county of Rogaland [7], but in 2013, virulent *D. nodosus* was diagnosed in 14 flocks in

* Correspondence: gry.groneng@vetinst.no
[1]Norwegian Veterinary Institute, P.O. Box 750 Sentrum, NO-0106 Oslo, Norway
Full list of author information is available at the end of the article

Table 1 Data used for estimating minimum, mode and maximum infection rate of severe footrot in Rogaland

	Rogaland excluding Rennesøy (minimum)		Whole of Rogaland (mode)		Rennesøy (maximum)	
Number of sheep flocks	2490		2597		107	
Year	Assumed infected	Predicted infected	Assumed infected	Predicted infected	Assumed infected	Predicted infected
2005	1	1	1	1	0	0
2006	ND	3	ND	3	1	1
2007	ND	9	ND	14	ND	4
2008	26	26	38	48	12	13
Regional percentage of infected flocks in 2008	1.0%		1.5%		11.2%	
Estimated infection rate (β)		**1.13**		**1.31**		**1.36**

ND = No data.
The estimates was based on data on the total number of sheep flocks and number of flocks assumed to be infected with severe footrot in the regions, from the introduction of the disease (2005 in Rogaland and 2006 in Rennesøy) until the initiation of the elimination programme in 2009. The predicted number of infected flocks in each region was the median value, of 2000 replicates of the model based on Equations 1–3. The infection rate is calculated using a constant yearly recovery rate of 5.3% and reversion rate of 1/3 of the infection rate.

the county of Aust-Agder, also situated in the southern part of Norway. By the end of 2013, 119 flocks in Norway had been diagnosed with severe footrot. Of these, 118 are now declared to be free from footrot, and measures have been implemented to eliminate severe footrot from the remainder [8]. Epidemiological and bacteriological investigations have indicated that virulent *D. nodosus* was introduced into a single flock in the county of Rogaland in 2005 through the purchase of sheep from abroad and thereafter spread locally [9,10].

The aim of this study was to estimate the potential spread of severe footrot in Norway if no elimination programme was implemented and estimate the importance of the different spreading routes of virulent *D. nodosus.* The developed model was based on the infection rate of the first diagnosed cases and the management and climatic factors specific to Norway.

Material and methods

A stochastic compartmental model can be used to simulate spread of disease within a population [11]. In a SILI-compartmental model, the susceptible(S), infected(I) and low susceptible(L) compartments and the transmission of flocks between these compartments describe the infection dynamics of the population. The susceptible flocks are not, and have not been, infected with the agent causing the disease. The infected flocks have at least one sheep infected with the agent causing disease and could infect susceptible or low susceptible flocks. The low susceptible flocks do not have any animals carrying the infection, and have a smaller contact network than the susceptible flocks, hence are less at risk of acquiring a disease than the susceptible flocks. The low susceptible flocks comprise of flocks with natural barriers towards other sheep flocks (called isolated flocks) and flocks that have recovered from the disease and by this increased their biosecurity measures (called recovered flocks). The latent period is assumed to be zero, and the immunity period for a flock is negligible.

In the model, flocks are transferred from one compartment to another at different rates. The infection rate (β) is the rate at which susceptible flocks become infected. This is dependent on the number of contacts, and the risk of transmission of disease per contact. The recovery rate (σ) is the rate of recovery of infected flocks, and which are accordingly assigned to the low susceptible compartment. The reversion rate (γ) is the rate at which low susceptible flocks become infected, and by this transferred to the infected compartment.

Spread within subpopulations

Subpopulations can be defined if the spread of disease is not uniform in the population [12], but highly reduced from one geographical area to another. Each subpopulation is then modelled with their own SILI-compartmental model with their own infection, recovery and reversion rate. These rates are based on specific values for each subpopulation that influence the spread of the disease in question.

Spread between subpopulations

Spread of disease is expected to be faster within the subpopulations than between two subpopulations as flocks within each subpopulation are expected to have more contact than flocks from two different subpopulations. Different types of contact between flocks in separate subpopulations may occur, leading to different transmission routes. Each transmission route between subpopulations are specified and quantified separately. Only susceptible flocks in the subpopulations are expected to be infected by other subpopulations as most of the low risk flocks have increased biosecurity and thereby will not be infected through the between subpopulation transmission route.

Model

Equations 1–3 and Figure 1 show the differential equations of the SILI-compartmental model for one subpopulation with the possible introduction of infection from other subpopulations. The equations give the number of flocks in the susceptible (1), infected (2), and low susceptible (3) compartments in a subpopulation for each year.

$$S_{i,y+1} = S_{i,y} - \min\left[\left(\beta_i \cdot S_{i,y} \cdot I_{i,y} + \sum_{j \neq i} \theta_{j,i,y} + \sum_{j \neq i} \tau_{j,i,y} + \sum_{j \neq i} \delta_{j,i,y}\right), S_{i,y}\right] \quad (1)$$

$$I_{i,y+1} = I_{i,y} - \sigma \cdot I_{i,y} + \min\left[\left(\beta_i \cdot S_{i,y} \cdot I_{i,y} + \sum_{j \neq i} \theta_{j,i,y} + \sum_{j \neq i} \tau_{j,i,y} + \sum_{j \neq i} \delta_{j,i,y}\right), S_{i,y}\right] + \gamma_i \cdot I_{i,y} \cdot L_{i,y} \quad (2)$$

$$L_{i,y+1} = L_{i,y} + \sigma \cdot I_{i,y} - \gamma_i \cdot I_{i,y} \cdot L_{i,y} \quad (3)$$

where i is the subpopulation receiving the infection, j is the subpopulation transmitting the infection and y is the time interval in years, S is the number of susceptible flocks, I is the number of infected flocks, L is the number of low susceptible flocks, β is the rate at which susceptible flocks become infected, σ is the rate at which infected flocks recover and hence become low susceptible flocks, γ is the rate at which low susceptible flocks become infected, θ, δ and τ is three possible ways of introduction of infection between subpopulations.

As the starting point for the simulations, the flocks infected with the disease was assigned to the infected compartment, the isolated flocks were assigned to the low susceptible compartment, and the remaining flocks were assigned to the susceptible compartment. Year was the time step and the model was run for the number of years desired.

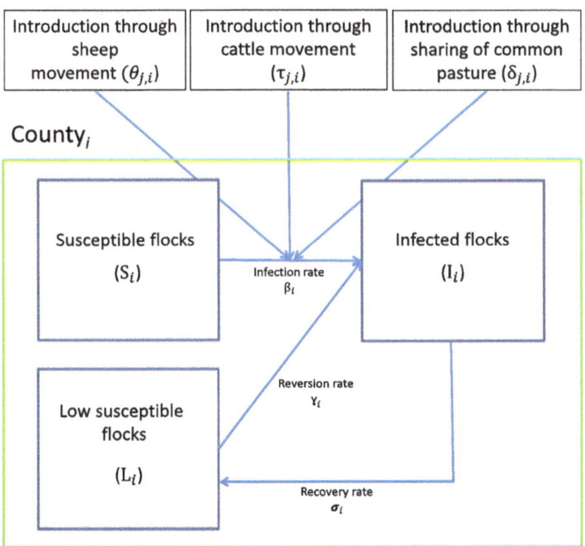

Figure 1 Susceptible - Infected – Low susceptible - Infected (SILI) model of severe footrot among sheep flocks. The simulation model was developed to estimate the potential spread of severe footrot in Norway if no elimination programme was initiated and to estimate the relative importance of the different spreading routes. The figure shows the transmission dynamics of severe footrot within one county (i) for one time step with possible introduction from other counties (j) through sheep movement, cattle movement and sharing of common pastures. The model was used to calculate all the 19 counties separately.

Adaptation of the model to footrot in Norwegian sheep flocks

A SILI-compartmental model was developed for estimating the spread of severe footrot in Norwegian sheep flocks without an elimination program. The isolated flocks in the low susceptible compartment were defined as sheep farms more than 3 km away from any other sheep farm. This was based on a study by Grøneng et al. [13] which showed that a geographic distance of more than 3 km between the main buildings of different sheep farms was not a significant risk factor in the univariable analysis. We interpret this as sheep farms with more than 3 km distance to the nearest sheep farm have a lower risk of contracting footrot.

The infection rate of footrot was calculated based on the rate of spread from the introduction of footrot in Norway in 2005 until the initiation of the elimination programme in 2009. At this time, severe footrot had only been detected in the county of Rogaland, but since different regions within the county possessed highly different rate of spread, the infection rate was expressed by a Pert distribution. Rogaland County excluding Rennesøy, Rogaland County with Rennesøy and the municipality of Rennesøy was the regions used to calculate the minimum (min), mode (mod) and maximum (max) infection rate respectively. The rates were then used in the Pert distribution.

To estimate the infection rate of the regions, the total number of sheep flocks and the number of flocks assumed to be infected with severe footrot in the region, from the introduction of the disease (2005 in Rogaland and 2006 in Rennesøy) until the initiation of the elimination programme in 2009 was used (Table 1). The infection rate was simulated based on Equations 1–3, with a constant annual recovery rate (σ) of 5.3% and a reversion rate (γ) of 1/3 of the infection rate (see below for descriptions of recovery and reversion rate). The assumed number of infected flocks was the number detected in the footrot outbreak in Norway, and the predicted median number of infected flocks was as close to this number as possible. The appurtenant infection rate was used in the model. The min, mod and max predicted median number of infected flocks and the appurtenant infection rates in parentheses were 26 (1.13), 48 (1.31) and 13

(1.36), respectively (Table 1). The Pert distribution for the infection rate for Rogaland was then ($\beta_{Rog} \sim$ Pert (1.13, 1.31, 1.36)).

The recovery rate was based on spread of severe footrot without an elimination programme and hence no compensation for sanitation or other measures to eliminate the disease. The recovered flocks have therefore either undergone sanitation procedure at their own cost or recovered from the disease spontaneously. Two of 38 flocks completed a successful sanitation procedure at the farmers own expense in 2008 (Vatn S, Healthy Feet project, personal communication), corresponding to a recovery rate of 5.3% per year. Some of the flocks might also recover from the disease with no intervention. Since it takes a long time for sheep in a flock to recover without human intervention [14], the percentage of these flocks is thought to be small and was not included. The recovery rate was assumed to be constant for all years.

Since none of the flocks which completed a successful sanitation procedure at the farmers own expense in 2008 was re-infected, the reversion rate could not be calculated based on data. The reversion rate was therefore sat based on knowledge of the infection dynamics. The susceptible flocks were assumed to have a three times higher infection rate than the low susceptible flocks, hence a reversion rate of ($\gamma = \beta/3$) was used.

Spread within subpopulations in Norway

Because of national maedi and scrapie legislation, sheep and goats are not allowed to be moved from one county to another without derogation. This gives a reduced spread from one county to another hence each of the 19 counties in Norway was assigned as a subpopulation. A SILI-compartmental model was constructed for each county. The number of sheep flocks, cattle herds and combined sheep and cattle flocks was allocated to each county from the Register of Production Subsidies of 31.07.2012 (Table 2). The register contains all holdings receiving production subsidies in Norway, hence includes >92% of the total number of sheep flocks; the ones missing are farms with very few sheep. The number was kept constant for all years.

The infection rate calculated earlier was only based on the rate of spread within the county of Rogaland. To calculate the rate of spread within each of the other counties, values which would interfere with the spread of footrot are quantified and used to adjust the minimum, mode and maximum within county infection rate for Rogaland.

One of the values expected to interfere with the infection rate of footrot was the climate within each county as this is an important factor for the survival of *D. nodosus* and for the initiation and development of ovine footrot [1,15]. In particular the precipitation and temperature are considered important for the spread of footrot [15,16]. The geo-coordinates of all sheep farm buildings in Norway (f) (the Agricultural Property Register, 2011) were linked to a mean value of precipitation $\left(\bar{p}_{f,\,i}\right)$ and temperature $(\bar{t}_{f,\,i})$ from May until October (Norwegian Meteorological Institute, data from 1971 till 2000). By summarising the mean daily precipitation in mm and mean daily temperature in degrees Celsius of the individual sheep farms in a county, and dividing by the number of sheep farms in that county ($N_{f,i}$), a climatic value (called Cl_i) was calculated for each of the 19 counties (Equation 4).

$$Cl_i = \frac{\sum_f \bar{p}_{f,\,i} + \sum_f \bar{t}_{f,\,i}}{N_{f,\,i}} \tag{4}$$

The fraction between the climatic factors in county i and the climatic factor in Rogaland was incorporated in Equation 5 to adjust the infection rate within each county.

Another value expected to interfere with the infection rate of footrot was the density of sheep farms within each county. Grøneng et al. [13] showed that a risk factor for contracting the disease is a sheep farm located less than 1 km from a sheep farm positive for severe footrot. The distances between farms were calculated based on the locations of the main building on each farm. Hence, for each sheep farm, the number of other sheep farms within 1 km (neighbour farms) was obtained. Based on this, the mean number of neighbour farms to the sheep farms within each county $(\bar{n}_{1km,i})$ was calculated (Table 2). The fraction between the mean number of sheep farms within 1 km in county i and the county Rogaland was used to adjust the infection rate in county i (Equation 5). By using the knowledge of the spread of disease in the county of Aust-Agder, the effect of the fraction between counties was adjusted. In 2013, 14 flocks in the county of Aust-Agder were diagnosed with severe footrot, and epidemiological investigations indicate that sheep moved from the county of Rogaland in 2006 were the source. The spread from the introduction in 2006 to 2013 was simulated based on Equations 1–3, and a value k, adjusting the effect of the density factor between Aust-Agder and Rogaland, was chosen so that the median value of 2000 replicates matched the number of infected flocks in Aust-Agder in 2013. A median of 14 (range 1–26) infected flocks was predicted for $k = 2.3$ (Equation 5).

For all counties except Rogaland, a county specific min, mod and max infection rate was estimated by

Table 2 Overview of demographic data, climatic rate and infection rate for modelling spread of severe footrot

County	N° of sheep flocks (nSh)	N° of cattle herds (nCa)	N° of combined flocks (*nShCa*)	N° of isolated flocks	Mean number of neighbouring flocks ($\bar{n}_{1km,i}$)	Climatic rate (Cl_i/Cl_{Rog})	Infection rate (β) (minimum, mode, maximum)
Østfold	160	360	43	49	0.2	0.61	0.04, 0.05, 0.05
Akershus	226	359	45	43	0.8	0.61	0.17, 0.19, 0.20
Oslo	8	5	4	6	0.0001*	0.67	0.01, 0.01, 0.01
Hedmark	669	1108	200	99	1.4	0.51	0.24, 0.28, 0.29
Oppland	1323	2224	324	60	1.6	0.51	0.28, 0.32, 0.34
Buskerud	552	593	111	53	1.5	0.56	0.29, 0.33, 0.35
Vestfold	129	225	29	25	0.3	0.69	0.07, 0.08, 0.09
Telemark	372	360	72	54	1.3	0.67	0.30, 0.35, 0.36
Aust-Agder	220	250	47	60	0.8	0.76	0.21, 0.24, 0.25
Vest-Agder	450	583	150	45	1.2	0.93	0.38, 0.44, 0.46
Rogaland	2597	2735	1297	20	3.3	1	1.13, 1.31, 1.36
Hordaland	1997	1457	603	37	2.3	1	0.79, 0.91, 0.95
Sogn og Fjordane	1617	1756	625	59	2.5	0.97	0.83, 0.96, 1.00
Møre og Romsdal	1053	1880	358	94	1.2	0.89	0.37, 0.42, 0.44
Sør-Trøndelag	728	1729	187	99	1.1	0.62	0.23, 0.27, 0.28
Nord-Trøndelag	524	1737	178	98	0.6	0.67	0.14, 0.16, 0.17
Nordland	1045	1366	272	169	0.8	0.73	0.20, 0.23, 0.24
Troms	522	442	92	92	0.8	0.5	0.14, 0.16, 0.16
Finnmark	123	192	26	42	0.5	0.38	0.07, 0.08, 0.08

*In the county of Oslo no flocks had any neighbouring flocks within 1 km, hence the value was set at 0.0001.

The data are displayed for all the 19 counties in Norway. The number of sheep and cattle flocks includes the number of combined flocks. The number of isolated flocks (no other flocks within 3 km), the mean number of neighbouring flocks (sheep farms within a distance of 1 km), and the climatic rate (Cl_i/Cl_{Rog}) was calculated on the basis of the geographical co-ordinates of the building of the sheep farms. The infection rate (β) was the rate of susceptible flocks becoming infected due to within county transmission.

adjusting the min, mod and max infection rate for Rogaland with the constant k, the mean number of sheep farms within 1 km and climatic value for the respective counties. These values were then used in a Pert distribution, where a new value was estimated for each county and each replicate (Equation 5).

$$\beta i \sim \text{Pert}\left(\beta_{Min,Rog} \cdot \sqrt[2.3]{\frac{\bar{n}_{1km,i}}{\bar{n}_{1km,Rog}} \cdot \frac{Cl_i}{Cl_{Rog}}},\ \beta_{Mod,Rog} \cdot \sqrt[2.3]{\frac{\bar{n}_{1km,i}}{\bar{n}_{1km,Rog}} \cdot \frac{Cl_i}{Cl_{Rog}}},\ \beta_{Max,Rog} \cdot \sqrt[2.3]{\frac{\bar{n}_{1km,i}}{\bar{n}_{1km,Rog}} \cdot \frac{Cl_i}{Cl_{Rog}}}\right) \quad (5)$$

where i is the county, and *Rog* is Rogaland County.

The recovery rate was not expected to differ between counties and was expected to be constant for every year. The reversion rate for each county was defined as one third of the infection rate ($\gamma_i = \beta_i/3$).

Spread between subpopulations in Norway

The spread of footrot between counties in Norway was modelled taking three potential transmission routes into consideration: 1) movement of sheep between counties, 2) movement of cattle between counties, and 3) introduction by sharing of common pastures (Figure 1).

Introduction from other counties through sheep movement (θ)

Although there is a general ban on movement of sheep from one county to another because of maedi and scrapie, derogations from the legislation can be authorised by the Norwegian Food Safety Authority. Two movements of sheep between counties were recorded in 2013 (MATS, the supervision system of the Norwegian Food Safety Authority). There may have been movements of sheep that have not been reported to the central Food Safety Authority, but these are believed to be minimal. We therefore assumed that some of the sheep in 0.05% of the flocks in a county would be moved to each of the neighbouring counties each year. In addition, some of the sheep in 0.025% of the flocks in a county would move sheep to each of the counties bordering on neighbouring counties each year. Thus the number of movements from county j to county i was estimated ($MSh_{j,i}$), and used to calculate the introduction of severe footrot to other counties (Equation 7). For Norway as a whole, this is equivalent to approximately 44 between county movements of sheep each year. As this is more than reported to the Norwegian Food Safety Authority, we believe the effect of moving sheep across county borders has been overestimated rather than underestimated.

Only movement of sheep that is infected with footrot can transmit the disease to other sheep flocks. This depends on the probability that sheep from an infected flock are moved $\left(\frac{I_j}{nSh_j} \cdot MSh_{j,i}\right)$, and also on the probability that at least one of the sheep moved is infected (*ProbMove*). The *ProbMove* is based on the number of sheep moved and the prevalence of infected sheep within the flock. The minimum *ProbMove* value was based on movement of one sheep from a flock with an infection prevalence of 0.01. The maximum *ProbMove* value was based on movement of five sheep from a flock with a prevalence of 0.65. The values were calculated to be 0.01 and 0.995 as shown in Equation 6. Consequently, a uniform distribution with a minimum and maximum value of the *ProbMove* was used (ProbMove ~ Unif (0.01, 0.995)) in Equation 7.

$$MaxProbMove = 1 - (1 - Prevalence)^{NumberMoveSheep} \quad (6)$$

The number of sheep moved was based on the knowledge that mostly rams are purchased, and since the sheep flocks are small, rarely more than two rams are acquired at the same time. The lowest prevalence was based on one infected sheep in a flock of 100 sheep. The highest prevalence was based on PCR examination of all sheep in three flocks infected with severe footrot, and the median of these values was used. This was chosen since only sheep from flocks with a veterinary health certificate may be moved across county borders. We therefore believe that flocks with a prevalence above 0.65 would not be allowed to move sheep because they would show pronounced clinical signs of footrot.

The introduction of severe footrot from other counties by sheep movement is shown in Equation 7, where the percentage of susceptible sheep flocks in county i $\left(\frac{S_i}{nSh_i}\right)$. was included in order to calculate the probability of an infected sheep arriving at a susceptible sheep flock. We expect that a sheep which is infected with footrot would infect a flock of susceptible animals.

$$\theta_{j,i} = \frac{I_j}{nSh_j} \cdot MSh_{j,i} \cdot ProbMove \cdot \frac{S_i}{nSh_i} \quad (7)$$

where i is the county receiving infectn, and j is the county transmitting the infection, I is the number of infected sheep flocks, nSh is the total number of sheep flocks, MSh is the number of flocks that have moved sheep, and S is the number of susceptible sheep flocks.

Introduction from other counties through cattle movement (τ)

Cattle that have been in contact with infected sheep may be carriers of virulent *D. nodosus* and transmit the infection to sheep [17,18]. Hence, virulent *D. nodosus* might be introduced to a new county by movement of cattle. The number of moved cattle aged >1 year (*MCa*) in 2007 was retrieved from the Norwegian National Cattle Register (Norwegian Food Safety Authority) (Table 2). Cattle aged <1 year were not included as calves are usually not in contact with sheep, and the probability of a calf being infected by its mother and remain infected until moved to another flock was expected to be minimal. Only information from 2007 was available. In cases where there was no registered movement between neighbouring counties in 2007, movement of one head of cattle was imputed. The register also included records of movement of cattle without information about which county they were moved from. These were included by giving the unknown county the mean number of cattle flocks, the mean number of combined flocks and the mean number infected for all the counties. The number of infected sheep flocks in a county that transmit the disease (I_j), the number of sheep flocks in the county j (nSh_j), the number of cattle flocks in counties i and j (nCa_i, nCa_j), and the number of combined cattle and sheep flocks in counties i and j ($nShCa_j$, $nShCa_i$) (Table 2) are used to calculate the probability of severe footrot being introduced from other counties by movement of cattle. The probability of a sheep infecting cattle (Sh2Ca) and vice versa (Ca2Sh) was also needed for the calculation. On the basis of a study by Knappe-Poindecker et al. [18], the value was found to be 0.1 (gelatin gel test showed five of fifty cattle to be positive after co-grazing with sheep), while a study by Rogdo et al. [19] found this probability to be 0.3 (18 of 58 cattle were PCR-positive for footrot with serogroup A). The probability of sheep infecting cattle and vice versa was given by a uniform distribution (Ca2Sh ~ *Unif* (0.1, 0.3), $Sh2Ca \sim Unif\,(0.1, 0.3)$), a new value was generated for each movement. The percentage of susceptible sheep flocks in county i $\left(\frac{S_i}{nSh_i}\right)$ was included to enable calculation of the probability of infected cattle entering a susceptible sheep flock. Equation 8 expresses the introduction of severe footrot from other counties through movement of cattle:

$$\tau_{j,i} = I_j \cdot \frac{nShCa_j}{nSh_j} \cdot Sh2Ca \cdot \frac{MCa_{j,i}}{nCa_j} \cdot \frac{nShCa_i}{nCa_i} \cdot Ca2Sh \cdot \frac{S_i}{nSh_i} \quad (8)$$

where i is the county receiving infection, and j is the county transmitting the infection.

Introduction from other counties through sharing of common pasture (δ)

In Norway, many sheep flocks are transported to common pastures during the summer. This is mainly pastures situated in mountain areas. This is an old tradition, and it is important both for reducing the farmer's feed expenses and for conserving the countryside. There are nearly 1000 common pasture groups in Norway, each with several members and a designated area for their sheep to graze (Norwegian Forest And Landscape Institute). The organisation of the pasture groups is quite complex, with some common pasture areas crossing county borders. Some pasture groups also have members from several counties. Information about common pastures that share borders with common pastures in other counties and common pastures that have members from different counties are included in the estimation of cross-county transmission on pasture. In these pastures there are no fences or other barriers, with the result that sheep from different counties can mix and transfer infection. The spread of severe footrot on common pasture was calculated in a same way as the within county infection rates (Equation 5) by adjusting the infection rate for Rogaland for differences in sheep flock density and climate. Since sheep flocks are free ranging on common pasture, it is difficult to estimate the mean number of flocks within 1 km, as was done when calculating the within county infection rates. But sheep flocks are often put on common pasture at different times and in different areas, and 1–2 ewes with their lambs tend to keep together within a small area and rarely be in contact with other sheep. Assuming maximum dispersion of flocks on common pasture, we calculated the mean number of flocks per 1 km^2 for each of the common pastures and used this as a proxy for the number for flocks within 1 km of each other. The higher the density of sheep flocks on common pasture, the higher the infection rate then will be. The mean number of flocks within 1 km^2 on the common pastures where flocks from county j and i can be in contact with each other ($\bar{N}_{1km^2,past\,j,i}$) was calculated as shown in Equation 9 by adding the density of common pastures in county j and i which have a common border (*Bpast*) to the density of common pasture which have members from both counties j and i (*Mpast*). This was used in Equation 10 to calculate the common pasture infection rates.

$$\bar{N}_{1km^2,past\,j,i} = \frac{\sum_{Bpast}\left(\frac{\left(N_{f(j)}/A_{past(j)} + N_{f(i)}/A_{past(i)}\right)}{2}\right) + \sum_{Mpast}\left(N_{f\,j,i}/A_{past(j,i)}\right)}{n_{Bpast} + n_{Mpast}} \quad (9)$$

where N_f is the number of sheep flocks on pasture, A_{past} is the geographic area of the pasture in km^2 and n is the number of pastures.

The climate of the common pastures (Cl_{past}) could not be calculated in the same way as the within county climate because we did not have specific geographical points, but rather large areas across which the sheep flocks were spread. The common pastures are often situated at a higher altitude than the general location of sheep farms, and the climate is often colder and dryer. Given this knowledge, we believe that the climate on common pasture has a lower value than the climate in any of the counties, so the climatic rate of common pasture (Cl_{past}/Cl_{Rog}) was assumed to be 0.3, lower than the lowest climate rate (Table 2). The climatic rate was constant for all years, and was used in the calculation of the common pasture infection rates as shown in Equation 10.

The common pasture infection rate was calculated in the same way as the within county infection rates (Equation 5) with a Pert distribution for each county and each iteration (Equation 10).

$$\beta_{past,j,\,i} \sim \text{Pert}\left(\beta_{Min,Rog}\cdot\sqrt[2.3]{\frac{\bar{N}_{1km^2,past,j,i}}{\bar{n}_{1km,Rog}}}\cdot 0.3,\;\beta_{Mod,Rog}\cdot\sqrt[2.3]{\frac{\bar{n}_{1km^2,past,j,i}}{\bar{n}_{1km,Rog}}}\cdot 0.3,\;\beta_{Max,Rog}\cdot\sqrt[2.3]{\frac{\bar{n}_{1km^2,past,j,i}}{\bar{n}_{1km,Rog}}}\cdot 0.3\right) \quad (10)$$

The introduction of severe footrot from other counties through sharing of common pasture was calculated on the basis of the common pasture infection rate ($\beta_{past,j,i}$), the percentage of infected flocks in county j $\left(\frac{I_j}{nSh_j}\right)$, and the percentage of susceptible flocks in county i $\left(\frac{S_i}{nSh_i}\right)$. The number of flocks from county i ($n_{past,i}$) and county j ($n_{past,j}$) on common pasture was also included to calculate the number of flocks in county i that were newly infected by sharing common pasture with county j (Equation 11).

$$\delta_{j,\,i} = \beta_{past,\,j,\,i}\cdot\frac{I_j}{nSh_j}\cdot n_{past,\,j}\cdot\frac{n_{past,\,i}}{(n_{past,\,j}+n_{past,\,i})}\cdot\frac{S_i}{nSh_i} \quad (11)$$

where i is the county receiving infection, and j is the county transmitting the infection.

Model for Norway

As the starting point for the simulations, one flock in the county of Rogaland was assigned to the infected compartment, the isolated flocks in each county were assigned to the low susceptible compartment in the respective counties, and the remaining flocks in each county were assigned to the susceptible compartments. When the probability of transferring flocks between compartments resulted in decimal number of flocks, the decimal number was converted to an integer by performing a Bernoulli trial with the decimal fraction as the probability. The county results were aggregated to give the results for Norway.

Scenarios

Basic scenario

The basic scenario was simulation of the spread of severe footrot without any elimination or control with input values as presented in Tables 1 and 2. For all the scenarios where input parameters were changed, the basic scenario was used as the reference.

Scenarios with different control measures

The disease can be controlled by reducing the within county or between county transmissions compared to the basic scenario. Scenarios with a 20%, 40%, 60% and 80% lower infection rate within the counties were modelled. Scenarios with 20%, 40%, 60%, 80% and 100% less movement of sheep between counties were modelled. Scenarios with 20%, 40%, 60%, 80% and 100% less movement of cattle between counties were modelled. Scenarios with 20%, 40%, 60%, 80% and 100% fewer flocks sharing common pasture were modelled.

Scenarios with increased between county transmission

Increased between county movement of both sheep and cattle, and an increased number of flocks on common pastures are scenarios that we might see in the future. Hence the importance of this factor is highlighted. A five-fold and ten-fold increase was modelled.

Sensitivity analyses

By increasing and decreasing the basic scenario parameters one by one, an indication of the robustness of the model and the sensitivity of the model parameters is found. The sensitivity analysis was performed by stepwise increasing and decreasing of the parameters, starting with 80%, then 60%, 40% and 20%. The analysis was continued until the number of infected flocks did not deviate by more than 5% compared to the basic model. Thus, only the 80% increase and decrease was performed for the parameters which showed little variance in the results compared to the basic scenario. The parameters included in the sensitivity analysis were the infection rate, recovery rate, reversion rate, climatic value, climatic rate on common pasture, number of farms within 1 km (neighbouring flocks) and number of farms within 3 km (isolated flocks).

Model simulations

The model was run from 2005 and 30 years onward. In addition, the basic scenario where the time interval was extended to the year 2100 was made. The intention was to capture the percentage of flocks in each of the compartments when the equilibrium state was reached. The model was run using R v2.15.1 [20] and the additional package deSolve [21]. For each simulation of a scenario, 2000 replicates were made.

Results

Basic scenario

In the basic scenario, severe footrot was estimated to have spread to six of the 19 counties and 16% of the sheep flocks in Norway by 2013, and 16 counties and 64% of the flocks were infected by 2035 (Figure 2). In 2100, severe footrot was estimated to be spread to all counties except Oslo, and to 76% of the sheep flocks.

The counties in the south-west of Norway were infected during the early years; after that, the remaining counties in southern Norway were infected, except Oslo, where none of the eight flocks were infected by 2035. Nor did the two northernmost counties, i.e. Troms and Finnmark, experience an introduction of severe footrot during the simulated period (Figures 3 and 4).

After the initial introduction of infection into a county, the model estimates that it takes four to twenty years before approximately 5% of the sheep flocks in the county are infected. Thereafter, one to nineteen years elapses before more than 30% of the sheep flocks in the county are infected. The steepest increase in the number of infected sheep flocks is observed in the five counties Rogaland, Hordaland, Vest-Agder, Sogn og Fjordane and Møre og Romsdal. Infected flocks in these counties increase from 5% to 60% within two to five years, while in the other counties it takes from eight to more than twenty years to reach this percentage (Figure 3).The counties of Rogaland and Finnmark have the highest and lowest percentages of infected flocks in 2100, at 88% and 7%, respectively, when the county of Oslo is excluded (0%). A state of equilibrium between the compartments are reached in the year 2068, when the number of infected flocks and low susceptible flocks stabilises at 76% and 24%, respectively.

Scenarios with different control measures

A 20% and 40% reduction in the infection rate results in 57% and 46% infected flocks respectively in 2035 (Figure 5). The exclusion of one of the between counties transmission routes at a time, while keeping the other two routes, reduces the number of infected flocks (Figure 5). The prohibition of common pasture reduces the number of infected flocks in 2035 by 9% compared to the basic scenario. The prohibition of movement of cattle reduces the number of infected flocks by 2%, and delays the introduction of severe footrot to one more county compared to the basic scenario, i.e. the county of Østfold is not infected by 2035 in this scenario. By concurrent exclusion of two between county transmission routes, the number of infected flocks is further reduced compared to the basic scenario. Excluding both the movement of cattle and common pasture results in a 20% decrease in the number of infected flocks in 2035 compared with the basic scenario.

Scenarios with increased between county transmission

A ten-fold increase in the movement of sheep, the movement of cattle, and the use of common pasture increase the number of infected flocks in 2035 by 3%, 9% and 17%, respectively. The spread of severe footrot is further extended (compared to the basic scenario) to the county of Troms in the scenarios with increased movement of cattle and increased use of common pasture, and also to the county of Oslo in the scenario with increased movement of cattle.

Sensitivity analysis

In the sensitivity analysis, the variables with a more than 5% decrease or increase in the number of infected flocks compared to the basic scenario in 2035 are listed underneath. When reducing the climatic value with 80, 60, 40 and 20%, the number of infected flocks was reduced to 3%, 30%, 44% and 55%, respectively. When increasing the climatic value with 80, 60, 40 and 20%, the number of infected flocks was increased to 81%, 78%, 73% and 70%, respectively. When reducing the number of neighbouring flocks with 80, 60 and 40%, the number of

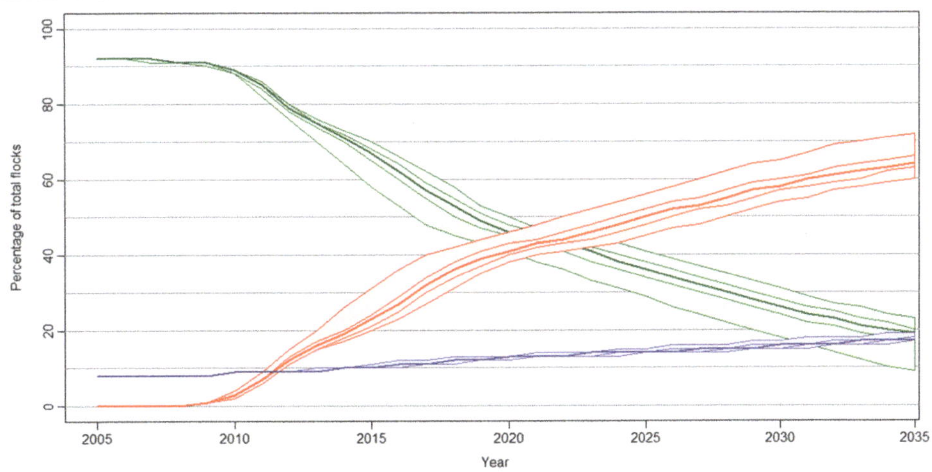

Figure 2 Simulated development of severe footrot in Norwegian sheep flocks without an elimination programme. The percentage of susceptible (green), infected (red) and low susceptible (purple) flocks are shown for each of the years 2005 – 2035 with the median value and 2.5, 25, 75 and 97.5 percentiles.

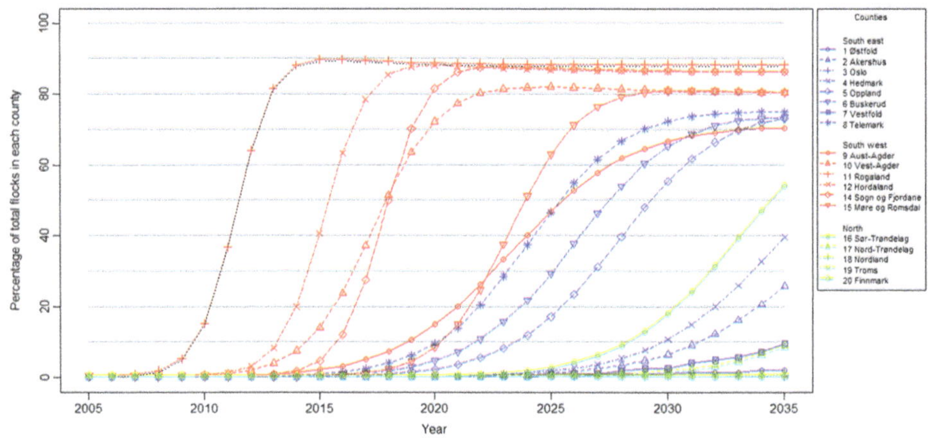

Figure 3 Simulated spread of severe footrot without an elimination programme in the 19 Norwegian counties. The median percentage of infected flocks within each county for each year in the period 2005 – 2035.

infected flocks was reduced to 38%, 48% and 55%, respectively. When increasing the number of neighbouring flocks with 80, 60 and 40%, the number of infected flocks was increased to 72%, 70% and 69%, respectively. When reducing the reversion rate by 80, 60 and 40%, the number of infected flocks was reduced to 44%, 53% and 58%, respectively. When increasing the reversion rate with 80, 60, 40 and 20%, the number of infected flocks was increased to 70%, 69% and 68%, respectively. When reducing the recovery rate by 80, 60 and 40%, the number of infected flocks was increased to 77%, 74% and 70%, respectively. When increasing the recovery rate by 80, 60 and 40%, the number of infected flocks was reduced to 53%, 56% and 59%, respectively. The variables which with an 80% increase or decrease deviated 5% or less from the basic scenario were; increased and decreased 3 km distance and increased and decreased climate on common pasture (Figure 6).

Discussion

A simulation model is a useful tool to predict the spread of disease in a population. But spread of an infectious

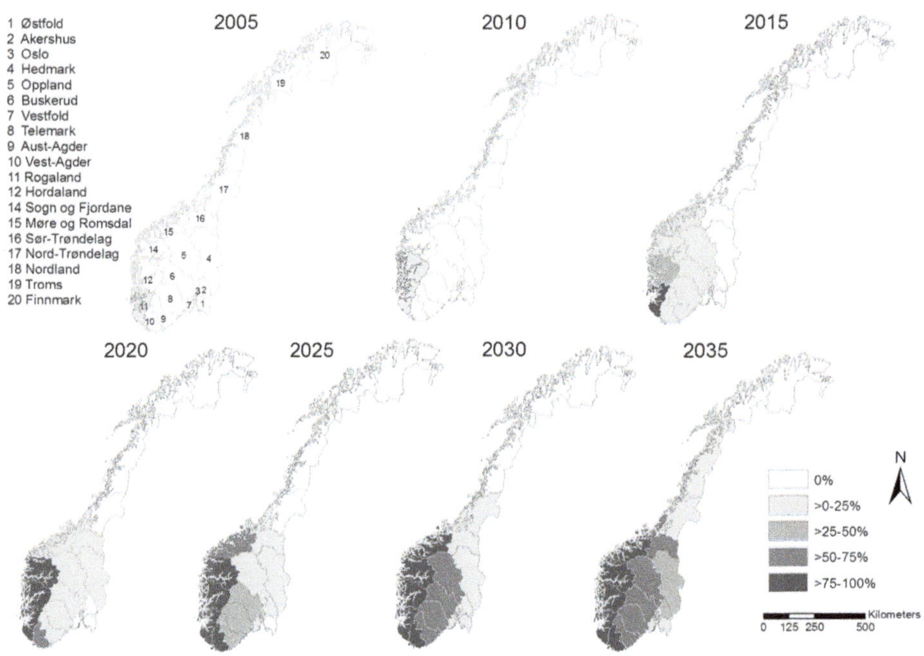

Figure 4 Simulated geographical spread of severe footrot in Norwegian sheep flocks without an elimination programme. The maps show the spread of severe footrot in the 19 counties of Norway at five-year intervals. The intensity of the grey shading shows the percentage of infected flocks in each of the counties.

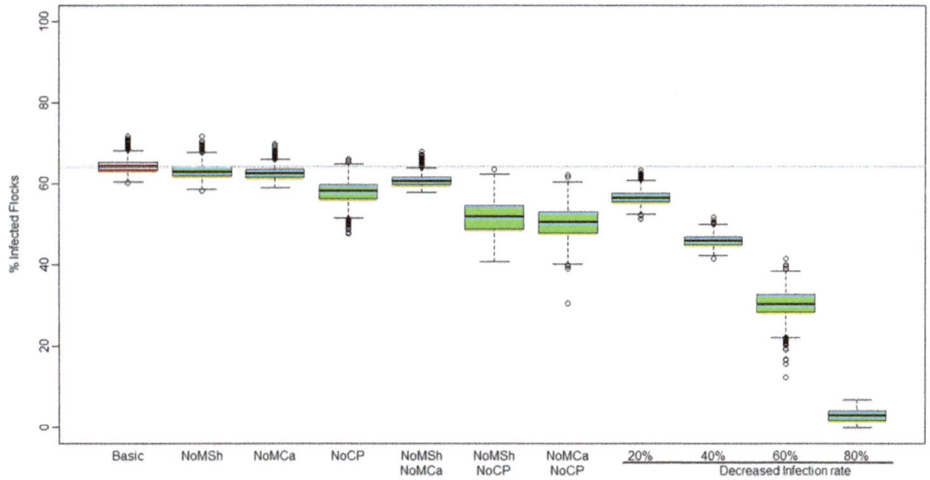

Figure 5 Estimated percentage of infected flocks in 2035 using different strategies for reducing severe footrot. The box-and-whiskers plot shows the distribution of the percentage of total flocks infected in Norway in 2035 based on 2000 replicates. The basic scenario is shown in red and various reduction strategies of the infection in green. The box represents the 25 and 75 percentiles and the black line inside the box represents the median value. Circles outside the whiskers are outliers. BasicS = Basic Scenario, NoMSh = exclusion of sheep movement, NoMCa = exclusion of cattle movement, NoCP = exclusion of common pasture, 20%, 40%, 60% and 80%: decrease in infection rate by 20%, 40%, 60% and 80%, respectively.

disease is a complex phenomenon with many interacting factors. Hence the development of a model must be based on knowledge of the specific disease in question and the routes of spread within the population as the model assumptions and the input variables used are important for obtaining a reliable result.

Most of the assumptions and input variables in this study have been based on observed parameters of the population, management and climate in Norway. In addition, the infection rate was based on observed values of the spread of footrot in Rogaland from introduction in 2005 until implementing the elimination program in 2009, and then adjusted to the other counties in Norway by using the observed spread in Aust-Agder. Data on spread for more than four years and more than two counties would have been desirable, but since an elimination program was implemented in Norway, such data was not available.

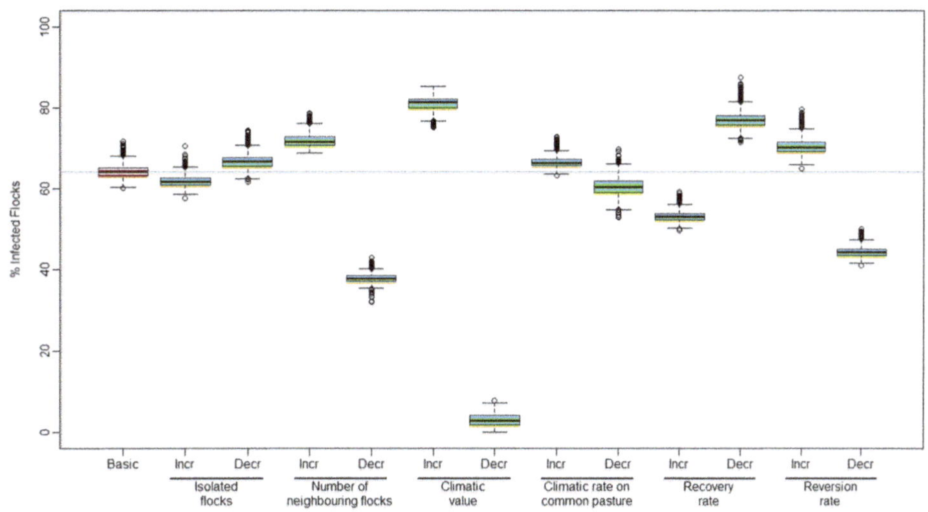

Figure 6 Sensitivity analysis of parameters used in a model for the spread of severe footrot. The box-and-whiskers plot shows the distribution of the estimated percentage of flocks infected with severe footrot in Norway in 2035 based on 2000 replicates. The basic scenario is shown in red and the 80% increase and decrease in the variables in the model is shown in green. The box represents the 25 and 75 percentiles and the black line inside the box represents the median value. Circles outside the whiskers are outliers. BasicS = Basic scenario, Incr = 80% increase in the variable and Decr = 80% decrease in the variable.

The sensitivity of the input parameters has also been examined. The variables found important in the sensitivity analysis were changes in the climatic value, the number of neighbouring flocks, the recovery, and the reversion rate. As expected, the climatic value is an important parameter for the spread of footrot. The values used in the model were based on observed mean precipitation and temperature for a 30 year period. More than a 20% increase or reduction of the observed value is not expected. Hence up to 14% decrease or 9% increase in the number of infected flocks compared to the basic scenario might be possible. The number of neighbouring flocks is also an important parameter. This value was based on the geographical coordinates of sheep farms. A higher or lower density of sheep farms might be possible, but we do not expect more than 20% change in this factor during the modelled 30 years. This would result in less than 5% deviation compared to the basic model. The recovery rate was based on data from the Healthy Feet project, and an increase or decrease in this value of more than 20% is not expected. With an increase/decrease of 20% the deviation from the basic scenario was less than 5%. The reversion rate is an important model parameter, and data on this value would have been desirable, but this is one of the few parameters in the model for which no data is available. A 40% change in this variable gives a more than 5% deviation in the result compared to the basic scenario. We cannot exclude the possibility that the reversion rate can have other values than the ones modelled. Low reversion rate is an advantage, and this can be achieved by good biosecurity measures. The rest of the variables did not change the outcome in the sensitivity analysis.

The reliability of the model can be assessed by comparing the infection dynamics in the model with what is expected based on knowledge of the disease and the spread in other populations.

Severe footrot was not introduced into the two northernmost counties in Norway in the period covered by the simulation. These counties are situated far from the county of Rogaland and to reach them the infection would have to cross several county borders that act as barriers for the transmission of the infection. In addition, the average temperature decreases going north in the country, resulting in a climate that is less favourable to the spread of footrot. A delayed introduction and spread to these counties, as predicted by the model, would accordingly be expected.

Another of the factors which increase the reliability of the model is the fact that the steepest increase in number of infected sheep flocks was seen in five counties that are all characterized by having a wet, warm climate and a relatively high density of sheep flocks compared to the other counties in Norway. These factors are known to enhance the development and spread of *D. nodosus*, resulting in a high within county infection rate, hence a steep increase is expected.

We also compared the modeled results with parameters from the UK, where footrot is endemic. In a study, 86% of the sheep farmers in the UK reported to have footrot within a twelve-month period, and more than 95% had experienced footrot at some time [22]. This is similar to the situation in Rogaland county which stabilised at 88%. The overall prevalence of infected flocks in Norway stabilised at a lower level, but this was as expected since the other counties with the exception of Hordaland, have a climate less favourable for footrot (Table 2).

Even though this model was based on the factors specific for Norway, a similar approach can be used to predict the spread of disease in other populations by estimating the input variables specific to the disease and the country or region in question.

Basic scenario

Extensive spread of severe footrot, in terms of both the number of infected flocks and the number of counties affected is predicted within 30 years (Figures 2, 3 and 4). This results in a large proportion of the Norwegian sheep population being affected by pain, lameness and welfare problems which would have a high economic cost for the sheep industry [23]. A comparison of the predicted number of infected flocks with the cumulative number of flocks diagnosed with severe footrot in 2013 appears to show that the footrot elimination programme initiated in 2009 was highly effective. This shows the importance of early implementation of an elimination programme for a newly introduced disease like severe footrot.

Scenarios with different control measures

The most effective way to reduce the spread of severe footrot was by decreasing the within county infection rate (Figure 5). This could be achieved by reducing contact between flocks or by reducing the environmental load of virulent *D. nodosus*, for example by footbathing, culling diseased sheep or eliminating severe footrot from the flock. In the event of an extensive outbreak of severe footrot, we believe that some farmers would implement control measures to reduce the welfare problem in their flock. A 20% or possibly a 40% decrease in the infection rate might be realistic, which would decrease the number of infected flocks in 2035 by 11% and 28%, respectively, compared with the basic scenario where no control measures are included.

The exclusion of one of the between counties transmission routes at a time, keeping the other two routes in the model, resulted in only a small decrease in the number of infected flocks in 2035. When two of the three transmission routes were excluded, a larger reduction in the number of infected flocks in 2035 was seen. When sheep movement was the only between county transmission route, the number of infected flocks decreased by 20%. Of the between county transmissions, this was the scenario with the largest deviation from the basic scenario. The low number of sheep moved across county borders is the main reason why the spread of disease is slowest for this route. National maedi and scrapie legislation prohibits the movement of sheep across county borders without derogation. This shows that keeping this transmission route only in the model at the current level limits the spread. This reflects the importance of the legislation in decreasing the spread of disease across county borders. With no such legislations, more sheep would be moved across the county borders and the spread of sheep diseases to other counties would be faster. The sheep industry in Norway supports the derogations for moving sheep across county borders, hence an increase is not expected.

Scenarios with increased between county transmission

Increased use of common pasture and movement of cattle gave the highest increase in the number of infected flocks of the between county transmissions. This shows the importance of the risk of spreading severe footrot by these means. But an extensive increase in these routes of transmissions is not expected as they are not restricted with legislations, and therefore not a major concern for the control of footrot in Norway.

The county-specific infection rates were based on the spread of severe footrot in Rogaland and adjusted to other counties by taking account of differences in climate and sheep density. The adjustment factors were fitted to the spread in Aust-Agder. We cannot exclude the possibility that other ways of generating the correction factors would be better. In view of the importance of the model results, data to validate the adjustment factors would have been beneficial, but such data does not exist for Norway.

In conclusion, a simulation model is a useful tool to estimate the spread of an infectious disease, but care must be taken so that model assumptions and values used are reasonable as the results are highly dependent on these. By using sensitivity analysis and assessing the consistency with spread in other populations, the reliability of the model can be assessed.

The spread of severe footrot in Norway without an elimination programme would have been extensive. Control measures decreasing the within county infection rate would delay the spread, but a ban on a single of the between county infection routes would not reduce the spread substantially. This shows the large effect, and the importance of initiating an elimination programme to prevent a large proportion of the Norwegian sheep population from being faced with pain, lameness and welfare problems. We cannot exclude the possibility of disease being introduced and spread by other means than those modelled, but we do believe that the model predicts a possible scenario for how the disease would develop in Norway without an elimination programme.

Competing interests

The authors declare that they have no competing interests.

Authors' contributions

GMG was main responsible for the design of the study, programming the simulation model, performing the statistical analysis and writing the manuscript. SV participated in the design of the study and contributed to writing the manuscript. ABK supervised the programming of the simulation model and the statistical analysis and contributed to writing the manuscript. ON participated in the design of the study and contributed to writing the manuscript. PH supervised the design of the study and contributed to writing the manuscript. All authors read and approved the final manuscript.

Acknowledgements

The authors would like to thank the Healthy Feet project for providing access to their data. We would also like thank Malin Jonsson and Chiek Er at the Norwegian Veterinary Institute for their technical support. The project was funded by the Research Levy on Agricultural Products, project number 199142/199.

Author details

[1]Norwegian Veterinary Institute, P.O. Box 750 Sentrum, NO-0106 Oslo, Norway. [2]Animalia - Norwegian Meat and Poultry Research Centre, P.O. Box 396 Løren, NO-0513 Oslo, Norway.

References

1. Beveridge WIB (1941) Foot-rot in sheep: a transmissible disease due to infection with *Fusiformis nodosus*. Studies on its cause, epidemiology and control. Council Sci Industr Res 140:1–56
2. Wassink GJ, King EM, Grogono-Thomas R, Brown JC, Moore LJ, Green LE (2010) A within farm clinical trial to compare two treatments (parenteral antibacterials and hoof trimming) for sheep lame with footrot. Prev Vet Med 96:93–103
3. Ley SJ, Waterman AE, Livingston A, Parkinson TJ (1994) Effect of chronic pain associated with lameness on plasma cortisol concentrations in sheep: a field study. Res Vet Sci 57:332–335
4. Palmer MA (1993) A gelatin test to detect activity and stability of proteases produced by *Dichelobacter (Bacteroides) nodosus*. Vet Microbiol 36:113–122
5. Meling S, Ulvund MJ. Flock health visits in 17 sheep flocks in Rogaland. In Proceedings of the 7th International Sheep Veterinary Congress: 12–16 June 2009; Stavanger. Edited by Stuen S, Ulvund MJ: 2009;148–49.
6. Øverås J (1994) Smittsom klauvsjuke hos sau. Et tilbakeblikk på import og utbrudd i Norge. Småfenytt 14:29–33 (in Norwegian)
7. Vatn S, Hektoen L, Høyland B, Reiersen A, Kampen AH, Jørgensen HJ (2012) Elimination of severe footrot from the Norwegian sheep population - A progress report. Small Ruminant Res 106:11–13
8. Healthy Feet Project: Statusrapport nr. 6 Friske føtter. Oslo: Animalia, Norwegian Meat and Poultry Research Centre; 2014. [http://www.fotrate.no/media/_Statusrapport_nr_6_Friske_fotter_endelig_mars_2014.pdf] Accessed 07 July 2014.
9. Gilhuus M, Vatn S, Dhungyel OP, Tesfamichael B, L'Abee-Lund TM, Jørgensen HJ (2013) Characterisation of *Dichelobacter nodosus* isolates from Norway. Vet Microbiol 163:142–148
10. Gilhuus M, Kvitle B, L'Abée-Lund TM, Vatn S, Jørgensen HJ (2014) A recently introduced *Dichelobacter nodosus* strain caused an outbreak of footrot in Norway. Acta Vet Scand 56:29
11. de Jong MCM (1995) Mathematical modelling in veterinary epidemiology: why model building is important. Prev Vet Med 25:183–193
12. Rohani P, Earn DJ, Grenfell BT (1999) Opposite patterns of synchrony in sympatric disease metapopulations. Science 286:968–971

13. Grøneng GM, Green LE, Kaler J, Vatn S, Hopp P (2014) A longitudinal study of the risks for introduction of severe footrot into sheep flocks in the south west of Norway. Prev Vet Med 113:241–248
14. Nieuwhof GJ, Conington J, Bishop SC (2009) A genetic epidemiological model to describe resistance to an endemic bacterial disease in livestock: application to footrot in sheep. Genet Sel Evol 41:19
15. Graham NPH, Egerton JR (1968) Pathogenesis of ovine foot-rot: the role of some environmental factors. Aust Vet J 44:235–240
16. Ridler A, Wilson D, Nixon N (2009) Effect of environmental and climatic conditions on footrot in sheep in the UK. In: Stuen S, Ulvund MJ (ed) Proceedings of the 7th International Sheep Veterinary Congress. Stavanger, Norway, pp 104–105
17. Ghimire SC, Egerton JR, Dhungyel OP (1999) Transmission of virulent footrot between sheep and goats. Aust Vet J 77:450–453
18. Knappe-Poindecker M, Gilhuus M, Jensen TK, Vatn S, Jørgensen HJ, Fjeldaas T (2014) Cross-infection of virulent *Dichelobacter nodosus* between sheep and co-grazing cattle. Vet Microbiol 170:375–382
19. Rogdo T, Hektoen L, Slettemeås JS, Jørgensen HJ, Østerås O, Fjeldaas T (2012) Possible cross-infection of *Dichelobacter nodosus* between co-grazing sheep and cattle. Acta Vet Scand 54:19
20. R Development Core Team. R: A Language and Environment for Statistical Computing. Vienna, Austria: R Foundation for Statistical Computing; 2012.
21. Soetaert K, Petzoldt T, Setzer RW (2010) Solving differential Equations in R: package deSolve. J Stat Softw 33:1–25
22. Wassink GJ, Grogono-Thomas R, Moore LJ, Green LE (2003) Risk factors associated with the prevalence of footrot in sheep from 1999 to 2000. Vet Rec 152:351–358
23. Nieuwhof GJ, Bishop SC (2005) Costs of the major endemic diseases of sheep in Great Britain and the potential benefits of reduction in disease impact. Anim Sci 81:23–29

4

Influence of the gestational stage on the clinical course, lesional development and parasite distribution in experimental ovine neosporosis

David Arranz-Solís[1†], Julio Benavides[2†], Javier Regidor-Cerrillo[1], Miguel Fuertes[2], Ignacio Ferre[1], Maria del Carmen Ferreras[2], Esther Collantes-Fernández[1], Andrew Hemphill[3], Valentín Pérez[2] and Luis Miguel Ortega-Mora[1*]

Abstract

Neospora caninum is considered one of the main causes of abortion in cattle, yet recent studies have also emphasised its relevance as an abortifacient in small ruminants. In order to gain deeper insight into the pathogenesis of ovine neosporosis, pregnant ewes were intravenously inoculated with 10^6 tachyzoites of the Nc-Spain7 isolate at days 40, 90 or 120 of gestation. Infection during the first term resulted in the death of all foetuses between days 19 and 21 post-infection, showing mainly necrotic lesions in foetal liver and the highest parasite DNA detection and burden in both placenta and foetal viscera. After infection at day 90, foetal death was also detected in all ewes, although later (34–48 days post-infection). In this group, lesions were mainly inflammatory. Foetal livers showed the lowest frequency of lesions, as well as the lowest parasite detection and burden. All ewes infected at day 120 delivered viable lambs, although 3 out of 9 showed weakness and recumbency. *Neospora* DNA was detected in all lambs but one, and parasite burden was similar to that observed in day 90 group. Lesions in this group showed more conspicuous infiltration of inflammatory cells and higher frequency in foetal brain and muscle when compared to both previous groups. These results highlight the crucial role that the stage of gestation plays on the course of ovine neosporosis, similar to that reported in bovine neosporosis, and open the doors to consider sheep as a valid model for exogenous transplacental transmission for ruminant neosporosis.

Introduction

Neospora caninum (Apicomplexa: Eimeriina: Sarcocystidae) is an obligate intracellular parasite, which is regarded as one of the most important infectious causes of abortion in cattle worldwide [1]. Since its discovery, *N. caninum* has been identified in various species of livestock, including cattle, sheep, goats, horses and deer [2]. Cattle can become infected by horizontal transmission via the ingestion of oocysts, or by vertical transmission (i.e. transplacentally) as a result of either a primary infection of the dam by oocysts (exogenous transplacental transmission) or recrudescence of a chronic infection (endogenous transplacental transmission) during pregnancy, with different clinical and epidemiological consequences [3].

Although cattle represent the most relevant and economically important target host, the presence of *Neospora* infection and transplacental transmission in small ruminants have been previously reported. In sheep, naturally occurring *N. caninum* transmission was first described in a congenitally infected lamb [4]. Subsequently *N. caninum* infections in sheep have been reported worldwide [5-8]. Nevertheless, *Toxoplasma gondii* is regarded as the primary parasite cause for both sheep and goat abortion [1,6,8], and the epidemiological, clinical and economic importance of neosporosis in small ruminants has been traditionally considered to be much less relevant compared to cattle [9,10]. However, recently acquired evidence suggests that *N. caninum* is an important abortifacient in small ruminants [6], or even the main

* Correspondence: luis.ortega@ucm.es
†Equal contributors
[1]SALUVET, Animal Health Department, Faculty of Veterinary Sciences, Complutense University of Madrid, Ciudad Universitaria s/n, 28040 Madrid, Spain
Full list of author information is available at the end of the article

cause of reproductive losses in some flocks [7,8]. Despite the obvious significance of ruminant neosporosis, there are still many aspects that require further studies, such as host-pathogen interactions, pathogenicity and immunological control. Previous experimental infections in pregnant ewes have shown that sheep are highly susceptible to infection, and display a similar pathogenesis and disease outcomes as reported for cattle [9,11,12]. It has been suggested that the time point of infection during gestation plays a key role in the pathogenesis of the disease [9,11-16]. However, it is complicated to compare the results from these studies, as they differ in experimental design, parasite isolate and infection dose, route of administration and time point of infection. Moreover, there are not reports on the outcomes of infection during different pregnancy periods within the same study and under the same experimental conditions. Clearly, the availability of well-defined ruminant infection models is a key factor for the evaluation of vaccine and drug candidates [17]. As an experimental animal model, sheep exhibit several advantages over cattle, including size, length of gestation and cost. Therefore, the aim of this study was to investigate the outcome of experimental infection by *N. caninum* in ewes under standardized conditions at an early, mid-term and late period of gestation. This allowed to evaluate the effect of the gestation period on the clinical course of disease, lesion development and parasite distribution in different organs, and to assess the validity of experimental infection in sheep as a model for exogenous transplacental transmission for ruminant neosporosis.

Material and methods

Ethics statement

All protocols involving animals were approved by the Animal Welfare Committee of the Livestock Health and Production Institute (IGM, ULE-CSIC), León, Spain, following proceedings described in Spanish and EU legislations (Law 32/2007, R.D. 1201/2005, and Council Directive 2010/63/EU). All animals used in this study were handled in strict accordance with good clinical practices and all efforts were made to minimize suffering.

Animals and experimental design

Animals used in this study came from the *Churra* sheep breed flock of ULE-CSIC, which is kept in dedicated animal facilities and free of *N. caninum* infection or any other abortifacient agent. Fifty pure *Churra* breed sheep aged 12 months were selected after checking by ELISA their seronegativity for *T. gondii*, *N. caninum*, Border disease virus (BDV), *Coxiella burnetii* and *Chlamydophila abortus*. These sheep were oestrus synchronized and mated with pure breed *Churra* tups for 2 days, after which the rams were removed from the ewes. Pregnancy and foetal viability were confirmed by ultrasound scanning (US) on day 40 after mating, and twenty-nine pregnant sheep were selected for the experiment.

Pregnant sheep ($n = 29$) were randomly distributed into five experimental groups. Twenty ewes were allocated in groups 1 (G1; $n = 6$), 2 (G2; $n = 7$) and 3 (G3; $n = 7$), which were inoculated intravenously (IV) with 10^6 culture-derived tachyzoites of the Nc-Spain7 bovine isolate [18] at day 40 (G1), 90 (G2) or 120 (G3) of gestation (dg), respectively. The nine remaining sheep were allocated in groups 4 (G4; $n = 6$) and 5 (G5; $n = 3$) as controls of infection and pregnancy, respectively. Two animals from G4 and one from G5 received an IV inoculum of phosphate-buffered saline (PBS) at each time point of infection (day 40, 90 or 120), thus two negative controls animals and one sentinel control were available for each time point. Ewes from G4 were culled at the average time points when abortion took place in their respective group, providing a negative control for further analyses (see below), and ewes from G5 were kept alive until the end of the experiment (Table 1).

Parasites

Tachyzoites of the Nc-Spain7 isolate were routinely maintained in cultured MARC-145 cells as described previously [19]. The experiment was carried out using similar

Table 1 Experimental design

Group	Number of pregnant ewes	Number of foetuses/lambs	Days of gestation at the time of inoculation	Inoculum (IV)	Animal euthanasia[a]
G1	6	11	40	Nc-Spain7 10^6 tachyzoites	Yes
G2	7	12	90	Nc-Spain7 10^6 tachyzoites	Yes
G3	7	9	120	Nc-Spain7 10^6 tachyzoites	Yes
G4	6	9	40-90-120[b]	PBS	Yes[b]
G5	3	4	40-90-120[c]	PBS	No[c]

IV: intravenous route.

[a]Animals were culled when fœtal death was detected or immediately after parturition.

[b]In G4, 2 ewes correspond to each period of inoculation (40, 90 and 120), and were culled at the average day of abortion of each group (i.e. 20 dpi for G1 and 40 dpi for G2) or at parturition (for G3).

[c]In G5, 1 ewe corresponds to each period of inoculation (40, 90 and 120). All three ewes gave birth to healthy lambs and were kept alive until the end of the experiment.

parasite passage numbers in MARC-145 cells cultures for all three days of inoculation (passage No. 12 for G1, No. 8 for G2 and No. 11 for G3). Inocula were prepared as described previously [19]. Briefly, tachyzoites were recovered from culture flasks when they were still largely intracellular and at least 80% of the parasitophorous vacuoles were undisrupted. Tachyzoite numbers were determined by Trypan blue exclusion followed by counting in a Neubauer chamber, and parasites were resuspended in PBS at the required dose of 10^6 tachyzoites in a final volume of 2 mL. Tachyzoites were administered to ewes within 30 min of harvesting from tissue culture.

Clinical monitoring and collection of samples

Following experimental infection, ewes were observed daily throughout the entire experimental period. Foetal viability was assessed by the transabdominal ultrasonography (US) monitoring of foetal heartbeat and movements. All ewes were checked upon once weekly for the two first weeks post-infection (pi), and then twice weekly until detection of foetal death. When foetal death occurred, or immediately after parturition, dams and lambs were first sedated with xylazine -Rompun- (Bayer, Mannhein, Germany) and then immediately euthanized by an IV overdose of embutramide and mebezonium iodide -T61- (Intervet, Salamanca, Spain). Animals from G4 were culled at 20 days post-inoculation (dpi) for G1, 40 dpi for G2 and at parturition for G3. Animals from G5 were examined once per month for pregnancy by US from the sixth week until lambing, and ewes were kept alive.

Post-mortem examination of the ewes and lambs was carried out immediately after euthanasia, and foetuses were immediately separated from the placenta. Samples for serological, histological and molecular studies were collected as follows: blood samples were taken on the day of necropsy by jugular vein-puncture in Vacutainer tubes (Becton Dickinson and Company, Plymouth, UK) without anticoagulant and were allowed to clot. Serum was obtained by centrifugation and samples were stored at −80 °C until analysis. After necropsy, five randomly selected placentomes were recovered from each placenta and were transversally cut in slices of 2–3 mm of thickness that were distributed for storage in 10% formalin for histopathological examinations, and the rest of the placentomes were stored at −80 °C for further parasite DNA detection by PCR. Brain (one half at −80 °C and one half in 10% formalin) and iliofemoral (uterine) and mesenteric lymph nodes from dams were collected for PCR and histopathological analysis. Foetal tissues (brain, heart, liver, lungs and a portion of semitendinosus skeletal muscle) were stored at −80 °C for DNA extraction and fixation in 10% formalin. Foetal thoracic and abdominal fluids or precolostral serum were also collected and maintained at −80 °C for serology. To prevent any transmission of colostral antibodies from dams, lambs were separated from their mothers immediately after birth, sampled for blood and euthanized. In order to avoid any accidental suckling from lambs born overnight, udders were covered with a piece of cloth one week before the expected date of delivery as a preventive measure.

Serological analyses: IFAT

Indirect fluorescent antibody test (IFAT) was used to detect specific IgG anti-*Neospora* antibodies in foetal fluids, precolostral sera, and sera from dams, according to the technique previously described by Álvarez-García et al. [20]. Foetal fluids, precolostral sera and sera from dams were diluted at two-fold serial dilutions in PBS starting at 1:8 (for foetal fluids and precolostral sera) and 1:200 (for sera from dams), up to the end point titre. Unbroken tachyzoite membrane fluorescence at a titre ≥ 8 for foetal fluids or precolostral sera and ≥ 200 for sera from dams was considered a positive reaction.

Histopathology and lesion scoring

After fixation in formalin for five days, maternal and foetal brains were cut coronally, embedded in paraffin wax, and were processed, with the rest of the samples, by standard procedures for haematoxylin and eosin (HE) staining. Conventional histological evaluation was carried out on all the sections. To quantify the lesions in the foetal viscera and placenta, the number and size of necrotic foci, as well as the total area of lesion in the examined tissue were calculated in HE stained sections. Necrotic lesions were chosen over inflammatory ones because the former were found in all the foetuses and placentas examined while the latter were found mainly in G2 and G3. In addition, necrotic lesions are more clearly demarcated than inflammatory ones. The number of sections studied varied according to the stage of gestation. Older foetuses had larger organs (brain and liver) and therefore more samples were evaluated in these cases: in the placenta, one section from each one of the five placentomes per placenta was studied; in the foetal liver, one section from one or two different samples; and in the foetal brain, one section from one, two or three different samples. Although lesions were found in other organs (i.e. lung, heart or skeletal muscle), brain and liver were the only ones showing lesions simultaneously in all three periods studied and were therefore the only ones to be evaluated by lesional scoring. Firstly, necrotic foci in each section were counted under the microscope. Subsequently, in order to compare between organs and animals, the total number of foci per square centimetre of studied tissue was calculated. The measurement of the total area studied (TAS) is explained in the next paragraph.

A computer-assisted morphometric analysis using imageJ software [21] was carried out to calculate the areas. Digital photomicrographs from each focus of necrosis at the placenta, liver and brain were taken at 10x magnification with a calibrated Motic 2 digital camera fitted to a BA310E Motic microscope. In the digital pictures, the perimeter of each necrotic focus was traced manually and measured automatically by the software, previously calibrated to the adequate magnification. Once every focus was measured, the average size of focus (ASF) for the placenta, liver and brain was calculated. The total area of lesion (TAL) in the placenta was calculated adding up the area of each focus found in the five placentomes studied per animal. TAL in the foetal brain and liver were similarly calculated, adding up the area of each individual lesion found in every section available from each organ.

For calculating the TAS, digital photographs of the whole section were taken with the same camera fitted to a macro tube and a focusable lens. TAS measurement was done through imageJ software as well. Instead of manually tracing the area, and in order to avoid the inclusion of empty areas into the measured area such as ventricles in the nervous organs or cutting artefacts, a thresholding detection procedure and automatic measurement was applied. Briefly, the colour picture was converted to 8-bit greyscale and the threshold was manually adjusted to detect any region containing tissue sections (grey to black in colour), excluding the empty areas (white). Then, the area of the threshold regions in the picture was automatically measured by the software, previously calibrated. When more than one section was available from the same organ (i.e. two or three samples of liver or brain from the same foetus), TAS was calculated adding up the TAS of each section.

Finally, the percentage of the section affected by lesions (%LES) resulted from the coefficient between TAL and TAS per organ. In order to compare groups, averages of these measurements (i.e. foci/cm^2, AF and %LES) obtained in the animals of each group were calculated.

DNA extraction and PCR for parasite detection and quantification in tissues

Genomic DNA was extracted from 50–100 mg of maternal and foetal tissue samples using the commercial Maxwell® 16 Mouse Tail DNA Purification Kit, developed for automated Maxwell® 16 System (Promega, Wisconsin, USA), following the manufacturer's recommendations. The concentration of DNA for all samples was determined by spectrophotometry and adjusted to 50–100 ng/μL.

Parasite DNA detection was carried out by a nested-PCR adapted to a single tube from the internal transcribed spacer (ITS1) region of *N. caninum*, using the external primers TgNN1-TgNN2 and internal primers NP1–NP2 as previously described [22-24]. Each reaction was performed in a final volume of 25 μL with 5 μL of sample DNA. PCR was carried out in five samples of the placentomes and three samples from the rest of tissues, except for the heart, lung and semitendinosus muscle from foetuses or lambs, in which either one, two or three samples were analysed. To avoid cross-contamination and false positive reactions, DNA extraction, PCR sample preparation and electrophoresis were performed in separate rooms employing different sets of instruments, aerosol barrier tips and disposable gloves. Moreover, both reactions without a template and DNA samples from the foetal-control group (G4) were included in each round of DNA extraction and PCR as negative controls. Positive PCR controls with *N. caninum* genomic DNA equivalent to 10, 1 and 0.1 tachyzoites in 100 ng of sheep DNA were also included in each batch of amplifications. Ten μL aliquots of the PCR products were visualized under UV light in 1.5% agarose/ethidium bromide gel to detect the *N. caninum*-specific 247 bp amplification product.

Placenta and foetal brain and liver samples that had tested positive by nested-PCR were adjusted to 20 ng DNA/μL and the parasite load was quantified using real-time PCR. Primer pairs from the *N. caninum* Nc-5 sequence [25] were used for parasite quantification, and primers from the β-actin gene [26] were used for the quantification of host DNA. Amplification reactions were performed as described by Collantes-Fernández et al. [25], in a final volume of 20 μL using Power SYBR® Green PCR Master Mix (Applied Biosystems, Foster City, CA, USA), 20 pmol of each primer and 100 ng of DNA in a ABI 7300 Real Time PCR System (Applied Biosystems). The *N. caninum* tachyzoite numbers were calculated by interpolating the average Ct values on two standard curves: 1) one curve equivalent to 5×10^5 to 5×10^{-1} tachyzoites with 10-fold serial dilutions in a solution of ovine genomic DNA; and 2) a curve of 320, 160, 80, 40, 20, 10, and 5 ng of genomic DNA for ovine DNA quantifications. Parasite numbers in tissue samples (parasite burden) was expressed as parasite number/mg ovine tissue. Standard curves for *N. caninum* and sheep DNAs showed an average slope of –3.38 and –3.34, respectively, and a $R^2 > 0.99$.

Statistical analysis

Occurrence of foetal death was analysed by the Kaplan–Meier survival method. Foetal survival curves of the infected groups were then compared by the Log-rank (Mantel-Cox) test. When statistically significant differences were found, Tukey's Multiple Range test was applied to examine all possible pairwise comparisons at each sampling time. Differences in PCR detection of parasite DNA were evaluated using the χ^2 or Fisher exact F-test. Differences in parasite burdens and histological scoring were analysed using the non-parametric Kruskal–Wallis test followed by Dunn's test for comparisons between groups, and the Mann–Whitney test for pairwise comparisons. Statistical significance for all analysis was established at $P < 0.05$. For statistical analysis, sentinel animals (G4) were mixed and considered as a unique control group. All statistical analyses were carried out using GraphPad Prism 5.0 software.

Results

Clinical observations

Foetal death was detected by US in all ewes (100%) from groups G1 (infection at 40 dg) and G2 (infection at 90 dg), although foetal death occurred significantly earlier in G1 (19–21 dpi) compared to G2 (34–48 dpi) ($P < 0.001$). In contrast, all ewes from G3 gave birth to a total of nine viable lambs between 142 and 155 dg. Three of 9 lambs were born prematurely prior to day 145, and exhibited weakness, recumbency and unresponsiveness to external stimuli. Foetal death was not detected in control groups; dams from the pregnancy control group (G5) gave birth to healthy lambs between 147 and 150 dg, and foetuses from the negative control group (G4) remained alive just before the euthanasia of their dams on day 20 pi (day 40 group), 40 pi (day 90 group) and at parturition (day 120 group).

Neospora-specific IgG responses

Neospora-specific IgG responses were analysed by IFAT in foetal fluids, precolostral sera and sera from dams collected immediately before necropsy and are summarized in Table 2. Individual values for each dam and foetus/lamb studied are detailed in Additional file 1. Seropositive titres were detected in all infected dams, ranging from 1:1600 to 1:3200 in G1, 1:3200 to 1:6400 in G2 and 1:200 to 1:1600 in G3 (Table 2). Foetal fluids from foetuses of G1 could not be collected due to the very low volume of liquid available. For G2, seropositive titres were detected in those foetuses dying from 42 dpi onwards, ranging from 1:16 to 1:64. Precolostral sera collected from lambs born after infection at day 120 of gestation (G3), specifically those three born prior day 145 of pregnancy, yielded positive titres ranging from 1:16 to 1:128 (Table 2). Specific IgG responses against parasite antigen were not detected in animals and foetuses/lambs from the two control groups (G4 and G5).

Pathology and lesion quantification

Gross lesions

At the time of necropsy, detachment of the placenta from the uterus was evident in one animal from G1 and three animals from G2. In G3, placenta and uterus could only be recovered from three animals, while in the remaining four animals from this group placentas were too autolytic when recovered after lambing, rendering proper examination impossible.

In G1, all foetuses examined showed a variable degree of abdominal haemorrhage and subcutaneous oedema (Figure 1A). One foetus from this group showed multifocal white spots in the lung (1–2 mm of diameter) and liver (of miliary size) (Figure 1B). No gross lesions were visible in any placenta from this group. In groups G2 and G3 there were macroscopic lesions in the placenta. In two animals, one from each group, multifocal white foci in the cotyledons were visible (Figure 1C). In three further animals from G2 and one from G3 there were focal aggregations of the cotyledonary villi (Figure 1D). No macroscopic lesions in any of the foetuses from these two groups were found, and no foetal lesions were detected in G4 and G5.

Microscopic lesions

The quantification of lesion size and number from placenta as well as foetal liver and brain is shown in Table 3 and Figure 2. Individual values for each foetus or placental sample studied are detailed in Additional file 2.

Placenta

All the placentas studied from infected animals showed multifocal non-purulent necrotic placentitis characterized by randomly distributed foci of necrosis in the placentome. The only difference between groups was the size and number of necrotic foci. In G1, the foci were well delimited, small (0.05 mm^2 in average) and affected

Table 2 Serological results in dams and foetuses/lambs

Group	Time of necropsy[a]	No. of dams with the stated sera titre					No. of foetuses/lambs with the stated FL/PCS titre						
		1/200	1/800	1/1600	1/3200	1/6400	NA	-	1/8	1/16	1/32	1/64	1/128
G1 (day 40)	19-21 dpi			4	2		11						
G2 (day 90)	34-48 dpi				4	3	3	1	1	1	3	3	
G3 (day 120)	142-155 dg	1	3	3				4	2*	1*		1	1

[a]Necropsies were carried out when foetal dead was detected or immediately after parturition.
*Lambs prematurely born showing weakness and unresponsiveness.
dpi: days post-infection; dg: days of gestation; NA: not available; FL: foetal liquid; PCS: precolostral serum.

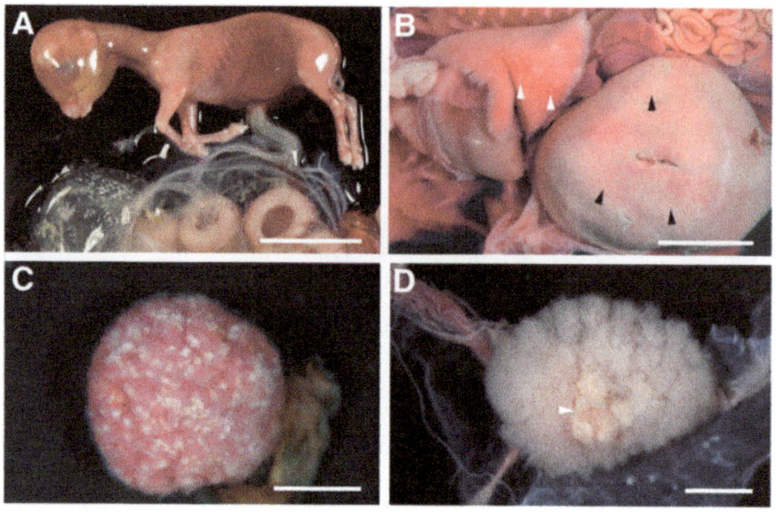

Figure 1 Macroscopic lesions in foetuses and placentas. A: haemorrhage in the abdominal region of a non-viable foetus from G1 (infection at 40 dg). Note the absence of gross lesions in the placentomes at the lower part of the image. Bar 3 cm. **B**: multiple minute white/yellowish foci of necrosis in the lung (white arrowheads) and liver (black arrowheads) in a non-viable foetus from G1 (infection at 40 dg). Bar: 1 cm. **C**: Multiple white foci of necrosis scattered in the surface of a cotyledon from a G2 placenta. Bar: 1.5 cm. **D**: Aggregation of cotyledonary villi (white arrowhead) in a placenta from G2. Bar: 1.5 cm.

the caruncular septa of the placentome, causing flattening or loss of the adjacent trophoblasts. The foetal mesenchyme in the vicinity of these foci showed hypercellularity when compared with non-affected regions. Inflammation was not a prominent feature, although occasional accumulation of lymphocytes was found between caruncles and foetal villi. Placentas from G2 showed necrotic foci of similar characteristics but larger (an average of 0.1 mm^2) than those in G1 ($P < 0.001$). They were almost exclusively located in the caruncular septa, although the largest could also affect the foetal mesenchyme. A number of these foci showed mineralization of the necrotic core area. Lesions in G3 placentas were also similar, only larger than those in previous groups (0.3 mm^2 in average) ($P < 0.001$ for G1 and $P < 0.05$ for G2). Some of the larger foci were made by the coalescence of several, smaller ones. Similarly to the other groups, inflammatory cells were not frequently observed, but when present lymphocytes were mainly distributed along the periphery of the lesion in the foetal mesenchyme (Figure 3). When analysing the percentage of damaged area in relation to the whole tissue section, there was a significant difference between placentas from G1 (0.25%) and those from G2 (9.07%) and G3 (5.74%) ($P < 0.001$).

Liver

Lesions were characterized by the presence of multiple foci of coagulative necrosis randomly distributed in the hepatic parenchyma (Figure 3). Differences in lesion size and severity were observed between groups. While in foetuses from G1 lesions coalesced forming large areas of necrosis, in G2 and G3 the necrotic foci were

Table 3 Lesion quantification and PCR detection and quantification of *N. caninum* in placenta and foetal liver and brain

Group	Foetal death (dpi)	Placenta				Liver				Brain			
		Histology$^{\alpha}$			PCR$^{\beta}$	Histology$^{\alpha}$			PCR$^{\beta}$	Histology$^{\alpha}$			PCR$^{\beta}$
		No. foci/cm^2	ASF (mm^2)	%LES		No. foci/cm^2	ASF (mm^2)	%LES		No. foci/cm^2	ASF (mm^2)	%LES	
G1 (day 40)	19-21	8.2^d	0.053^d	0.25%^{d}	6/6 (7888^c)	82.3^c	0.041	3.37%^{c}	11/11^a (6318^c)	1.68	0.038	0.05%	11/11 (1697^c)
G2 (day 90)	34-48	73.0^c	0.113^d	9.07%^{c}	7/7 (308.5^d)	0.2^d	0.044	0.02%^{d}	5/12^b (0.01^d)	3.14	0.047	0.18%	10/12 (0.25^d)
G3 (day 120)	Born*	18.7^d	0.304^c	5.74%^{c}	7/7 (190.8^d)	4.2^d	0.047	0.16%^{d}	4/9^b (0.01^d)	3.50	0.063	0.25%	6/9 (0.01^d)

*All lambs from this group gave birth to viable lambs between days 142 and 155 of gestation.
$^{\alpha}$Average values of histological scoring for each group.
$^{\beta}$Fractions represent the number of positive animals/total number of animals checked by nested-ITS1 PCR, and figures within brackets represent the median values of parasite burden (tachyzoites/mg tissue).
^{a,b}Fractions determined for positive animals followed by unlike superscripts differ significantly by Fisher's exact test.
^{c,d}Values followed by unlike superscripts differ significantly by Dunn's test for pairwise comparisons.
dpi: days post infection when abortion occurred; ASF: Average size of focus; %LES: Percentage of section affected by lesions.

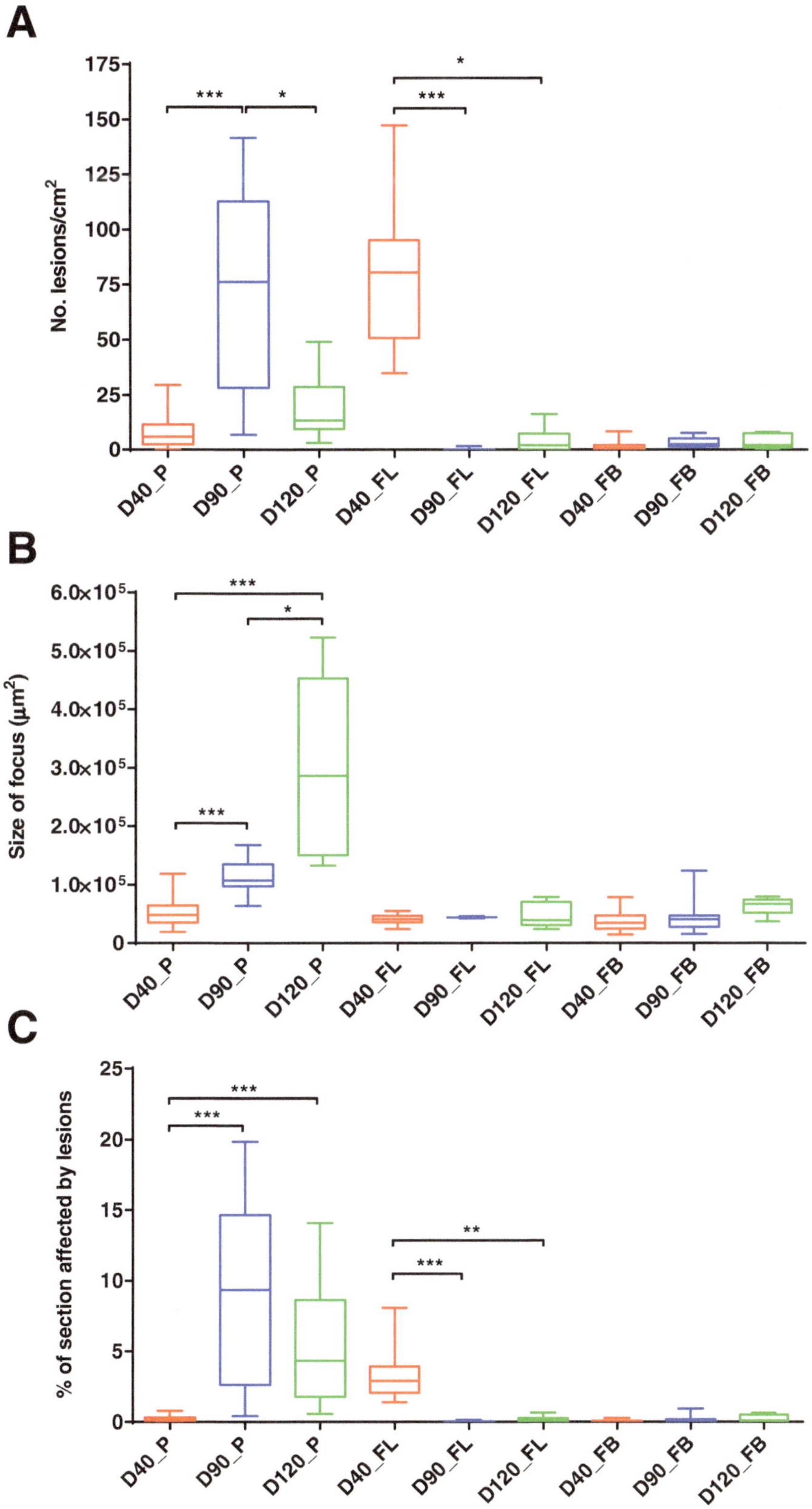

Figure 2 Box-plot graphs of histological scores. Number of lesions per centimetre square **(a)**, size of focus **(b)** and lesions rates **(c)** in placenta (P), foetal liver (FL) and foetal brain (FB) from animals inoculated with 10^6 Nc-Spain7 tachyzoites at days 40 -G1- (D40), 90 -G2- (D90) and 120 -G3- (D120) of gestation. Box-plot graphs represent the median percentage, the lower and upper quartiles (boxes) and minimum and maximum values (whiskers). (*) indicates $P < 0.05$, (**) $P < 0.01$ and (***) $P < 0.001$ significant differences between infected groups in each tissue.

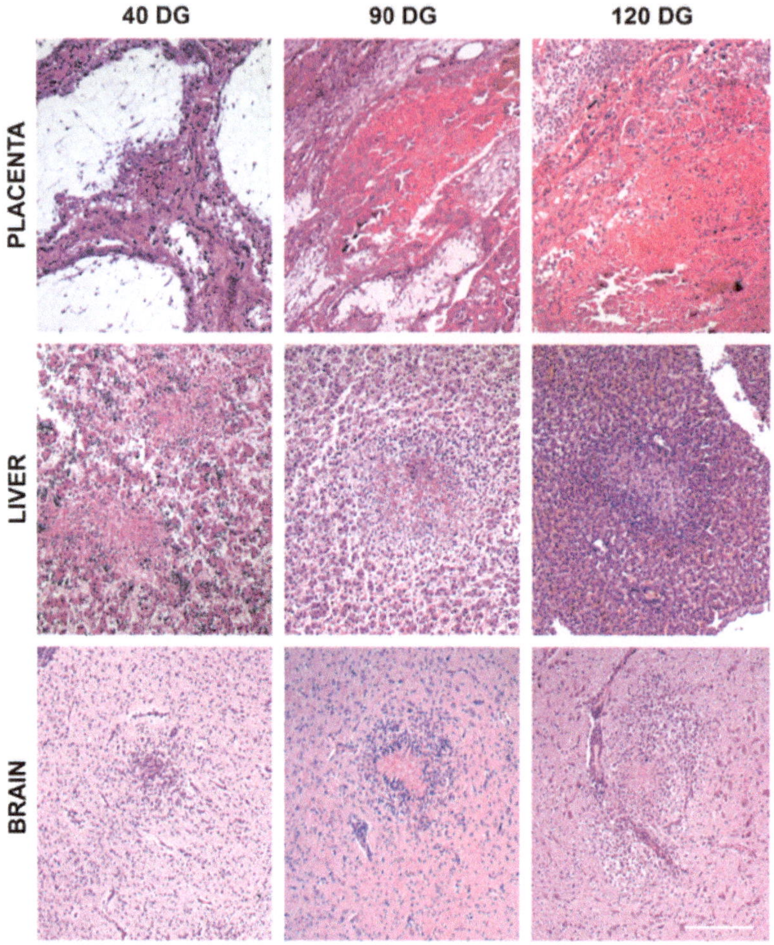

Figure 3 Comparison of the characteristic microscopic lesions found in placenta and foetal liver and brain. Pictures show the histological changes measured for the quantification of lesions. When necrotic areas and infiltration of inflammatory cells coexisted, mainly at the liver and brain of G2 and G3, only the area showing necrosis was measured. All the pictures were taken at the same magnification. Bar 200 μm.

individually well-demarcated. Inflammation was not seen in samples from G1, but there was a mild infiltration surrounding the necrotic areas formed mainly by lymphocytes. When comparing the number and size of lesions among the groups, it should be highlighted that only two foetuses from G2 had necrotic foci in the liver, while liver lesions were found in all foetuses from G1 and all but 2 in G3. There were no significant differences in the size of lesions when they were present, but the amount increased drastically in G1, which exhibited the highest percentage of affected parenchyma ($P < 0.01$).

Brain

The common lesion in all the groups was multifocal non-purulent necrotizing encephalitis characterized by the presence of randomly distributed glial foci. While in G1 necrosis was rarely observed, lesions in G2 and G3 were characterized by large necrotic foci surrounded by mononuclear cells, consistent with microglia and lymphocytes, forming a palisade. Besides the increase on the necrotic component, lesions in G2 and G3 were also larger than those found in G1, although differences in the total damaged area were not statistically significant (Figure 3).

Other organs

Foetuses from G1 showed multiple areas of necrosis randomly distributed in the lung but also in the heart and skeletal muscle (Additional file 3A). Occasionally, and mainly in the heart, these foci showed central mineralization. There was no evident infiltration related to these lesions. However, in the foetuses from G2 and G3, lesions were mainly found in the skeletal muscle, characterized by a multifocal non-purulent myositis (Additional file 3B), although occasional neutrophils could be identified among the muscular fibres. The latter were seen as unaffected, healthy fibres or exhibited degenerative changes characterized by loss of striation, hyper-eosinophilic cytoplasm and rarely mineralization. No obvious signs of fibre regeneration were found. Milder

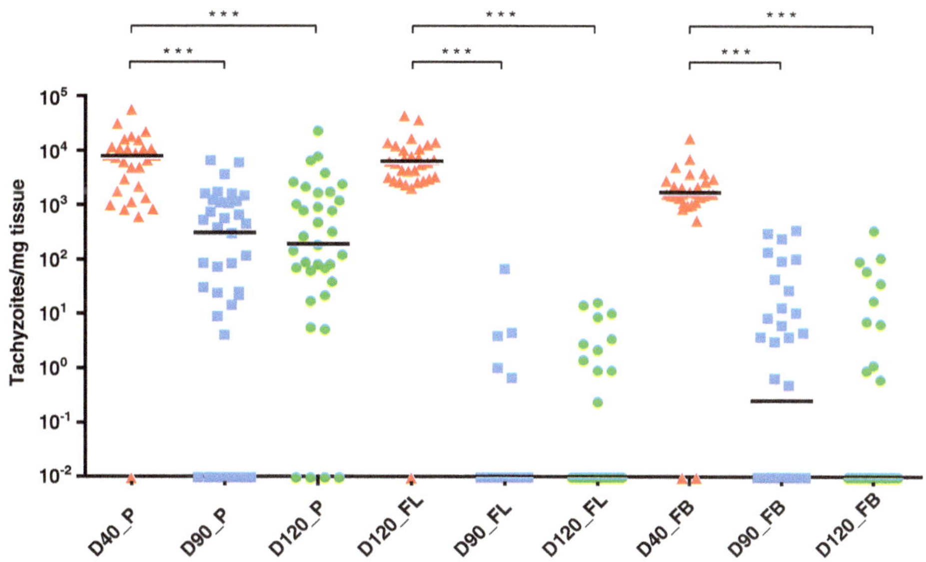

Figure 4 Dot-plot graph of *N. caninum* burdens. Parasite burdens were quantified by real-time PCR in placenta (P) and foetal liver (FL) and brain (FB) from animals inoculated with 10^6 Nc-Spain7 tachyzoites at days 40 -G1- (D40), 90 -G2- (D90) and 120 -G3- (D120) of gestation. Each dot represents individual values of parasite burden (number of parasites per mg of host tissue), and medians are represented as horizontal lines. Taking into account that the *N. caninum* detection limit by real-time PCR is 0.1 parasites, negative samples (0 parasites) were represented on the log scale as < 0.1 (i.e. 10^{-2}). (***) indicates $P < 0.001$ significant differences between infected groups in each tissue.

lesions were occasionally found in the heart, mainly in G3. No evident lesion was found in the lungs of G2 or G3.

No significant microscopic lesion was seen in the placenta or foetuses of G4 and G5.

Parasite distribution and burden in placental and foetal tissues

Maternal tissues

N. caninum DNA was detected in both mesenteric and iliofemoral lymph nodes of ewes from all three infected groups. Parasite DNA was more often detected in lymph node samples from G1 compared to G2 and G3 ($P <$ 0.05). 5/6 mesenteric and 4/6 iliofemoral lymph nodes from G1 harboured parasite DNA, compared to G2 (1/7 and 2/7, respectively) and G3 (2/7), although significant differences were only found between mesenteric lymph nodes from G1 and G2 ($P < 0.05$). Parasite DNA was not detected in any brain sample of dams from any group.

Placental and foetal tissues

Neospora DNA was widely detected in placentomes from all ewes in the three infected groups (Additional file 4), with 97% of the placentome samples analysed being positive in G1 (29/30), 83% in G2 (29/35) and 89% in G3 (31/35), with no statistical significances between them. Nevertheless, the mean parasite burden, measured as number of tachyzoites per mg of tissue, was significantly higher in placentomes from G1 compared to both G2 and G3 ($P < 0.001$) (Figure 4, Table 3).

Regarding foetal tissues, the highest percentage of detection was observed in the brain, liver, heart and skeletal muscle of foetuses from G1 (100%, 11/11), whereas the lowest corresponded to the liver and heart of foetuses from G2 (41.6%, 5/12). In addition, significant differences were observed between G1 and G2 when comparing detection percentage in liver ($P < 0.01$), heart ($P < 0.01$) and skeletal muscle ($P < 0.05$), and also between G1 and G3 for liver samples ($P < 0.05$). Moreover, parasite burdens were significantly higher in brain and liver from G1 compared to G2 and G3 ($P < 0.001$) (Figure 4). When comparing parasite burdens in foetuses from G3, those which were prematurely born before day 145 showed a statistically higher parasite burden in both foetal brain and liver compared to the 6 remaining foetuses born after day 145 ($P < 0.01$) (data not shown). As expected, all placental and foetal samples from G4 and G5 were negative.

Discussion

Whereas *N. caninum* is established as one of the most important infectious causes of abortion in cattle worldwide [1], its epidemiological, clinical and economic relevance for reproductive failure in small ruminants has remained elusive. However recent studies in small ruminants suggest that neosporosis may be a more important cause of reproductive disorders than it has traditionally been considered, at least in certain scenarios. Recent serological surveys have shown high prevalences in asymptomatic sheep and goats from some flocks [1] and evidence has accumulated that points towards *N. caninum* as a cause of natural abortion and reproductive failure in sheep and goats [6-8,27].

The aim of this study was to characterize the clinical, parasitological and lesional parameters in experimental ovine neosporosis at early (40 dg), mid (90 dg) and late (120 dg) stages of pregnancy, to better understand the pathogenesis of *N. caninum* infection. To our knowledge, this is the first study in which all three periods of gestation have been tested within the same experiment under the same conditions (isolate, breed, dose and route of administration). In addition, and in the absence of broadly accepted international guidelines on models for ruminant neosporosis [17], there is a need to establish a suitable and economically viable experimental model for the disease. With this in mind, sheep have been evaluated as suitable experimental model for neosporosis in this study.

Experimental infection was carried out using the *N. caninum* Nc-Spain7 isolate [18], which is a well-characterized highly virulent isolate. Indeed, this isolate caused 100% foetal death upon experimental infection of pregnant cows during the first trimester of gestation [22,28]. The intravenous route of inoculation used in this study was chosen so as to mirror parasitaemia produced in natural infections [29]. Finally, the inoculation dose, 10^6 tachyzoites, was a 1:10 dilution of that commonly used in cattle (i.e. 10^7 tachyzoites) [30-33], considering the weight difference between cattle and sheep (aprox. 10:1).

Clinical observations revealed that infection during the first (G1) and second (G2) term of gestation produced foetal death in all ewes, although it happened significantly earlier in the G1. On the other hand, infection during the last term of gestation (G3) resulted in the birth of viable lambs, although some of them were born prematurely and showed evident weakness that, most probably, would have compromised their viability. Infection during the first period of gestation (G1) showed similar results to those reported in previous experiments carried out at early gestation in both cattle [28,30,34] and sheep [9], where foetal death and abortion were observed. In the current study, lesions and parasite burden found in both dams and foetuses confirm that the parasite readily disseminates in pregnant sheep, crosses the placenta and subsequently induces foetal damage. In this group, high parasite burdens were found in all studied placentomes, but only mild lesions were observed, which might be attributed to the short period of time that occurred between infection and abortion (19–21 days), thus limiting the development of histological lesions. The only placenta studied in previous experimental infections at 45 dg also showed mild lesions [9]. Interestingly, these findings are in clear contrast with the widespread necrosis and inflammation reported in placenta from cattle infected at 70 dg [22,35,36], which suggests that there could be differences between cattle and sheep regarding the initial infection dynamics. It has already been suggested that the lack of mature immune response at this stage of foetal development would allow the parasite to cross the placenta and colonise foetal viscera and multiply with ease [22,36]. Indeed, the highest frequency of detection and parasite burden in the current study were detected in foetuses from this group (G1), where *N. caninum* was widely detected in the brain, liver, heart and semitendinosus muscle of all foetuses. There was a good correlation between parasite burden and frequency of lesions in the foetal liver, which most probably represents the gateway for the parasite to invade the foetus through the umbilical vein. This correlation did not occur in the brain, where there was a high parasite burden, though not as high as in the liver, but the histological lesions were much less frequent. While the reason for this difference is not clear, it is known that antigen levels required to produce lesions in the immune privileged brain are, at least, ten times higher than those needed in other organs, and inflammatory reactions require more time to develop [37]. Thus, the low frequency of lesions in the brain at this stage may be caused by the short period of time since infection. The contrast between mild lesions in the placenta and severe multifocal necrosis in the foetal liver may suggest that the abortion at this stage of gestation is consequence of the foetal lesions, similarly as suggested to occur in bovine neosporosis at early gestation [22,36].

Previous studies addressing the infection in ewes during mid-gestation (mainly at day 90) have reported a variety of results, which could be attributed to the different time points chosen for infection as well as the isolate, dose, breed and the employed route of administration [9,11,12,38]. Nevertheless, all of them reported high rates, of even 100%, of abortion. Conversely, the most commonly reported outcome in cattle after experimental infection at mid-gestation is the delivery of live, although congenitally infected, calves [39-41]. However, abortion has also been reported [31,42] and it is actually at this stage when most of the abortions in natural infection occur [2,17]. Considering the findings from the current study and previous experimental infections, it seems that infection of sheep at mid-gestation generally results in more dramatic consequences than in cattle, as most of the ewes aborted or, less frequently, produced weak lambs. Although these differences may be related to the species, similarly to the discrepancy between sheep and cattle regarding the placental damage at early gestation, it is also possible that the doses used in this and previous experiments (even up to 10^8) have been excessively aggressive for the infected sheep. This suggestion is supported by the fact that previous studies employing lower doses obtained more variable outcomes, ranging from few aborted foetuses to birth of weak or healthy lambs [11,12]. Nevertheless, information concerning parasite dose and isolate virulence is limited. Hence, in order to address the standardization of a pregnant model in sheep, further experiments would be desirable to compare outcomes from different inoculation doses and various *N. caninum* isolates. Our study confirmed that around 90 dg the foetal immune system is undergoing development according to specific antibodies detected in foetal fluids, and the lower parasite burden found in this group compared to G1 (day 40). This suggests a partial, yet insufficient, control of the infection.

The finding of more severe lesions in the placenta found at G2 despite the lower parasite burden suggests that the inflammatory response developed in this organ has been effective in controlling the parasite, maybe because of the longer period of time elapsed since infection, but has also damaged the organ as a "bystander effect". Indeed, the highest ewe serum titres were found in this group, probably due to the longer time before abortion occurred. In foetal samples, parasite detection (both frequency and burden) were lower in comparison to G1, but the frequency of lesions in the brain and skeletal muscles were higher. This, together with the shift from necrotic to inflammatory characteristic of the lesions, was most likely also a consequence of the maturation of foetal immune response. The dramatically smaller number of lesions in the liver compared to G1 may be consequence of the longer period of time elapsed since infection. The liver is probably the first foetal organ reached by the parasite through the umbilical vein, so the three additional weeks compared to G1 may have given the organ time to clear the lesions, as it has been previously observed [9].

With regard to infection at late pregnancy (G3), all ewes delivered live lambs, although three of them were born before day 145 and showed weakness and unresponsiveness. These results are in accordance with those previously described for both pregnant cattle [43-45] and sheep [12], in which the delivery of live, but congenitally infected, calves or lambs with no obvious clinical signs is the most common consequence of experimental infection during the third term of gestation. However, although infection of the placenta and foetuses (i.e. transplacental infection) occurred in all sheep from this group, the three lambs prematurely born showed both higher parasite burden and number of lesions in brain and liver compared to the other six lambs born after day 145. In addition, parasites could only be detected in the lymph nodes from the dams that delivered these three premature animals. In the remaining lambs, parasite detection was higher when compared to that observed in G2, except for one of the twin lambs delivered at day 155 of gestation, which was completely negative by PCR. This could be attributed to the difference in time at necropsy between the two groups, since lambs from G3 were studied two weeks earlier than those from G2, giving therefore less time to the immune response, already mature in both cases, to control the infection. Sera from G3 lambs collected before suckling showed a range of titres from negative to 1:128. Four of the 6 lambs born apparently healthy after day 145 of gestation were seronegative. Despite this, 3 of these 4 lambs were infected as proven by PCR. Moreover, as lambs were culled soon after birth, we do not know what would have happen thereafter, and can only hypothesise that those lambs with negative sera titres would have survived as persistently infected animals, whereas those prematurely born with high parasite detection and showing weakness and recumbency may have not survived long after delivery, as they were too weak to be nourished by the mother.

Finally, the quantification of histological lesions in the placenta and foetuses has shown to be very useful in adding to the interpretation of the results from this experiment. In a similar approach, Buxton et al. [14] described how the number of necrotic foci in the placenta increased with the time post-infection up to a maximum, around 40 days pi, from where the organ recovered and the number of foci decreased sharply. These observations correlates with our results, suggesting that: a) there is a relation between the time post-infection and the severity of the lesions and b) lesions may regress in the affected organs. The latter has been described to occur in the placenta [14] and, according to the present results, also in the foetal liver, but not in the foetal brain.

In the light of the results from this study, we suggest that the experimental infection of sheep had similar outcomes, in term of abortions and birth of weak or clinically healthy lambs, to those described in natural bovine or ovine neosporosis. Despite a number of differences, which trigger further investigations of ovine neosporosis, the use of an ovine model seems reasonably valid for assessments of both, vaccines and drug candidates for bovine neosporosis. In addition, this model is uniquely suited to investigate the pathogenesis of ovine neosporosis, a disease with increasing relevance. Further studies would be desirable in order to achieve a better and well-established *N. caninum* infection model in sheep [17].

Additional files

Additional file 1: Individual serological titres in dams and foetuses/lambs at the time of necropsy. [a]Necropsies were carried out when foetal dead was detected or immediately after parturition. *Lamb prematurely born showing weakness and unresponsiveness. dpi: days post-infection; dg: days of gestation; NA: not available; FL: foetal liquid; PCS: precolostral serum.

Additional file 2: Individual quantification of lesions in the placenta, foetal liver and brain. [a]Necropsies were carried out when foetal dead was detected or immediately after parturition. *Lamb prematurely born showing weakness and unresponsiveness. dpi: days post-infection; dg: days of gestation; NA: not available.

Additional file 3: Sections of skeletal muscle from non-viable foetuses. A: large area of coagulative necrosis in the skeletal muscle of a foetus from G1. Note the scarcity of inflammatory cells related to this lesion. B: diffuse infiltration of mixed inflammatory cells among muscular fibres. With this lesions, note the coexistence of degenerated (arrows) and preserved (arrowheads) fibres. Both pictures were taken at the same magnification. Bar: 200 µm.

Additional file 4: Individual frequency of parasite DNA detection. [a]Necropsies were carried out when foetal dead was detected or immediately after parturition. *Lamb prematurely born showing weakness and unresponsiveness. dpi: days post-infection; dg: days of gestation; MLN: mesenteric lymph node; ULN: uterine lymph node; FL: foetal liquid; PCS: precolostral serum; STM semitendinosus muscle; plus (+++, ++, +) and minus (–) signs represent PCR detection in >67%, 66-34%, <33% and 0% of samples analysed, respectively.

Competing interests
The authors declare that they have no competing interests.

Authors' contributions
JB, JRC, IF, AH and LMO conceived the study and participated in its design; DAS and JB wrote the manuscript, with results interpretation and discussion inputs from JRC, ECF, VP, AH and LMO; DAS and IF prepared the inocula and carried out the infections; DAS and JRC performed PCR and qPCR analysis, serological assays, statistical analysis and interpreted the results. JB, MF, MFE and VP participated in inoculation and clinical examination of animals, performed necropsies and sampling of the animals, carried out histopathological analyses and interpreted the results. All authors read and approved the final manuscript.

Acknowledgments
We gratefully acknowledge Esperanza Selva from the SALUVET group (Complutense University of Madrid, Spain), Mario Ferrero, Melchor Molero, Ivan Panero, Miguel Fernández and Carmen Espiniella from IGM (CSIC-ULE) and Idoia Badiola, from Agropal S. C. for their excellent technical assistance. David Arranz Solís is supported by a fellowship from the Spanish Ministry of Economy and Competitiveness (MINECO), as part of the Program of Training of Researcher Staff (FPI, grant number BES-2011-043433). This work was supported by the Swiss National Foundation (SNF grant No. 310030_146162), research grant LE253U13 from Junta de Castilla y León (Spain) and Iberoamerican science and technology programme for development (CYTED).

Author details
[1]SALUVET, Animal Health Department, Faculty of Veterinary Sciences, Complutense University of Madrid, Ciudad Universitaria s/n, 28040 Madrid, Spain. [2]Livestock Health and Production Institute (ULE-CSIC), 24346 León, Spain. [3]Institute of Parasitology, Vetsuisse Faculty, University of Bern, CH-3012 Bern, Switzerland.

References
1. Dubey JP, Schares G (2011) Neosporosis in animals–the last five years. Vet Parasitol 180:90–108
2. Dubey JP, Schares G, Ortega-Mora LM (2007) Epidemiology and control of neosporosis and *Neospora caninum*. Clin Microbiol Rev 20:323–367
3. Williams DJ, Hartley CS, Bjorkman C, Trees AJ (2009) Endogenous and exogenous transplacental transmission of *Neospora caninum* - how the route of transmission impacts on epidemiology and control of disease. Parasitology 136:1895–1900
4. Dubey JP, Hartley WJ, Lindsay DS, Topper MJ (1990) Fatal congenital *Neospora caninum* infection in a lamb. J Parasitol 76:127–130
5. Kobayashi Y, Yamada M, Omata Y, Koyama T, Saito A, Matsuda T, Okuyama K, Fujimoto S, Furuoka H, Matsui T (2001) Naturally-occurring *Neospora caninum* infection in an adult sheep and her twin fetuses. J Parasitol 87:434–436
6. Moreno B, Collantes-Fernández E, Villa A, Navarro A, Regidor-Cerrillo J, Ortega-Mora LM (2012) Occurrence of *Neospora caninum* and *Toxoplasma gondii* infections in ovine and caprine abortions. Vet Parasitol 187:312–318
7. West DM, Pomroy WE, Collett MG, Hill FI, Ridler AL, Kenyon PR, Morris ST, Pattison RS (2006) A possible role for *Neospora caninum* in ovine abortion in New Zealand. Small Rumin Res 62:135–138
8. González-Warleta M, Castro-Hermida JA, Regidor-Cerrillo J, Benavides J, Álvarez-García G, Fuertes M, Ortega-Mora LM, Mezo M (2014) *Neospora caninum* infection as a cause of reproductive failure in a sheep flock. Vet Res 45:88
9. Buxton D, Maley SW, Wright S, Thomson KM, Rae AG, Innes EA (1998) The pathogenesis of experimental neosporosis in pregnant sheep. J Comp Pathol 118:267–279
10. Givens MD, Marley MS (2008) Infectious causes of embryonic and fetal mortality. Theriogenology 70:270–285
11. Weston JF, Howe L, Collett MG, Pattison RS, Williamson NB, West DM, Pomroy WE, Syed-Hussain SS, Morris ST, Kenyon PR (2009) Dose-titration challenge of young pregnant sheep with *Neospora caninum* tachyzoites. Vet Parasitol 164:183–191
12. McAllister MM, McGuire AM, Jolley WR, Lindsay DS, Trees AJ, Stobart RH (1996) Experimental neosporosis in pregnant ewes and their offspring. Vet Pathol 33:647–655
13. Dubey JP, Lindsay DS (1990) *Neospora caninum* induced abortion in sheep. J Vet Diagn Invest 2:230–233
14. Buxton D, Maley SW, Thomson KM, Trees AJ, Innes EA (1997) Experimental infection of non-pregnant and pregnant sheep with *Neospora caninum*. J Comp Pathol 117:1–16
15. Buxton D, Wright S, Maley SW, Rae AG, Lunden A, Innes EA (2001) Immunity to experimental neosporosis in pregnant sheep. Parasite Immunol 23:85–91
16. Jenkins MC, Tuo WB, Dubey JP (2004) Evaluation of vaccination with *Neospora caninum* protein for prevention of fetal loss associated with experimentally induced neosporosis in sheep. Am J Vet Res 65:1404–1408
17. Benavides J, Collantes-Fernández E, Ferre I, Pérez V, Campero C, Mota R, Innes E, Ortega-Mora LM (2014) Experimental ruminant models for bovine neosporosis: what is known and what is needed. Parasitology 141:1471–1488
18. Regidor-Cerrillo J, Gómez-Bautista M, Pereira-Bueno J, Aduriz G, Navarro-Lozano V, Risco-Castillo V, Fernández-García A, Pedraza-Diaz S, Ortega-Mora LM (2008) Isolation and genetic characterization of *Neospora caninum* from asymptomatic calves in Spain. Parasitology 135:1651–1659
19. Regidor-Cerrillo J, Gómez-Bautista M, Del Pozo I, Jiménez-Ruiz E, Aduriz G, Ortega-Mora LM (2010) Influence of *Neospora caninum* intra-specific variability in the outcome of infection in a pregnant BALB/c mouse model. Vet Res 41:52
20. Álvarez-García G, Collantes-Fernández E, Costas E, Rebordosa X, Ortega-Mora LM (2003) Influence of age and purpose for testing on the cut-off selection of serological methods in bovine neosporosis. Vet Res 34:341–352
21. Schneider CA, Rasband WS, Eliceiri KW (2012) NIH Image to ImageJ: 25 years of image analysis. Nat Methods 9:671–675
22. Regidor-Cerrillo J, Arranz-Solís D, Benavides J, Gómez-Bautista M, Castro-Hermida JA, Mezo M, Pérez V, Ortega-Mora LM, González-Warleta M (2014) *Neospora caninum* infection during early pregnancy in cattle: how the isolate influences infection dynamics, clinical outcome and peripheral and local immune responses. Vet Res 45:10
23. Hurtado A, Aduriz G, Moreno B, Barandika J, García-Pérez AL (2001) Single tube nested PCR for the detection of *Toxoplasma gondii* in fetal tissues from naturally aborted ewes. Vet Parasitol 102:17–27
24. Buxton D (1998) Protozoan infections (*Toxoplasma gondii, Neospora caninum* and *Sarcocystis* spp.) in sheep and goats: recent advances. Vet Res 29:289–310
25. Collantes-Fernández E, Zaballos A, Álvarez-García G, Ortega-Mora LM (2002) Quantitative detection of *Neospora caninum* in bovine aborted fetuses and experimentally infected mice by real-time PCR. J Clin Microbiol 40:1194–1198
26. Gutierrez J, O'Donovan J, Proctor A, Brady C, Marques PX, Worrall S, Nally JE, McElroy M, Bassett H, Fagan J, Maley S, Buxton D, Sammin D, Markey BK (2012) Application of quantitative real-time polymerase chain reaction for the diagnosis of toxoplasmosis and enzootic abortion of ewes. J Vet Diagn Invest 24:846–854
27. Howe L, Collett MG, Pattison RS, Marshall J, West DM, Pomroy WE (2012) Potential involvement of *Neospora caninum* in naturally occurring ovine abortions in New Zealand. Vet Parasitol 185:64–71
28. Caspe SG, Moore DP, Leunda MR, Cano DB, Lischinsky L, Regidor-Cerrillo J, Álvarez-García G, Echaide IG, Bacigalupe D, Ortega Mora LM, Odeon AC, Campero CM (2012) The *Neospora caninum*-Spain 7 isolate induces

placental damage, fetal death and abortion in cattle when inoculated in early gestation. Vet Parasitol 189:171–178

29. Dubey JP, Buxton D, Wouda W (2006) Pathogenesis of bovine neosporosis. J Comp Pathol 134:267–289
30. Williams DJ, Guy CS, Smith RF, Ellis J, Bjorkman C, Reichel MP, Trees AJ (2007) Immunization of cattle with live tachyzoites of *Neospora caninum* confers protection against fetal death. Infect Immun 75:1343–1348
31. Almería S, Araujo R, Tuo W, López-Gatius F, Dubey JP, Gasbarre LC (2010) Fetal death in cows experimentally infected with *Neospora caninum* at 110 days of gestation. Vet Parasitol 169:304–311
32. Rosbottom A, Guy CS, Gibney EH, Smith RF, Valarcher JF, Taylor G, Williams DJ (2007) Peripheral immune responses in pregnant cattle following *Neospora caninum* infection. Parasite Immunol 29:219–228
33. Rojo-Montejo S, Collantes-Fernández E, Pérez-Zaballos F, Rodríguez-Marcos S, Blanco-Murcia J, Rodríguez-Bertos A, Prenafeta A, Ortega-Mora LM (2013) Effect of vaccination of cattle with the low virulence Nc-Spain 1H isolate of *Neospora caninum* against a heterologous challenge in early and mid-gestation. Vet Res 44:106
34. Rojo-Montejo S, Collantes-Fernández E, Blanco-Murcia J, Rodríguez-Bertos A, Risco-Castillo V, Ortega-Mora LM (2009) Experimental infection with a low virulence isolate of *Neospora caninum* at 70 days gestation in cattle did not result in foetopathy. Vet Res 40:49
35. Macaldowie C, Maley SW, Wright S, Bartley P, Esteban-Redondo I, Buxton D, Innes EA (2004) Placental pathology associated with fetal death in cattle inoculated with *Neospora caninum* by two different routes in early pregnancy. J Comp Pathol 131:142–156
36. Rosbottom A, Gibney EH, Guy CS, Kipar A, Smith RF, Kaiser P, Trees AJ, Williams DJ (2008) Upregulation of cytokines is detected in the placentas of cattle infected with *Neospora caninum* and is more marked early in gestation when fetal death is observed. Infect Immun 76:2352–2361
37. Matyszak MK (1998) Inflammation in the CNS: balance between immunological privilege and immune responses. Prog Neurobiol 56:19–35
38. Innes EA, Lunden A, Esteban I, Marks J, Maley S, Wright S, Rae A, Harkins D, Vermeulen A, McKendrick IJ, Buxton D (2001) A previous infection with *Toxoplasma gondii* does not protect against a challenge with *Neospora caninum* in pregnant sheep. Parasite Immunol 23:121–132
39. Barr BC, Rowe JD, Sverlow KW, BonDurant RH, Ardans AA, Oliver MN, Conrad PA (1994) Experimental reproduction of bovine fetal *Neospora* infection and death with a bovine *Neospora* isolate. J Vet Diagn Invest 6:207–215
40. Gondim LFP, McAllister MM, Anderson-Sprecher RC, Bjorkman C, Lock TF, Firkins LD, Gao L, Fischer WR (2004) Transplacental transmission and abortion in cows administered *Neospora caninum* oocysts. J Parasitol 90:1394–1400
41. Almería S, De Marez T, Dawson H, Araujo R, Dubey JP, Gasbarre LC (2003) Cytokine gene expression in dams and foetuses after experimental *Neospora caninum* infection of heifers at 110 days of gestation. Parasite Immunol 25:383–392
42. Dubey JP, Rommel M (1992) Abortions caused by protozoa in agricultural animals. Dtsch Tierarztl Wochenschr 99:355–362 (in German)
43. Benavides J, Katzer F, Maley SW, Bartley PM, Cantón G, Palarea-Albaladejo J, Purslow CA, Pang Y, Rocchi MS, Chianini F, Buxton D, Innes EA (2012) High rate of transplacental infection and transmission of *Neospora caninum* following experimental challenge of cattle at day 210 of gestation. Vet Res 43:83
44. Gibney EH, Kipar A, Rosbottom A, Guy CS, Smith RF, Hetzel U, Trees AJ, Williams DJ (2008) The extent of parasite-associated necrosis in the placenta and foetal tissues of cattle following *Neospora caninum* infection in early and late gestation correlates with foetal death. Int J Parasitol 38:579–588
45. Williams DJ, Guy CS, McGarry JW, Guy F, Tasker L, Smith RF, MacEachern K, Cripps PJ, Kelly DF, Trees AJ (2000) *Neospora caninum*-associated abortion in cattle: the time of experimentally-induced parasitaemia during gestation determines foetal survival. Parasitology 121:347–358

Different clinical, virological, serological and tissue tropism outcomes of two new and one old Belgian type 1 subtype 1 porcine reproductive and respiratory virus (PRRSV) isolates

Ilias S Frydas[1*], Ivan Trus[1], Lise K Kvisgaard[2], Caroline Bonckaert[1], Vishwanatha RAP Reddy[1], Yewei Li[1], Lars E Larsen[2] and Hans J Nauwynck[1*]

Abstract

In this study, the pathogenic behavior of PRRSV 13V091 and 13V117, isolated in 2013 from two different Belgian farms with enzootic respiratory problems shortly after weaning in the nursery, were compared with the Belgian strain 07V063 isolated in 2007. Full-length genome sequencing was performed to identify their origin. Twelve weeks-old pigs were inoculated intranasally (IN) with 13V091, 13V117 or 07V063 (9 pigs/group). At 10 days post inoculation (dpi), 4 animals from each group were euthanized and tissues were collected for pathology, virological and serological analysis. 13V091 infection resulted in the highest respiratory disease scores and longest period of fever. Gross lung lesions were more pronounced for 13V091 (13%), than for 13V117 (7%) and 07V063 (11%). The nasal shedding and viremia was also most extensive with 13V091. The 13V091 group showed the highest virus replication in conchae, tonsils and retropharyngeal lymph nodes. 13V117 infection resulted in the lowest virus replication in lymphoid tissues. 13V091 showed higher numbers of sialoadhesin$^-$ infected cells/mm^2 in conchae, tonsils and spleen than 13V117 and 07V063. Neutralizing antibody response with 07V063 was stronger than with 13V091 and 13V117. It can be concluded that (i) 13V091 is a highly pathogenic type 1 subtype 1 PRRSV strain that replicates better than 07V063 and 13V117 and has a strong tropism for sialoadhesin$^-$ cells and (ii) despite the close genetic relationship between 13V117 and 07V063, 13V117 has an increased nasal replication and shedding, but a decreased replication in lymphoid tissues compared to 07V063.

Introduction

Porcine reproductive and respiratory syndrome (PRRS) is a devastating disease that continuously hits swine industry all over the world [1]. A recent economic analysis in the US demonstrated that the amount of total annual losses increased from $560 million in 2005 to $664 million in 2011 [2]. The disease first appeared in the US in the late eighties and then a few years later in Europe and Asia [3]. The causative agent is a positive single-stranded enveloped RNA virus classified together with lactate dehydrogenase virus (LDV), simian hemorrhagic fever virus (SDHF) and equine arteritis virus (EAV) in the family of the *Arteriviridae* within the order of the *Nidovirales* [4]. PRRSV causes reproductive failure in late-term gestation sows with an increased number of stillborn, mummified and weak-born piglets. Respiratory disorders are characterized mainly by dyspnea and tachypnea in young animals [5,6].

The PRRSV genome is approximately 15 kb in length and contains nine open reading frames (ORFs) [3]. Open reading frames 1a and 1b constitute 75% of the viral genome and encode viral replicase polyproteins, which are processed by self-encoded proteases into 14 non-structural proteins (nsp) [3]. Major (GP5, M, N) and minor (GP2, GP3, GP4, ORF5a-protein, E) structural proteins are being encoded at the 3' end of the genome by ORFs 2a, 2b, 3, 4, 5, 5a, 6 and 7 [7]. Like with other

* Correspondence: ilias.frydas@ugent.be; hans.nauwynck@ugent.be
[1]Laboratory of Virology, Department of Virology, Immunology and Parasitology, Faculty of Veterinary Medicine, Ghent University, Salisburylaan 133, B-9820 Merelbeke, Ghent, Belgium
Full list of author information is available at the end of the article

nidoviruses, transcription of the PRRSV genome is characterized by the formation of a 3'-co-terminal nested set of subgenomic messenger RNAs, each of them with a common 5'-leader sequence [8].

Two distinct genotypes were identified, and designated as European type 1 (prototype LV-Lelystad, GenBank: M96262) and American type 2 (prototype VR2332, GenBank: AY150564), with 40% differences at the nucleotide level [7]. A large genetic variability has been shown within both subtypes [9]. Genetic heterogeneity is one of the main reasons why current commercial attenuated and inactivated vaccines provide incomplete protection against heterologous strains and as a result there is an urgent need for a novel generation of vaccines [10,11].

Starting from 2006, new highly pathogenic strains emerged, causing large-scale outbreaks in Eastern Europe (type 1, prototype Lena, GenBank: JF802085), and Southeastern Asia (type 2, prototype JXA1, GenBank: EF112445). These isolates are characterized by high viral loads in blood and tissues, high fever, severe general clinical signs and increased mortality [12-14]. A common genetic characteristic of highly pathogenic strains of both PRRSV type 1 and 2 is a discontinuous 30-amino acid deletion in the non-structural protein 2 (nsp2) (Lena: aa 710–739, JXA1: aa 534–563) [13,14]. However, this deletion is most probably not solely responsible for differences in virulence, as nsp2 is the most divergent one in PRRSV [7]. In Europe, highly virulent strains from Eastern Europe clearly differed from the circulating low virulent Western European strains and taxonomically they were designated as different type 1 subtypes (LV-like strains: subtype 1, Lena-like strains: subtype 3) [4]. Subtype 3 strains are constrained in Eastern Europe and up till now, there were no reports of highly pathogenic strains emerging in Western Europe [4].

In the present study, the virulence and pathogenicity of three PRRSV strains from Belgium were evaluated: two isolates (13V091 and 13V117) from 2013, originating from farms experiencing uncommon long-lasting anorexia, fever and respiratory problems within the first two weeks after weaning during an enzootic PRRSV infection, and the well-characterized Belgian strain 07V063 (GenBank: GU737264) from 2007 that was used as a reference [15,16]. Full-length genome sequencing was performed to characterize these PRRSV isolates.

Materials and methods

Viruses

PRRSV 13V091 and 13V117 were isolated from sera of pigs that showed severe respiratory problems in two Belgian farms. Virus isolation was performed as described before [12]. Briefly, porcine alveolar macrophages (PAM) were cultured in RPMI 1640 + GlutaMax modified medium (Gibco Invitrogen), supplemented with 10% fetal calf serum (FCS), 1% non-essential amino acids (Gibco Invitrogen), 1 mM sodium pyruvate and a mixture of antibiotics. Subsequently, cells were inoculated with ten-fold serial dilutions of sera and when cytopathic effect (CPE) was observed after three days, cells were fixed and stained with immunohistochemistry (IPMA) [10]. The monoclonal antibody (mAb) 13E2 against the nucleocapsid protein of PRRSV was used as primary antibody to identify PRRSV [17]. After isolation, 13V091 and 13V117 were grown in PAM and used for sequencing and pathogenesis studies. The viral stocks were confirmed to be free from Mycoplasma, porcine parvovirus, porcine circoviruses and swine influenza viruses. The 07V063 strain was enclosed as a reference. A 2nd-3rd passage of 13V117, 13V091 and 07V063 was used for the animal inoculations.

Experimental design

Thirty-six twelve-week-old pigs, originating from a PRRSV-negative farm, were randomly divided in 4 groups of 9 animals. Relevant pathogens (PRRSV, SIV, PCV2) were not detected in the animals. Experiments were conducted in a biosafety level 2 (BSL-2) facility and were approved by the Ethical Committee of the University of Ghent (EC 2010/090). The pigs of groups 13V091, 13V117 and 07V063 were inoculated intranasally (IN) with 2 mL containing 10^5 tissue culture infectious dose with 50% end point ($TCID_{50}$) of the respective viruses (1 mL per nostril). Group CON consisted of animals mock-inoculated with PBS. Rectal temperature and clinical observations were monitored daily, starting from the third day before challenge until the 21st day post inoculation (dpi). Body temperature over 40.0 °C was considered as fever. The scoring system was used before and is fully described in previous studies [12,14]. Breathing, sneezing, coughing, nasal discharge, liveliness, ear discoloration, presence of peri-ocular oedema and diarrhea were taken into account. Detailed list and parameters of the clinical scores is shown in Additional file 1. In all groups, blood samples and nasal swabs were taken at 0, 3, 5, 7, 10, 14, 21, 28, 35 and 42 dpi. Plasma and nasal secretions were collected and stored at −70 °C for virus titration. At 10 dpi, 4 pigs from each group were euthanized and two samples were collected from the following tissues: nasal mucosa (septum and conchae), pharynx, tonsils, lymph nodes (pharyngeal, bronchial, mediastinal, inguinal), lungs (apical, cardiac and diaphragmatic lobes from both sides) and spleen. Lungs were examined macroscopically. One sample was embedded in methocel and was snap frozen for double immunofluorescense (IF) stainings, and the second sample was stored at −70 °C for virus titration.

Gross pathology and bacteriology

After euthanasia, individual lungs were collected, and to all lung lobes macroscopic lesions were given a score to estimate the percentage of lungs affected by pneumonia using the evaluation system adapted from Halbur et al. [18].

Samples from lungs (cardiac left) and lymph nodes (bronchial) were collected after euthanasia and bacteriological analysis was performed. Each sample was inoculated on Columbia agar or Columbia CAN agar supplemented with 5% sheep blood (Oxoid, Hampshire, UK) with a *Staphylococcus pseudintermedius* streak for the growth support of NAD-dependent bacteria (*Actinobacillus, Haemophilus spp.*). Plates were incubated for 48 h in a 5% CO_2-enriched environment at 35 ± 2 °C and phenotypic identification of isolated bacteria was performed as earlier described [19].

Virus titration

Nasal secretions and 20% suspensions of the collected tissues were titrated on PAM as previously described [10]. Nasal swabs were collected using Aluminium Rayon sterile plain swabs (160C, Copan Italia S.p.A., Italy). After swabbing, the swabs were brought into transportation medium consisting of phosphate buffer saline (PBS), 10% fetal calf serum (FCS) and a mixture of antibiotics. Afterwards, the swabs were vortexed, and the diluted secretions were titrated [12]. Tissue suspensions were titrated on PAM in quadruplicate and a final $TCID_{50}$ was determined after subjecting the cells to a PRRSV-specific immunoperoxidase staining to analyze the presence of PRRSV-positive cells.

Serology

Serum samples were examined for the presence of PRRSV-specific antibodies using IPMA plates as described before [10]. In these plates, LV-infected MARC-145 cells were used to detect PRRSV-specific antibodies. Virus neutralizing antibody titers were detected with a seroneutralization (SN) test on MARC-145 cells after propagation of PRRSV strains on this cell line. Two fold dilution series of sera were made and an equal volume containing 100 $TCID_{50}$ PRRSV of the homologous strains was added to each dilution and the mixture was further incubated for 1 h at 37 °C. Afterwards, the serum-virus mixture was transferred to suspension cultures of MARC-145 cells and the cells were analyzed for cytopathic effect (CPE) at ten days post inoculation. The virus neutralizing antibody titers were determined as the reciprocal of the highest dilution that inhibited CPE in 50% of the wells [16]. Samples that tested negative in IPMA were given a numerical value of 1.7 and in SN test a numerical value of 0.5.

Quantification and identification of PRRSV-positive cells

To quantify and identify viral antigen and sialoadhesin (Sn) positive cells in the different tissues, several 9 μm cryosections were made at a distance of 50 μm between each other and fixed in 100% methanol at −20 °C for 15 min. Mouse monoclonal antibodies were used against the PRRSV N protein (13E2, 1:25, IgG_{2a}) and porcine sialoadhesin (41D3, 1:2, IgG_1) [18]. Isotype-specific secondary antibodies conjugated with FITC and Alexa Fluor 594 (1:500, Invitrogen) were used to reveal the different antigens. Cell nuclei were stained with Hoechst 33342 (Invitrogen) and to confirm the specificity of each antibody, negative isotype-specific control monoclonal antibodies were used: 13D12 against gD of PRV (IgG_1), and 1C11 against gB of PrV (IgG_{2a}) [20]. Countings were made in 5 sections with 5 fields per section measured in a blind way. Results were expressed per mm^2, and analysis was performed using a Leica TCS SPE laser-scanning confocal microscope (Leica Microsystems GmbH, Wetzlar, Germany).

Sequencing

Total RNA was extracted from 140 μL PAM culture supernatant of a 2nd passage of 13V091 and a 3rd passage of 13V117 strain using the QIAcube 230 volt robot and the QIAamp® Viral RNA Mini kit (QIAGEN, cat. No. 52906). The QIAamp Viral RNA body fluid standard program was used as the extraction protocol with the elution volume of 60 μL. The RNA was screened for PRRSV using the previously published Kleiboeker modified type 1 assay [21]. PCR products covering the whole PRRSV genome in two fragments were produced from full genome cDNA as described elsewhere [22]. The PCR fragments for each virus were pooled in equimolar concentration (165 ng in total) and sequenced by the Ion Torrent PGM sequencer using the 318v2 chip (DMAC, Technical University of Denmark). After initial removal of adaptors and low quality sequences, the quality of the output data (FastQ) files was examined using the applicant FastQC (v. 0.10.1). The reads were trimmed accordingly to the FastQC report. *De novo* assembly was performed using the commercial software CLC Genomics v. 4.6.1 (CLCBIO, Aarhus, Denmark) and the genetic comparability of the obtained contigs was found using the NCBI's Basic Local Alignment Search Tool (BLASTn). The most similar sequence to the newly sequenced virus found by NCBI BLASTn was used as reference sequence for mapping reads to a reference. The final consensus sequence was found by alignment of contigs derived from *de novo* assembly and the sequence obtained from mapping to a reference. The consensus sequence from each virus was aligned to other publicly available full genome PRRS type 1 viruses using MUSCLE (Multiple Sequence Comparison by Log-Expectation). Gaps were either confirmed or closed by specifically designed primers surrounding the gaps and sequenced by cycle sequencing (LGC Genomics GmbH, Germany). All alignments and phylogenetic analysis, were performed by the commercial software CLC DNA workbench v. 6.9 (CLCBIO, Aarhus, Denmark). The phylogenetic trees were constructed using the Neighbor Joining algorithm, nucleotide/protein distance measure: Kimura80/Kimura Protein model, and Bootstrap analysis of 1000 replicates.

Statistics

All data were analyzed with GraphPad Prism 6 software (GraphPad Software Inc., San Diego, CA, USA). Serological titers (IPMA and SN) as well as viral loads were log-transformed prior to the analyses. Gross pathology scores and area under the curve (AUC) were analysed using the non-parametric Kruskal-Wallis test with Dunn's post-test. Statistical analysis of continuous data was performed using two-way analysis of variance (ANOVA) with Tukey's post-test. All results shown represent means and standard deviation (SD). Results with *P*-values < 0.05 were considered significantly different.

Results

Clinical signs and body temperature

Clinical scores in respiratory functions, liveliness and presence of conjuctivitis are summarized in Figure 1. Daily registration of clinical scores for each individual animal is shown in Additional file 2. Animals from the control group did not display clinical signs during the whole study. The 13V091 group exhibited significantly ($P < 0.05$) higher mean scores from 3 till 10 and at 14 dpi compared to the 13V117 group, and from 2 till 8 dpi compared to the 07V063 group. All 13V091-infected animals scored positive for clinical signs at least at one time point during the experiment. Respiratory symptoms were observed from the beginning of the experiment with a peak at 4 dpi (8 out of 9 animals) and lasted until 15 dpi (1 out of 4 animals). The 13V117 group showed significantly ($P < 0.05$) higher mean scores compared to the 07V063 group at 2 and 4 dpi. Animals scored positive from 2 till 6 dpi but not all the animals showed respiratory disorders. A peak was observed at 4 dpi (4 out of 9 animals). In the 07V063 group, 2 animals showed clinical scores from 2 till 4 dpi and from 7 till 11 dpi. Loss of appetite was not observed in any group but visible growth retardation was marked in the 13V091 group compared to the other groups. Diarrhea was also apparent in the 13V091 group between 13 and 21 dpi. Nasal discharge, coughing or ear discoloration was never observed.

Body temperature data are represented for each group in Figure 2. Detailed daily registration of body temperature for each individual animal is presented in Additional file 2. The mean body temperature of group 13V091 was significantly higher ($P < 0.05$) from 3 till 7 and at 13 dpi compared to the 13V117 group and from 3 till 5 dpi compared to the 07V063 group. In the 13V091 group, 8 out of 9 animals showed fever at least at one day during the experiment, whereas in the 13V117 and the 07V063 group, only 5 and 6 out of 9 animals showed fever, respectively. AUC values of individual pigs were calculated, and afterwards the AUC means per group were calculated and compared. The mean AUC value of increased body temperature with a threshold at 39.5 °C was significantly ($P < 0.05$) higher in the 13V091 group (6.0 ± 4.2) compared to the 13V117 (1.2 ± 1.3) and control groups (0.2 ± 1.3) but not to the 07V063 group (3.5 ± 3.4). 13V091-infected animals showed the highest mean number of fever days (5.1 ± 4.2 days) which was significantly different

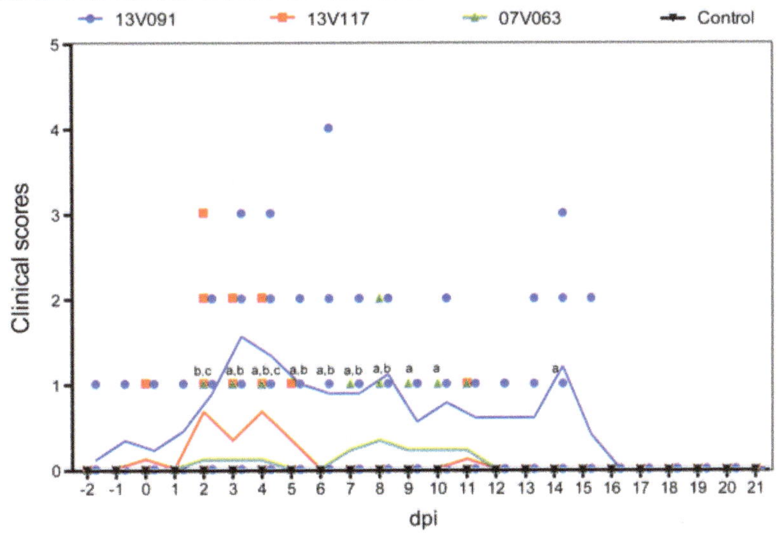

Figure 1 Clinical scores in pigs inoculated with PRRSV 13V091, 13V117 and 07V063 are summarized. Lines represent the mean value in each group. Letters denote significant statistical differences ($P < 0.05$) between viral strains (a: 13V091 and 13V117, b: 13V091 and 07V063, c: 13V117 and 07V063).

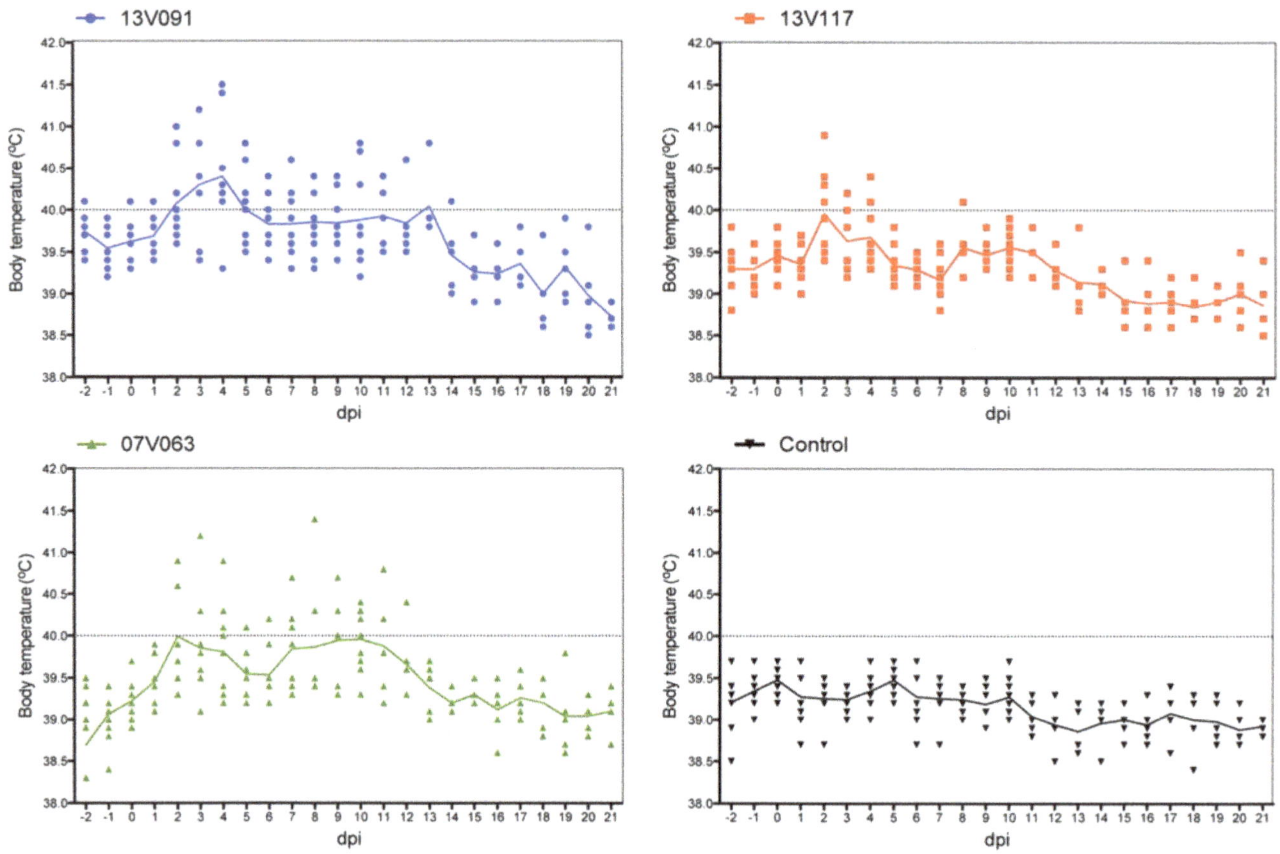

Figure 2 Body temperature of pigs upon inoculation with PRRSV 13V091, 13V117 and 07V063. Temperature ≥ 40 °C was considered as fever. Lines represent the mean value in each group.

($P < 0.05$) from the 13V117 group (1.1 ± 1.1 days) but not from the 07V063 group (3.4 ± 3.3 days).

Gross pathology and bacteriology

At 10 dpi, four pigs per group were euthanized and necropsied. Swollen pharyngeal, bronchial, mediastinal and inguinal lymph nodes were observed in the 13V091 and 07V063 infected animals. 13V091 induced a pneumonia that was characterized by tissue consolidation, haemorrhagic spots and multifocal red tanned lesions in both sides (Figure 3A). 13V117-infected animals showed also tissue consolidation and single spotted lesions located mainly at the cardiac lobe. In 07V063-infected pigs, tissue consolidation and multifocal bilateral red-tanned lesions, concentrated mainly at the cranial and cardiac lobes, were observed. No gross pulmonary lesions were found in negative control pigs, and no pleuritis and no Mycoplasma-related lesions were observed in all animals of the experiment. 13V091-infected pigs showed the highest mean percentage of lungs with gross lesions (12.9 ± 3.6%), which was significantly higher ($P < 0.05$) than the 13V117 group (6.5 ± 1.4%) and the control group (4.7 ± 2.4%) but was not different from the 07V063 group (11.3 ± 9.4%) (Figure 3B). Finally, samples from the cranial left part of the lungs and the bronchial lymph nodes of euthanized pigs were sent for bacteriological analysis. No specific bacterial pathogens were isolated.

Virological analysis

Titration of nasal swabs in the 13V091 group showed significantly higher mean titers ($P < 0.05$) at 5 dpi compared to the 13V117 group, and at 3 and 5 dpi compared to the 07V063 group. Group 13V117 exhibited significantly higher mean titers than group 07V063 at 3 and 5 dpi (Figure 4). The highest mean AUC value was observed in the 13V091 group (16.9 ± 3.7), which was significantly higher ($P < 0.05$) than the 13V117 (13.3 ± 4.3) and the 07V063 group (8.2 ± 4.3). Virus was detected for the first time at 3 dpi and two animals remained positive up till 14 dpi for the 13V091 and 07V063 groups, whereas in the 13V117 group one animal remained positive until 21 dpi. The 13V091 group showed the highest mean duration of nasal shedding (5.8 ± 2.4 days), which was not significantly different from the nasal shedding duration of the 13V117 (5.4 ± 2.4 days) and 07V063 (3.3 ± 1.9 days) group.

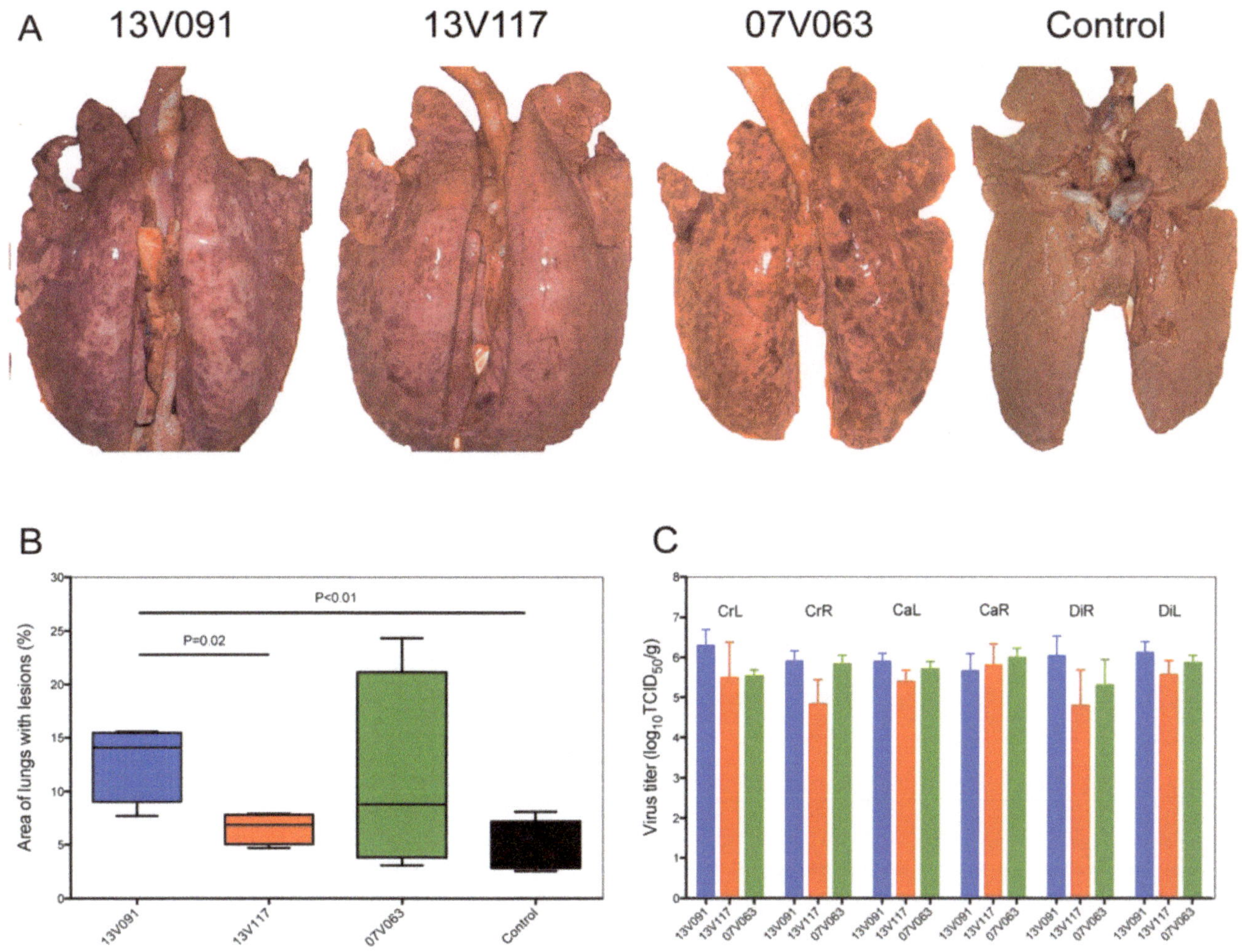

Figure 3 Lung compartment analysis of animals infected with different PRRSV strains and euthanized at 10 dpi. Representative gross pulmonary lesions **(A)**, mean macroscopic lesion scores **(B)** and virus titers in different lung compartments **(C)** are presented. CrL: Cranial Left, CrR: Cranial Right, CaL: Cardiac Left, CaR: Cardiac Right, DiL: Diaphragmatic Left, DiR: Diaphragmatic Right. Whiskers denote the standard deviation (SD) and $P < 0.05$ values represent statistically significant comparisons.

Viremia was first detected at 3 dpi and lasted until 14 dpi for the 13V091 group. Two pigs in the 13V117 and 07V063 groups remained positive until the 35th and 28th dpi, respectively. The 13V091 group showed significantly higher ($P < 0.05$) mean virus titers at 5 dpi compared to the 13V117 group, and at 5 and 10 dpi compared to the 07V063 group. The 13V117 group exhibited significantly higher mean titers at 5 and 7 dpi compared to the 07V063 group (Figure 5). Control animals did not show viremia during the experiment. 13V091 showed the highest duration (8.8 ± 1.9 days) compared to 13V117 (8.1 ± 1.8 days) and 07V063 (6.9 ± 0.7 days). The average AUC value of the 13V091 (22.2 ± 9.3) and the 13V117 group (25.1 ± 8.4), were slightly higher than that of the 07V063 group (18.7 ± 10.5) ($P > 0.05$).

Serology

PRRSV-specific antibodies were first detected with IPMA in all PRRSV-infected groups as early as 7 dpi (Figure 6A). The highest mean antibody titers ranged from $2^{12.9}$ to $2^{14.1}$ for all groups and were reached at 21–35 dpi. No significant difference was observed between the infected groups at any time point. Control animals remained seronegative during the whole experiment.

In 07V063-infected animals, homologous SN titers appeared at 28 dpi in three out of five pigs, and reached a maximum mean titer at 49 dpi (2^3) when all animals were positive. In the 13V091 group, SN titers against the homologous strain could be detected in three pigs at 28 dpi (2^1) and the titers remained at a similar level until 49 dpi when all the animals became positive and the group showed a mean titer of $2^{1.4} \pm 2^{0.4}$ (Figure 6B).

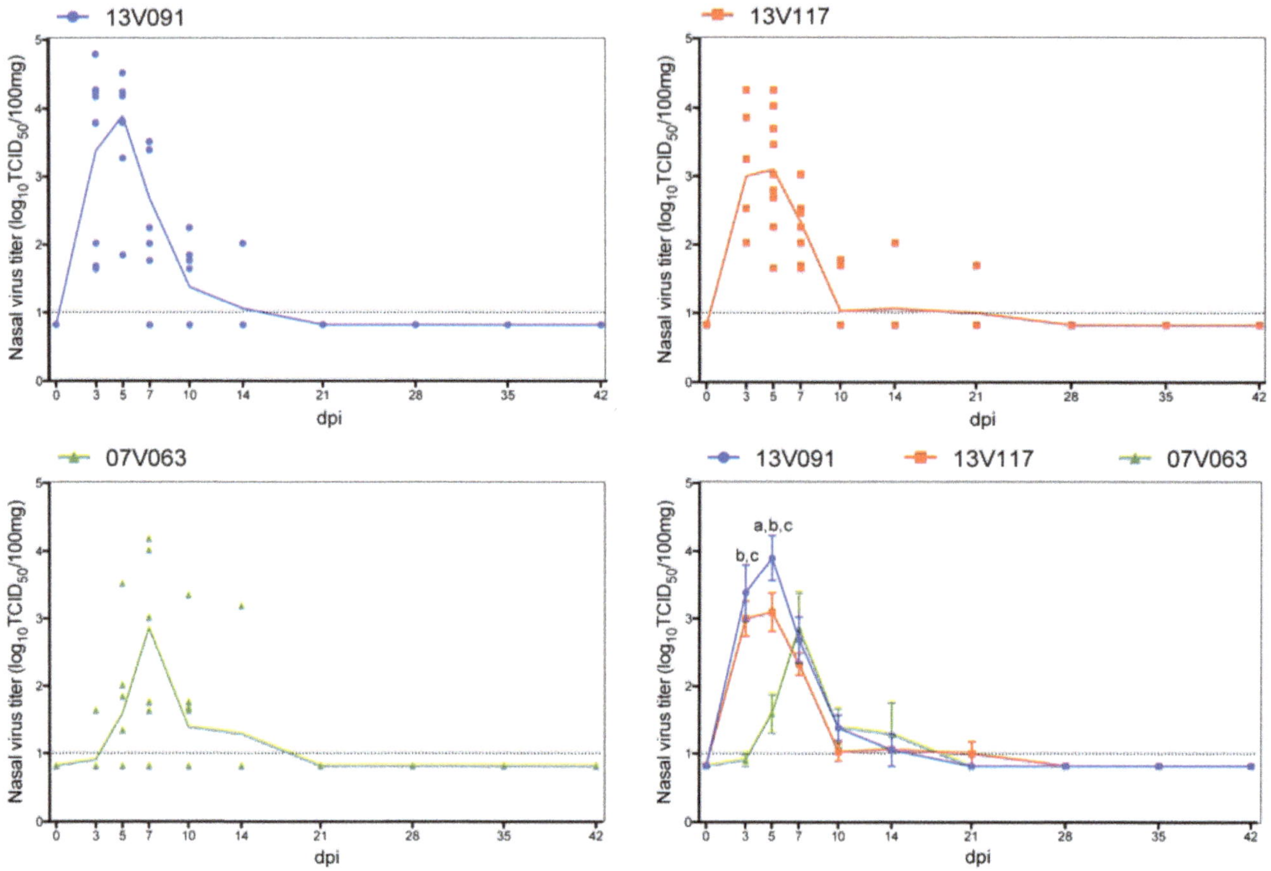

Figure 4 Virus titers in nasal secretions of pigs inoculated with PRRSV 13V091, 13V117 and 07V063. Lines represent the mean value in each group. Whiskers denote the standard deviation (SD). The dotted line gives the detection limit for virus titration. Letters denote significant statistical differences ($P < 0.05$) between viral strains (a: 13V091 and 13V117, b: 13V091 and 07V063, c: 13V117 and 07V063).

13V117-infected animals did not show any SN titer against the homologous strain until 42 dpi when one pig out of five was positive (2^1). At 49 dpi, one additional pig became positive (2^2).

PRRSV titers in different organs

Respiratory tract

Tissues from animals euthanized at 10 dpi were collected for PRRSV titration. In the conchae, 13V091-infected animals showed higher ($P > 0.05$) mean virus titers (5.1 ± 0.9 $log_{10}TCID_{50}/g$) than 13V117 (3.8 ± 2.1 $log_{10}TCID_{50}/g$) and 07V063 infected animals (3.7 ± 2.2 $log_{10}TCID_{50}/g$) (Figure 7A). In the 13V091-infected animals, septum and pharynx displayed titers of 2.6 ± 1.2 and 3.5 ± 1.6 $log_{10}TCID_{50}/g$ respectively, which were slightly higher than the ones in the 13V117 group (septum: 2.2 ± 1.3 $log_{10}TCID_{50}/g$, pharynx: 3.0 ± 1.4 $log_{10}TCID_{50}/g$) and the 07V063 group (septum: 1.2 ± 0.1 $log_{10}TCID_{50}/g$, pharynx: 3.3 ± 1.1 $log_{10}TCID_{50}/g$), but not significantly different. Slightly higher titers for the 13V091 group were found after titration of lung compartments (Figure 3C), and values from all strains ranged from 4.8 to 6.2 $log_{10}TCID_{50}/g$. Samples from the pigs of the control group were negative for virus isolation.

Lymphoid tissues

Average viral titers in tonsils (5.7 ± 0.5 $log_{10}TCID_{50}/g$) and retropharyngeal lymph nodes (RPLN) (5.2 ± 0.4 $log_{10}TCID_{50}/g$) in the 13V091 group, were significantly higher ($P < 0.05$), than in the 13V117 group (tonsils: 4.0 ± 2.0 $log_{10}TCID_{50}/g$, RPLN: 3.0 ± 1.8 $log_{10}TCID_{50}/g$), but not from the 07V063 group (tonsils: 4.8 ± 1.0 $log_{10}TCID_{50}/g$, RPLN: 4.5 ± 2.0 $log_{10}TCID_{50}/g$). Virus titration of bronchial (BLN), mediastinal (MLN) and inguinal (ILN) lymph nodes of the 13V091 (BLN: 3.8 ± 0.4 $log_{10}TCID_{50}/g$, MLN: 4.4 ± 0.7 $log_{10}TCID_{50}/g$, ILN: 4.4 ± 0.8 $log_{10}TCID_{50}/g$) and 07V063 groups (BLN: 4.5 ± 0.8 $log_{10}TCID_{50}/g$, MLN: 3.4 ± 0.8 $log_{10}TCID_{50}/g$, ILN: 4.2 ± 0.1 $log_{10}TCID_{50}/g$), showed significantly ($P < 0.05$) higher titers compared to the 13V117 group (BLN: 1.6 ± 0.5 $log_{10}TCID_{50}/g$, MLN: 1.7 ± 0.5 $log_{10}TCID_{50}/g$, ILN: 2.5 ± 0.7 $log_{10}TCID_{50}/g$) (Figure 7C). Finally, in spleen, the

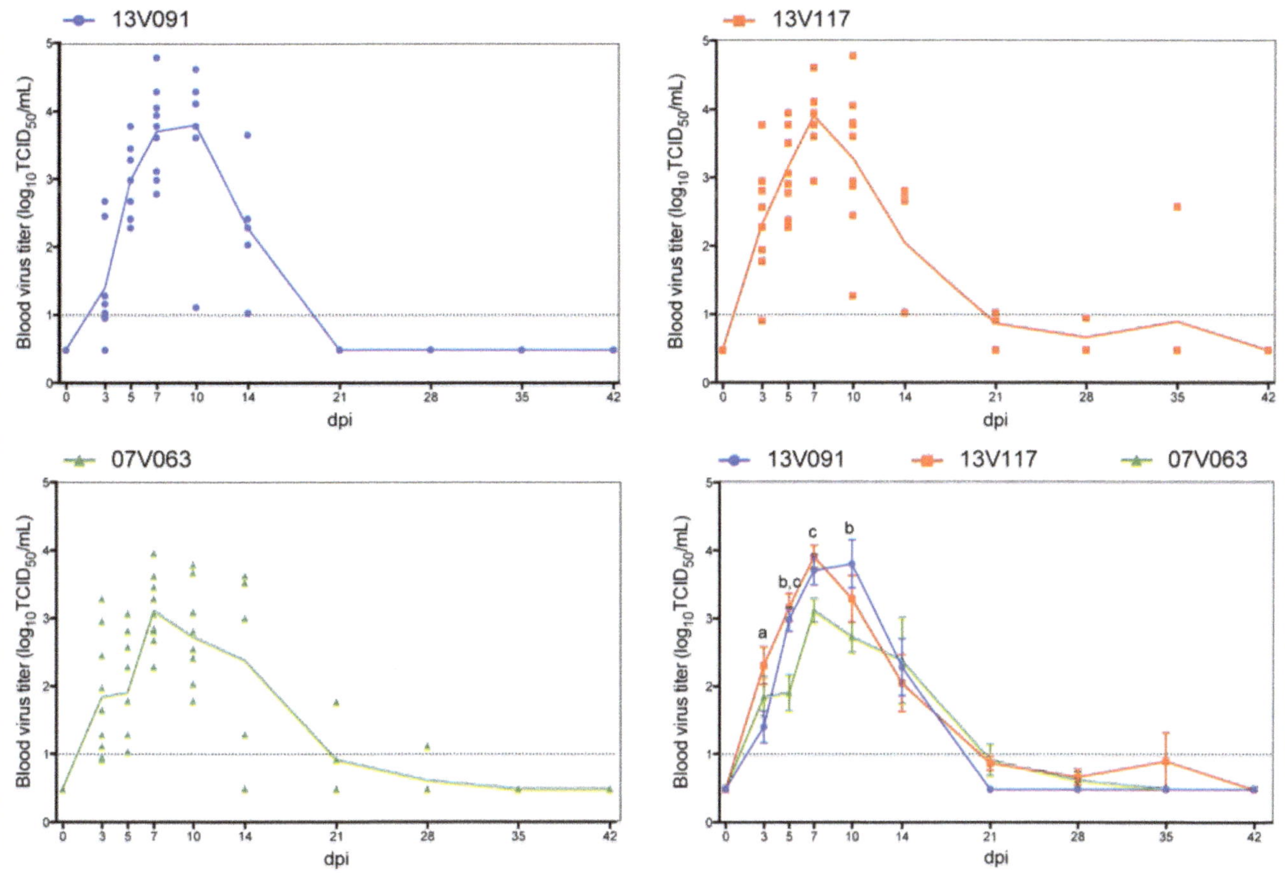

Figure 5 Viremia in pigs inoculated with PRRSV 13V091, 13V117 and 07V063. Patterns represent individual animals. Lines represent the mean value. Whiskers denote the standard deviation (SD). The dotted line gives the detection limit for the virus titration. Letters denote significant statistical differences ($P < 0.05$) between viral strains (a: 13V091 and 13V117, b: 13V091 and 07V063, c: 13V117 and 07V063).

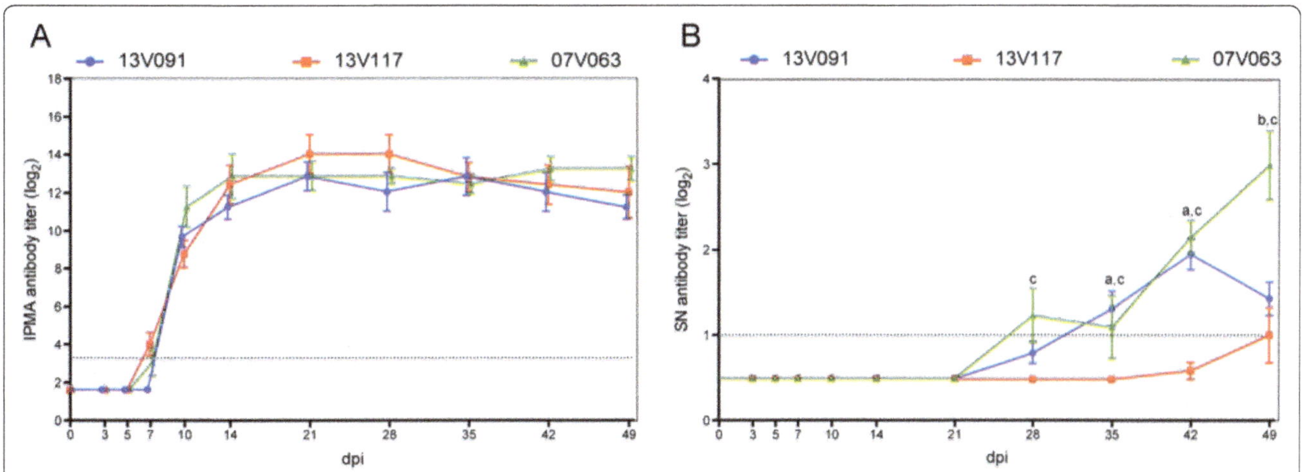

Figure 6 Antibody response, IPMA (A) and SN (B) in pigs inoculated with PRRSV 13V091, 13V117 and 07V063. Whiskers denote the standard deviation (SD). Dotted lines denote detection limits. Letters denote significant statistical differences ($P < 0.05$) between viral strains (a: 13V091 and 13V117, b: 13V091 and 07V063, c: 13V117 and 07V063).

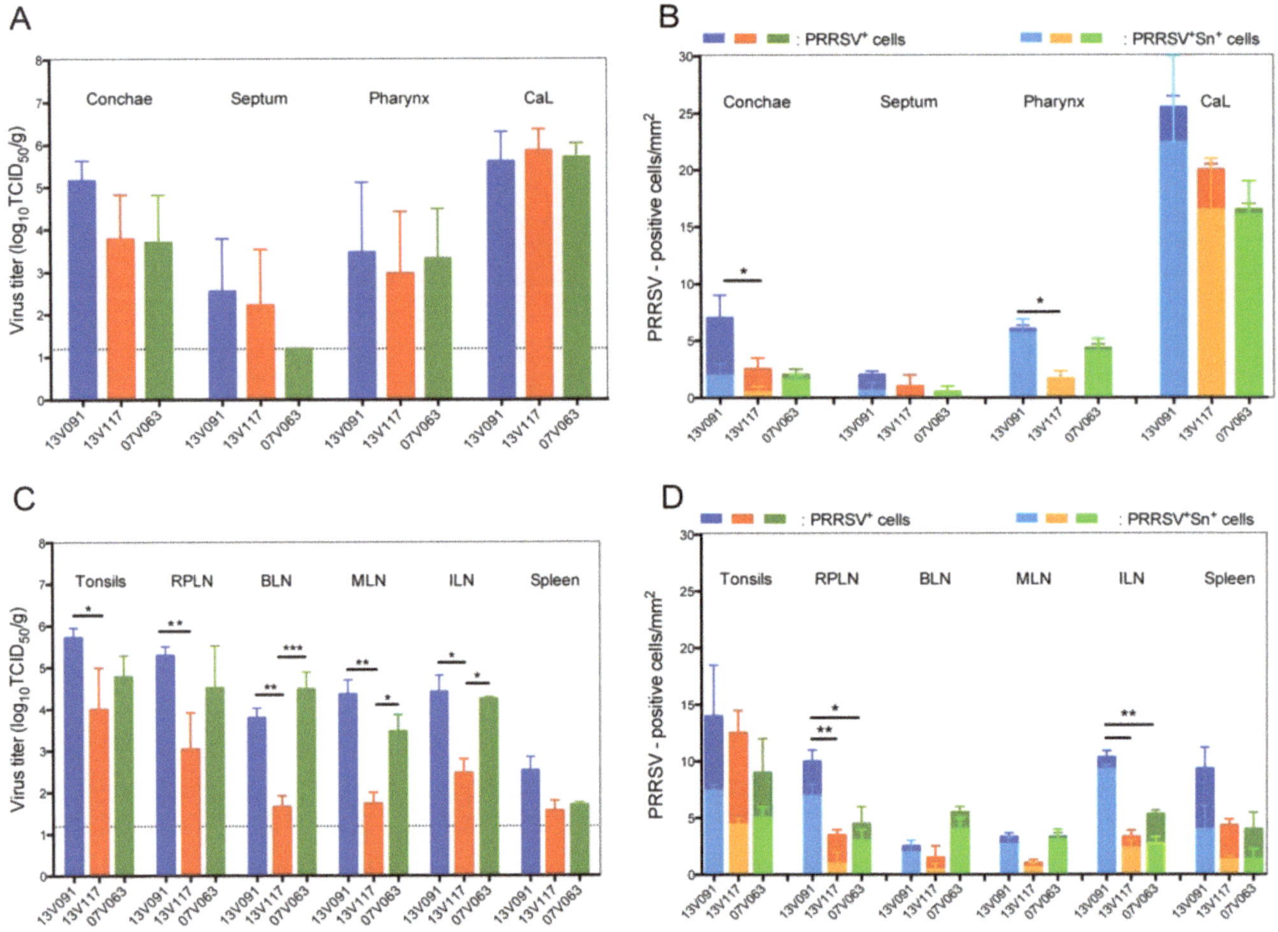

Figure 7 Virus titers (A and C), and quantification and identification of PRRSV-infected cells (B and D). Different parts of the respiratory system and lymphoid tissues from animals inoculated with PRRSV 13V091, 13V117 and 07V063, and euthanized at 10 dpi were analyzed. Dark colors represent PRRSV⁺ cells, whereas lighter colors in the subcolumns represent PRRSV⁺Sn⁺ cells. CaL denotes the cardiac left part of the lungs. Whiskers denote the standard deviation (SD) and asteriscs (*) represent statistically significant comparisons (*$P < 0.05$, **$P < 0.01$, ***$P < 0.001$).

13V091 group showed the highest titers (2.5 ± 0.6 log_{10} $TCID_{50}/g$) of the PRRSV-infected groups ($P > 0.05$).

Immunofluorescence

Respiratory tract

Double IF stainings were performed for the quantification and identification of PRRSV cells. In conchae, 13V091 showed higher amounts of PRRSV$^+$ cells/mm^2 (8.0 ± 1.4) compared to 13V117 (2.5 ± 0.7) and 07V063 (4.3 ± 0.7) (Figure 7B). Tissues from the septum displayed also a higher amount of PRRSV$^+$ cells/mm^2 in the 13V091 (2.2 ± 1.4) group, compared to the 13V117 (0.8 ± 0.9) and 07V063 (0.6 ± 0.3) groups. In the pharynx, a higher ($P < 0.05$) number of PRRSV$^+$ cells/mm^2 (6.0 ± 1.7) was found with 13V091 than with 13V117 (1.7 ± 1.2) but not from 07V063 (4.3 ± 1.2). Finally, immunofluorescence stainings from the left cardiac lobe of the lung showed higher amounts of PRRSV$^+$ cells/mm^2 for 13V091 (25.5 ± 9.1) compared to 13V117 (20.3 ± 5.4) and 07V063 (16.5 ± 2.3). The number of infectious virus particles per infected cell in the left cardiac lung lobe was calculated according to the ratio: pfu per gram of tissue/cells per mm^2 after converting $TCID_{50}/g$ to pfu/g [23]. 07V063 showed the highest number (21 200) of infectious virus particles per infected cell compared to 13V091 (15 300) and 13V117 (8600).

The Sn phenotype of PRRSV$^+$ cells in the nasal mucosa, tonsils and lungs is shown in Figure 8. Identification of PRRSV$^+$ cells in the nasal mucosa based on Sn, revealed that the 13V091 and 13V117 strains were able to replicate more efficiently in Sn$^-$ cells compared to the 07V063 strain. In conchae, 87.5% of 13V091-infected cells were Sn$^-$, while that percentage was 80.0% with the 13V117 and only 17% with the 07V063 strain (Figure 7B). In the septum, half (48%) of the 13V091-infected cells and the few 13V117-infected cells (0.8 ± 0.9/mm^2) were Sn$^-$, whereas all 07V063-infected cells were Sn$^+$. In the pharynx and lungs, all isolates showed

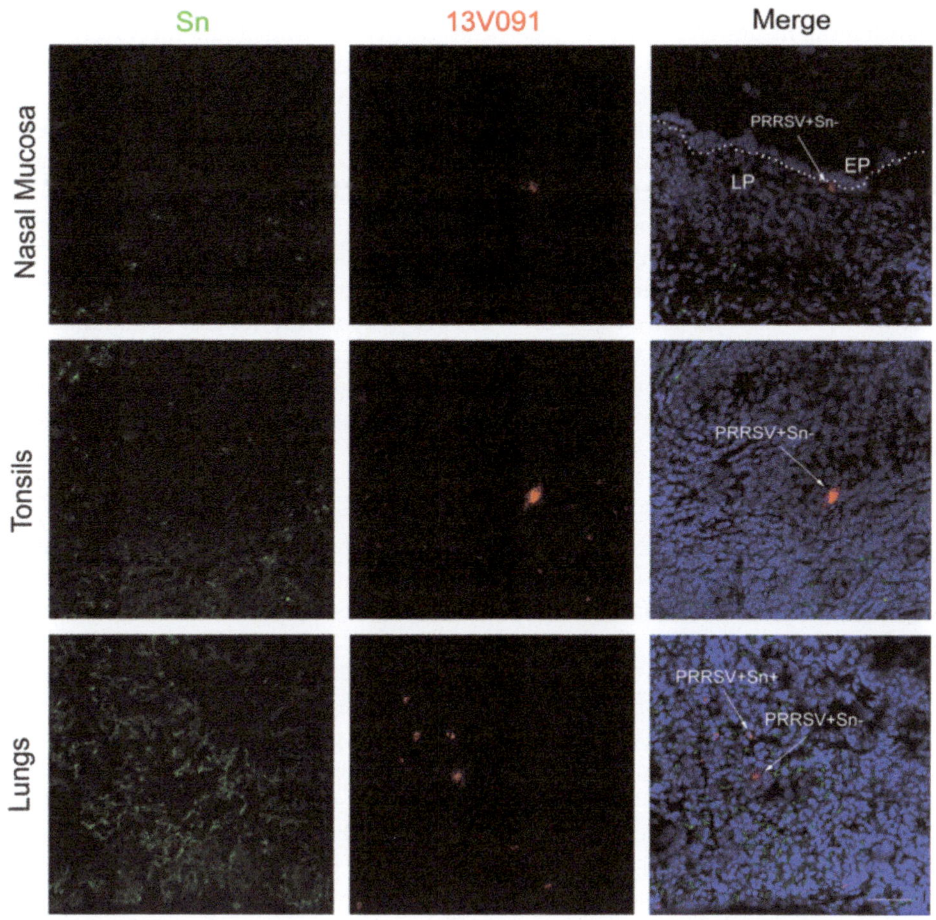

Figure 8 Confocal microscope double immunofluorescence images of 13V091-infected nasal mucosa, tonsils and lungs are illustrated. Tissue samples were sectioned (9 μm) and co-immunostained for Sn (green) and PRRSV N-protein (red) at 10 dpi. White arrows show PRRSV$^+$Sn$^+$ and PRRSV$^+$Sn$^-$ cells. Scale bar 50 μm.

a restricted cell tropism, as the percentage of PRRSV$^+$Sn$^+$ cells ranged from 80.7% to 100% (Figure 7B).

Lymphoid tissues

In tonsils, a higher amount of PRRSV$^+$ cells/mm^2 was found in 13V091-infected tissues (14.0 ± 5.6), compared to 13V117 (12.5 ± 2.1) and 07V063 (9.0 ± 5.7) -infected tissues (Figure 7D). In BLN, a higher amount of PRRSV$^+$ cells/mm^2 was observed in the 07V063 group (5.5 ± 2.2) than in the 13V091 (2.6 ± 0.8) and 13V117 (1.5 ± 0.7) groups, whereas in RPLN, 10.0 ± 2.8 (13V091), 2.5 ± 0.6 (13V117) and 4.5 ± 3.5 (07V063) PRRSV$^+$ cells/mm^2 were found. Finally, in MLN, infection with the 13V091 and 07V063 strains resulted in 3.4 ± 1.5 and 3.3 ± 2.3 PRRSV$^+$ cells/mm^2 respectively, while infection with the 13V117 strain gave only 1.1 ± 0.8 PRRSV$^+$ cells/mm^2. The amount of PRRSV$^+$ cells in ILN was higher ($P < 0.05$) with the 13V091 strain (10.3 ± 0.5) compared to the 13V117 (3.3 ± 2.1) and 07V063 (5.3 ± 0.6) strains. In spleen, the highest amount of PRRSV$^+$ cells/mm^2 was displayed by 13V091 (9.3 ± 6.7) while 13V117 showed 4.3 ± 3.5 and 07V063 4.0 ± 2.8 PRRSV$^+$ cells/mm^2.

The highest percentage of infected cells that were Sn$^-$, ranged from 45% to 64% in tonsils, 20% to 68% in the different lymph nodes and 64% to 71% in the spleen.

PRRSV genome sequencing and phylogenetic analysis

The full genomes of 13V091 and 13V117 were 15020 and 15014 nucleotides (nt) long (excluding the polyA tail), respectively. A NCBI BLASTn search showed that the two viruses belong to the PRRSV type 1 genotype. Pairwise nucleotide comparisons of the complete genomes showed that 13V117 shared 91.55% identity to Lelystad virus and 99.81% identity to 07V063, whereas 13V091 only shared 86.69% identity to the Lelystad virus and 85.03% to the 07V063 strain. The nucleotide (nt) similarity between 13V091 and 13V117 was 84.38%. 13V091, 13V117 and 07V063 showed deletions in ORF1a, in the region encoding the non-structural protein 2 (nsp2). 13V117 had a 84 nt deletion following the nucleotide position 2345 in

LV. 13V091 had three discontinuous deletions of 3, 45, and 27 nucleotides following the nt positions 1919, 2384, and 2492 in LV, respectively. The first deletion of 3 nt has also been found in five strains isolated in Asia (GenBank: FJ349261, KF287128-31). The deletions of 45 and 27 nucleotides were located in the highly variable region of nsp2 close to the deletion seen in 13V117. A partial amino acid alignment representing the highly variable region of nsp2 is shown in Additional file 3. The 13V091 strain, also harbored a 3 nt deletion in the region of the genome encoding the structural proteins. This deletion affected both ORF3 and ORF4 as the coding regions of these two genes overlap, but did not disturb the open reading frame [24].

Phylogenetic analysis of the complete genomes of the two viruses to 33 published PRRSV type 1 sequences showed that 13V091 grouped alone, and 13V117 grouped with 07V063 (Figure 9). Phylogenetic analysis of 171 complete PRRSV type 1 ORF5 sequences showed that 13V117 grouped with 07V063 and with viruses isolated in Denmark, China, Korea, and Spain, whereas 13V091 grouped with viruses isolated in Romania. The phylogenetic analysis of ORF5 is presented in Additional file 4. The phylogenetic tree of ORF7 was constructed from 154 sequences and showed 13V117 to group with 07V063 and viruses from Hong Kong, Korea, and Thailand. 13V091 grouped with an Italian isolated virus.

To investigate the impact of the high genetic diversity of 13V091 and 13V117, a pairwise amino acid comparison of the case viruses to three other type 1 viruses was performed and is shown in Additional file 5. From the comparison, it was clear that both 13V091 and 13V117 showed a high level of diversity on the protein level to the LV virus, the subtype 1 prototype and to Lena, the subtype 3 prototype virus. 13V091 was also different from 13V117 and 07V063, where the percentage identity for nsp2, GP3, GP4 and GP5 ranged from 77% to 88%. Finally, full-genome analysis revealed that 13V117 and 07V063 only differed by 8 amino acids located in nsp1, nsp2, nsp7 nsp9, GP3 and GP4, respectively.

Discussion

PRRSV is one of the most economically important pathogens in swine industry worldwide [2]. The virus continues to evolve genetically and antigenically despite the efforts for control and eradication [7]. Genetically, PRRSV strains are divided into European type 1 and North-American type 2 strains [8]. Type 1 strains are subdivided in four subtypes (1, 2, 3 and 4). In the recent past, highly pathogenic type 1 subtype 3 strains emerged in Eastern Europe but there was no indication of an invasion of these strains in Western Europe, a region that is dominated by type 1 subtype 1 isolates [4]. Up till now, no highly pathogenic type 1 subtype 1 strains have been isolated. Continuous monitoring of emerging PRRSV isolates is of great importance in order to prevent new outbreaks and provide novel insights for vaccine development. In the current study, the pathogenicity and the virulence of two new Belgian PRRSV isolates designated 13V091 and 13V117 originating from animals experiencing severe respiratory disorders were compared clinically, virologically and genetically with the mild-pathogenic PRRSV strain 07V063.

PRRSV 13V091 appeared to be more pathogenic than the 13V117 and 07V063 strains. Animals infected with 13V091 showed the longest duration of fever (5.1 ± 4.2) and the highest clinical scores (1.6 ± 0.3) due to dyspnea, tachypnea and respiratory distress. Macroscopic analysis of lungs of pigs euthanized at 10 dpi showed that 13V091 strain caused the most severe multifocal gross lesions compared to the 13V117 and 07V063 isolates. Percentage of lung lesions of 13V091 was also higher than that of the type 1 strains that were used in a recent study from Spain [25]. In another Korean study, three new subtype 1 strains were compared with the prototype LV, and it was found that at 10 dpi only one of them (SNUVR100744, GenBank: JX988618) showed a higher percentage (>25%) of affected lung surface than 13V091 (12.9 ± 3.6) [26]. The clinical and pathological outcome of 13V091 showed some similarities with the highly pathogenic subtype 3 strain (Lena, GenBank: JF802085) [12,14]. In the latter study, Lena showed clinical score values ranging from 0.5 to 2 from 3 to 14 dpi, whereas in our results 13V091 showed a clinical score from 0.6 to 1.6 during the same timeframe. Previous in vivo studies with the Lena strain, induced fever from 2 till 13 dpi [14], and from 2 till 28 dpi [12]. In the current study, 13V091 induced fever from 2 till 14 dpi.

The clinical outcome can be fully attributed to PRRSV and not to PRRSV-related pathogens (SIV, PCV2). Experiments were performed in BSL-2 facilities and pathogenic bacteria were not isolated from all the euthanized pigs. Furthermore, no Mycoplasma-related lung lesions were observed in all animals. Co-infections are important because they enhance the impact of PRRSV leading to porcine respiratory disease complex (PRDC) [27]. In a previous study with highly pathogenic PRRSV strains that showed mortality, bacteria like *Arcanobacterium pyogenes* and *Streptococcus suis* were isolated from the lungs [12].

Transmission of PRRSV via airborne route is an important characteristic after the appearance of highly pathogenic viral strains [28]. In a previous study, virus titers in nasal secretions of a highly pathogenic strain (Lena) showed a titer of 2.5 to 5.6 $\log_{10}TCID_{50}/100$ mg from 3 to 14 dpi [12]. In the current study, during the same timeframe, viral titers of 2.0 to 4.8 and 1.8 to 4.3 $\log_{10}TCID_{50}/100$ mg were detected for 13V091 and 13V117 respectively. These results indicate that both

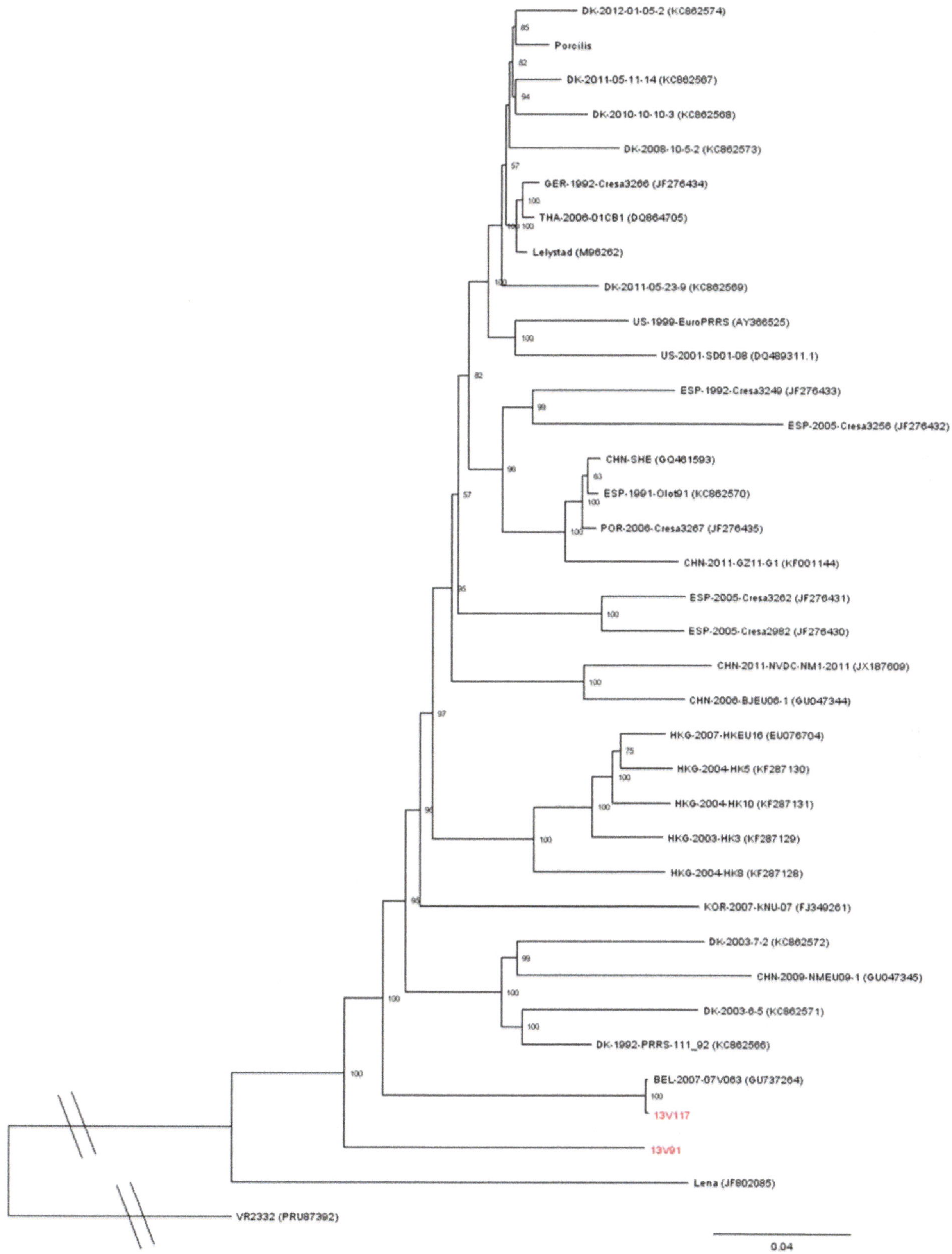

Figure 9 Phylogenetic analysis of complete genome nucleotide sequences of PRRSV type 1 is presented. The tree was constructed by the Neighbor Joining algorithm with Bootstrap 1000 replicates. Bootstrap values are shown in percent. 13V091 and 13V117 are highlighted in red.

new strains although not as pathogenic as Lena, have the potential to be transmitted via airborne route in the early stages of infection based on the high virus titers in the nasal secretions. It has been speculated, that recent outbreaks in the USA and China were due to virus isolates that can replicate and spread more efficiently [29]. The location of virus replication and an expanded cell tropism may strongly support this hypothesis. In typical swine herds, animals are in close nose-to-nose contact with each other, and during the last years several studies were performed evaluating the efficiency of different isolates to spread via airborne route [30]. A PRRSV strain that is able to replicate in the nasal mucosa and produce progeny virus, will be more likely to spread to another pig via airborne route compared to a virus strain that mainly replicates the lungs such as typical LV-like strains. In addition, presence of other nose pathogens such as *Bordetella bronchiseptica* and *Chlamydia suis* may cause intensive sneezing, which may facilitate virus spread [31].

In this study, different PRRSV strains showed a different tissue tropism. Animals infected with the 13V091 strain, showed the highest replication efficiency based on virus titration and PRRSV-positive cell counting. Furthermore, 13V091 showed significantly higher numbers of $PRRSV^+$ cells compared to 13V117 and 07V063 in the upper respiratory tract, tonsils and draining lymph nodes (conchae, septum, pharynx, RPLN). Respective virus titers of 13V091 were 10 to 1000 times higher than 13V117, and 10 times higher than 07V063. In the upper respiratory tract, 13V091 and 13V117 showed an expanded cell tropism as they were shown to replicate in Sn^- macrophages with a different degree of efficiency. It is important to mention that in the nasal mucosa (conchae, septum), the same distribution pattern of $PRRSV^+Sn^-$ cells was observed for 13V091 and 13V117, with cells being located within the epithelium, and just underneath the basement membrane. Large round cells with large cytoplasm was the morphology of $PRRSV^+Sn^-$ and $PRRSV^+Sn^+$ cells located in the lamina propria, whereas $PRRSV^+Sn^-$ cells located within the epithelium and just underneath the basement membrane were smaller with large elongated filopodia. Together with the disability of Lelystad virus to grow in Sn^- cells and the strong ability of a highly pathogenic PRRSV strain (Lena) to replicate extremely efficiently in Sn^- cells of the nasal mucosa, this indicates that in Western Europe there is an increase of PRRSV tropism for Sn^- nasal macrophages in time, which reaches the level of virulent/pathogenic subtype 3 strains [32].

In our study, 13V091 showed a higher replication rate and produced more progeny virus in the lungs compared to 13V117 and 07V063. Viral loads of type 1 subtype 1 strains of our study in lungs, are in agreement with the results of Labarque et al., where LV reached a mean titer of $10^{6.2}$ $TCID_{50}$/g in lung tissues at 9 dpi [10]. It was shown before, that PRRSV replication in the lungs is correlated with the number of the susceptible Sn^+ macrophages that are present at the time of infection and that only 2% of susceptible macrophages are infected [10]. In the present study, 13V117 and 07V063 showed a similar number of viral antigen positive cells and virus titers in the left cardiac lung lobe (13V117: 20.3 cells/mm^2 and $10^{5.4}$ $TCID_{50}$/g, 07V063: 16.5 cells/mm^2 and $10^{5.7}$ $TCID_{50}$/g). Analysis of the virus production per infected cell showed that 13V091 and 07V063 were able to produce more infectious virus particles per infected cell than 13V117 in a ratio of 1:2 and 1:2.4 respectively. Thus, not only the number of susceptible cells, but also the strain-dependent replication efficiency is important for PRRSV lung pathogenesis. Differences in replication level within distinct lung lobes were not observed with all the tested strains, which correlate with two other studies with the Lelystad (LV) virus, where no difference in replication levels of distinct lung lobes was observed at 10 dpi [10,18].

Virus replication in BLN and MLN showed that 13V091 and 07V063 produced similar amounts of virus, which were up to 1000 times higher than 13V117. High viral loads of 13V091 and 07V063 in the lungs and the draining lymph nodes (BLN, MLN) can be explained by the mobilization of Sn^+ cells from lungs to LN. In addition, strains with an expanded cell tropism like 13V091, may use the Sn^- monocytic cells that are infiltrating after 9 dpi to increase their transportation and replication efficiency in the correspondent tissues [10].

In the spleen, 13V091 showed the highest replication level compared to the other tested isolates and the virus production reached $10^{2.8}$ $TCID_{50}$/g at 10 dpi, which was similar to LV (10^3 $TCID_{50}$/g) at 8 dpi [33]. More than 60% of PRRSV-infected cells were of Sn^- phenotype. The lower replication level observed in spleen compared to lungs and lymph nodes might be explained by the low expression of Sn and presence of other receptor(s). In rats, it was shown that Sn expression on splenic macrophages is reduced 25-fold compared to lymph node macrophages mainly due to masking of Sn by endogenous ligands [34].

In our study, PRRSV-specific antibodies for all strains appeared at 7 dpi and reached a plateau at 14 dpi, which is in agreement with previous studies using other PRRSV strains [10,35]. The late induction and the low titers of neutralizing antibodies observed in the current study is in agreement with other studies that used the LV and the 07V063 strains, where only low titers of Nabs were observed after 25 dpi for LV ($2^{1-3.6}$), and after 35 dpi for 07V063 ($2^{1-2.2}$) [10,16]. A correlation between the appearance of neutralizing antibodies (Nabs) and the virus elimination from blood was mentioned before, but the exact degree of Nabs contribution in viral clearance is still questionable [35-37]. Only in the 07V063 group Nabs appeared at the same time with the elimination of viremia, an observation that was reported before for the 07V063 strain [16]. In 13V091 and 13V117, Nabs appeared later and at lower titers, and at that time the virus was already eliminated from blood. Based on these observations, it is obvious that neutralizing antibodies are not the sole immunological tool to eliminate PRRSV, and their role in clearance of primary viremia and prevention of reinfection is not clear [38]. The presence of additional glycosylation sites at the neutralizing epitopes, and the sensitivity of the SN test, might contribute for the late development of Nabs observed in 13V091 and 13V117 compared to 07V063. Analysis of glycosylation sites on PRRSV structural proteins based on Lelystad virus, revealed one additional glycosylation site for 13V091 into GP3 protein at the amino acid position 253 [39]. No additional or different glycosylation sites were observed within 13V117 and 07V063. Addition of newly acquired sugar moieties to the sugar tree of 13V117 may make the virus unrecognizable and mask the neutralizing epitopes that reduce or eliminate the binding affinity of the antibodies. This mechanism of immune evasion has been well described for HIV-1 [40]. MARC-145 cells and PRRSV strains adapted on this cell line are generally used in SN tests. This cell type is not the natural cell-target for PPRSV and does not express Sn, and CD163 is not present at detectable levels. Both Sn and CD163 are main factors for PRRSV entry and replicaton, and are major targets for viral entry mediators (GP5-M for Sn and GP2-GP3-GP4 for CD163) [41,42]. Therefore, primary target cells like alveolar macrophages or cell lines that express Sn and CD163 like $PK15^{Sn\text{-}CD163}$ cells should be preferably used for all the contemporary PRRSV strains that have a main tropism for PAM [43]. Newly emerging isolates with a tropism for additional receptors might need another SN test based on primary monocytic cells from nasal mucosa or lymph nodes that express the new receptors to search for neutralizing antibodies. New SN tests might help to better understand the function of virus Nabs, with regard to the degree of viral clearance.

To study the evolutionary relationship of 13V091 and 13V117 with other PRRSV strains, the complete genome sequence was compared with other type 1 European strains and the prototype type 2 strain VR-2332. 13V091 showed a high genetic diversity to all, currently, publicly available complete genomes of type 1 viruses and was located "alone" in the phylogenetic tree between 13V117 and 07V063, and the highly pathogenic subtype 3 strain Lena. The phylogenetic analysis of ORF5 and ORF7 showed that 13V091 and 13V117 grouped with other type 1 subtype 1 sequences, thus, it can be concluded that both isolates belong to PRRSV type 1 subtype 1.

By coincidence, 13V117 showed an extremely high genetic similarity to 07V063. Despite the fact that genome comparison revealed only eight different amino acids, the virological, clinical and pathological changes induced by these two viruses were quite different. 13V117 replicated efficiently in the nasal mucosa, induced a high viremia but had problems to replicate in lymphoid tissues. In addition, 13V117-infected animals showed breathing problems between 2 and 7 dpi. On the other hand, animals from the 07V063 group, showed a restricted replication in the nasal mucosa, a ten-fold lower viremia but an extensive replication in the lymphoid tissues. Only two pigs had mild breathing problems. Pairwise alignments revealed that the following eight amino acid differences were observed between 07V063 and 13V117: V140M in nsp1, H786L and G1300S in nsp2, S2192N in nsp7a, M72I and M266V in nsp9, N253H in GP3 and Q72P in GP4. Nsp1 is a cysteine protease that plays an important role in the cleavage of ORF1 proteins and for virion biogenesis [44]. Nsp2 is the papain-like proteinase 2 (PLP2) that is encoded from ORF1a and is responsible for the cleavage of the nsp2-3 junction [7]. It is the most variable non-structural protein between PRRSV subtypes, and it contains a hypervariable region (HVR) in which deletions are commonly found among PPRSV isolates; a cluster of immunodominant B- and T-cell epitopes was also identified [7]. Deletions in nsp2 have also been found for 13V091 and 13V117. Recent data support the hypothesis that these deletions are not necessarily related to virulence, but other studies support that changes in the nsp2 region might be related with plaque appearance and the cytolytic activity of the isolate [45,46]. Nsp7a is a 149 aa protein that plays an important role in the induction of host humoral immune response and has been found to induce specific antibodies as early as 14 dpi till 202 dpi [47]. Nsp9 is the RNA-dependent RNA polymerase (RdRp) encoded by ORF1b. It mediates the genome replication and the synthesis of subgenomic mRNAs, and is one of the most conserved proteins within nidoviruses [7]. GP3 is a heavily glycosylated membrane protein with a hydrophobic C-terminal domain [39]. The single amino-acid change in GP3 between 07V063 and 13V117 is located within the neutralizing antigenic region in the C-terminal domain, that has been found to be recognised by neutralizing antibodies against LV [39]. GP4 is a membrane protein with an N-glycosylated ectodomain that forms a heterotrimer with GP2 and GP3, and interacts with GP5 [42]. The single amino acid difference between 07V063 and 13V117 is located at the ectodomain of GP4 within the most immunogenic region that was identified, in all envelope proteins, but is also part of a neutralizing antibody region (NAR) named ES12 found to induce high virus neutralizing antibody titers at 42 dpi in all the 6 tested animals of the study [42,48]. In our results, only one animal in the 13V117 group showed low virus neutralizing antibody titers at 42 dpi, whereas at the same timepoint all animals in the 07V063 group developed virus neutralizing antibody titers (mean titer: $2^{2.16}$). Whether these single amino acid substitutions have an effect on virus pathogenesis and immune response by changing the glycan shielding, or the possible immune decoy epitopes remains to be clarified. A distinct PRRSV population was reported that emerged by one single amino acid change in the GP5 ectodomain after infection in pigs [49]. Furthermore, it was reported for lactate dehydrogenase virus (LDV) in mice that a small number of mutations in ORF5 can alter the tropism and the interaction of virus with neutralizing antibodies favoring viral persistence [50]. Viral persistence may also be favored by a single amino acid change in the C-terminus region of a viral protein if this modification, creates a novel motif selecting the retainment of virions to the endoplasmatic reticulum (ER) [49]. Production of viral infectious clones of the 07V063 and 13V117 isolates and site-directed mutations will shed new light in this field.

In summary: (1) two new PRRSV strains designated 13V091 and 13V117 were isolated from pigs showing respiratory distress. Pathogenic and genetic studies showed that 13V091 is the most pathogenic type 1 subtype 1 strain isolated up till now showing fever, breathing problems, high virus titers in nasal secretions, an increased percentage of lung lesions in young animals and an expanded cell tropism to Sn^- cells in nasal mucosa and other lymphoid tissues. (2) Despite the fact that 13V117 and 07V063 have only eight amino acid differences in their genomes, they showed contrasting clinical and virological outcomes. 13V117 was able to induce fever, high viremia, and respiratory problems at the early stages of infection and it was able to replicate in the nasal mucosa but not in the lymph nodes, whereas 07V063 showed only fever, a 10-fold lower viremia, low virus titers in nasal excretions, but higher virus titers in lymphoid tissues.

These are important findings in order to evaluate the virulence and the pathogenesis caused by different type 1 subtype 1 PRRSV strains, to control the respiratory disease caused by PRRSV in young animals, and to develop novel vaccines for the newly emerged PRRSV isolates.

Additional files

Additional file 1: List of clinical scoring. All the parameters were scored for each individual animal and a sum of total scoring was taken into account.

Additional file 2: Detailed clinical scoring and body temperature of all animals. Daily registration of clinical scores (CS) and body temperature (BT) for each individual animal of PRRSV-infected and control groups is shown.

Additional file 3: Partial amino acid alignment of the highly diverse region of nsp2 is presented. The numbering is counted from the first amino acid in the poly protein 1a (pp1a) encoded from ORF1a. Grey squares represent deletions.

Additional file 4: Phylogenetic analysis of ORF5. The tree was constructed by the Neighbor Joining algorithm with Bootstrap 1000 replicates. Bootstrap values above 69% are shown in percent. 13V091 and 13V117 are highlighted in red.

Additional file 5: Pairwise amino acid comparisons between different type 1 PRRSV strains. Each open reading frame was translated into amino acid sequences and compared.

Competing interests
The authors declare that they have no competing interests.

Authors' contributions
ISF performed the experiments, analyzed the data and wrote the manuscript. IT, CB, VR and YL helped in performing the experiments. LK performed the sequencing of viral strains. LL coordinated the work and helped in writing the manuscript. HJN designed the study, coordinated the work and helped in writing the manuscript. All authors read and approved the final manuscript.

Acknowledgements
The authors want to acknowledge Michel Loicq and Martin Fockedey for providing field material for the isolation of the new strains 13V091 and 13V117. Carine Boone, Chantal Vanmaercke and Zeger Vandenabeele are acknowledged for their excellent technical assistance. This work was funded by the European Union Seventh Framework Programme (FP7/2007-2013) under grant agreement n° 245141.

Author details
[1]Laboratory of Virology, Department of Virology, Immunology and Parasitology, Faculty of Veterinary Medicine, Ghent University, Salisburylaan 133, B-9820 Merelbeke, Ghent, Belgium. [2]National Veterinary Institute, Technical University of Denmark, Frederiksberg C, Denmark.

References
1. Nieuwenhuis N, Duinhof TF, van Nes A (2012) Economic analysis of outbreaks of porcine reproductive and respiratory syndrome virus in nine sow herds. Vet Rec 170:225
2. Holtkamp DJ, Kliebenstein JB, Neumann EJ, Zimmerman JJ, Rotto HF, Yoder TK, Wang C, Yeske PE, Mowrer CL, Haley CA (2013) Assessment of the economic impact of porcine reproductive and respiratory syndrome virus on United States pork produces. J Swine Health Prod 21:72–84
3. Yun SI, Lee YM (2013) Overview: Replication of porcine and respiratory syndrome virus (PRRSV). J Microbiol 51:711–723
4. Stadejek T, Stankevicius A, Murtaugh MP, Oleksiewicz MB (2013) Molecular evolution of PRRSV in Europe. Vet Microbiol 165:21–28
5. Terpstra C, Wensvoort G, Pol JM (1991) Experimental reproduction of porcine epidemic abortion and respiratory syndrome (mystery swine disease) by infection with Lelystad virus: Koch's postulates fulfilled. Vet Q 13:131–136
6. Mengeling WL, Lager KM, Vorwald AC (1994) Temporal characterization of transplacental infection of porcine fetuses with porcine reproductive and respiratory virus. Am J Vet Res 55:1391–1398
7. Snijder EJ, Kikkert M, Fang Y (2013) Arterivirus molecular biology and pathogenesis. J Gen Virol 94:2141–2163
8. Nelsen CJ, Murtaugh MP, Faaberg KS (1999) Porcine reproductive and respiratory syndrome virus comparison: divergent evolution on two continents. J Virol 73:270–280
9. Shi M, Lam TT, Hon CC, Hui RK, Faaberg KS, Wennblom T, Murtaugh MP, Stadejek T, Leung FC (2010) Molecular epidemiology of PRRSV: a phylogenetic persperctive. Virus Res 154:7–17
10. Labarque GG, Nauwynck HJ, Van Reeth K, Pensaert MB (2000) Effect of cellular changes and onset of humoral immunity on the replication of porcine reproductive and respiratory syndrome virus in the lungs of pigs. J Gen Virol 81:1327–1334

11. Zuckermann FA, Garcia EA, Luque ID, Christopher-Hennings J, Doster A, Brito M, Osorio F (2007) Assessment of the efficacy of commercial porcine reproductive and respiratory syndrome virus (PRRSV) vaccines based on measurement of serologic response, frequency of gamma-IFN-producing cells and virological parameters of protection upon challenge. Vet Microbiol 123:69–85
12. Karniychuk UU, Geldhof M, Vanhee M, Van Doorsselaere J, Saveleva TA, Nauwynck HJ (2010) Pathogenesis and antigenic characterization of a new East European subtype 3 porcine reproductive and respiratory syndrome virus isolate. BMC Vet Res 6:30
13. Tian K, Yu X, Zhao T, Feng Y, Cao Z, Wang C, Hu Y, Chen X, Hu D, Tian X, Liu D, Zhang S, Deng X, Ding Y, Yang L, Zhang Y, Xiao H, Qiao M, Wang B, Hou L, Wang X, Yang X, Kang L, Sun M, Jin P, Wang S, Kitamura Y, Yan J, Gao GF (2007) Emergence of fatal PRRSV variants: unparalleled outbreaks of atypical PRRS in China and molecular dissection of the unique hallmark. PLoS One 2:e526
14. Weesendorp E, Morgan S, Stockhofe-Zurwieden N, Popma-De Graaf DJ, Graham SP, Rebel MJ (2012) Comparative analysis of immune responses following experimental infection of pigs with European porcine reproductive and respiratory syndrome virus strains of different virulence. Vet Microbiol 59:20–32
15. Karniychuk UU, Saha D, Vanhee M, Geldhof M, Cornillie P, Caij AB, De Regge N, Nauwynck HJ (2012) Impact of a novel inactivated PRRS virus vaccine on virus replication and virus-induced pathology in fetal implantation sites and fetuses upon challenge. Theriodology 78:1527–1537
16. Geldhof MF, Vanhee M, Van Breedam W, Van Doorsselaere J, Karniychuk UU, Nauwynck HJ (2012) Comparison of the efficacy of autogenous inactivated porcine reproductive and respiratory syndrome virus (PRRSV) vaccines against homologous and heterologous challenges. BMC Biotechnol 8:182
17. Van Breedam W, Costers S, Vanhee M, Cagnon AC, Rodriguez-Gomez MI, Geldhof M, Verbeeck M, Van Doorsselaere J, Karniychuk U, Nauwynck HJ (2011) Porcine reproductive and respiratory syndrome virus (PRRSV)-specific mAbs: supporting diagnostics and providing new insights into the antigenic properties of the virus. Vet Immunol Immunopathol 141:246–257
18. Halbur PG, Paul PS, Frey ML, Landgraf J, Eernisse K, Meng XJ, Lum MA, Andrews JJ, Rathje JA (1995) Comparison of the pathogenicity of two US porcine reproductive and respiratory syndrome virus isolates with that of the Lelystad virus. Vet Pathol 32:648–660
19. Quinn P, Carter M, Markey B, Carter G (1994) Clinical Veterinary Microbiology. Mosby, Edinburgh, pp 254–259
20. Nauwynck HJ, Pensaert MB (1995) Effect of specific antibodies on the cell-associated spread of pseudorabies virus in monolayers of different cell types. Arch Virol 140:1137–1146
21. Wernike K, Bonilauri P, Dauber M, Errington J, Leblanc N, Revilla-Fernandez S, Hjulsager C, Isaksson M, Stadejek T, Beer M, Hoffmann B (2012) Porcine reproductive and respiratory syndrome virus: interlaboratory ring trial to evaluate real-time reverse transcription polymerase chain reaction detection methods. J Vet Diagn Invest 24:855–866
22. Kvisgaard LK, Hjulsager CK, Fahnoe U, Breum SO, Ait-Ali T, Larsen LE (2013) A fast and robust method for full genome sequencing of Porcine Reproductive and Respiratory Syndrome Virus (PRRSV) Type 1 and Type 2. J Virol Methods 193:697–705
23. Flint SJ, Enquist LW, Racaniello VR, Skalka AM (2008) Principles of Virology, vol 2. ASM press, Washington
24. Martinez-Lobo FJ, Diez-Fuertez F, Segales J, Garcia-Artiga C, Simarro I, Castro JM, Prieto C (2011) Comparative pathogenicity of type 1 and 2 isolates of porcine reproductive and respiratory syndrome virus (PRRSV) in a young pig infection model. Vet Microbiol 154:58–68
25. Han K, Seo HW, Park C, Oh Y, Kang I, Han HJ, Kim SH, Chae C (2013) Comparative pathogenicity of three Korean and on Lelystad Type 1 porcine reproductive and respiratory syndrome virus (Pan-European subtype 1) isolates in experimentally infected pigs. J Com Pathol 149:331–340
26. Choi YK, Goyal SM, Joo HS (2003) Retrospective analysis of etiologic agents associated with respiratory disease in pigs. Can Vet J 44:735–7
27. Otake S, Dee S, Corzo C, Oliveira S, Deen J (2010) Long-distance airborne transport of infectious PRRSV and Mycoplasma hyopneumoniae from a swine population infected with multiple viral variants. Vet Microbiol 145:198–208
28. Murtaugh MP, Stadejek T, Abrahante JE, Lam TY, Leung CC (2010) The ever expanding diversity of porcine reproductive and respiratory syndrome virus. Virus Res 154:18–30
29. Cutler TD, Wang C, Hoff SJ, Kittawornrat A, Zimmerman JJ (2011) Median infectious dose (ID_{50}) of porcine reproductive and respiratory syndrome virus isolate MN-184 via aerosol exposure. Vet Microbiol 151:229–237
30. Thanawongnuwech R, Thacker EL (2003) Interleukin-10, interleukin-12, and interferon-gamma levels in the respiratory tract following Mycoplasma hyopneumoniae and PRRSV infection in pigs. Viral Immunol 16:357–367
31. Frydas IS, Verbeeck M, Cao J, Nauwynck HJ (2013) Replication characteristics of porcine reproductive and respiratory syndrome virus (PRRSV) European subtype 1 (Lelystad) and subtype 3 (Lena) strains in nasal mucosa and cells of the monocytic lineage: indications for the use of new receptors of PRRSV (Lena). Vet Res 44:73
32. Pol JM, van Dijk JE, Wensvoort G, Terpstra C (1991) Pathological, ultrastructural and immunohistochemical changes caused by Lelystad virus in experimentally induced infections of mystery swine disease (synomym: Porcine epidemic abortion and respiratory syndrome (PEARS)). Vet Q 13:137–143
33. Nakamura K, Yamaji T, Crocker PR, Suzuki A, Hashimoto Y (2002) Lymph node macrophages, but not spleen macorphages, express high levels of unmasked sialoadhesin: implication for the adhesive properties of macrophages in vivo. Glycobiology 12:209–216
34. Xiao Z, Batista L, Dee S, Halbur P, Murtaugh MP (2004) The level of virus-specific T-cell and macrophage recruitment in porcine reproductive and respiratory syndrome virus infection in pigs is independent of virus load. J Virol 78:5923–5933
35. Díaz I, Darwich L, Pappaterra G, Pujols J, Mateu E (2005) Immune responses of pigs after experimental infection with a European strain of Porcine reproductive and respiratory syndrome virus. J Gen Virol 86:1943–1951
36. Mateu E, Diaz I (2008) The challenge of PRRS immunology. Vet J 177:345–351
37. Van Gorp H, Van Breedam W, Van Doorsselaere J, Delputte PL, Nauwynck HJ (2010) Identification of the CD163 protein domains involved in infection of the porcine reproductive and respiratory syndrome virus. J Virol 84:3101–3105
38. Vanhee M, Van Breedam W, Costers S, Geldhof M, Noppe Y, Nauwynck HJ (2011) Characterization of antigenic regions in the porcine reproductive and respiratory syndrome virus by the use of peptide-specific serum antibodies. Vaccine 29:4794–4804
39. Kwong P, Doyle M, Casper D, Cicala C, Leavitt SA, Majeed S, Steenbeke TD, Venturi M, Chaiken I, Fung M, Katinger H, Parren PW, Robinson J, Van Ryk D, Wang L, Burton DR, Freire E, Wyatt R, Sodroski J, Hendrickson WA, Arthos J (2002) HIV-1 evades antibody-mediated neutralization through conformational masking of receptor-binding sites. Nature 420:678–682
40. Van Breedam W, Van Gorp H, Zhang JQ, Crocker PR, Delputte PL, Nauwynck HJ (2010) The M/GP(5) glycoprotein complex of porcine reproductive and respiratory virus binds the sialoadhesine receptor in a sialic acid-dependent manner. PLoS Pathog 6:e1000730
41. Das PB, Dinh PX, Ansari IH, de Lima M, Osorio FA, Pattnaik AK (2010) The minor envelope glycoproteins GP2a and GP4 of porcine reproductive and respiratory syndrome virus interact with the receptor CD163. J Virol 84:1731–1740
42. Delrue I, Van Gorp H, Van Doorsselaere J, Delputte PL, Nauwynck HJ (2010) Susceptible cell lines for the production of porcine reproductive and respiratory syndrome virus by stable transfection of sialoadhesin and CD163. BMC Biotechnol 10:48
43. Nedialkova DD, Ulferts R, Born E, Lauber C, Gorbalenya AE, Ziebuhr J, Snijder EJ (2009) Biochemical characterization of arterivirus nonstructural protein 11 reveals the nidovirus-wide conservation of a replicative endoribonuclease. J Virol 83:5671–5682
44. Zhou L, Zhang J, Zeng J, Yin S, Li Y, Zheng L, Guo X, Ge X, Yang H (2009) The 30-amino-acid deletion in the Nsp2 of highly pathogenic porcine reproductive and respiratory syndrome virus emerging in China is not related to its virulence. J Virol 83:5156–5167
45. Brockmeier SL, Loving CL, Vorwald AC, Kehrli ME, Baker RB, Nicholson TL, Lager KM, Miller LC, Faaberg KS (2012) Genomic sequence and virulence comparison of four Type 2 porcine reproductive and respiratory syndrome virus strains. Virus Res 169:212–221
46. Brown E, Lawson S, Welbon C, Gnanandarajah J, Li J, Murtaugh MP, Nelson EA, Molina RM, Zimmerman JJ, Rowland RR, Fang Y (2009) Antibody response to porcine reproductive and respiratory syndrome virus (PRRSV) nonstructural proteins and implications for diagnostic detection and differentiation of PRRSV types I and II. Clin Vaccine Immunol 16:628–635

47. Oleksiewicz MB, Bøtner A, Toft P, Normann P, Storgaard T (2001) Epitope mapping porcine reproductive and respiratory syndrome virus by phage display: the nsp2 fragment of the replicase polyprotein contains a cluster of B-cell epitopes. J Virol 75:3277–3290
48. Rowland RR, Steffen M, Ackerman T, Benfield DA (1999) The evolution of porcine reproductive and respiratory syndrome virus: quasispecies and emergence of a virus subpopulation during infection of pigs with VR-2332. Virology 259:262–266
49. Chen Z, Rowland RR, Anderson GW, Palmer GA, Plagemann PG (1997) Coexistence in lactate dehydrogenase-elevating virus pools of variants that differ in neuropathogenicity and ability to establish a persistent infection. J Virol 71:2913–2920
50. Kvisgaard LK, Hjulsager CK, Kristensen CS, Lauritsen KT, Larsen LE (2013) Genetic and antigenic characterization of complete genomes of Type 1 Porcine Reproductive and Respiratory Syndrome Virus (PRRSV) isolated in Denmark over a period of 10 years. Virus Res 178:197–205

6

Genetic subgroup of small ruminant lentiviruses that infects sheep homozygous for *TMEM154* frameshift deletion mutation A4$^{\Delta}$53

Michael L Clawson[1*], Reid Redden[2], Gennie Schuller[1], Michael P Heaton[1], Aspen Workman[1], Carol G Chitko-McKown[1], Timothy PL Smith[1] and Kreg A Leymaster[1]

Abstract

Small ruminant lentivirus (SRLV) infections of sheep are influenced by genetics on both the host and pathogen sides. Genetic variation in the ovine transmembrane 154 (*TMEM154*) gene associates with infection susceptibility, and distinct SRLV genetic subgroups infect sheep in association with their *TMEM154* diplotypes. In this study, a novel SRLV subgroup was identified that naturally infected sheep with various *TMEM154* diplotypes, including those homozygous for a rare frameshift mutation (A4 delta53), which is predicted to abolish TMEM154 protein function. Thus, these SRLVs may infect sheep that lack functional TMEM154, and may not be restricted by *TMEM154* diplotypes in establishing infections.

Introduction, methods and results

Small ruminant lentiviruses (SRLVs) are genetically diverse retroviruses that infect monocytes, macrophages, dendritic cells, and microglial cells of domestic sheep, goats, and wild ruminants [1-4]. Infections persist for the lifetime of the host, causing chronic inflammation and a slow progression to disease [5,6]. Common symptoms of SRLV infection in sheep include interstitial pneumonia with dyspnea, indurative mastitis, and cachexia [7]. There are no available preventative vaccines or cures for SRLVs, and the disease affects sheep and goats in the U.S. and around much of the world [8-11].

In sheep, there is a strong genetic component to the relative risk of SRLV infection on both the host and pathogen sides [12,13]. On the host side, genetic variation in the ovine transmembrane 154 (*TMEM154*) gene associates with SRLV infection susceptibility [12,14]. The biological function of TMEM154 is unknown; however, it is predicted to be a type I membrane protein based on its amino acid sequence. Twelve non-synonymous SNPs have been detected in regions of *TMEM154* that encode predicted leader or extracellular domains of the protein, giving rise to 12 haplotypes that each encode different isoforms (Table 1) [12]. Haplotypes 1, 2, and 3 are the most common haplotypes found in sheep, and all three have an effect on SRLV susceptibility. Sheep with a copy of either haplotype 2 or 3, both of which encode a glutamate amino acid residue at position 35 (E35) of the extracellular portion of TMEM154, have an increased risk of SRLV infection. Conversely, sheep homozygous for haplotype 1, which encodes a lysine residue at position 35 (K35), have a decreased risk of infection (Table 1) [12,15].

On the pathogen side, two SRLV subgroups defined by genetic variation within segments of proviral *gag* and *env* genes, associate with alleles of the ovine *TMEM154* E35K polymorphism [13]. SRLV subgroup 1 associates with homozygous and hemizygous *TMEM154* K35 genotypes with the K allele encoded by haplotype 1, and subgroup 2 associates with hemi-and homozygous *TMEM154* E35 genotypes with the E allele encoded by haplotypes 2 or 3 (Table 1) [13]. Thus, some SRLVs have adapted to infect sheep with distinct *TMEM154* E35K genotypes and can influence *TMEM154* E35K susceptibility to infection.

The biology responsible for *TMEM154* E35K associations with SRLV infection susceptibility, and SRLV subgroup associations with *TMEM154* E35K genotypes is unknown. While a portion of TMEM154 is predicted to

* Correspondence: mike.clawson@ars.usda.gov
[1]United States Department of Agriculture (USDA) Agricultural Research Service (ARS), U.S. Meat Animal Research Center (USMARC), State Spur 18D, Clay Center, NE 68933, USA
Full list of author information is available at the end of the article

Table 1 Ovine *TMEM154* haplotypes and their associations with infection susceptibility and SRLV subgroups

Haplotype	Amino acid at position indicated												Allelic effect[b]	SRLV association
	4[a]	13	14	25	31	33	35	44	70	74	82	102		
1	R	A	L	T	E	D	K	T	N	I	E	I	Less-susceptible	Subgroup 1
2	R	A	L	T	E	D	E	T	I	I	E	I	Highly-susceptible	Subgroup 2
3	R	A	L	T	E	D	E	T	N	I	E	I	Highly-susceptible	Subgroup 2
4	A	P[c]	F[c]	P[c]	R[c]	T[c]	N[c]	W[c]	NA[d]	NA	NA	NA	Unknown	Unknown, can be infected by Subgroup 4 (this study)
6	R	A	L	T	E	D	E	T	N	I	Y	NA	Unknown	Unknown
9	R	A	L	T	E	N	E	T	N	I	E	I	Unknown	Unknown
10	R	A	H	T	E	D	K	T	N	I	E	I	Unknown	Unknown
11	R	A	L	I	E	D	E	T	N	I	E	I	Unknown	Unknown
12[e]	R	A	L	T	E	D	E	T	N	F	E	I	Unknown	Unknown
13	R	V	L	T	E	N	E	T	N	I	E	I	Unknown	Unknown
14	R	A	L	T	E	D	E	T	N	I	E	T	Unknown	Unknown
15[e]	R	A	L	T	Q	D	E	T	N	F	E	I	Unknown	Unknown

[a]Numbers refer to amino acid positions in [GenBank:HM355886].
[b]Does not account for SRLV subgroups.
[c]Result of frameshift mutation at amino acid position 4.
[d]Not applicable due to preceding premature stop codon.
[e]Haplotype observed in wild sheep.

extend from the host cell into the external milieu, it is not known if TMEM154 serves as a receptor, or co-receptor for SRLV attachment to the host cell, affects viral processing within the cell, or exit from it, or has a different biological function regarding SRLV infection. It is also not known if genetic variation in proviral *gag* and/or *env* directly causes SRLV subgroups to associate with *TMEM154* E35K genotypes, or is in linkage disequilibrium with causal alleles elsewhere in the SRLV genome. However, given that SRLV subgroups and *TMEM154* E35K genotypes associate with each other through apparent coevolution, TMEM154 is implicated as having a critical role in SRLV infections, leading us to hypothesize that sheep lacking functional TMEM154 may be completely resistant to SRLV infection.

TMEM154 A4Δ53 is a frameshift mutation that is predicted to abolish protein function [12]. With leader peptide, the ovine TMEM154 precursor protein encoded by haplotypes 1, 2, and 3 is 191 amino acids, and yields a mature protein of 161 amino acids once the predicted leader peptide has been removed [12]. *TMEM154 A4Δ53* is part of haplotype 4, and encodes a single nucleotide deletion at amino acid position four of the precursor protein which results in an extensive change of amino acid coding at and downstream of amino acid four, and the first of multiple premature stop codons starting at amino acid position 54 (Table 1). Consequently, a truncated 53 amino acid protein with little homology to other TMEM154 isoforms results from the mutation, and sheep that are homozygous for *TMEM154 A4Δ53* constitute natural TMEM154 "knockouts". Although generally rare, the *TMEM154 A4Δ53* allele has been found in multiple sheep breeds in the U.S., and in sheep from Turkey, Iran, Spain, France, and India [12,16]. Thus, sheep homozygous for *TMEM154 A4Δ53* are distributed throughout multiple geographical regions that may have their own distinct SRLV populations.

As part of a research surveillance program, a flock of approximately 250 sheep at North Dakota State University was sampled for SRLV infection and *TMEM154* diplotypes. The flock was comprised of multiple breeds including Columbia, Dorset, Hampshire, and Katahdin. Members of the flock were approved for research use by the animal care and use committee of the North Central Region-Sustainable Agriculture Research and Education program (Project Number FNC13-929). *TMEM154* diplotypes were scored using a commercially run matrix-assisted laser desorption/ionization-time-of-flight mass spectrometry (MALDI-TOF MS) assay (GeneSeek, Lincoln, NE, USA) [16], and SRLV infection status was determined serologically using a commercially run competitive enzyme linked immunosorbent assay (cELISA), (GeneSeek [17]). Over 50% of the flock was infected, including a Hampshire ewe and a Katahdin ewe that were both *TMEM154* "4,4" diplotypes, and thus homozygous for *TMEM154 A4Δ53* (Table 2).

The MALDI-TOF MS genotyping results for both of the *TMEM154* "4,4" ewes, were confirmed with Sanger sequencing of *TMEM154* DNA and cDNA amplified from their blood. The sequencing was conducted on PCR-generated amplicons of *TMEM154* exons 1 and 2, and *TMEM154* cDNA that was RT-PCR amplified with

Table 2 SRLV-infected sheep sampled for proviral *gag* sequence

Animal ID	Breed	Age	*TMEM154* diplotype	SRLV *gag* GenBank #
6004	Dorset	7	1,1	KP120553
7006	Dorset	6	1,1	KP120547
7056	Columbia	6	1,1	KP120545
8344	Columbia	5	1,1	KP120540
9032	Columbia	4	1,1	KP120543
261	Dorset	3	1,2	KP120554
6012	Dorset	7	1,2	KP120549
7028	Dorset	6	1,2	KP120539
9451	Dorset	4	1,2	KP120541
256	Hampshire	3	1,4	KP120542
6542	Hampshire	7	1,4	KP120544
7434	Hampshire	6	1,4	KP120546
8539	Katahdin	5	1,4	KP120555
9322	Hampshire	4	1,4	KP120548
15	Hampshire	3	2,4	KP120552
1150	Hampshire	2	4,4	KP120550
8540	Katahdin	5	4,4	KP120551

previously described reagents and conditions [12,16]. The sequences were produced with an ABI 3730 capillary sequencer (PE Applied Biosystems, Foster City, CA, USA) and assembled into complete contigs with Phred and Phrap [18,19], Polyphred (version 6.10), and Consed software [20], and visually genotyped. By DNA and cDNA sequence, both ewes were homozygous for *TMEM154 A4Δ53* and had *TMEM154* "4,4" diplotypes [GenBank: KP142216 - KP142219]. Thus, the *TMEM154* DNA and corresponding mRNA sequences were identical, with no evidence of alternate splicing of *TMEM154* at the transcript sequence level.

To verify the infection status of the two seropositive ewes with *TMEM154* "4,4" diplotypes, and to characterize the SRLVs they were infected by, nested PCR for SRLV proviral *gag* was conducted on blood DNAs isolated from the two animals (Table 2). Additionally, the PCR was conducted on blood DNAs from 15 seropositive ewes of the same flock with other *TMEM154* diplotypes, to determine if similar SRLVs had infected sheep with or without *TMEM154* "4,4" diplotypes (Table 2). Previously described reagents, conditions, and methods were used for the PCR [13]. The amplicons were Sanger sequenced and assembled with Phred, Phrap, Polyphred (version 6.10), and Consed software [18-20]. All 17 seropositive ewes were confirmed positive for SRLV infection by proviral *gag* amplification and sequence.

In addition to the recent classification of SRLV subgroups 1 and 2 that associate with sheep *TMEM154* E35K genotypes, SRLVs from around the world have been typed into major genotype groups A-E, and into subtypes within the genotype groups based on *gag* and/or *pol* variation [13,21-23]. To characterize the SRLVs infecting the North Dakota sheep, their *gag* sequences were compared to 1) those of SRLVs from North America and elsewhere in the world, and 2) the top ten closest blast matches to the *gag* sequence from one of the infected *TMEM154* "4,4" ewes in a Neighbor-Net phylogenetic network (Figure 1) and a Neighbor-Joining tree (Figure 2), (see Additional file 1 for sequence information). The network was constructed as SRLVs can have recombinant genomes [24,25], including those that comprise subgroups 1 and 2 [13], and the network accounted for recombinant sequences. The

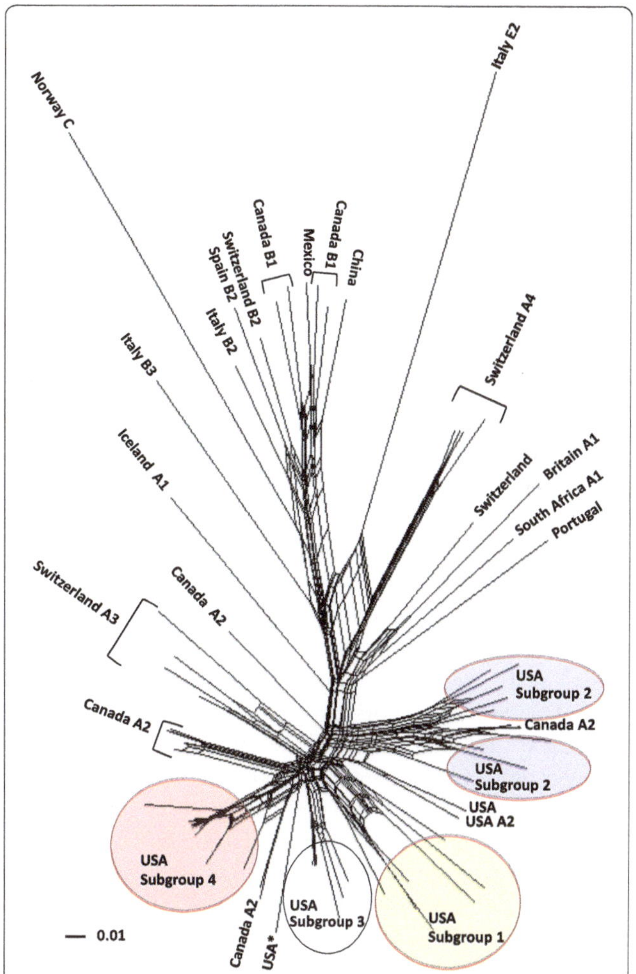

Figure 1 Neighbor-Joining network of SRLV partial *gag* sequences. The sequences were either produced in this study or were available from GenBank, and with amplification primer sites excluded correspond to nucleotide positions 1290–1771 of reference sequence [GenBank: NC_001452]. Capital letters and numbers following the country of origin represent genotypes and subtypes, respectively. The asterisk represents the one sequence [GenBank:KP120539] that originated from a ewe of the North Dakota State University flock that did not cluster within USA subgroup 4. The scale bar represents substitutions per site.

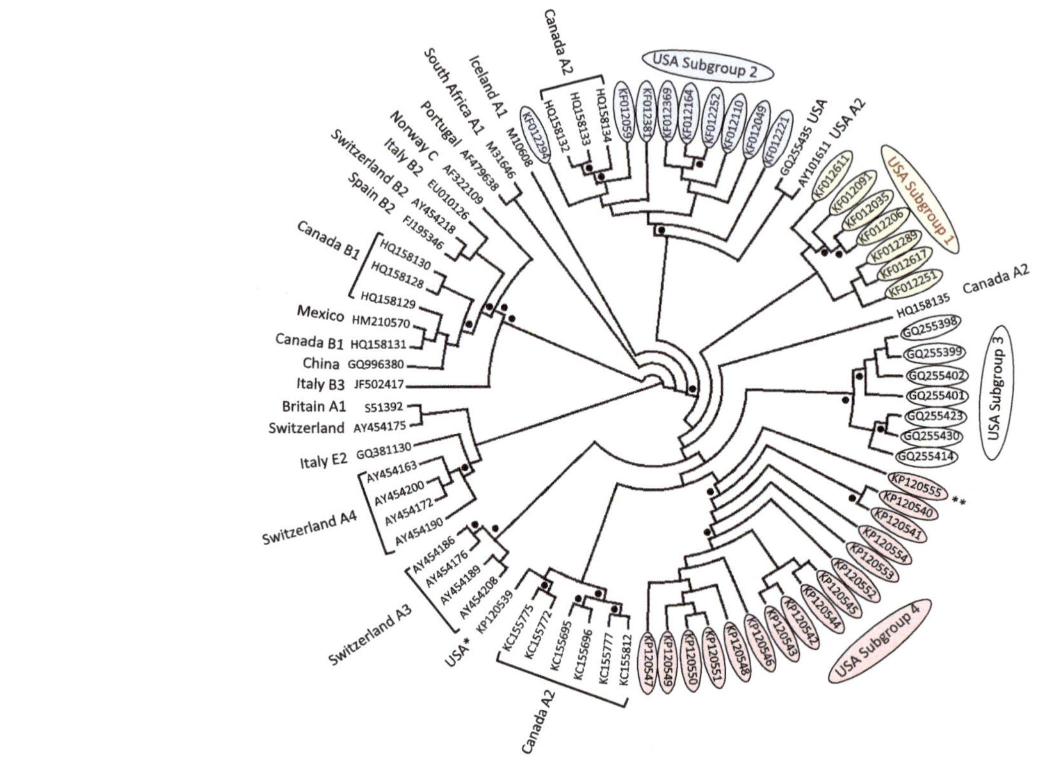

Figure 2 Bootstrapped Neighbor-Joining tree of SRLV partial *gag* sequences. The tree was produced from the same alignment used to produce the network in Figure 1. Like Figure 1, capital letters and numbers following the country of origin represent genotypes and subtypes, respectively. Outer taxonomic numbers represent GenBank accession numbers. Black dots represent bootstrap values greater than 80%. The single asterisk represents the one sequence that originated from an ewe of the North Dakota State University flock that did not cluster within USA subgroup 4. The double asterisk represents one sequence that clusters with subgroup 4 sequences but is not supported within the clade with a bootstrap equal to or greater than 80%. USA subgroups 1 and 2 both contain recombinant sequences that impact bootstrap support [13]. The tree is drawn as a circular cladogram and does not have a scale bar.

Neighbor-Joining tree was constructed to evaluate clade support with bootstraps, although Neighbor-Joining trees do not account for recombinant sequences. The network was constructed in SplitsTree (version 4.12.3) [26]. The tree was constructed in PHYLIP [27] using the programs Seqboot, Dnadist, Neighbor, and Consense, and viewed in Dendroscope [28]. Both the network and the tree were produced from a *gag* alignment generated with ClustalW in MacVector (version 12.0.6), with an F84 model of substitution and a transition/transversion ratio of two. The tree was bootstrapped with 1000 pseudoalignments. Sequence representatives of SRLV subgroups 1 and 2 were included in the analyses, as were those of what we describe as subgroup 3, which infected a flock of sheep in the Western United States [29], and has not been tested for an association with *TMEM154* genotypes.

Of the North Dakota proviral *gag* sequences, 16 of 17 sequences clustered together in both the Neighbor-Net phylogenetic network and the Neighbor-Joining tree, indicating that a distinct SRLV subgroup infected members of the flock (USA Subgroup 4, Figures 1 and 2). Additionally, within the Neighbor-Joining tree, 15 of 16 sequences within the clade were supported by a bootstrap value greater than 80%, delineating a clear genetic distinction of these strains from all others in the tree as a subgroup (USA Subgroup 4, Figure 2). The *gag* sequences from both of the infected *TMEM154* "4,4" diplotype ewes placed in this subgroup, as did the sequences from ewes with *TMEM154* "1,1", "1,2", "1,4", and "2,4" diplotypes (Figure 2, Table 2). This demonstrates that SRLVs of subgroup 4 are not restricted to infecting only sheep with *TMEM154* "4,4" diplotypes. Both the network and the tree show that USA subgroups 1, 2, 3, and 4 either contain or are flanked by genotype A, subtype A2 sequences. Additionally, the Neighbor-Joining tree has two bootstrap values greater than 80% that collectively support the clustering of all four USA subgroups with A2 sequences, with subtype A3 sequences from Switzerland comprising a related but separate clade (Figure 2). This indicates that all four USA subgroups are members of the A2 subtype.

The one SRLV *gag* sequence from a member of the North Dakota flock that was distinct from subgroup 4 originated from an ewe with a *TMEM154* 1,2 diplotype that was born in 2007, most likely in South Dakota. This ewe was introduced into the North Dakota flock in 2009. It is possible that she was infected with an SRLV prior to her introduction to the North Dakota flock.

Discussion

Subgroup 4 SRLVs can infect sheep with *TMEM154* "4,4" diplotypes that are homozygous for the *TMEM154 A4Δ53* mutation, as well as sheep that do not have haplotype 4. This indicates that subgroup 4 SRLVs do not require functional TMEM154 to infect sheep, and may be able to infect sheep with any *TMEM154* diplotype. The mechanism(s) or host receptors that subgroup 4 SRLVs use to infect sheep in the absence of functional TMEM154 are unknown. Additionally, whether or not other SRLV subgroups infect cells in the same manner as subgroup 4 members at low frequency is also unknown. Additional barriers to infection that are independent of the *TMEM154* locus may be required to prevent infection of sheep by subgroup 4 SRLVs.

All four SRLV subgroups that have been identified in the U.S. place within the A2 subtype. SRLV genotype A is highly diverse with 15 subtypes currently known [23]. To better understand the context of ovine *TMEM154* allele associations with SRLV infection susceptibility, it would be interesting to know if SRLV members of other A subtypes, genotypes B-E, and any circulating recombinant forms vary by an association with *TMEM154* alleles, including an ability to infect sheep with TMEM154 "4,4" diplotypes. Additionally, it would be beneficial to obtain full-length genomic sequences from members of the SRLV subgroups to identify viral alleles that are biologically responsible for *TMEM154* associations, potential interactions, or lack thereof. Ultimately, knowledge at this level could lead to precision control of ovine SRLV infection through genetic management of both the host and the pathogen.

Additional file

Additional file 1: *gag* sequences used for phylogenetic trees of Figures 1 and 2. Table containing the following information for the *gag* sequences used to construct the phylogenetic trees of Figures 1 and 2; GenBank accession number, genetic subgroup affiliation, phylotype, production in this study, country of origin.

Competing interests

The authors declare that they have no competing interests.

Authors' contributions

Conceived and designed the experiments; MLC, RR, GS, MPH, AW, GPH, CGCM, TPLS, KAL. Performed the experiments; GS. Contributed reagents/materials/analysis tools; MLC, RR, GS, MPH, KAL. Analyzed the results; MLC, RR, GS, MPH, AW, GPH, CGCM, TPLS, Wrote the manuscript; MLC. Revised the manuscript with critical intellectual content; MLC, RR, GPS, MPH, AW, GPH, CGCM, TPLS, KAL. All authors read and approved the final manuscript.

Acknowledgments

This work was supported by the Agricultural Research Service and by funding from the North Central Region–Sustainable Agricultural Research and Education program. We thank Jan Watts for secretarial support. The use of product and company names is necessary to accurately report the methods and results; however, the United States Department of Agriculture (USDA) neither guarantees nor warrants the standard of the products, and the use of names by the USDA implies no approval of the product to the exclusion of others that may also be suitable. The USDA is an equal opportunity provider and employer.

Author details

[1]United States Department of Agriculture (USDA) Agricultural Research Service (ARS), U.S. Meat Animal Research Center (USMARC), State Spur 18D, Clay Center, NE 68933, USA. [2]Department of Animal Sciences, North Dakota State University, Fargo, ND 58108-6050, USA.

References

1. Leroux C, Cruz J, Mornex J-F (2010) SRLVs: A genetic continuum of lentiviral species in sheep and goats with cumulative evidence of cross species transmission. Curr HIV Res 8:94–100
2. Patton KM, Bildfell RJ, Anderson ML, Cebra CK, Valentine BA (2012) Fatal *Caprine arthritis encephalitis virus*-like infection in 4 rocky mountain goats (*Oreamnos americanus*). J Vet Diagn Invest 24:392–396
3. Erhouma E, Guiguen F, Chebloune Y, Gauthier D, Lakhal LM, Greenland T, Mornex JF, Leroux C, Alogninouwa T (2008) Small ruminant lentivirus proviral sequences from wild ibexes in contact with domestic goats. J Gen Virol 89:1478–1484
4. Ryan S, Tiley L, McConnell I, Blacklaws B (2000) Infection of dendritic cells by the Maedi-Visna lentivirus. J Virol 74:10096–10103
5. Pépin M, Vitu C, Russo P, Mornex J-F, Peterhans E (1998) Maedi-visna virus infection in sheep: a review. Vet Res 29:341–367
6. Blacklaws BA, Harkiss GD (2010) Small ruminant lentiviruses and human immunodeficiency virus: cousins that take a long view. Curr HIV Res 8:26–52
7. Pritchard GC, Dawson M (2000) Maedi-visna. In: Martin WB, Aitken ID (ed) Diseases of Sheep, 3rd edition. Oxford: Blackwell Science, Osney Mead, Oxford, UK, pp 187–191
8. Gudnadóttir M, Demosthenous A, Hadjisavvas T (2013) Vaccination delays maedi-visna lentivirus infection in a naturally-infected sheep flock. BMC Vet Res 9:16
9. Keen JE, Hungerford LL, Littledike ET, Wittum TE, Kwang J (1997) Effect of ewe ovine lentivirus infection on ewe and lamb productivity. Prev Vet Med 30:155–169
10. Reina R, Berriatua E, Luján L, Juste RA, Sánchez A, de Andrés D, Amorena B (2009) Prevention strategies against small ruminant lentiviruses: an update. Vet J 182:31–37
11. Clements JE, Zink MC (1996) Molecular biology and pathogenesis of animal lentivirus infections. Clin Microbiol Rev 9:110–117
12. Heaton MP, Clawson ML, Chitko-McKown CG, Leymaster KA, Smith TP, Harhay GP, White SN, Herrmann-Hoesing LM, Mousel MR, Lewis GS, Kalbfleisch TS, Keen JE, Laegreid WW (2012) Reduced lentivirus susceptibility in sheep with TMEM154 mutations. PLoS Genet 8:e1002467
13. Sider LH, Heaton MP, Chitko-McKown CG, Harhay GP, Smith TPL, Leymaster KA, Laegreid WW, Clawson ML (2013) Small ruminant lentivirus genetic subgroups associate with sheep *TMEM154* genotypes. Vet Res 44:64
14. White SN, Mousel MR, Herrmann-Hoesing LM, Reynolds JO, Leymaster KA, Neibergs HL, Lewis GS, Knowles DP (2012) Genome-wide association identifies multiple genomic regions associated with susceptibility to and control of ovine lentivirus. PLoS One 7:e47829
15. Leymaster KA, Chitko-McKown CG, Clawson ML, Harhay GP, Heaton MP (2013) Effects of *TMEM154* haplotypes 1 and 3 on susceptibility to ovine progessive pneumonia virus following natural exposure in sheep. J Anim Sci 91:5114–5121
16. Heaton MP, Kalbfleisch TS, Petrik DT, Simpson B, Kijas JW, Clawson ML, Chitko-McKown CG, Harhay GP, Leymaster KA, Consortium ISG (2013) Genetic testing for TMEM154 mutations associated with lentivirus susceptibility in sheep. PLoS One 8:e55490

17. Herrmann LM, Cheevers WP, McGuire TC, Adams DS, Hutton MM, Gavin WG, Knowles DP (2003) Competitive-inhibition enzyme-linked immunosorbent assay for detection of serum antibodies to caprine arthritis-encephalitis virus: diagnostic tool for successful eradication. Clin Diagn Lab Immunol 10:267–271
18. Ewing B, Hillier L, Wendl MC, Green P (1998) Base-calling of automated sequencer traces using phred I Accuracy assessment. Genome Res 8:175–185
19. Ewing B, Green P (1998) Base-calling of automated sequencer traces using phred II Error probabilities. Genome Res 8:186–194
20. Gordon D, Abajian C, Green P (1998) Consed: a graphical tool for sequence finishing. Genome Res 8:195–202
21. Shah C, Boni J, Huder JB, H-R. V, Muhlherr J, Zanoni R, Miserez R, Lutz H, Schupbach J: Phylogenetic analysis and reclassification of caprine and ovine lentiviruses based on 104 new isolates: evidence for regular sheep-to-goat transmission and worldwide propagation through livestock trade. Virology 2004, 319:12–26
22. Grego E, Bertolotti L, Quasso A, Profiti M, Lacerenza D, Muz D, Rosati S (2007) Genetic characterization of small ruminant lentivirus in Italian mixed flocks: evidence for a novel genotype circulating in a local goat population. J Gen Virol 88:3423–3427
23. Kuhar U, Barlič-Maganja D, Grom J (2013) Phylogenetic analysis of small ruminant lentiviruses detected in Slovenia. Vet Microbiol 162:201–206
24. L'Homme Y, Leboeuf A, Arsenault J, Fras M (2015) Identification and characterisation of an emerging small ruminant lentivirus circulating recombinant form (CRF). Virology 475:159–171
25. Santry LA, de Jong J, Gold AC, Walsh SR, Menzies PI, Wootton SK (2013) Genetic characterization of small ruminant lentiviruses circulating in naturally infected sheep and goats in Ontario, Canada. Virus Res 175:30–44
26. Huson DH, Bryant D (2006) Application of phylogenetic networks in evolutionary studies. Mol Biol Evol 23:254–267
27. PHYLIP (Phylogeny Inference Package) version 3.69: [http://evolution.genetics.washington.edu/phylip.html]
28. Huson DH, Richter DC, Rausch C, Dezulian T, Franz M, Rupp R (2007) Dendroscope: an interactive viewer for large phylogenetic trees. BMC Bioinformatics 8:460
29. Herrmann-Hoesing LM, Broughton-Neiswanger LE, Gouine KC, White SN, Mousel MR, Lewis GS, Marshall KL, Knowles DP (2010) Evaluation of a caprine arthritis-encephalitis virus/maedi-visna virus indirect enzyme-linked immunosorbent assay in the serological diagnosis of ovine progressive pneumonia virus in U.S. sheep. Clin Vaccine Immunol 17:307–310

Piscine orthoreovirus (PRV) replicates in Atlantic salmon (*Salmo salar* L.) erythrocytes ex vivo

Øystein Wessel[1*], Christel Moræus Olsen[1], Espen Rimstad[1] and Maria Krudtaa Dahle[2]

Abstract

Piscine orthoreovirus (PRV) is a reovirus that has predominantly been detected in Atlantic salmon (*Salmo salar* L.). PRV is associated with heart and skeletal muscle inflammation (HSMI) in farmed Atlantic salmon, and recently erythrocytes were identified as major target cells. The study of PRV replication and pathogenesis of the infection has been impeded by the inability to propagate PRV in vitro. In this study we developed an ex vivo cultivation system for PRV in Atlantic salmon erythrocytes. PRV was successfully passaged to naïve erythrocytes using lysates of blood cells from infected salmon. During cultivation a significant increase in viral load was observed by RT-qPCR and flow cytometry, which coincided with the formation of cytoplasmic inclusions. The inclusions resembled viral factories and contained both PRV protein and dsRNA. In addition, the erythrocytes generated an antiviral immune gene activation after PRV infection, with significant up-regulation of IFN-α, RIG-I, Mx and PKR transcripts. Supernatants from the first passage successfully transmitted virus to naïve erythrocytes. This study demonstrates that PRV replicates in Atlantic salmon erythrocytes ex vivo. The ex vivo infection model closely reflects the situation in vivo and can be used to study the infection and replication mechanisms of PRV, as well as the antiviral immune responses of salmonid erythrocytes.

Introduction

Piscine orthoreovirus (PRV) has a double-stranded RNA (dsRNA) genome and belongs to the family *Reoviridae* [1]. PRV primarily infects Atlantic salmon (*Salmo salar* L.) and is associated with heart and skeletal muscle inflammation (HSMI), an important disease of farmed Atlantic salmon in Norway [1,2]. The virus is ubiquitously present in both diseased and apparently healthy individuals [3]. PRV is widespread in farmed salmonids in Europe, North and South America and present in several species of wild salmonids [4-6]. However, PRV has only been associated with disease in farmed Atlantic salmon. The study of viral replication and pathogenesis of the infection has been hindered by the inability to propagate PRV efficiently in cell cultures.

Phylogenetically PRV branches off the common root of the genera *Orthoreovirus* and *Aquareovirus*, but clusters more closely with the orthoreoviruses, although it is a fish virus [7-9]. Among orthoreoviruses, mammalian orthoreovirus (MRV) has been studied extensively and used as a model system for investigations of virus-host interactions, which has generated a wealth of information regarding replication cycle, protein functions and virion structure [10]. Even if nucleotide and protein sequence identities between the mammalian orthoreoviruses and PRV are low, important structural motifs and key amino acid are conserved in homologous proteins [7,9]. Currently PRV studies have been restricted to bioinformatic analyses [4,9], RT-qPCR screenings, field epidemiology [3,6] or laborious and costly in vivo challenge studies [11,12]. There have been a number of attempts to culture PRV in vitro. Cytopathic effects (CPE) have been observed in several cell lines including epithelioma papulosum cyprini (EPC), fathead minnow (FHM) and GF-1 derived from orange-spotted grouper [11,13]. However, increase in PRV titer has not been shown in any of these cell lines. An efficient in vitro cultivation system would be a highly desired tool of PRV research.

The association between PRV and HSMI has been strengthened in recent studies. The high viral RNA loads in the heart and the presence of viral antigens in cardiomyocytes correlate with development of the cardiac lesions observed in HSMI [11,14]. However, an explanation for high viral load in both farmed and wild salmon

* Correspondence: oyfi@nmbu.no
[1]Department of Food Safety and Infection Biology, Norwegian University of Life Sciences, Oslo, Norway
Full list of author information is available at the end of the article

without HSMI lesions is lacking [3,6], and in Canada PRV is present without HSMI being diagnosed [5]. This underlines the importance to study the PRV pathogenesis. We have recently demonstrated high viral loads in blood prior to PRV presence in cardiomyocytes and shown that red blood cells (RBC) are major target cells for PRV [12,14]. At peak infection phase more than 50% PRV positive erythrocytes were detected in individual fish. Despite the massive PRV infection of RBC, clinical anemia is not associated with HSMI or a PRV infection [15]. The study of PRV infection in erythrocytes will be important to understand the pathogenesis of PRV infection and its implications on Atlantic salmon health.

In MRV infected cells, viral-inclusions are present in distinct areas of the cell during replication; these are recognized as viral factories [16]. The cytoplasmic inclusions observed in PRV infected RBC resemble the globular viral factories of MRV type 3 prototype strain Dearing (T3D) [17,18]. The PRV inclusions contain reovirus-like particles as demonstrated by transmission electron microscopy (TEM) [12]. Inclusions and virus-like particles have previously been reported in erythrocytes of salmonid fish, suggesting that such infections are common [19-22]. The most commonly reported is erythrocytic inclusions body syndrome (EIBS) [23]. However, these findings have not been associated with any specific viral agent. The reovirus-like particles and intraerythrocytic inclusions observed in PRV infected RBC may resemble some of those described as EIBS [24-26]. Piscine erythrocytes, in contrast to mammalian erythrocytes, are nucleated cells containing organelles and capable of protein production [27,28]. Therefore, piscine erythrocytes are potentially able to support viral replication.

Recent studies have indicated that piscine erythrocytes may have immune functions [29]. Rainbow trout erythrocytes stimulated with Poly(I:C) respond by expression of genes encoding pathogen receptors (including toll-like receptors (TLRs)), interferon alpha (IFN-α) and immune cell recruiting mediators like CC chemokine (CCL) 4 [30]. Erythrocytes from Atlantic salmon have been shown to respond to infectious salmon anemia virus (ISAV) by production of IFN-α [31]. An important trigger of interferon production is recognition of dsRNA, either in endosomal compartments by the transmembrane receptor TLR3, or in the cytoplasm by RNA helicases like Retinoic-acid inducible gene (RIG)-I and Melanoma differentiation-associated protein (MDA)-5 [32,33]. In addition, cytosolic dsRNA bind dsRNA-activated kinases like PKR and PKZ and induce partial translational shutdown [34,35]. In order to bypass these antiviral responses, dsRNA viruses have developed counter-mechanisms. These include avoiding the exposure of the dsRNA genome by performing transcription and replication within the viral core, masking the viral RNA by dsRNA-binding viral proteins, inhibiting the dsRNA signaling pathway, or by producing non-polyadenylated viral mRNA which can omit the translational shutdown [36]. All these mechanisms have been demonstrated for MRV [37,38], and it is likely, due to structural similarities, that PRV counteracts antiviral mechanisms in similar ways. Recently, it was shown that PRV protein σ3 binds dsRNA in a sequence independent manner, thus sharing this function with MRV σ3 [39].

Through in vivo challenge experiments we have recently found that RBC is an important target cell for PRV infection in salmon [12], and we hypothesized that PRV can replicate in Atlantic salmon erythrocytes cultures ex vivo. In this study, supernatant from lysed blood cells collected from in vivo PRV infected salmon were passaged to RBC isolated from naïve salmon and cultured ex vivo. The viral propagation was monitored by RT-qPCR, flow cytometry, and immunofluorescence microscopy. The ability of the recipient erythrocytes to elicit an innate antiviral response was also assessed. Finally, a supernatant from the first passage was used to passage PRV to naïve RBC.

Materials and methods

Blood samples

Heparinized blood (0.5 mL) was collected from the caudal vein of six naïve Atlantic salmon (F1-F6). The fish had an average weight of 40 g and originated from a naïve population kept in a fresh water tank at VESO aquatic research facility (Vikan, Norway). The fish were anesthetized prior to sampling by bath immersion (2–5 min) in benzocaine chloride (0.5 g/10 L water) and euthanized after sampling using benzocaine chloride (1 g/5 L water) for 5 min. The RBC were isolated from the blood samples as described below and used as recipient erythrocytes in the first passage. Three weeks later heparinized blood samples were collected from six fish (F11-F16) of the same fish population. RBC were isolated and used as recipient erythrocytes in the second passage.

Isolation of naïve RBC

We diluted the heparinized blood 1:15 in phosphate-buffered saline (PBS) and isolated the RBC using a Percoll gradient as previously described [12]. The cells were counted using Countess (Invitrogen, Eugene, Oregon, USA) and resuspended to a concentration of 3×10^7 cells/mL in Leibovitz's L15 medium (Life Technologies, Carlsbad, CA, USA) supplemented with fetal calf serum (2%) and gentamicin (50 μg/mL). All recipient RBCs (first passage F1-F6; second passage F11-F16) were confirmed PRV-negative by RT-qPCR and flow cytometry before initiation of the study (described below).

Preparation of inoculums

The PRV inoculum was prepared from a batch of pooled heparinized blood samples collected 6 weeks post challenge (wpc) from cohabitant fish of a PRV challenge experiment (VESO, Vikan, Norway). We centrifuged the pooled blood sample at 2000 *g* for 10 min at 4 °C, removed the plasma and diluted the blood pellet 1:10 in L15 with gentamicin (50 μg/mL). The diluted blood was then sonicated on ice by 8 × 10 s pulses at 25 Hz with 30 s rest in between, and the lysed blood was centrifuged at 2000 *g* for 5 min at 4 °C to remove cellular debris. The resulting supernatant was used as PRV inoculum in the first passage. Similarly, a negative control inoculum was prepared as described above, using heparinized blood collected from naïve fish. The control inoculum was confirmed PRV negative by RT-qPCR. The PRV inoculum used had a Ct-value of 22.3.

Ex vivo setup; 1st passage

In the first PRV passage, RBC isolated from six naïve fish were inoculated and cultured ex vivo for 21 days. The culture experiment was performed in 24-deepwell microtiter plates with pyramidal bottom (AB Ninolab, Stockholm, Sweden) to allow easy centrifugation and washing of the cells. The plates were closed using Mikro-Flask sandwich cover and clamp system by Duetz (Applikon, Foster City, CA, USA) to minimize evaporation and prevent well to well contamination. Incubation was performed at 15 °C in an Ecotron incubation shaker (Infors HT, Basel Switzerland) shaken at 225 rpm to ensure that the RBC was kept in a homogenous suspension.

The cultivation setup included four identical PRV infected plates and four control plates that were sequentially harvested at 1, 7, 14 and 21 days post infection (dpi). On each plate, RBC isolated from fish F1-F6 was plated at 3×10^7 RBC per well in 1 mL medium. The wells were subsequently inoculated with 100 μL of either the PRV-infected inoculate or the control inoculate described above. Following 24 h of incubation the plates were centrifuged at 500 *g* for 5 min at 4 °C to remove the supernatant and washed in Leibovitz's L15 medium (Life Technologies). Finally, the RBC was resuspended to a final concentration of 10×10^6 RBC/mL in 3 mL Leibovitz's L15 medium (Life Technologies) supplemented with fetal calf serum (2%) and gentamicin (50 μg/mL). The 1 dpi samples were sampled immediately after resuspension and the remaining plates were incubated until harvested at 7, 14 and 21 dpi respectively. The 0 dpi samples were collected prior to inoculation.

At each time point a sample of 2 mL (20×10^6 RBC) was collected from each well for RNA isolation and subsequent RT-qPCR analysis to assess the viral load in the RBC and the supernatant. In addition, the immune response of infected RBC was assayed. The remaining 1 mL (10×10^6 RBC) was used for PRV detection by flow cytometry analysis and immunofluorescence/confocal microscopy to study viral inclusions. The number of cells were counted using Countess (Invitrogen) in order to determine the amount of cell lysis. Details for all analyses are described below.

Ex vivo setup; 2nd passage

In the second PRV passage, RBC isolated from six fish were infected with supernatant from the first passage and cultured ex vivo for 21 days. A pool of supernatant was prepared from the 21 dpi samples of the first passage after centrifugation at 1000 *g* for 5 min at 4 °C and used as inoculum.

The cultivation setup included two identical PRV infected plates that were sequentially harvested at 14 and 21 dpi. On each plate, RBC isolated from fish F11-F16 was plated at 3×10^7 RBC per well in 1 mL media as for the first passage. The cells were subsequently inoculated with 100 μL of a 10-fold dilution of the supernatant from the first passage. The RBC were incubated for 24 h, centrifuged, washed and resuspended in growth medium to a final concentration of 10×10^6 RBC/mL. The plates were cultured under identical conditions as those of the first passage and harvested at 14 and 21 dpi. The 0 dpi samples had been collected prior to inoculation.

At each time point a sample of 2 mL (20×10^6 RBC) was collected from each well for RNA isolation and RT-qPCR analysis to detect PRV in the RBC fraction and 1 mL was used for flow cytometry analysis and immunofluorescence microscopy. Details for the analyses are described below.

RNA isolation

The 2×10^6 cells (2 mL) harvested from each culture were pelleted at 1000 *g* for 5 min at 4 °C and total RNA was isolated from the RBC pellet and the supernatant. The RBC pellet was homogenized in Isol-RNA Lysis Reagent (5 PRIME, Hilden, Germany) using 5 mm steel beads and TissueLyser II (Qiagen) for 2 × 5 min at 25 Hz. After addition of chloroform and centrifugation, the aqueous phase was collected and proceeded with automated RNA isolation using RNeasy Mini QIAcube Kit (Qiagen) as described by the manufacturer. For the supernatant samples, a combination of Trizol LS (Invitrogen) and RNeasy Mini spin column (Qiagen) was used. Briefly, 100 μL supernatant was mixed and incubated with Trizol LS before adding chloroform, separating the phases by centrifugation, and then proceeding with the RNeasy Mini spin column as recommended by the manufacturer, eluting isolated RNA in 50 μL RNase-free water. RNA was quantified using a NanoDrop ND-1000 spectrophotometer (Thermo Fisher Scientific, Wilmington, DE, USA).

RT-qPCR; PRV detection

The Qiagen OneStep kit (Qiagen) was used for RT-qPCR. The input was 100 ng (5 μL of 20 ng/uL) total RNA from RBC per reaction and 5 μL purified RNA solution from the cell free samples, i.e. supernatants and inoculums. RT-qPCR targeted PRV segment S1 using the following conditions: 400 nM primer, 300 nM probe, 400 nM dNTPs, 1.26 mM MgCl2, 1:100 RNase Out (Invitrogen) and 1 × ROX reference dye with the following cycle parameters: 30 min at 50 °C, 15 min at 94 °C, 35 cycles of 94 °C/15 s, 54 °C/30 s and 72 °C/15 s in a Mx3005P (Stratagene, La Jolla, CA, USA). The samples were run in duplicate, and a sample was defined as positive if both parallel samples had a Ct < 35. Primers and probe are listed in Table 1.

qPCR; Antiviral response

Reverse transcription was performed using 200 ng RNA per sample, and a mixed input from representative samples was used to prepare a seven point concentration standard curve. The RNA was denaturated at 95 °C for 5 min prior to cDNA synthesis, using the Quantitect reverse transcription kit with integrated genomic DNA removal (Qiagen). Quantitative PCR (qPCR) was run in duplicate on cDNA corresponding to 10 ng RNA input. The antiviral response gene expression analysis was performed using 2 × Maxima SYBR Green qPCR Master Mix (Thermo Fisher scientific, Waltham, MA, USA) and 500 nM specific primers targeting Atlantic salmon IFNα, myxovirus resistance (Mx), RIG-I and PKR respectively.

Table 1 Primers and probe used in this study

Primer/probes	Primer sequence (5′ → 3′)	Accession #
σ3 S1-659 Fwd	TGCGTCCTGCGTATGGCACC	GU994022
σ3 S1-801 Rev	GGCTGGCATGCCCGAATAGCA	
σ3 S1-693 Probe	*FAM*-ATCACAACGCCTACCT-*MGBNFQ*	
IFNα Fwd	ACTGAAACGCTACTTCAAGAAGTTGA	AY216595
IFNα Rev	GCAGATGACGTTTTGTCTCTTTCCT	
Mx Fwd	GATGCTGCACCTCAAGTCCTATTA	BT043721.1
Mx Rev	CACCAGGTAGCGGATCACCAT	
RIG-I Fwd	ACGCCTTGAAGAGCTGGATA	FN178459
RIG-I Rev	CTGGCTGGACTTGTGTCCTC	
PKR Fwd	CAGGATGCAACACCATCATC	EF523422.1
PKR Rev	GGTCTTGACCGGTGACATCT	

The quencher and reporter dye of the probes are in italic. Accession numbers are shown in the right column.

The assays were run 40 cycles of 94 °C/15 s, 60 °C/30 s in a Mx3005P device (Stratagene). Primers used are listed in Table 1.

Flow cytometry

RBC sampled during the first and second passage were screened for PRV by flow cytometry. The RBC were stained intracellularly using a rabbit polyclonal antibody against PRV putative outer capsid protein σ1 (Anti-σ1, #K275) as previously described [12]. The corresponding zero serum (Anti-σ1 Zero #K275) [14] was used as negative control serum. The cells were analyzed on a Gallios Flow Cytometer (Beckman Coulter, Miami, FL, USA) counting 30 000 cells per sample. The data were analyzed using the Kaluza software (Becton Dickinson). The forward/side gate was set to adjust for variation in background staining. The arithmetic mean fluorescence intensity (MFI) was calculated for all PRV infected (green) and control (grey) samples at each time point, in addition to the ΔMFI. The differences were calculated statistically using Wilcoxon matched pairs signed rank test due to the small sample size ($n = 6$).

Immunofluorescence microscopy

The PRV σ1 stained RBC used in flow cytometry were also assayed by immunofluorescence microscopy. The nuclei were stained with Hoechst 33342 (Invitrogen) before they were transferred to Countess chamber slides (Invitrogen). Photographs were taken by an inverted fluorescence microscope (Olympus IX81), at 20× and 40× magnification.

Confocal microscopy

Smears of RBC were dried before fixation for 5 min in ice cold methanol. Slides were rehydrated in PBS and blocked in PBS with 5% skimmed milk before sequentially staining with a mouse monoclonal antibody against dsRNA (J2; 1:200) (Scicons, Hungary) and rabbit anti-σ1 (1:750) with washing in-between. Secondary antibody; goat anti-mouse Alexa Fluor 488 and goat anti-rabbit Alexa Fluor 594 (1:1000) were obtained from Molecular Probes (Invitrogen). The nucleus was counterstained with Hoechst 33342 (Invitrogen) and coverslips were mounted with Fluoroshield (Sigma-Aldrich). The images were generated on an inverted Zeiss LSM 710 confocal laser scanning microscope (CLSM) (Carl Zeiss, Oberkochen, Germany), using lasers of 405 nm, 488 nm and 594 nm to excite the respective stains. In post-production, the original color of dsRNA (Alexa Flour 488) and PRV-σ1 protein (Alexa Flour 594) was switched to match the immunofluorescence pictures, in which PRV-σ1 protein was colored green.

Data analysis

The PRV RT-qPCR results from 1 dpi were compared to paired samples collected at 7, 14 and 21 dpi in the first. For the immune gene analysis of IFNα, Mx, RIG-I and PKR the fold increase at 1, 7, 14 and 21 dpi was calculated, assigning the qPCR results from the uninfected paired samples as 1. In the second passage, the results from the undiluted and the 10 fold diluted inoculum was compared at each time point. The differences were analyzed statistically using Wilcoxon matched pairs signed rank test due to the small sample size ($n = 6$). All statistical analysis described were performed with GraphPad Prism (GraphPad Software inc., USA) and p-values of $p \leq 0.05$ were considered as significant.

Results

A blood cell lysate prepared from PRV infected fish was used as inoculum in the first passage of PRV to naïve erythrocytes. The inoculum had Ct value of 22.3. The recipient naïve RBC were confirmed negative for PRV by both RT-qPCR and flow cytometry before onset of the study and they were cultured ex vivo for 21 dpi.

Increased PRV RNA shown by RT-qPCR

Following inoculation with PRV containing lysate, there was an increase in the PRV titer in both RBC and supernatant during the first passage (Figure 1). At 1 dpi, after removal of the inoculum and washing of the cells, the mean Ct value was 21.2 ± 0.6 in the RBC fraction. A significant increase in viral load was observed from 1 dpi to 14 dpi when the Ct was 14.6 ± 0.9 ($p < 0.05$), and it stayed on this level until the end of the first passage at 21 dpi (Ct 14.9 ± 0.7). Similarly, in the supernatant there was a significant increase in mean Ct-value from 1 dpi (Ct 33.4 ± 1.1) to 21 dpi (Ct 27.0 ± 1.8) ($p < 0.05$).

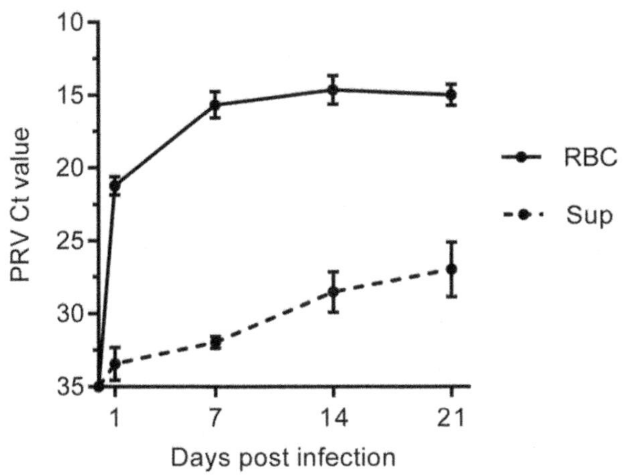

Figure 1 PRV load in 1st passage of culturing. Mean PRV Ct value with SD ($n = 6$) as detected by RT-qPCR in red blood cells (RBC) and supernatant (Sup) at 1, 7, 14 and 21 days post infection.

Increased PRV protein shown by flow cytometry

The infected RBC were stained intracellularly with a PRV σ1-antibody and analyzed by flow cytometry to determine the level of viral protein during the first passage. At 1 dpi the RBC population observed in the PRV-infected cultures had shifted to the right compared to the uninfected controls (Figure 2A; 1 dpi), indicating cell association of PRV. At 7 dpi the main population partly overlapped the control culture, but a distinct right shoulder, constituting RBC with higher PRV σ1 content, was evident in infected cultures (Figure 2A; 7 dpi). At 14 dpi a broader right shoulder was observed, and the entire PRV infected population had shifted to the right indicating a general increased amount of PRV σ1 protein (Figure 2A; 14 dpi). At 21 dpi the PRV infected cells were separated into two populations; a PRV high and low positive population (Figure 2A; 21 dpi).

The pattern described above was observed in all infected cultures and was accompanied by elevated mean fluorescence intensity (MFI) (Figure 2B). The detection of PRV σ1, as measured by ΔMFI, was significantly increased from each time point to the next during the first passage ($p < 0.05$) (Figure 2C). Whereas the main increase in viral load detected by RT-qPCR appeared during the early phases from 1 dpi to 7 dpi, the most prominent increase in viral protein was observed in later phases from 7 to 21 dpi (Figure 2D).

Development of erythrocytic PRV inclusions

PRV infected erythrocytes from passage one were inspected by immunofluorescence (IF) microscopy. At 1 dpi PRV positive staining was observed as small cytoplasmic granules within infected RBC (Figure 3A; 1 dpi). At 7 dpi a similar granular staining pattern was detected, including positive cells with increased fluorescence intensity (Figure 3A; 7 dpi). At 14 dpi positive cells with prominent large inclusion was observed. (Figure 3A; 14 dpi). The cellular morphology of the PRV infected cells varied, as both elongated ellipsoidal RBC and erythrocytes with rounded cell shape and nucleus was observed. At 21 dpi the number of cells with large inclusions was numerous (Figure 3A; 21 dpi). The large inclusions were also visible in phase contrast and co-localized with the immunofluorescent staining of PRV. The staining pattern observed by IF, i.e. increasing amounts of PRV σ1, was in line with the flow cytometry observations.

We showed that the erythrocytic inclusions contained both dsRNA and PRV σ1 protein by double staining of smears of infected RBC. The dsRNA staining partly or completely co-localized with the PRV σ1 as observed by confocal imaging (Figure 3B). Fixation with methanol was necessary for detection of dsRNA in the co-lolcalization experiments. This fixation technique reduced the signal to noise ratio compared to the method used for

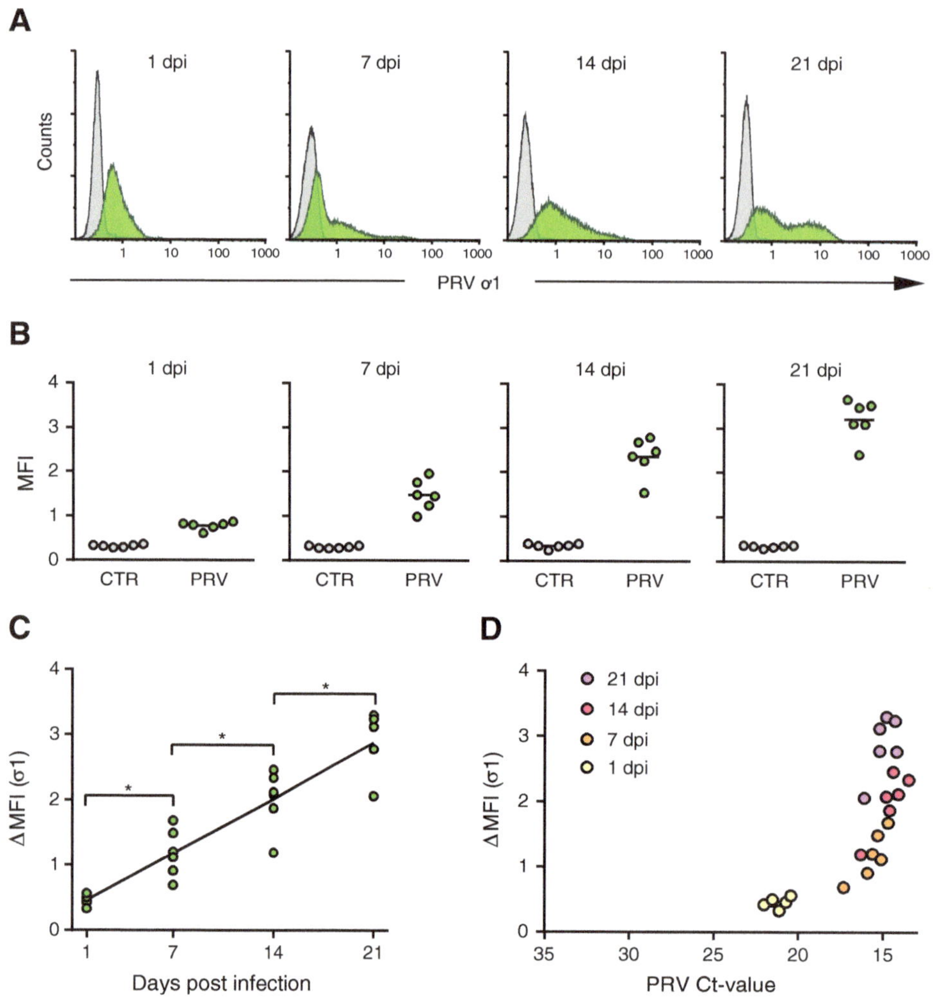

Figure 2 Detection of PRV σ1 protein by flow cytometry in the 1st passage. (A) Results from intracellular staining for PRV σ1 protein from PRV infected culture (green) and control culture (grey) at 1, 7, 14 and 21 days post infection (dpi). The fluorescence intensity (PRV σ1) is shown on the X-axis and cell count on the y-axis counting 30 000 cells per sample. The results of one individual are presented to illustrate the staining pattern. **(B)** Plot of the arithmetic mean fluorescence intensity (MFI) for all PRV infected (green) and control (grey) cultures ($n = 6$) at each time point. **(C)** The amount of PRV σ1 protein detected presented by ΔMFI (MFI Infected – MFI Control) at 1, 7, 14 and 21 dpi. Data were analyzed using Wilcoxon matched pairs signed rank test. *$p < 0.05$. **(D)** The correlation between the amount of PRV nucleic acid and PRV σ1 protein detected during the cultivation is illustrated by plotting PRV Ct-values (X-axis) against the ΔMFI for PRV σ1 (Y-axis) color coding the different time points; 1 dpi (yellow), 7 dpi (orange), 14 dpi (red) and 21 dpi (purple).

flow cytometry and standard immunofluorescence microscopy (Figure 3A).

Ex vivo infected RBC elicit an antiviral immune response

In order to determine if the PRV infected RBC responded to PRV infection by antiviral gene expression, the mRNA levels of IFN-α, Mx, RIG-I and PKR were analyzed. IFN-α was significantly up-regulated at 1 dpi (Figure 4A). A significant up-regulation at 1 and 7 dpi was observed for Mx (Figure 4B), RIG-I (Figure 4C) and PKR (Figure 4D). These latter three genes followed a similar expression pattern with peak expression detected at 7 dpi, before the expression levels returned to baseline.

Successful passage of PRV

Tenfold dilutions of the supernatant from passage 1 were used as inoculums in passage 2. The undiluted and 10-fold diluted inoculums were measured to Ct values of 27.0 and 31.6 respectively. Following inoculation there was an increase in viral load from 1 dpi until 14 dpi, and similar to passage 1 the increase leveled off thereafter (Figure 5A). The peak viral load was significantly higher in RBC given the undiluted compared to the 10 fold diluted inoculum at 14 dpi (Ct 20.5 ± 0.6 and Ct 22.9 ± 0.3 respectively) and 21 dpi (Ct 21.2 ± 0.7 and Ct 23.0 ± 0.6 respectively) ($p < 0.05$). In line with passage 1, PRV σ1 positive RBC were observed at 14 and 21 dpi by IF microscopy (Figure 5B). However, the number of positive

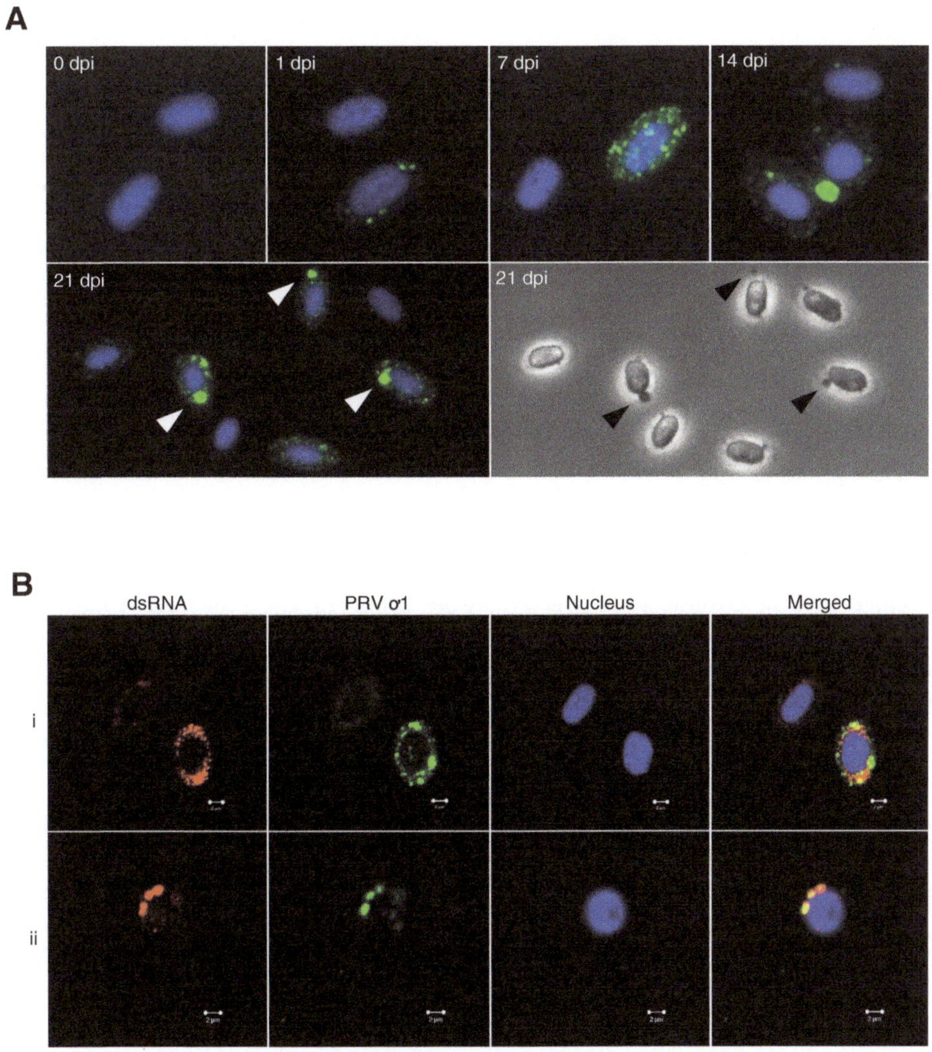

Figure 3 Immunofluorescence and confocal microscopy of PRV infected RBC. (A) Fluorescent labeling of the PRV σ1-protein (green) in ex vivo infected RBC. The nuclei were stained with Hoechst (blue). Non-infected cells are shown at 0 dpi, and infected cells are shown at 1, 7 14 and 21 dpi. Large PRV inclusions at 21 dpi (marked by arrowheads) can also be observed in phase contrast. **(B)** Confocal images of ex vivo infected RBC at 21 dpi, stained with anti-dsRNA (red) and anti-PRV-σ1 (green). The nuclei were stained with Hoechst (blue). dsRNA was detected within PRV inclusions, and either partly (i) or completely (ii) co-localized with PRV σ1. Scale bar 2 μm.

cells was much lower, and the PRV positive population was below the detection level for flow cytometry (data not shown).

Discussion

In this study we demonstrated that PRV replicates in Atlantic salmon erythrocytes ex vivo. PRV obtained from infected fish were passaged to naïve erythrocytes. A significant increase in viral load was detected and viral factories containing PRV proteins and dsRNA was formed within infected RBC. Supernatant from the first passage was successfully passaged to naïve erythrocytes. In addition, we demonstrated that ex vivo infected RBC generated an innate antiviral immune response.

During the first passage, a significant increase in PRV load in the RBC fraction was observed by RT-qPCR and flow cytometry. At 1 dpi the mean Ct-value was relatively low, indicating that the added PRV efficiently associated with RBC. The results of flow cytometry corroborated this as the entire RBC population shifted to the right, suggesting that all RBC were PRV positive at this time point. The increase in the amount of viral RNA was most prominent in the early phase and plateaued at 14 dpi. The peak Ct-values were similar to those observed in previous in vivo challenge trials [12]. On the other hand, the viral load as detected by flow cytometry increased until 21 dpi, indicating a continuous production of PRV proteins within infected RBC. During ex vivo cultivation, PRV infected RBC formed two

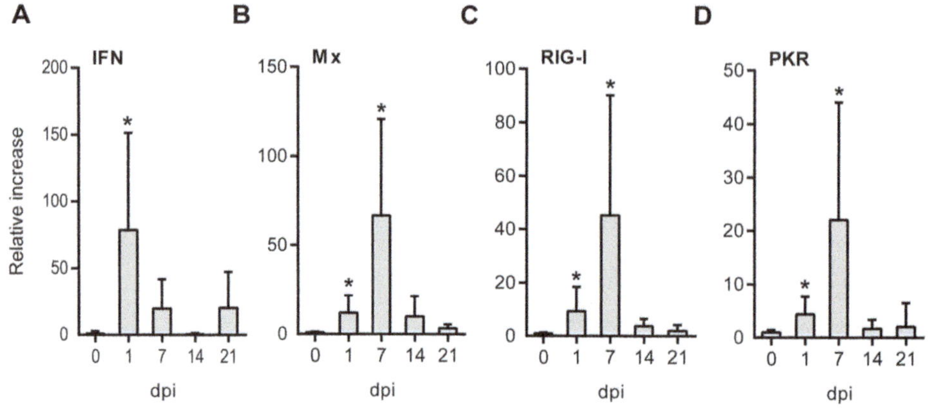

Figure 4 Erythrocytic antiviral responses to PRV infection. Expression of genes involved in antiviral responses was measured by RT-qPCR. The expression levels in infected RBC relative to the paired non-infected controls were calculated for each sample ($n = 6$) at 1, 7, 12 and 21 dpi. The relative increase (and SD) for IFNα **(A)**, Mx **(B)**, RIG-I **(C)** and PKR **(D)** is shown. Data were analyzed using Wilcoxon matched pairs signed rank test. $^*p < 0.05$.

distinct populations observed by flow cytometry. This is similar to that observed during in vivo challenge experiments in which low and high PRV positive RBC populations are found during peak PRV infection [12].

The amount of PRV protein detected by flow cytometry were in line with the PRV staining observed by immunofluorescence microscopy. The PRV staining was observed as cytoplasmic inclusions similar to those observed during in vivo studies [12], and developed over time from small numerous granules to large distinct inclusions. At 14 dpi and 21 dpi, many RBC with one or two very large inclusions were observed, probably reflecting the high PRV positive RBC population. The inclusions were shown to contain both dsRNA and PRV σ1 protein, although the degree of co-localization varied between cells. For MRV, the viral replication process takes place in cytoplasmic inclusions called viral factories [16]. These viral factories are shown to contain large amounts of both viral proteins and dsRNA and are essential for successful replication [16,40]. The globular inclusions detected in PRV infected RBC resembles the shape of the viral factories observed in MRV type 3 Dearing (T3D) infected cells [12,17,18]. Thus, both content and morphology of PRV inclusions are similar to the viral factories of orthoreoviruses.

A significant increase in PRV load was observed in the supernatant, which successfully passaged PRV to naïve erythrocytes. This indicates that infectious viral progeny is produced during the ex vivo cultivation. RBC with PRV inclusions were observed in the second passage,

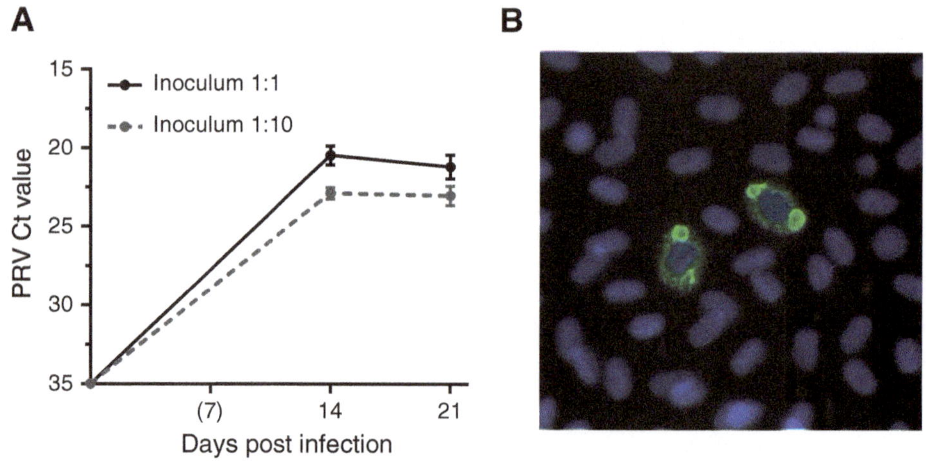

Figure 5 RT-qPCR and PRV σ1 staining from the 2nd passage. (A) Mean PRV Ct value (and SD) detected by RT-qPCR in red blood cells (RBC) at 14 and 21 dpi ($n = 6$) during the second passage. Results are shown for cultures infected with undiluted and diluted (1:10) inoculum from the 1st passage. **(B)** Immunofluorescence microscopy picture showing the PRV σ1-protein (green) in cells at 14 dpi infected by undiluted inoculum. Cell nuclei stained with Hoechst (blue).

however, the number of positive cells was low and below detection level for flow cytometry. In previous in vivo experiments, the threshold of detection by flow cytometry appeared to be corresponding to a Ct-value of about 20 [12], thus slightly below the level obtained in the second passage. The viral titer of the inoculum was significantly higher in passage 1 (Ct-value 22.3) compared to passage 2 (Ct-value 27.0). This could explain the difference in virus outcome between the passages.

The amount of PRV within infected RBC was substantial; however, it was not accompanied by cell lysis (data not shown). The low, but increasing viral load detected in the supernatant suggests a slow but steady release of virus. This correlates well with in vivo observations where neither a PRV infection or an HSMI outbreak is associated with anemia [15]. However, HSMI is associated with circulatory disturbances, and a swollen spleen with high viral load is a common finding [12,41]. Orthoreovirus infections commonly results in cell lysis and release of progeny particles is thought to follow cell death and disruption of the plasma membrane [10]. However, non-lytic persistent infections have also been demonstrated in cell cultures [42-46]. The release mechanism of PRV remains to be shown. Although the present study suggests salmon RBC can tolerate high amounts of PRV, it is not known how it affects other important erythrocyte functions, such as oxygen transport.

Viral replication in erythrocytes is not well documented in the literature. Mature mammalian erythrocytes are not nucleated and thus not able to support a viral replication [47]. However, it is demonstrated that MRV can bind erythrocytes by the σ1 protein [48,49], and amino acid residues involved in this binding are partly conserved in the PRV σ1 protein [7,9]. In contrast to mammalian RBC, piscine erythrocytes are nucleated and retain ribosomes and a number of organelles while in circulation, thus competent to perform transcription and protein synthesis [27,30]. Differences in the content of PRV protein in RBC were observed during the present ex vivo infection and in previous in vivo experiments, indicating that the susceptibility of RBC varies [12]. During maturation and ageing of erythrocytes there is an inverse relationship between loss of cytoplasmic organelles and increase in hemoglobin content [50,51] accompanied by a reduced aerobic metabolic rate [52]. Both total RNA content and protein synthesis is higher in young erythrocytes [28]. It is a possibility that the putative differences in PRV susceptibility of erythrocytes is correlated to maturation.

PRV is the first virus shown to replicate in salmonid erythrocytes. However, there have been several reports of different viral inclusions in salmonid erythrocytes [19-22]. The most commonly reported is erythrocytic inclusions body syndrome (EIBS) [23], which have been associated with a transient anemia in freshwater Pacific salmon [53]. In contrast, EIBS has not been linked to anemia in Atlantic salmon [54]. No specific viral agent has been characterized for these findings. Interestingly, EM images of PRV and PRV inclusions strongly resemble some of those reported for EIBS [12,24-26]. Blood smears collected from experimentally PRV infected fish have been shown to stain positive by pinacyanol chloride [12]; the most commonly used method in detection and characterization of EIBS. However, a report suggested the EIBS agent to be enveloped, whereas PRV is a reovirus which is non-enveloped [55]. The present study demonstrated that erythrocytic PRV inclusions contain dsRNA, whereas a previous report suggested the EIBS agent to be a single stranded RNA virus based on acridine orange staining [26]. Pinacyanol chlorid and acridine orange are not agent specific staining methods, in contrast to the dsRNA MAb and PRV σ1 specific antibody used in the present study. Whether EIBS represents one viral agent or several related or non-related viral agents is not known and should be sorted out.

Prior studies have shown that salmon erythrocytes can elicit antiviral responses to Poly(I:C) stimulation [30]. We observed that PRV infection ex vivo induced gene expression of IFNα, Mx, RIG-I and PKR, indicating the mobilization of an antiviral response. The production of Mx, which is an interferon target gene [56,57], indicate that interferon is also produced at the protein level following PRV infection. Expression of RIG-I and PKR in particular indicate that the induced response may specifically target dsRNA viruses. This response may have the ability to inhibit or moderate further PRV infection and replication in the RBC cultures, leading to suboptimal viral production, and indicating that viral propagation in RBC ex vivo can be optimized further.

RBC is a major target cell for PRV in vivo and thus the study of PRV infection in erythrocytes will be central to progress our understanding of PRV infection and its implications on Atlantic salmon health. The lack of available cell lines supporting PRV replication has restricted studies of PRV infection and pathogenesis. The present study demonstrated an ex vivo infection model using primary naïve erythrocytes, which could be used to propagate PRV. The advantage of using RBC would be that it closely mimics the in vivo situation; therefore, the ex vivo cultivation model will likely benefit future studies of PRV infection, replication and release from RBC. In addition, it could be used to study the antiviral immune response of erythrocytes in salmonid fish.

Abbreviations

CCL: CC chemokine ligand; Ct: Cycle threshold; dpi: Days post infection; dsRNA: Double-stranded RNA; EIBS: Erythrocytic inclusion body syndrome; EPC: Epithelioma papulosum cyprinid; FHM: Fathead minnow; HSMI: Heart and skeletal muscle inflammation; IFN-α: Interferon alpha; ISAV: Infectious salmon anemia virus; MDA: Melanoma differentiation-associated; MFI: Mean fluorescence intensity; MRV: Mammalian orthoreovirus; MX: Myxovirus resistance; PBS: Phosphate-buffered saline; PRV: Piscine orthoreovirus; RBC: Red blood cells; RIG: Retinoic-acid inducible gene; RT-qPCR: Real-time quantitative polymerase chain reaction; T3D: Type 3 Dearing; TEM: Transmission electron microscopy; TLR: Toll-like receptor.

Competing interests

A patent application for the ex vivo propagation of PRV in RBC has been sent to the Norwegian Patent Office 30.08.2013 as patent application number NO 20131163. This may become public on 28.02.2015. The patent application has also been filed internationally as PCT/EP2014/068293. We have received no reimbursements, fees, funding, or salary linked to this patent application.

Authors' contributions

ØW participated in the overall design of the study, performed sampling, RBC isolation, RT-qPCR analysis, flow cytometry and immunofluorescence microscopy, interpretation of the data and drafted the manuscript. CMO helped in blood smear staining and confocal microscopy and in interpretation of the overall data. ER participated in the overall design of the study, helped in interpretation of the data and drafting the manuscript. MKD participated in the overall design of the study, qPCR analysis, helped in interpretation of the data, drafting the manuscript and coordination of the study. All authors read and approved the final manuscript.

Acknowledgements

Thanks to the team at VESO Vikan, including Marie Løvoll and Christian Wallace, for conducting the challenge experiment, and to Randi Faller and Even Thoen at the Norwegian Veterinary Institute for technical assistance and confocal imaging respectively.

Author details

[1]Department of Food Safety and Infection Biology, Norwegian University of Life Sciences, Oslo, Norway. [2]Section of Immunology, Norwegian Veterinary Institute, Oslo, Norway.

References

1. Palacios G, Løvoll M, Tengs T, Hornig M, Hutchison S, Hui J, Kongtorp RT, Savji N, Bussetti AV, Solovyov A, Kristoffersen AB, Celone C, Street C, Trifonov V, Hirschberg DL, Rabadan R, Egholm M, Rimstad E, Lipkin WI (2010) Heart and skeletal muscle inflammation of farmed salmon is associated with infection with a novel reovirus. PLoS One 5:e11487
2. Kongtorp RT, Kjerstad A, Taksdal T, Guttvik A, Falk K (2004) Heart and skeletal muscle inflammation in Atlantic salmon, *Salmo salar* L.: a new infectious disease. J Fish Dis 27:351–358
3. Løvoll M, Alarcon M, Bang JB, Taksdal T, Kristoffersen AB, Tengs T (2012) Quantification of piscine reovirus (PRV) at different stages of Atlantic salmon *Salmo salar* production. Dis Aquat Organ 99:7–12
4. Kibenge MJ, Iwamoto T, Wang Y, Morton A, Godoy MG, Kibenge FS (2013) Whole-genome analysis of piscine reovirus (PRV) shows PRV represents a new genus in family *Reoviridae* and its genome segment S1 sequences group it into two separate sub-genotypes. Virol J 10:230
5. Marty GD, Morrison DB, Bidulka J, Joseph T, Siah A. Piscine reovirus in wild and farmed salmonids in British Columbia, Canada: 1974–2013. J Fish Dis, in press.
6. Garseth AH, Fritsvold C, Opheim M, Skjerve E, Biering E (2013) Piscine reovirus (PRV) in wild Atlantic salmon, *Salmo salar* L., and sea-trout, *Salmo trutta* L., in Norway. J Fish Dis 36:483–493
7. Key T, Read J, Nibert ML, Duncan R (2013) Piscine reovirus encodes a cytotoxic, non-fusogenic, integral membrane protein and previously unrecognized virion outer-capsid proteins. J Gen Virol 94:1039–1050
8. Nibert ML, Duncan R (2013) Bioinformatics of recent aqua- and orthoreovirus isolates from fish: Evolutionary gain or loss of FAST and fiber proteins and taxonomic implications. PLoS One 8:e68607
9. Markussen T, Dahle MK, Tengs T, Løvoll M, Finstad ØW, Wiik-Nielsen CR, Grove S, Lauksund S, Robertsen B, Rimstad E (2013) Sequence analysis of the genome of piscine orthoreovirus (PRV) associated with heart and skeletal muscle inflammation (HSMI) in Atlantic salmon (*Salmo salar*). PLoS One 8:e70075
10. Schiff LA, Nibert ML, Tyler KL (2007) Orthoreoviruses and their replication. In: Knipe DM, Howley PM, Fields BN (ed) Fields virology, 5th edition, vol 2. Wolters Kluwer/Lippincott Williams & Wilkins, Philadelphia, pp 1853–1915
11. Mikalsen AB, Haugland Ø, Rode M, Solbakk IT, Evensen Ø (2012) Atlantic salmon reovirus infection causes a CD8 T cell myocarditis in Atlantic salmon (*Salmo salar* L.). PLoS One 7:e37269
12. Finstad OW, Dahle MK, Lindholm TH, Nyman IB, Lovoll M, Wallace C, Olsen CM, Storset AK, Rimstad E (2014) Piscine orthoreovirus (PRV) infects Atlantic salmon erythrocytes. Vet Res 45:35
13. Kongtorp RT, Taksdal T (2009) Studies with experimental transmission of heart and skeletal muscle inflammation in Atlantic salmon, *Salmo salar* L. J Fish Dis 32:253–262
14. Finstad ØW, Falk K, Løvoll M, Evensen Ø, Rimstad E (2012) Immunohistochemical detection of piscine reovirus (PRV) in hearts of Atlantic salmon coincide with the course of heart and skeletal muscle inflammation (HSMI). Vet Res 43:27
15. Kongtorp RT, Taksdal T, Lyngøy A (2004) Pathology of heart and skeletal muscle inflammation (HSMI) in farmed Atlantic salmon *Salmo salar*. Dis Aquat Organ 59:217–224
16. Fields BN, Raine CS, Baum SG (1971) Temperature-sensitive mutants of reovirus type 3: Defects in viral maturation as studied by immunofluorescence and electron microscopy. Virology 43:569–578
17. Broering TJ, Parker JS, Joyce PL, Kim J, Nibert ML (2002) Mammalian reovirus nonstructural protein μNS forms large inclusions and colocalizes with reovirus microtubule-associated protein μ2 in transfected cells. J Virol 76:8285–8297
18. Parker JS, Broering TJ, Kim J, Higgins DE, Nibert ML (2002) Reovirus core protein μ2 determines the filamentous morphology of viral inclusion bodies by interacting with and stabilizing microtubules. J Virol 76:4483–4496
19. Landholt ML, MacMillan JR, Patterson M (1977) Detection of an intra-erythrocytic virus in rainbow trout (*Salmo gairdneri*). Fish Health News 6:4–6
20. Hedrick RP, McDowell T, Groff JM (1987) Another erythrocytic virus from salmonid fish? Am Fish Soc Fish Health Sect Newsl 15:5
21. Thorud KE, Lunder T, Wiik S, Engeland E (1990) Electron microscopic observations of EIBSV-like particles and two intraerythrocytic virus-like particles different from EIBSV in Atlantic salmon, *Salmo salar*, in Norway. Bull Eur Ass Fish Pathol 104:95–97
22. Evelyn TPT, Traxler GS (1978) Viral erythrocytic necrosis: natural occurrence in Pacific salmon and experimental transmission. J Fish Res Board Can 35:903–907
23. Leek SL (1987) Viral erythrocytic inclusion body syndrome (EIBS) occurring in juvenile spring chinook salmon (*Oncorhynchus tshawytscha*) reared in freshwater. Can J Fish Aquat Sci 44:685–688
24. Lunder T, Thorud K, Holt RA, Rohovec JS (1990) Particles similar to the virus of erythrocytic inclusion body syndrome, EIBS, detected in Atlantic salmon (*Salmo salar*) in Norway. Bull Eur Assoc Fish Pathol 10:21–23
25. Michak P, Smith CE, Hopper K (1992) Erythrocytic inclusion body syndrome: a light and electron microscopic study of infected erythrocytes of chinook *Oncorhynchus tshawytscha* and coho *O. kisutch* salmon. Dis Aquat Organ 12:229–233
26. Rodger HD (2007) Erythrocytic inclusion body syndrome virus in wild Atlantic salmon, *Salmo salar* L. J Fish Dis 30:411–418
27. Claver JA, Quaglia AIE (2009) Comparative morphology, development, and function of blood cells in nonmammalian vertebrates. J Exot Pet Med 18:87–97
28. Lund SG, Phillips MC, Moyes CD, Tufts BL (2000) The effects of cell ageing on protein synthesis in rainbow trout (*Oncorhynchus mykiss*) red blood cells. J Exp Biol 203:2219–2228
29. Morera D, Mackenzie SA (2011) Is there a direct role for erythrocytes in the immune response? Vet Res 42:89
30. Morera D, Roher N, Ribas L, Balasch JC, Donate C, Callol A, Boltana S, Roberts S, Goetz G, Goetz FW, MacKenzie SA (2011) RNA-Seq reveals an integrated immune response in nucleated erythrocytes. PLoS One 6:e26998
31. Workenhe ST, Kibenge MJ, Wright GM, Wadowska DW, Groman DB, Kibenge FS (2008) Infectious salmon anaemia virus replication and induction of alpha interferon in Atlantic salmon erythrocytes. Virol J 5:36
32. Jacobs BL, Langland JO (1996) When two strands are better than one: the mediators and modulators of the cellular responses to double-stranded RNA. Virology 219:339–349

33. Saito T, Gale M, Jr (2008) Differential recognition of double-stranded RNA by RIG-I-like receptors in antiviral immunity. J Exp Med 205:1523–1527
34. Taghavi N, Samuel CE (2012) Protein kinase PKR catalytic activity is required for the PKR-dependent activation of mitogen-activated protein kinases and amplification of interferon beta induction following virus infection. Virology 427:208–216
35. Taghavi N, Samuel CE (2013) RNA-dependent protein kinase PKR and the Z-DNA binding orthologue PKZ differ in their capacity to mediate initiation factor eIF2alpha-dependent inhibition of protein synthesis and virus-induced stress granule formation. Virology 443:48–58
36. Zinzula L, Tramontano E (2013) Strategies of highly pathogenic RNA viruses to block dsRNA detection by RIG-I-like receptors: Hide, mask, hit. Antiviral Res 100:615–635
37. Qin Q, Carroll K, Hastings C, Miller CL (2011) Mammalian orthoreovirus escape from host translational shutoff correlates with stress granule disruption and is independent of eIF2alpha phosphorylation and PKR. J Virol 85:8798–8810
38. Holm GH, Zurney J, Tumilasci V, Leveille S, Danthi P, Hiscott J, Sherry B, Dermody TS (2007) Retinoic acid-inducible gene-I and interferon-beta promoter stimulator-1 augment proapoptotic responses following mammalian reovirus infection via interferon regulatory factor-3. J Biol Chem 282:21953–21961
39. Wessel Ø, Nyman IB, Markussen T, Dahle MK, Rimstad E (2015) Piscine orthoreovirus (PRV) σ3 protein binds dsRNA. Virus Res 198:22–29
40. Silverstein SC, Schur PH (1970) Immunofluorescent localization of double-stranded RNA in reovirus-infected cells. Virology 41:564–566
41. Kongtorp RT (2008) Heart and skeletal muscle inflammation (HSMI) in Atlantic salmon, *Salmo salar*: pathology, pathogenesis and experimental infection. PhD. Norwegian School of Veterinary Science, Oslo
42. Ahmed R, Fields BN (1982) Role of the S4 gene in the establishment of persistent reovirus infection in L cells. Cell 28:605–612
43. Ahmed R, Graham AF (1977) Persistent infections in L cells with temperature-sensitive mutants of reovirus. J Virol 23:250–262
44. Bell TM, Ross MG (1966) Persistent latent infection of human embryonic cells with reovirus type 3. Nature 212:412–414
45. Danis C, Mabrouk T, Garzon S, Lemay G (1993) Establishment of persistent reovirus infection in SC1 cells: absence of protein synthesis inhibition and increased level of double-stranded RNA-activated protein kinase. Virus Res 27:253–265
46. Wetzel JD, Chappell JD, Fogo AB, Dermody TS (1997) Efficiency of viral entry determines the capacity of murine erythroleukemia cells to support persistent infections by mammalian reoviruses. J Virol 71:299–306
47. Parmley RT (1988) Mammals. In: Rowley HM, Ratcliffe NA (ed) Vertebrate blood cells. Cambridge University Press, Cambridge, pp 337–424
48. Dermody TS, Nibert ML, Bassel-Duby R, Fields BN (1990) A σ1 region important for hemagglutination by serotype 3 reovirus strains. J Virol 64:5173–5176
49. Weiner HL, Ramig RF, Mustoe TA, Fields BN (1978) Identification of the gene coding for the hemagglutinin of reovirus. Virology 86:581–584
50. Sekhon SS, Beams HW (1969) Fine structure of the developing trout erythrocytes and thrombocytes with special reference to the marginal band and the cytoplasmic organelles. Am J Anat 125:353–373
51. Lane HC, Weaver JW, Benson JA, Nichols HA (1982) Some age related changes of adult rainbow trout, *Salmo gairdneri* Rich., peripheral erythrocytes separated by velocity sedimentation at unit gravity. J Fish Biol 21:1–14
52. Phillips MC, Moyes CD, Tufts BL (2000) The effects of cell ageing on metabolism in rainbow trout (*Oncorhynchus mykiss*) red blood cells. J Exp Biol 203:1039–1045
53. Piacentini SC, Rohovec JS, Fryer JL (1989) Epizootiology of erythrocytic inclusion body syndrome. J Aquat Anim Health 1:173–179
54. Rodger HD, Richards RH (1998) Observational study of erythrocytic inclusion bodies in farmed Atlantic salmon, *Salmo salar* L., in the British Isles. J Fish Dis 21:101–111
55. Arakawa CK, Hursh DA, Lannan CN, Rohovec JS, Winton JR (1989) Preliminary characterization of a virus causing infectious anemia among stocks of salmonid fish in the Western United States. In: Ahne W, Kurstak E (ed) Viruses of Lower Vertebrates. Springer, Berlin, pp 442–450
56. Staeheli P, Danielson P, Haller O, Sutcliffe JG (1986) Transcriptional activation of the mouse Mx gene by type I interferon. Mol Cell Biol 6:4770–4774
57. Jorgensen JB, Johansen A, Hegseth MN, Zou J, Robertsen B, Collet B, Secombes CJ (2007) A recombinant CHSE-214 cell line expressing an Mx1 promoter-reporter system responds to both interferon type I and type II from salmonids and represents a versatile tool to study the IFN-system in teleost fish. Fish Shellfish Immunol 23:1294–1303

8

Structural insight in the inhibition of adherence of F4 fimbriae producing enterotoxigenic *Escherichia coli* by llama single domain antibodies

Kristof Moonens[1,2†], Imke Van den Broeck[1,2†], Emmanuel Okello[1,2,3], Els Pardon[2], Maia De Kerpel[1,2], Han Remaut[1,2] and Henri De Greve[1,2*]

Abstract

Enterotoxigenic *Escherichia coli* that cause neonatal and post-weaning diarrhea in piglets express F4 fimbriae to mediate attachment towards host receptors. Recently we described how llama single domain antibodies (VHHs) fused to IgA, produced in *Arabidopsis thaliana* seeds and fed to piglets resulted in a progressive decline in shedding of F4 positive ETEC bacteria. Here we present the structures of these inhibiting VHHs in complex with the major adhesive subunit FaeG. A conserved surface, distant from the lactose binding pocket, is targeted by these VHHs, highlighting the possibility of targeting epitopes on single-domain adhesins that are non-involved in receptor binding.

Introduction, methods and results

F4 fimbriae are expressed on the cell surface of enterotoxigenic *E. coli* (ETEC) to mediate attachment towards carbohydrate receptors localized on the enterocytes of piglets [1]. ETEC strains are responsible for significant death and morbidity in neonatal and post-weaned piglets by causing severe, watery diarrhea [2], resulting worldwide in severe economic losses in pig industry. Clinical symptoms are generated by the action of enterotoxins: the heat-labile enterotoxin (LT) and/or two unrelated heat-stable enterotoxins (STa and STb) [3]. F4 fimbriae are assembled by the conserved chaperone-usher pathway [4] and composed out of a major adhesive subunit FaeG, resulting in the exposure of many hundreds consecutive binding surfaces along the flexible F4 fimbrial structure. In the final quaternary structure fimbrial subunits complement the incomplete immunoglobulin-like fold of one another by donating an N-terminal donor strand *in trans* to the preceding subunit [4]. Three naturally occurring serological variants of F4 fimbriae ($F4_{ab}$, $F4_{ac}$ and $F4_{ad}$) exist that differ in the primary sequence of FaeG, with each variant featuring a related but yet different binding and hemagglutination profile [5,6]. The FaeG structure was earlier determined and shows a conserved immunoglobulin-like fold, typical for fimbrial subunits, on which a subdomain comprising two short β-strands and two α-helices is grafted [7]. Most of the variability is localized on and around this additional subdomain and recently we elucidated the co-complex structure between $FaeG_{ad}$ and lactose (Moonens *et al.*, under review), demonstrating the glycan ligand is interacting in a binding site located on the additional subdomain. A commercial vaccine containing F4 fimbriae is currently available on the market and provides maternal passive immunity against *E. coli* induced neonatal diarrhea [8]. To this date no commercial vaccine or prevention strategy against post-weaning diarrhea caused by F4 fimbriated ETEC is yet available. Within our research group anti-ETEC antibodies were generated by fusing four different variable domains of llama heavy chain-only antibodies (V1-4), raised against $FaeG_{ntd/dsc,\ ac}$ and panned against all three $FaeG_{ntd/dsc}$ variants (first variant ac, than ad and finally ab), to the Fc domain of a porcine immunoglobulin IgA. The resulting four VHH-IgA constructs were subsequently expressed in *Arabidopsis thaliana* seeds and fed to piglets [9]. The oral feed-based passive immunization strategy protected piglets as demonstrated by the progressive decline in shedding of F4 positive ETEC bacteria, the significantly lower

* Correspondence: hdegreve@vub.ac.be
†Equal contributors
[1]Structural & Molecular Microbiology, Structural Biology Research Center, VIB, Brussels, Belgium
[2]Structural Biology Brussels, Vrije Universiteit Brussel, Pleinlaan 2, 1050 Brussels, Belgium
Full list of author information is available at the end of the article

immune responses of the piglets to F4 fimbriae which suggest a reduced exposure to the ETEC pathogen, and a significantly higher body weight in comparison with control piglets [9]. It was demonstrated as well that seed extracts containing VHH-IgA antibodies could inhibit the attachment of F4 positive ETEC strains to porcine gut villous enterocytes in vitro [9].

Using X-ray crystallography we investigated the mechanism of action of the isolated VHHs that inhibit the F4 fimbriae-mediated binding. Stable self-complementing FaeG constructs of all three variants ($FaeG_{ab}$, $FaeG_{ac}$ and $FaeG_{ad}$), in which the N-terminal donor strand was swapped to the C-terminus via a short tetrapeptide DNKQ linker, were expressed and purified as described earlier [10]. Complexes between the different purified VHHs [11] and the self-complementing variants of FaeG were produced by incubating them together with excess VHH and separating the complex by size exclusion chromatography. Crystals were obtained for the complexes of $FaeG_{ac}$-V1, $FaeG_{ac}$-V2 and $FaeG_{ad}$-V3 in respectively condition A10 of the Clear Strategy Screen I HTS-96 (Molecular Dimensions), C4 of the JBScreen Basic HTS (Jena Bioscience) and E12 of the Morpheus Screen HT-96 (Molecular Dimensions) using the sitting drop damp diffusion method. Diffraction data were indexed using XDS [12] (Table 1) and further prepared and scaled using respectively Pointless and Scala [13]. The phase problem was solved with the molecular replacement method by Phaser [13] with the coordinates of the self-complementing $FaeG_{ad}$ (PDB identifier 3HLR) and a llama single domain antibody as search models. The resulting models of the co-complexes were further improved by manually building in the molecular graphics program COOT [14] and refined using Refmac5.5 [13] (Table 1). All three inhibitory VHHs interact with conserved epitopes on the FaeG surface (Figure 1A). V1 and V2 interact with nearly similar epitopes constituted of residues of the conserved immunoglobulin-like core domain and

Table 1 Crystal parameters and data processing statistics

Complex	$FaeG_{ac}$-V1	$FaeG_{ac}$-V2	$FaeG_{ad}$-V3
Wavelength	0.98	0.98	0.98
Beamline	Soleil - Proxima 1	Soleil - Proxima 1	Diamond - IO3
Space group	P 3 2 1	P 3 2 1	$P\ 2\ 2_1\ 2_1$
a, b, c (Å)	145.5, 145.5, 38.9	145.8, 145.8, 37.9	79.8, 95.2, 113
α, β, γ (°)	90, 90, 120	90, 90, 120	90, 90, 90
Resolution (Å)	47.62 – 1.55 (1.63 – 1.55)	47.74 - 1.89 (2.0 - 1.89)	29.54 – 2.61 (2.67 – 2.61)
R_{meas} (%)^{a,b}	4.9 (56.9)	12.3 (198.4)	10.5 (117)
No. of unique reflections^{b}	68481 (9923)	36784 (5212)	26553 (1559)
Average I/σI	24.8 (4.2)	14.3 (1.4)	16.1 (1.1)
CC (1/2)	100 (92.2)	99.9 (79.6)	99.8 (49)
Multiplicity^{b}	11.2 (10.9)	20.2 (19.3)	10.6 (3.8)
Completeness (%)^{b}	99.9 (99.0)	99.7 (97.7)	98.3 (79.6)
Wilson B-factor	24.9	35.6	63.4
R_{work}/R_{free}(%)$^{c,\ d}$	16.9/19.3	18.9/22.7	20.5/24.5
Average B-factor (Å^2)	20.2	28.3	35.7
R.m.s. deviations			
Bond lengths (Å)	0.026	0.021	0.012
Bond angles (°)	2.715	2.150	1.607
No. Atoms (except H)			
Protein	2778	2752	5293
Water	305	105	29
Residues in allowed regions	100	98.6	98.7
(%) of Ramachandran plot			
PDB entry	4WEM	4WEN	4WEU

$^{a}R_{meas} = \Sigma h\ (nh/nh\text{-}1)\ \Sigma I\ |Ihl - < Ih > |/\ \Sigma h\ \Sigma I < Ih>$, where *nh* = the number of observations for reflection **h**,Ihl = the intensity for observation **I** of reflection **h**, and < Ih > = the average intensity for reflection **h**.
[b]Statistics for outer resolution shell are given in parenthesis.
$^{c}R_{work} = \Sigma hkl\ ||Fobs| - |Fcalc|| / \Sigma hkl\ |Fobs|$.
$^{d}R_{free}$ is defined as above but calculated for 5% of randomly chosen reflections that were excluded from the refinement.

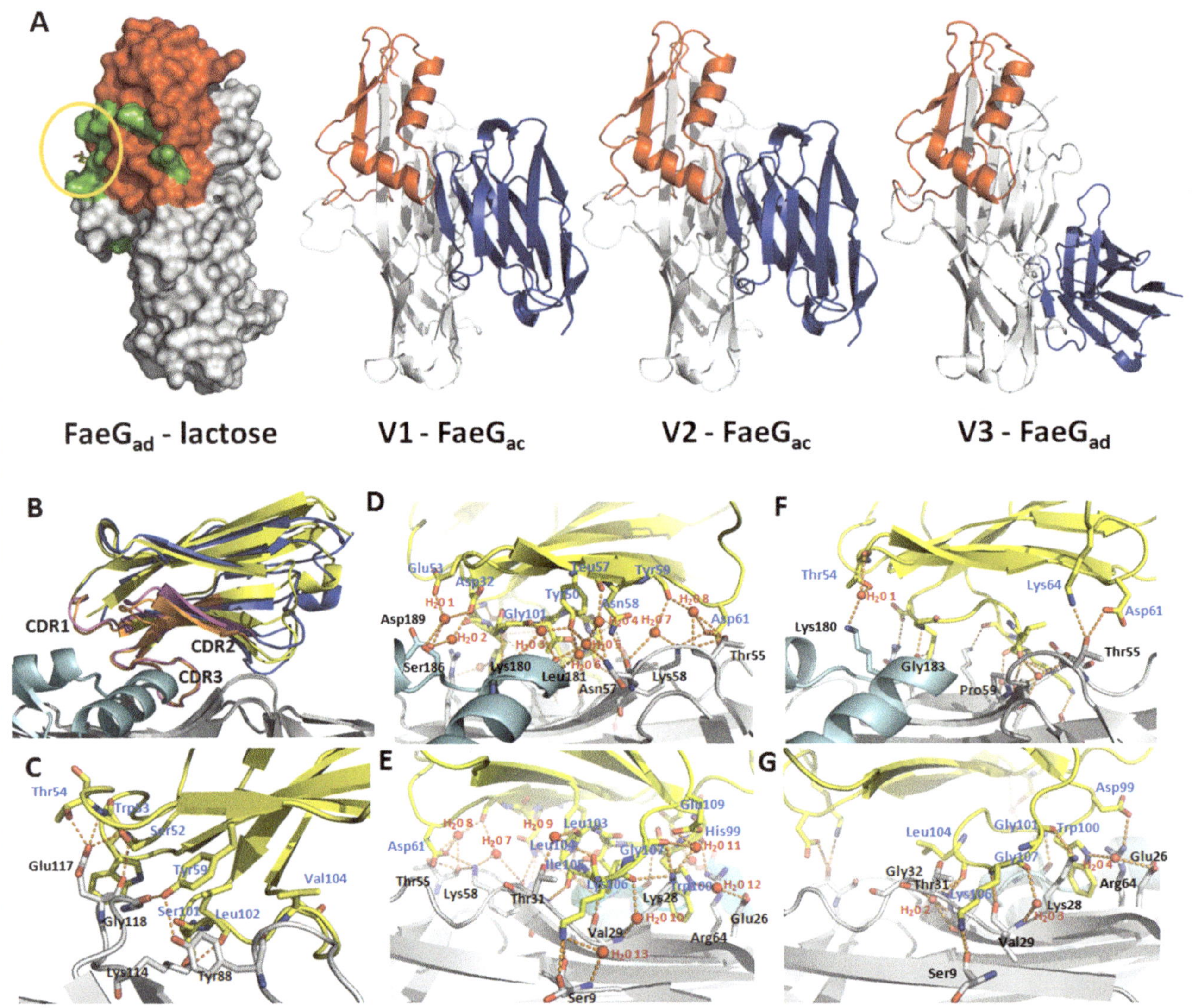

Figure 1 Crystal structures of inhibitory VHHs in complex with the major adhesive subunit FaeG. (A) From left to right, molecular surface representation of the structure of FaeG$_{ad}$ in complex with lactose (stick representation), co-complex structure of V1 with FaeG$_{ac}$, co-complex structure of V2 with FaeG$_{ac}$ and finally the co-complex structure between V3 and FaeG$_{ad}$. The orientation of FaeG in each panel is identical, the additional binding domain grafted onto the FaeG immunoglobulin-like core is colored red and the VHH in the last three panels is colored in blue. Variation between the different FaeG variants is colored on the molecular surface of FaeG$_{ad}$ in green. The lactose binding site on the surface of FaeG$_{ad}$ is indicated by a yellow circle for clarity. **(B)** Comparison of the binding conformation of V1 (yellow) and V2 (blue). The different CDR regions of the VHHs are indicated and colored in orange (V1) and purple (V2). In V2 the CDR2 is shifted upwards and located at a further distance from the FaeG surface, whereas the conformation of the CDR3 is near identically traced. **(C)** Close-up on the interactions formed in the complex between V3 and FaeG$_{ad}$. **(D-G)** Interactions formed between V1 and FaeG$_{ac}$ **(D,E)** and V2 and FaeG$_{ac}$ **(F,G)** in different orientations. In each panel FaeG is colored gray and the additional variable subdomain in cyan. VHHs are depicted in yellow and water molecules are represented as red spheres. Interacting residues of the VHH and FaeG adhesin are labeled respectively blue and black and shown as stick model with nitrogen atoms colored blue and oxygen atoms in red. Hydrogen bonds are depicted as orange dashed lines.

conserved residues of the additional variable subdomains (Figure 1A). V3, in contrast, is only interacting with a patch of amino acids located on the Ig-like conserved core domain (Figure 1A). The heavy chain-only antibodies V3 and V4 only differ in one amino acid substitution (Lys 100 Arg), and analysis of the crystal structure of V3 in complex with FaeG$_{ac}$ revealed Lys100 is not involved in any stabilizing interactions. When comparing the structures of the FaeG-VHH complexes with the recently determined FaeG$_{ad}$-lactose structure (Moonens et al., under review) it is obvious that the binding of the different VHHs onto FaeG$_{ad}$ does not target the lactose binding site and hence the F4$_{ad}$ fimbriae are not obstructed in their carbohydrate binding capability (Figure 1A). All VHHs are targeting conserved patches on FaeG, and since the specificity of the different FaeG variants has been localized on the additional binding domain [15] we can conclude that the inhibitory mechanism of the VHHs is not governed by directly interfering with the carbohydrate binding site.

The strength of the interaction between the different VHHs and FaeG variants was determined using surface plasmon resonance (Figure 2). The surface of a CM5 sensor chip (GE Health Care) was activated, the different VHHs immobilized on flow channel 2 via primary amine groups and finally residual unreacted active ester groups were deactivated, all according to manufacturer's protocol. As a control, flow channel 1 was as well activated and deactivated. The different FaeG variants were flowed over the chip surface in a two-fold dilution series in HBS buffer (10 mM HEPES, 150 mM NaCl, 1 mM EDTA, 0.005% Tween20, pH 7.4) at a flow rate of 10 μL/min at 25°C. The obtained sensorgrams of the subtracted (Fc2 - Fc1) signals were fitted using a Langmuir binding isotherm with a 1:1 stoichiometry, from which the kinetic rate constants k_a and k_d were obtained (BIAeval software; Biacore AB). Affinities varied from low μM for V1 and V3, to high nM for V2 (Figure 2B). These experimentally determined affinities differ significantly from the low nM dissociation constants by which VHHs typically recognize their target antigens [16,17]. This discrepancy may arise because of the VHH selection procedure. The earlier described anti-FaeG VHHs were selected consecutively against all three FaeG variants and instead of selecting binders that demonstrated the highest affinity towards only one FaeG variant, most likely VHHs with moderate affinity against all three variants were obtained during the selection procedure. Even amongst the conserved surfaces of the different FaeG variants small structural perturbations are observed. A panning procedure selecting binders against all FaeG variants would select VHHs interacting with an averaged FaeG structure, but not necessarily with high affinity.

A

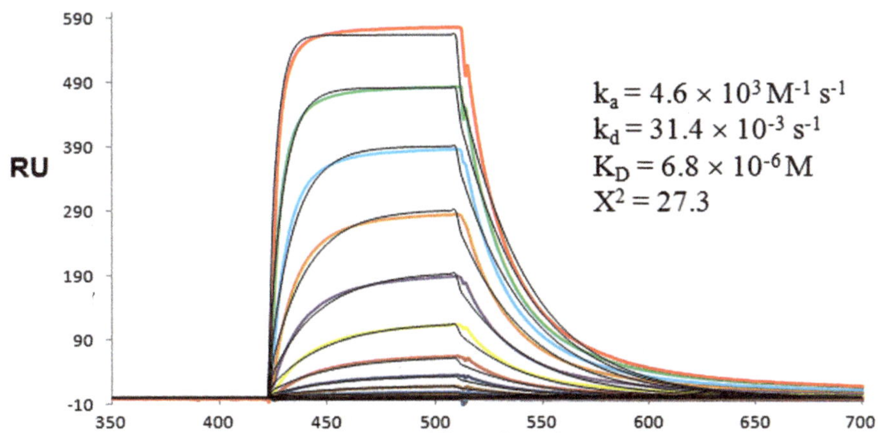

B

	FaeG variant	k_a ($s^{-1}M^{-1}$)	k_d (s^{-1})	K_A (M^{-1})	K_D (M)	Chi^2
V1	ab	2.8×10^3	7.8×10^{-3}	3.6×10^5	2.8×10^{-6}	60.4
	ac	4.6×10^3	31.4×10^{-3}	1.4×10^5	6.8×10^{-6}	27.3
	ad	2.2×10^3	5.2×10^{-3}	4.3×10^5	2.3×10^{-6}	48.7
V2	ab	16.8×10^3	1.1×10^{-3}	15.0×10^5	0.1×10^{-6}	115
	ac	14.0×10^3	1.4×10^{-3}	9.9×10^5	0.1×10^{-6}	34.5
	ad	3.0×10^3	1.4×10^{-3}	2.2×10^5	0.5×10^{-6}	96.4
V3	ab	0.4×10^3	2.1×10^{-3}	1.8×10^5	5.5×10^{-6}	168.0
	ac	4.7×10^3	36.5×10^{-3}	1.3×10^5	7.7×10^{-6}	49.4
	ad	52.5×10^3	301.0×10^{-3}	1.7×10^5	5.7×10^{-6}	91.0

Figure 2 Interaction between inhibitory VHHs and the different FaeG variants. (A) Typical set of sensorgrams obtained when assaying the interaction between inhibitory VHHs and FaeG (here depicted is the interaction between V1 and FaeG variant ac). Sensorgrams were obtained by injecting varying concentrations of FaeG (50 μM to 1.5 nM) over covalently immobilized VHHs. The curves were fitted using a 1:1 Langmuir binding model. Fitted curves are shown in black, while the original data is represented by the colored curves. **(B)** Overview on the association (k_a) and dissociation (k_d) rate constants, and association (K_A)/dissociation (K_D) constants of the interaction between the different VHHs and FaeG variants.

The detailed interactions between the inhibitory VHHs and the major adhesive subunit FaeG of F4 fimbriae are shown in Figure 1B-G. The interaction between V3 and $FaeG_{ad}$ is mediated mainly by direct hydrogen bonds between the amino acid stretches Ser52-Thr54, Tyr59 and Ser101-Val104 of V3, that correspond with respectively the complementarity determining regions CDR2 and CDR3, with the amino acid residues Tyr88, Lys114 and Glu117-Gly118 from $FaeG_{ad}$ (Figure 1C). Since V1 and V2 are targeting overlapping epitopes, we superimposed the two structures of V1-$FaeG_{ac}$ and V2-$FaeG_{ac}$. The two VHHs are directed in an identical orientation to interact with the FaeG adhesin (Figure 1A). Only the conformation of the CDR2 is significantly altered and is more distant from the FaeG molecular surface in the V2-$FaeG_{ac}$ co-complex structure (Figure 1B). In the V1-$FaeG_{ac}$ structure a large amount of water molecules, eight in total, are observed in the interaction interface formed by the CDR2 region and those are all involved in inter molecular hydrogen bond formation between V1 and $FaeG_{ac}$ (Figure 1D). In addition, only four direct hydrogen bonds are formed between the $FaeG_{ac}$ and CDR2 of V1 (Figure 1D). In contrast, the V2-$FaeG_{ac}$ co-complex structure in the same interface exhibits only one water molecule and three direct hydrogen bond interactions (Figure 1F). As there is no sequence conservation between the CDR2s of V1 (SEG**G**ILN) and V2 (TNT**G**VTE) this difference in binding mode is not so surprising. The VHH-FaeG interaction surface on the other side is bordered by the CDR3 region that is nearly conserved amongst V1 (**AA**SH**WGTLLIKGI**E**H**) and V2 (**AA**TD**WGTLLIKGI**D**H**). Again more water molecules are observed in the interaction interface between V1-$FaeG_{ac}$ compared to V2-$FaeG_{ac}$ (5 versus 3 water molecules); however more direct interactions (6 direct hydrogen bonds) are formed in both complexes (Figures 1E and G). Unexpectedly although in the V1-$FaeG_{ac}$ complex many more direct and indirect interactions are formed the affinity between V1 and $FaeG_{ac}$ is 70 times lower compared to the affinity of V2 for $FaeG_{ac}$ (Figure 2B). The inclusion of more water molecules in the V1-$FaeG_{ac}$ complex binding interface might have an unfavorable effect on the interaction, thereby reducing affinity.

Discussion

Crosslinking of bacteria by antibodies, like for example in *Vibrio cholera* [18] and *Streptococcus mutans* that causes dental carries [19], has been shown to be important for mediating protection. In contrast the neutralizing activity of polyclonal IgM in the attachment of influenza virus to

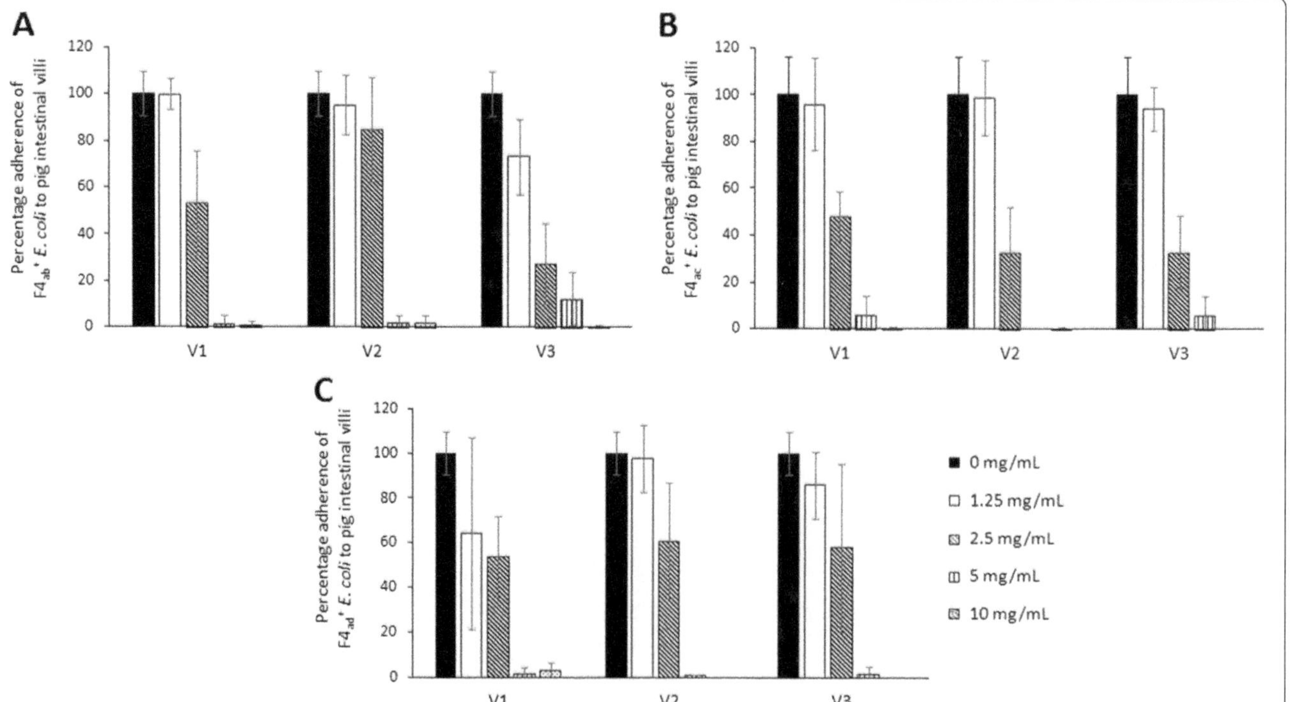

Figure 3 VHH inhibition of the adherence of F4 fimbriated *E. coli* to piglet enterocytes *in vitro*. Quantitative analysis of bacterial adherence to piglet enterocytes of strains expressing $F4_{ab}$ **(A)**, $F4_{ac}$ **(B)** and $F4_{ad}$ **(C)** fimbriae. A two-fold dilution series of monomeric VHHs was added to 4×10^8 $F4^+$ cells and incubated during one hour with an average of 50 villi. Villi were examined by phase-contrast microscopy at a magnification of 600x and the number of bacterial cells adhering to 250 μm villi length (5 repeated reads for each test sample) were counted and plotted as a percentage of wild type binding.

target cells is due to steric hindrance [20]. When the four VHHs were covalently coated on magnetic beads, specific agglutination with the three variants of $F4^+$ bacteria was observed [9]. In a hemagglutination based assay purified monovalent VHH were unable to inhibit the interaction of guinea red blood cells and F4 fimbriated bacteria (results not shown). However, in an in vitro adherence assay the VHHs were able to prevent the attachment of F4 fimbriated bacteria to piglet enterocytes (Figure 3). The inhibition of adherence by VHHs was fully reversible by the addition of monomeric FaeG, demonstrating the specificity of the VHHs. Concentrations of VHH were identical in both experiments and these results indicate the VHHs are able to abrogate binding towards enterocyte based receptors but cannot prevent the cross-linking of red blood cells by F4 fimbriated bacteria. With crystallographic evidence we demonstrated the different VHHs contact conserved patches on the FaeG surface that are non-involved in carbohydrate binding. We conclude the mechanism of inhibition is mostly attributed to steric hindrance of the interaction between F4 fimbriae and enterocyte based receptors and to a lesser extent cross linking of F4 expressing bacterial cells.

VHHs possess a range of advantages compared to more commonly employed prophylactic treatments. They recognize their target antigen often with high affinity, whereas organic compounds often require several intensive rounds of structure-based chemical optimization to attain a reasonable binding affinity. However in this study the measured affinity of anti-F4 VHHs was relatively weak, probably due to the VHH panning procedure that selected out reasonable binders against all three FaeG variants. The binding site interface contains many water molecules, a peculiar binding mode that potentially could facilitate recognition and interaction with all three FaeG variants but at the cost of affinity. Since the receptor binding subdomain is highly variable, during the selection rounds VHHs interacting at a conserved surface will be selected since they recognize all three variants. However more often anti-adhesives target the carbohydrate binding site to efficiently prevent the interaction between the bacterial cell and host receptors [21]. In future this understanding will help to further enhance the prophylaxis treatment against F4 fimbriated ETEC by selecting specific VHHs with increased affinity and inhibitory capacity by selecting them against the carbohydrate binding site and against solely one FaeG variant at a time. Recently we could completely inhibit the in vitro attachment of F18 fimbriae positive *E. coli* to piglet enterocytes by raising VHHs against the carbohydrate binding site of the F18 fimbrial adhesin FedF [22]. Krüger et al. demonstrated single-chain Fv (scFv) antibody fragment expressing lactobacilli could markedly reduce the *Streptococcus mutans* bacteria counts and caries scores in a rat model [23]. Likewise, expression of VHHs on lactobacilli can provide an alternative approach for in vivo passive immunity against F4 fimbriated ETEC. Nevertheless, although the selected VHHs (V1, V2, V3 and V4) against the three F4 variants do not exhibit a high affinity and target mainly the conserved immunoglobulin-like core domain of the FaeG subunit variants, they are protecting weaned piglets against infection by F4 positive ETEC strains regardless of the F4 variant that is expressed by the ETEC strain.

Competing interests

The authors declare that they have no competing interests.

Authors' contributions

HDG conceived the study. EP isolated the single domain antibodies (VHHs) from an immunized llama. KM, MDK and IVDB purified the anti-FaeG VHHs and the FaeG self-complementing subunit variants, isolated the complexes and performed the crystallizations. IVDB and KM obtained the diffraction data and solved the structures. KM and IVDB performed the surface plasmon resonance. EO performed the in vitro adherence assay. KM, IVDB, HR and HDG interpreted the results and wrote the manuscript. All authors read and approved the final manuscript.

Acknowledgements

K.M. was a doctoral fellow of the Fonds voor Wetenschappelijk Onderzoek (FWO) – Vlaanderen. H.R. is supported by a VIB Young PI project grant and the Odysseus program of the FWO-Vlaanderen. E.P. is supported by grant 7/40 of the Interuniversity Attraction Poles (IAP) Program of the Belgian Science Policy Office. E.O. received a PhD fellowship of VLIR-UOS. This research was granted by FWO project G030411N and equipment grant UABR/09/005 from the Hercules Foundation. We are grateful to the beamline staff of Proxima1 (Soleil, France) and (Diamond, Oxfordshire, UK) for support with data collection and processing.

Author details

[1]Structural & Molecular Microbiology, Structural Biology Research Center, VIB, Brussels, Belgium. [2]Structural Biology Brussels, Vrije Universiteit Brussel, Pleinlaan 2, 1050 Brussels, Belgium. [3]College of Veterinary Medicine, Animal Resources and Bio-security, Makerere University, P.O. Box 7062, Kampala, Uganda.

References

1. Fairbrother JM, Nadeau E, Gyles CL (2005) *Escherichia coli* in postweaning diarrhea in pigs: an update on bacterial types, pathogenesis, and prevention strategies. Anim Health Res Rev 6:17–39
2. Nagy B, Fekete PZ (1999) Enterotoxigenic *Escherichia coli* (ETEC) in farm animals. Vet Res 30:259–284
3. Nagy B, Fekete PZ (2005) Enterotoxigenic *Escherichia coli* in veterinary medicine. Int J Med Microbiol 295:443–454
4. Busch A, Waksman G (2012) Chaperone-usher pathways: diversity and pilus assembly mechanism. Philos Trans R Soc Lond B Biol Sci 367:1112–1122
5. Orskov I, Orskov F, Sojka WJ, Wittig W (1964) K antigens K88ab(L) and K88ac (L) in *E. coli*. A new O antigen: 0147 and a new K antigen: K89(B). Acta Pathol Microbiol Scand 62:439–447
6. Guinée PA, Jansen WH (1979) Behavior of *Escherichia coli* K antigens K88ab, K88ac, and K88ad in immunoelectrophoresis, double diffusion, and hemagglutination. Infect Immun 23:700–705
7. Van Molle I, Joensuu JJ, Buts L, Panjikar S, Kotiaho M, Bouckaert J, Wyns L, Niklander-Teeri V, De Greve H (2007) Chloroplasts assemble the major subunit FaeG of *Escherichia coli* F4 (K88) fimbriae to strand-swapped dimers. J Mol Biol 368:791–799
8. Hur J, Lee JH (2012) Comparative evaluation of a vaccine candidate expressing enterotoxigenic *Escherichia coli* (ETEC) adhesins for colibacillosis with a commercial vaccine using a pig model. Vaccine 30:3829–3833
9. Virdi V, Coddens A, De Buck S, Millet S, Goddeeris BM, Cox E, De Greve H, Depicker A (2013) Orally fed seeds producing designer IgAs protect weaned

piglets against enterotoxigenic *Escherichia coli* infection. Proc Natl Acad Sci U S A 110:11809–11814

10. Van Molle I, Moonens K, Garcia-Pino A, Buts L, De Kerpel M, Wyns L, Bouckaert J, De Greve H (2009) Structural and thermodynamic characterization of pre- and postpolymerization states in the F4 fimbrial subunit FaeG. J Mol Biol 394:957–967
11. Pardon E, Laeremans T, Triest S, Rasmussen SG, Wohlkönig A, Ruf A, Muyldermans S, Hol WG, Kobilka BK, Steyaert J (2014) A general protocol for the generation of nanobodies for structural biology. Nat Protoc 9:674–693
12. Kabsch W (2010) XDS. Acta Crystallogr D Biol Crystallogr 66:125–132
13. Collaborative Computational Project Nm (1994) The CCP4 suite: programs for protein crystallography. Acta Crystallogr D Biol Crystallogr 50:760–763
14. Emsley P, Cowtan K (2004) Coot: model-building tools for molecular graphics. Acta Crystallogr D Biol Crystallogr 60:2126–2132
15. Zhang W, Fang Y, Francis DH (2009) Characterization of the binding specificity of K88ac and K88ad fimbriae of enterotoxigenic *Escherichia coli* by constructing K88ac/K88ad chimeric FaeG major subunits. Infect Immun 77:699–706
16. Lo AW, Moonens K, De Kerpel M, Brys L, Pardon E, Remaut H, De Greve H (2014) The molecular mechanism of Shiga toxin Stx2e neutralization by a single-domain antibody targeting the cell receptor-binding domain. J Biol Chem 289:25374–25381
17. Muyldermans S (2013) Nanobodies: natural single-domain antibodies. Annu Rev Biochem 82:775–797
18. Corthésy B, Spertini F (1999) Secretory immunoglobulin A: from mucosal protection to vaccine development. Biol Chem 380:1251–1262
19. Ma JK, Hunjan M, Smith R, Kelly C, Lehner T (1990) An investigation into the mechanism of protection by local passive immunization with monoclonal antibodies against *Streptococcus mutans*. Infect Immun 58:3407–3414
20. Outlaw MC, Dimmock NJ (1990) Mechanisms of neutralization of influenza virus on mouse tracheal epithelial cells by mouse monoclonal polymeric IgA and polyclonal IgM directed against the viral haemagglutinin. J Gen Virol 71:69–76
21. Lo AW, Moonens K, Remaut H (2013) Chemical attenuation of pilus function and assembly in Gram-negative bacteria. Curr Opin Microbiol 16:85–92
22. Moonens K, De Kerpel M, Coddens A, Cox E, Pardon E, Remaut H, De Greve H (2014) Nanobody mediated inhibition of attachment of F18 fimbriae expressing *Escherichia coli*. PLoS One 9:e114691
23. Krüger C, Hu Y, Pan Q, Marcotte H, Hultberg A, Delwar D, van Dalen PJ, Pouwels PH, Leer RJ, Kelly CG, van Dollenweerd C, Ma JK, Hammarström L (2002) In situ delivery of passive immunity by *lactobacilli* producing single-chain antibodies. Nat Biotechnol 20:702–706

9

Tritrichomonas foetus infection, a cause of chronic diarrhea in the domestic cat

Chaoqun Yao[1,3*] and Liza S Köster[2,3]

Abstract

Tritrichomonas foetus is a very intriguing trichomonad protozoan with respect to its varied choice of residence in the different host species. It is an obligate parasite of the reproductive and the gastrointestinal tract of bovine and feline host respectively, leading to trichomonosis. Bovine trichomonosis is a sexually transmitted disease whereas feline trichomonosis is a disease with a purported fecal-oral route of spread. Further, the trichomonad is a commensal in the nasal passages, stomach, cecum and colon of swine host. Advances have been exponential in understanding the trichomonad biology and specifically feline trichomonosis since late 1990s and early 2000s when *T. foetus* was soundly determined to be a causative agent of chronic diarrhea in the domestic cat. It is a challenging task, even for a skilled investigator not to mention the busy clinical veterinarian, to keep up with the vast volume of information. Here we comprehensively reviewed the trichomonad biology, clinical manifestations, pathogenesis, host immunity, world map of distribution, risk factors, diagnosis and treatment. Risk factors associated with *T. foetus*-positive status in the domestic cat include young age, purebred, history of diarrhea, co-infections with other enteral pathogens. In addition, molecular similarity of bovine and feline isolates of *T. foetus* in DNA sequence was concisely discussed. The data presented serve as an information source for veterinarians, and investigators who are interested in biology of *T. foetus* and feline trichomonosis.

Table of contents

* Correspondence: chyao@rossvet.edu.kn
[1]Department of Biomedical Sciences, Ross University School of Veterinary Medicine, P.O. Box 334, Basseterre, St. Kitts, West Indies
[3]One Health Center for Zoonoses and Tropical Veterinary Medicine, Ross University School of Veterinary Medicine, P.O. Box 334, Basseterre, St. Kitts, West Indies
Full list of author information is available at the end of the article

1. Introduction

The genus *Tritrichomonas* belongs to the family Trichomonadidae. Among a few species of veterinary importance in the genus is *Tritrichomonas foetus. Tritrichomonas foetus* is fascinating both biologically and in its clinical manifestations in addition to being occasionally diagnosed in immunocompromised human beings [1]. It resides in the urogenital tract of cattle and causes bovine trichomonosis, a sexually transmitted disease with no approved treatment, throughout many geographic regions worldwide (bovine isolate) [2]. The same trichomonad species was soundly confirmed in 2003 to be the causative agent of chronic diarrhea in the domestic cat (feline isolate) [3,4] although the discovery of protozoan in these animals was made decades ago, as early as in 1928 [5]. Similar to other trichomonads such as human parasite *Trichomonas vaginalis*, *T. foetus* has only trophozoite stage although a pseudocyst stage is described [6-9]. Trophozoites reproduce asexually by longitudinal binary fission; no sexual reproduction has been ever discovered. They are pear- or spindle-shaped with three anterior flagella and one posterior flagellum. An undulating membrane extends along the whole length of the body and emerges as the posterior flagellum. The axostyle extends to the length of the cell and usually projects posteriorly. The size approximates 10-25 μm in length and 3-15 μm in width (Figure 1).

Tritrichomonas foetus has been a topic of review, especially on the clinical aspects of feline trichomonosis [10-15]. The major purpose of the current manuscript is to comprehensively review trichomonad biology, geographic distributions with compiling a world map of distribution, risk factors, host immunity and pathogenesis of the feline isolate. Of course it would not be complete without briefly going over clinical signs, diagnosis, treatment and prognosis of feline trichomonosis.

2. Molecular studies

Feline isolates found in the gastrointestinal (GI) tract of the domestic cat and bovine isolates in the urogenital tract of cattle are morphologically indistinguishable. An identity of 100% has been found within each of both feline and bovine isolates among more than 5000 base pair (bp) at 11 loci by DNA sequencing [16-19]. Nevertheless, there are minor, but consistent differences among these loci, ranging from 0.3% of internal transcribed spacer (ITS) and cysteine protease (CP) 7 and 8 to 1.9% of CP6 gene [16-19] (see Table 1 for details of each locus). Lately, 0.7% difference were found among eight protease inhibitors covering a total of 4674 bp, with individual sequence length ranging from 297 to 1145 bp by a transcriptomical approach. Further, CP8 and CP7 were the most transcribed gene in bovine and feline isolate, respectively [20]. Based on the molecular sequence differences along with disparity of experimental cross-infections and divergence in pathogenicity Walden et al. proposed a new name for the feline isolate. They named it *T. blagburni*, a new trichomonad species [21]. However, these authors did not show a clear separation of feline from bovine isolate, a requirement for naming a new species. The new nomenclature, if holding up, still waits to be accepted, which may take a while, especially among veterinarians. Nevertheless, comparative transcriptomics revealed near identical functional category distribution of expressed genes with no indication of molecular level divergence, which strongly suggested feline and bovine isolates were taxonomically two isolates of one species [20]. It is not our intension, nor the scope of this manuscript deals with such a debate on taxonomical status of the pathogen causing chronic diarrhea in the domestic cat. Consequently, the name of *T. foetus* is kept in the current review as well as in the title referring the feline isolate unless otherwise stated in order to be consistent with literature and to avoid confusion among readers.

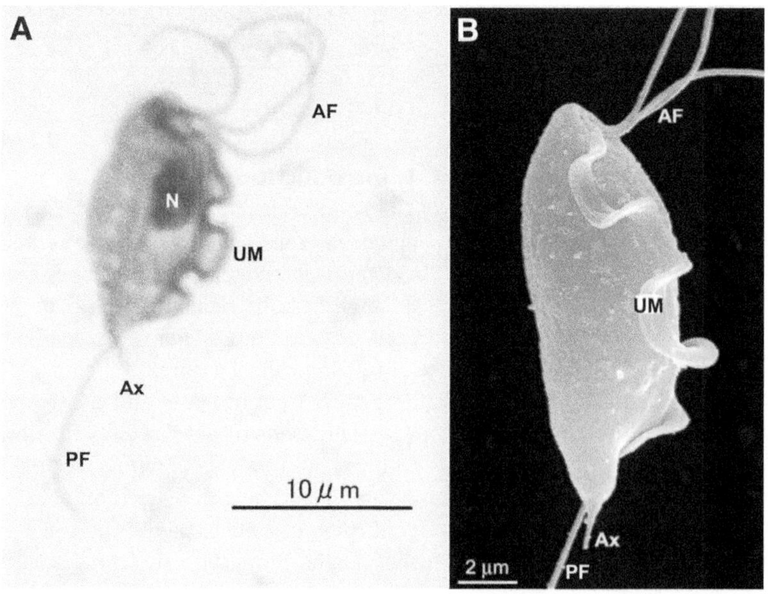

Figure 1 ***Tritrichomonas foetus*** **trophozoites. A**: Giemsa-stain. **B**: scanning electron microscopy. AF: anterior flagella; Ax: axostyle; N: nucleus; PF: posterior flagellum; UM: undulating membrane. A and B: reproduced from Figure 1 of Doi et al. ([80]) and Figure 1b of Midlej et al. [81], respectively, with permission.

Table 1 Genetic similarity in percentage (%) between feline isolates and bovine isolates of *Tritrichomonas foetus*

	Bovine isolates*														
Feline isolates[#]	**ITS (2)**	**ITS-2 (10)**	**EF-1α (10)**	**CP8 (2)**	**CP1 (8)**	**CP2 (8)**	**CP4 (8)**	**CP5 (8)**	**CP6 (8)**	**CP7 (8)**	**CP8 (8)**	**CP9 (8)**	**MDH1 (8)**	**ITS1 + 2 (8)**	**Refs**
ITS (4, 327)	99.7														[17]
ITS-2 (4, 368)		99.7													[16]
EF-1α (4, 783)			99.4												[16]
CP8 (4, 663)				99.7											[19]
CP1 (7, 503)					99.4										[18]
CP2 (7, 669)						96.7									[18]
CP4 (7, 273)							99.3								[18]
CP5 (7, 361)								99.2							[18]
CP6 (7, 318)									98.1						[18]
CP7 (7, 373)										99.7					[18]
CP8 (7, 907)											99.4				[18]
CP9 (7, 289)												99.3			[18]
MDH1 (7, 562)													99.6		[18]
ITS1 + 2 (7, 297)														99.7	[18]

CP, cysteine protease; MDH, malate dehydrogenase; ITS, internal transcribed spacer; EL, elongation factor.
*number of cattle isolates.
[#]first number - number of cat isolates; second number - length of sequence in base pair (bp).

In addition it is worth briefly describing another trichomonad, *T. suis*. The latter localizes at the nasal passages, stomach, cecum and colon of the domestic pig, and is morphologically indistinguishable from *T. foetus*. No differences have been found between *T. suis* and *T. foetus* bovine isolates at the molecular level such as random amplified polymorphic DNA (RAPD) [22-24], restriction fragment length polymorphism (RFLP) [24], and ITS-1 - 5.8S-rRNA - ITS-2 sequences [25,26]. Consequently they have been suggested synonyms, i.e. the same species [24,27]. Further sequence analysis of more than 5000 bp at 11 loci reveals 100% identity in all loci except elongation factor (EL)-1α and CP8 with 99.4% and 99.7%, respectively (Table 2). Together these molecular data confirm that *T. suis* and *T. foetus* bovine isolate are the same species, which makes *T. foetus* even more fascinating.

3. Survival of trophozoites in the environment and possible transmission route

Tritrichomonas foetus like many other trichomonad protozoa has only trophozoites stage. Under the experimental conditions four pathogen-free and four *Cryptosporidium* sp. infected cats were inoculated via orogastric intubation with 2×10^6 axenic *T. foetus*. All cats were persistently carrying the protozoan for the entire study period of over 200 days and experienced diarrhea that was self-resolved in seven weeks [28]. It is plausible that trophozoites are transmitted by a fecal-oral route from an infected cat to an uninfected one. By doing so trophozoites have to overcome challenges they face and survive in: 1) the environment they encounter during the period between being discharged from one host and being ingested by the next; and 2) the hostile gastric niche of the new host after ingestion and before moving down to the intestine. A few studies have been done on these areas.

In an experiment that normally formed cat feces that were first mixed with saline in a 1:1 ratio, resulting in no form, loose, puddles or piles, were spiked with 10-fold serially diluted trophozoites (2×10^2 – 2×10^5/gram feces) and stored at room temperature (23-25 °C) for various length periods of time. An accumulative rate of more than 80% of positive culture for feces stored for 6 and 24 h was obtained in both InPouch™ and in Modified Diamond's Medium (MDM) [29]. It would be more relevant to find out how long the organisms would survive in diarrheic feces, which is currently unavailable. In another experiment cat food was spiked, the pathogens were cultivable for five consecutive days when MDM was used [30]. Similarly *T. foetus* trophozoites survived more than 3 h in feline urine and sauced cat food, 2 h on ground cat food although only half an hour in tap or distilled water [31]. These data collectively suggest that transmission is not solely limited to close contact between cats. Contamination of food and water by the trichomonads, although less likely in the latter, may be an important route for transmission. Further, garden slugs common in Sydney, Australia were fed cat foods spiked with 10^6 *T. foetus* feline isolate trophozoites per gram. One hundred percent and 83% of the Leopard slugs and the Yellow cellar slugs shed viable *T. foetus* in their feces, respectively, which was cultivable in MDM. Therefore slugs may facilitate the transmission of *T. foetus* among cats [30] as a vector. It is also plausible that these slugs may serve as transport hosts upon accidental ingestion by cats, which needs to be confirmed.

4. Clinical signs associated with gastrointestinal tract infection

Gastrointestinal disease has been demonstrated in cats experimentally infected with *T. foetus*, an organism not considered part of the normal feline microbiome [3,28,32]. It is possible to isolate *T. foetus* from a healthy cat as subclinical shedding does occur [33]. Infection can be demonstrated as early as 2 to 7 days after orogastric inoculation [28]. In experimental infection, *T. foetus* is limited to the ileum, cecum and colon [28]. Clinical signs vary from subclinical to intractable large bowel diarrhea [3]. Typical clinical signs in natural infections are chronic or intermittent large bowel diarrhea reported in about 61% to 64% of infected cats, with many cats having no reported diarrhea in the 6 months preceding diagnosis [34,35]. The feces has been described as yellow-green in color and malodorous with typical signs of colitis including fresh blood, mucous, fecal incontinence, tenesmus and flatulence [3,36]. The consistency of the feces has been described most commonly as semi-formed to cow pat [28]. An objective fecal scoring system has been used in studies: a scale of 1 to 5 based on consistency, with a score of 1 representing watery feces and a score of 5 is dry and firm feces. Trichomonad infected cats fecal score have been described to range from 3 to 5 [33]. Up to as many as 20% of infected cats have reported systemic signs including anorexia, depression, vomiting and weight loss with a case report describing a kitten as pyrexic and experimental infections reporting vomiting and fever [34,36,37]. In a study examining experimental infection ($n = 8$), only two cats demonstrated clinical signs of disease, fecal blood and mucous at nine days post-infection (dpi), and fever with vomiting 21 dpi [32]. Interestingly, motile trichomonads were observed in intestinal content culture in only three of the eight cats infected, none of which showed clinical signs. Mortality is extremely rare and only reported in kittens. The first report of mortality was in the study that first described natural and experimental trichomonosis in kittens in 1928 with a feline isolate [5]. All nine kittens

Table 2 Genetic similarity in percentage (%) between *Tritrichomonas suis* and bovine isolates of *T. foetus*

	Bovine isolates of *T. foetus**													Refs.
T. suis#	ITS-2 (10)	EF-1α (10)	CP8 (2)	CP1 (8)	CP2 (8)	CP4 (8)	CP5 (8)	CP6 (8)	CP7 (8)	CP8 (8)	CP9 (8)	MDH1 (8)	ITS1 + 2 (8)	
ITS-2 (4, 368)	100.0													[16]
EF-1α (4, 783)		99.4												[16]
CP8 (4, 663)			99.7											[19]
CP1 (4, 503)				100.0										[18]
CP2 (4, 669)					100.0									[18]
CP4 (4, 273)						100.0								[18]
CP5 (4, 361)							100.0							[18]
CP6 (4, 318)								100.0						[18]
CP7 (4, 373)									100.0					[18]
CP8 (4, 907)										100.0 (3); 99.9 (1)				[18]
CP9 (4, 289)											100.0			[18]
MDH1 (4, 562)												100.0		[18]
ITS1 + 2 (4, 297)													100.0	[18]

CP, cysteine protease; MDH, malate dehydrogenase; ITS, internal transcribed spacer.
*number of cattle isolates.
#first number - number of cat isolates; second number - length of sequence in base pair (bp).

diagnosed with naturally acquired infection, and five of the six experimentally infected kittens, wasted and died within five to ten days and four to nine days of diagnosis respectively [5]. The second report that documents mortality was a prevalence study examining *T. foetus* infection in cats with diarrhea in a shelter colony in Italy [38]. One 7-month old kitten housed in this shelter with confirmed *T. foetus* infection succumbed to suspected septic shock despite having started ronidazole therapy two days prior [38].

Clinical signs are reported to persist for 5 to 24 months (median 9 months) from the time of diagnosis [33]. More than half of the cats that go into clinical remission will have PCR evidence of trichomonad infection (asymptomatic carrier), and many of these cats will relapse for a short duration, often with worse diarrhea [33]. Not surprisingly, the number of other cats in the same household will negatively impact the time from diagnosis to resolution of clinical signs [33]. Infection with *T. foetus* is not unlikely in single-cat households even in cats that have lived in isolation for years, as they can acquire the infection in the early stages of their lives [34]. Trichomonad infections can occur as co-infections, most notably *Giardia* species and coccidia [3,34,35,39]. More severe diarrhea has been reported in four cats experimentally infected with *T. foetus* and *Cryptosporidium* species, despite the latter organism having a tropism for the small intestines [28]. In surveys of naturally acquired trichomonad infections the severity of diarrhea has not reported to be worsened by co-infection with enteric parasites [35].

5. Infection in the urogenital tract

In addition to the GI tract *T. foetus* is also found in the urogenital tract of the domestic cat at least once. Dahlgren et al. reported the first case of *T. foetus* in the uterus of a cat with pyometra [40]. In this case wet mounts made directly from the fluid collected from the surgically removed uterus revealed microscopically numerous motile flagellated protozoa. They were 13–17 × 5–7 μm in size with undulating membrane, suggesting *T. foetus*. Further, PCR detected an expected size band product of 343 bp in length using primers PRF3 and PRF4. The PCR product was sequenced and the sequence was 100% identical to *T. foetus* feline isolate sequences, which confirmed the identity of the protozoan causing feline pyometra as *T. foetus* [40]. *T. foetus* was also found in the feces of three other cats in the same household, one of which had chronic diarrhea [40]. These authors were unable to conclude that the infection was sexually transmitted even though the female mated repeatedly with *T. foetus*-positive male with chronic diarrhea [40].

In a comprehensive study Gray et al. used parallel samples collected in USA from both the urogenital tract as a result of ovariohysterectomy or castration and feces of purebred cats [41]. Direct microscopy, Immunohistochemical analysis and PCR were used to test each sample for the presence of *T. foetus* among the two sets of samples. *Tritrichomonas foetus* infections were detected by PCR in 25% (15/61) cats and 67% catteries (22/33). Nevertheless, *T. foetus* was never detected in the urogenital tract of any cats, including the 15 *T. foetus*-positive cats in feces. These authors concluded that no evidence of urogenital tract colonization by *T. foetus* was detected and that urogenital tract infection with *T. foetus* very unlikely plays an important role in overall disease transmission [41]. Collectively this data demonstrates that infection of the urogenital tract by *T. foetus* does occur and may cause pyometra, but it is a rare event especially among the healthy cats presenting to clinics for ovariohysterectomy or castration.

6. Pathogenesis

In the above mentioned experiment, four pathogen-free and four *Cryptosporidium* sp. infected cats were inoculated with axenic *T. foetus*. All cats experienced self-resolved diarrhea for weeks. *Tritrichomonas foetus* was isolated from the ileum, cecum, and colon during necropsy. It was further shown that protozoa and its surface-located antigen were detected on surface epithelia and within superficial detritus of the cecal and colonic mucosa (Figure 2) [28]. Similarly in naturally infected cats the parasites were generally present in close proximity to the mucosal surface and less frequently in the lumen of colonic crypts. Mild-to-moderate lymphoplasmacytic and neutrophilic colitis, crypt epithelial cell hypertrophy, hyperplasia and increased mitotic activity, loss of goblet cells were associated with the presence of trichomonads in colon [42]. Consequently in both experimental and natural infections the predilection sites for *T. foetus* trophozoites are the epithelial surface and crypts of cecum and colon.

Burgess et al. found that *T. foetus* bovine isolate was highly cytotoxic to Hela cells, a human cervical cell line, and early bovine lymphosarcoma (BL-3) but displayed low levels of cytotoxicity against Vero cells [43]. The latter are African green monkey kidney cells [43]. This isolate also adheres to bovine vaginal epithelial cells (BVECs) in an in vitro assay. The adhesion process was first initiated by the posterior flagellum followed by the body. IgG_1 antibodies inhibited adherence, whereas IgG_2 did not [44]. Furthermore, purified lipophosphoglycan (LPG) of *T. foetus* bovine isolate inhibited the binding of *T. foetus* to BVECs by competing with the protozoa in specific receptor – ligand interactions [45]. Adhesion of *T. foetus* resulted in extensive damage of BVEC monolayers [45]. This cytopathic effect was the results of apoptosis induced by *T. foetus*. A painstaking research pinpointed that CP8 of 30 kDa was the major player in *T. foetus* inducing BVEC

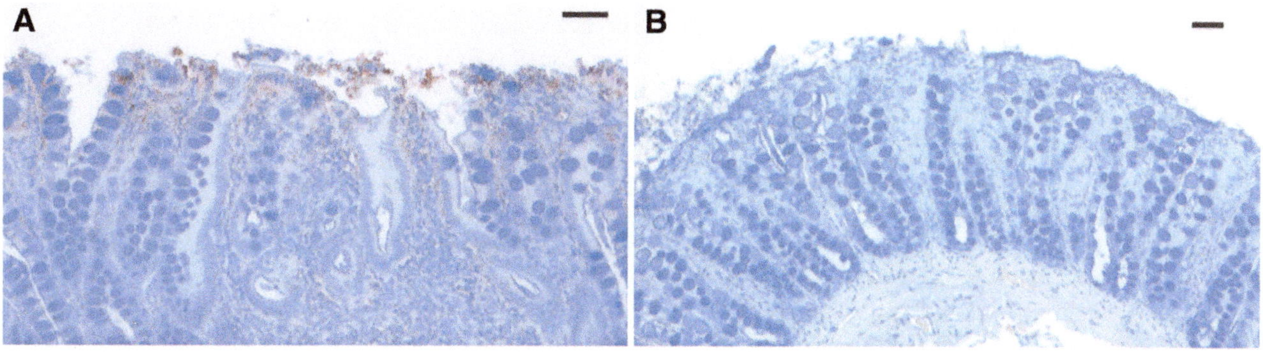

Figure 2 ***Tritrichomonas foetus*** **antigens in colonic mucosal biopsy specimens.** Immunolabeled trichomonads (red stained organisms) in panel **A** are located on surface enterocytes and within superficial mucus and detritus of the cecal mucosa. Panel **B** is a negative control omitting primary antibody. Bar = 100 μm. Reproduced with permission [28].

apoptosis [46]. Collectively the data from multiple research groups demonstrate that *T. foetus* bovine isolate causes cell death of BVECs by means of apoptosis, in which CPs such as CP8 plays a pivotal role. It is not clear whether the same occurs in vivo in infected cows and heifers, which waits to be confirmed.

In an in vitro analysis Tolbert et al. demonstrated that feline *T. foetus* trophozoites adhere to monolayers of the porcine intestinal epithelial cell line (IPEC)-J2 cells [47] (Figure 3). The reason for using a porcine jejunal cell line was the unavailability of epithelial cell line of feline origin. It is worthy of noting that *T. suis*, a synonym of *T. foetus* resides in the GI tract of pigs without causing clinical signs as mentioned in the section of molecular studies. So IPEC-J2 may represent the second best in vitro model. These authors showed that adhesion was via specific receptor – ligand interaction, required viable trichomonad cells and was independent of cytoskeletal activity of the trophozoites [47]. Lately the same authors elegantly demonstrated that feline *T. foetus* trophozoites progressively destroyed IPEC-J2 cell monolayer via apoptosis. The protozoan promoted a direct contact – dependent activation of intestinal epithelial cell apoptosis signaling. This pathologic effect depended upon *T. foetus* – cell associated cysteine proteases [48]. Effect of bovine *T. foetus* on epithelial cultured cells was investigated using clonal populations of the protozoan. Five clonal populations destroyed epithelial monolayers at different degrees, ranging from 25% to 55% despite similar cytoadhesion levels and whole-cell protease activity. They also showed various degrees of contact – dependent and contact – independent cytotoxicity. Contact – independent cytotoxicity was strictly related to the degree of enzyme activation of an extracellular protease [49]. Furthermore, it was shown that extracellular proteinases such as CP8 of *T. foetus* bovine isolate cleaved C3b (the bigger fragment of two C3 component in the original paper designed as

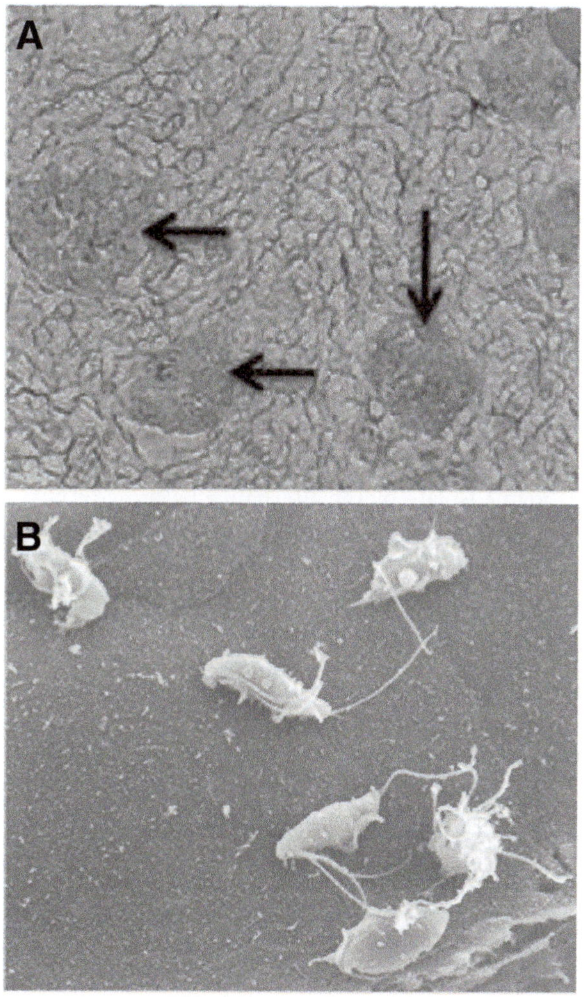

Figure 3 Scanning electron microscopy of ***Tritrichomonas foetus*** **adhesion to porcine intestinal epithelial cell (IPEC)-J2 monolayers.** **A**. Aggregates of trophozoites adhering to IPEC-J2 monolayers (arrows). **B**. Six trophoziotes adhering to a single IPEC-J2 cell. Reproduced with permission [47].

C3a) to small fragments, which could play a role in evasion of complement killing in vivo as a result of preventing completion of complement activation cascade [50].

Taken together, the pathogenesis of *T. foetus* on the intestinal epithelial cells is both contact – dependent and contact – independent. In the former, cytopathic effect is mainly via apoptosis induced by cell-associated proteases, whereas extracellular proteases are the major players in contact – independent cytotoxicity. Extracellular proteases may also play a role in evading complement killing. Consequently proteases are a major player although other uncharacterized molecules may also contribute to pathogenesis of this intriguing trichomonad. Consistent with the notion, 483 and 445 bovine and feline isolates of *T. foetus* transcripts were determined to be proteases by a transcriptomical approach. Among these 389 and 346 were CP, respectively [20].

7. Host immunity

There is significant paucity of literature on immunity of feline hosts to microbial infections in general and to *T. foetus* infections in the GI tract in specific. The latter is understandable provided that the trichomonad has been ascribed to be causative agents only in last 15 or so years. In general IgA is a pivotal player in mucosal secretion of cat's GI tract [51,52]. Consequently IgA profile in the GI tract among different age groups of various breeds is crucial to understand host immunity against and susceptibility to microbial infections. Unfortunately this information is very scarce at present. It was found very low concentrations of hyperimmune serum (up to 1:640 dilution, the highest available title in the experiments) promoted significant enhancement of killing of *T. foetus* bovine isolate by the alternative pathway of bovine complement [53]. Nevertheless, extracellular proteinases such as CP8 of *T. foetus* bovine isolate cleaved C3b to small inactive fragments, which may counteract this host defense system [50].

8. Epidemiology

8.1. Geographic distribution

Although *T. foetus* was reported in nine kittens with diarrhea as early as 1928 [5] its status as an etiological pathogen of chronic diarrhea of the domestic cat was only confirmed very recently. Gookin et al. established an association between diarrhea and *T. foetus* infections in the domestic cat in the USA [3]. They further determined that this trichomonad was the etiological agent of feline trichomonal diarrhea using rRNA gene sequence analysis; restriction enzyme digest mapping; and light, transmission, and scanning electron microscopy [4].

Tritrichomonas foetus has been diagnosed in the domestic cat in many geographic regions. To the best of our knowledge its geographic distribution has covered four continents including Europe (Austria, Finland, France, Germany, Greece, Italy, Netherland, Norway, Poland, Spain, Sweden, Switzerland, and UK), North America (Canada and USA), Australia/Oceania (Australia and New Zealand), and Asia (Japan and South Korea) (Figure 4). In some regions only case reports were available, whereas in others survey data were generated (Table 3). Many of the survey data were collected from diarrheic cats, show cat, cats in catteries, or cats presenting to veterinarians and veterinary clinics. Consequently there is a bias associated with such samples, i.e., a bias resulting in higher positive rate than cross-sectional samples that would have been collected from pet owners under the most scenarios. For instance in New Zealand, 22 samples of show cats revealed a positive rate of 82%. In USA diarrheic cats had positive rate as low as 6% in one study [54], and as high as 40% in another [55]. Figure 4 shows the different geographic regions of the world where surveys have been conducted and/or cases have been reported.

8.2. Risk factors

Odds ratio (OR) is commonly used to quantitatively gauge risk factors. An OR is a measure of association between an exposure and an outcome [56]. In this section OR will be used either directly taken from the original publications or calculated by us if data allow to do so. Risk factors discussed in the section include age and breed of the animals, a history of diarrhea, co-infection with other enteral protozoa and housing conditions etc.

8.2.1. Age

An association between age of infected cats and *T. foetus* infections has been probed in many studies, of which several were showed in Table 4. A common notion is that cats of one year old or younger are more susceptible to *T. foetus*. However, data presented in Table 4 did not show a clear picture at all. OR for cats ≤ 1 year old generated from data collected from France and UK were 2.5 ($P = 0.057$) and 13.4 ($P < 0.01$), respectively [57,58]. Further, Galian et al. reported a positive association between age and *T. foetus* prevalence among 1391 fecal samples submitted to a diagnostic laboratory originated from 15 countries in the European Union [59]. They found 10.4%, 5.5%, 2.5%, 3.5% and 0% *T. foetus*-positive cats among age groups ≤1 year old, 2-7, 8-11, 12-15 and ≥15 years old, respectively [59]. However, data from Germany yielded a contradicted picture with younger cats marginally less susceptible with OR 0.9 ($P < 0.05$) [35]. Also no association was found from data collected from Canada, Norway, and USA [60-62] (Table 4). Collectively data from multiple countries do not consistently support a notion that *T. foetus* infections occur more often in the domestic cat of one year old or younger.

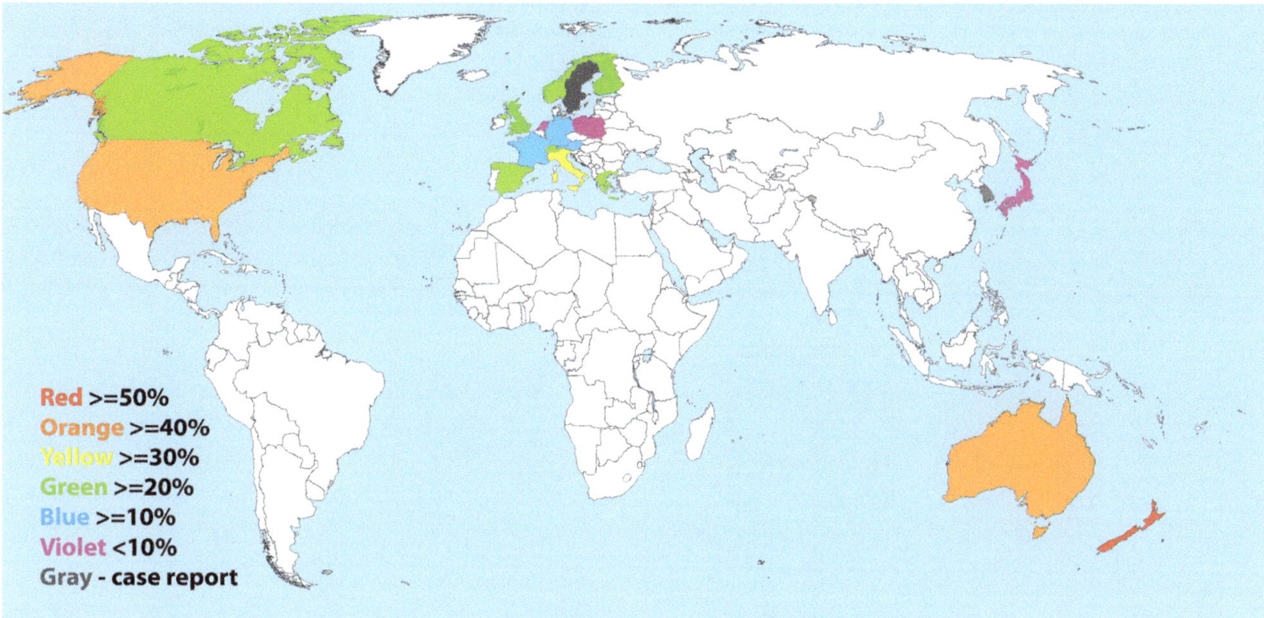

Figure 4 Geographical distribution of surveys for and case report of *Tritrichomonas foetus* detected positive cats worldwide. The prevalence of *T. foetus* infection of each regional study is reported although is not representative of the true prevalence of the entire country. Highest rate is used in countries with more than one regional report on prevalence.

A metadata analysis on OR of cat of one year old or younger was performed by the current authors on available data in publications, which all happened to originate from various European countries (Table 5). The cats in this age group had an OR of 2.1 (1.7-2.6) than older animals. Therefore, young age is a risk factor for *T. foetus* infection.

8.2.2. Breed

There are many different pure breed and crossbreeds of the domestic cat throughout the world. Some breeds are more popular than the others in certain geographic regions. Many veterinarians have observed that purebreds present more often to clinics than crossbreds due to *T. foetus* infections. Among six sets of data all except one found this is true (Table 4). The only exception might be due to a small sample size. In this case, 20 *T. foetus*-positive samples were found in 140 show cats [58]. Purebreds have a much higher OR to be *T. foetus* positive than non-purebreds, which range from 26.3 in Canada [61] to >999.9 in UK [57]. Further analysis showed that a few breeds with a higher OR, such as 7.3 for Siamese and Bengal in UK [57], and 25.9 for Norwegian Forest in Germany [35]. Abyssinians, Siamese and Bengal were found more likely to be *T. foetus* positive in a survey carried out in USA [54]. Collectively purebred is a risk factor for *T. foetus* infections in general, and Abyssinians, Siamese, Bengal and Norwegian Forest in specific. Nevertheless, it is worthy of mentioning that some studies sampled purebred cats from cat breeding centers with a densely housed population. Under this scenario increased incidence of infection might be due to the reliance on close and direct contact among animals.

8.2.3. History of diarrhea

History of diarrhea can be the *T. foetus* positive cat itself, or the other cats sharing the same household in the past, say 6 months. In the former, two studies showed OR 3.2 ($P < 0.05$) in Germany [35] and 3.5 ($P < 0.05$) in USA [60]. Third study in Canada showed an OR 1.7 without statistical significance [61]. For the latter, two investigations resulted in ORs of 4.4 ($P < 0.01$) in Canada [61] and 3.2 in Germany ($P < 0.01$) [35]. Therefore, history of diarrhea in the past six months, no matter whether it is the presenting cat itself or its playmates, rendered a cat a threefold higher chance of having a *T. foetus*-positive status.

8.2.4. Co-infection with other enteric protozoa

Enteral protozoa of the domestic cat include, but are not limited to, *T. foetus*, *Giardia duodenalis*, *Cryptosporidium* spp. *Toxoplasma gondii*, *Isospora* spp. and *Sarcocystis* spp. Co-infection of these is not unusual. For example, five of 16 *T. foetus* positive cats were *Giardia* sp. positive in Australia [63]; five of 18 *T. foetus* positive cats were *Giardia* sp. positive in New Zealand [64]; ten, six and one of 36 *T. foetus* positive cats were *Giardia* sp., *Isospora* sp., and *Cryptosporidium* sp. positive, respectively, three were

Table 3 Cases and prevalence of feline trichomonosis throughout the world

Country	Year	Sources (cat examined)	Diagnosis	Case report	Prevalence (%)	Refs
Australia		Vet Clinic	M;C;PCR;S	16		[63]
Australia	2006-2010	Vet Clinic	M: PCR	13		[82]
	2008-2009	Cattery (59)	PCR		42.4	
Australia	2006-2007	Cattery (82)	C;PCR		0	[83]
		Shelter (52)			0	
Austria & Germany		Fecal samples (31)	PCR,S		19.4	[84]
Austria	1997-2008	Necropsy (96); Organ samples (6)	chromogenic in situ hybridization; PCR; S		2.9	[71]
Canada		Cats with chronical diarrhea (1)	PCR	1		[85]
Canada	2011-2012	Cat Clinic (140)	C;PCR		0.7	[61]
		Cat show (55)			23.6	
		Humane Society (46)			0	
European Union – 15 countries	2009-2010	Diarrheic cats (1840)	PCR,S		9.0	[59,86]
Finland	2008-2010	Diagnostic samples (60)	PCR		28.3	[87]
France	2009-2010	Cat show (140)	C;S		14.3	[58]
Germany		Diarrheic cats (3)	M, PCR, S	3		[88]
Germany	2008	Cat shows (230)	C;PCR;S		15.7	[35]
Greece		Fecal samples (30)	PCR		20.0	[89]
Italy	2008-2010	Pet (181), sheltered cats (54), stray cats (28)	C		0	[90]
Italy		Healthy pets (146)	PCR		2.1	[65]
Italy	2006	Rescued Cats (74)	M;C;PCR		32.4	[38]
Japan	2008	Animal Hospitals (147)	C;PCR;S		8.8	[80]
Netherland	2006	Diarrheic cats (53)	PCR		2	[91]
		Cattery (47)			4	
		pet (54)			0	
New Zealand	2006	Cat shows (22)	C;PCR		81.8	[64]
Norway	2006	Vet Clinic	M; PCR;S	3		[40]
Norway	2009	Cat show (52)	C; PCR;S		21.2	[62]
Poland		Vet Clinics (135)	C;PCR		7.3	[92]
South Korea	2008	Vet Clinic	M;C;PCR	2		[93]
Spain		Cattery (20)	M;C;PCR		25.0	[94]
Sweden		Diarrheic cats (1)		1		[95]
Switzerland	2007	Diarrheic cats (45)	C;PCR;S		24.4	[96]
Switzerland	2007-2008	Vet Clinic (105)	C;PCR		25.7	[97]
UK	2004	Diarrheic cats (1)	M; PCR	1		[36]
UK	2006	Diarrheic cats (111)	PCR		14.4	[57]
UK	2010 - 2012	Diarrheic cats (1882)	PCR		18.8	[66]
UK		Vet Clinic (163)	PCR		20.0	[98]
USA		Diarrheic cats (26)	M;C;PCR	26		[33]
USA		Diarrheic cats (32)	M;C	32		[3]
USA		Diarrheic cats (1)	M;C;PCR	1		[75]
USA		Diarrheic cats (4)	C; PCR	4		[74]
USA		Diarrheic cats (4)	C; PCR	4		[78]
USA	2006-2009	Vet Clinic (104)	PCR	104		[34]

Table 3 Cases and prevalence of feline trichomonosis throughout the world *(Continued)*

USA		Diarrheic cat (7)	M;C;PCR	7		[42]
USA		nondiarrheic cats (53)	C;PCR		0.0	[54]
		Diarrheic cats (170)			5.9	
USA		Fecal samples (173)	C;PCR		9.8	[39]
USA		Catteries (61)	M; PCR		24.6	[41]
USA	2001	Cat show (117)	M;C;PCR		30.8	[60]
USA	2009-2012	Diarrheic cats (68)	PCR		39.7	[55]

C: Culture; M: Microscopy; PCR: polymerase chain reaction; S: Sequencing.

co-infected by all except *Cryptosporidium* sp. in a survey carried out in Germany [35]. In a survey of 146 fecal samples in Italy, co-infections were not found although 15, 11, 3, and 3 were positive for *T. gondii, G. duodenalis, Cryptosporidium* sp. and *T. foetus*, respectively [65]. A detail analysis of enteropathogen co-infection in UK cats with diarrhea was carried out. There was greater co-occurrence than random of *G. duodenalis* with either *T. foetus* or *Cryptosporidium* sp. respectively. Further a greater three-way co-occurrence existed among these three enteral protozoa [66]. These data collectively show that these enteral protozoa render greater risk for the domestic cat to be infected with *T. foetus* even though they may locate at different niches than *T. foetus*.

8.2.5. Others

A few other factors have been analyzed for and found their association with *T. foetus*-positive status occasionally. One is sex. Among seven studies only one demonstrated being a male kitten is a great risk factor ($P < 0.01$) [41]. Another one is housing with more than one other cat. One of four surveys showed sharing house with more than five cats had an OR 4.6 ($P < 0.01$) [61]. The third one is food, one of three investigations resulted in an OR 5.4 for feeding raw food diet ($P < 0.01$) [61]. What causes this disparity is beyond the scope of this manuscript. Plausible reasons include small sample sizes and confounding factors.

9. Diagnosis

Tritrichomonas foetus infection should be suspected in a cat with recent (<6 months) clinical signs of chronic large bowel diarrhea, with highest risk in densely housed young, purebred, show cats [3,60]. There are no differences in the signalment between *Giardia* sp. and *T. foetus* infected cats and co-infections are common enough (12%) to warrant testing for *T. foetus* despite the diagnosis of other enteric protozoal infection, although *Giardia* sp. is a small bowel parasite and the clinical signs should distinguish the infections. There have been no hematological or biochemical abnormalities reported in the literature. Diagnosis of a trichomonad infection is made by either the demonstration of the trophozoite on a saline diluted direct fecal smear (14.7% sensitivity), culture by inoculating MDM (26.4% sensitivity) or the commercially available InPouch™ TF medium (InPouch TF; BioMed Diagnostics, Inc, White City, OR USA) (58.8% sensitivity) or the extraction of DNA in feces and the amplification of *T. foetus* rDNA by the use of PCR [13,60]. Fecal samples include either a voided stool or collected by manual extraction with the aid of fecal loops or by a colon flush technique. The technique of colon flush is demonstrated in a video clip the North Carolina (NC) State University, College of Veterinary Medicine (CVM) website (Colon Flush Technique [67]). Fecal wet preparation is viewed under 40 × magnification. The motile characteristic of *T. foetus* differ from *Giardia* sp. in that it has a forward motility in contrast to a falling leaf motility of *Giardia* sp. as demonstrated in a video clip from the NC State University CVM website (*T. foetus* vs. *Giardia* [68]). Failing to distinguish the two trophozoites on microscopy, *Giardia* sp. can be confirmed by fecal enzyme-linked immunosorbent assay for *Giardia*-specific antigen [60]. In cases where *T. foetus* is suspected despite negative microscopy or fecal culture, when a faster turn-around time than culture is required, or for confirmation of an organism visible on microscopy, *T. foetus* cannot precisely be distinguished microscopically from *Pentatrichomonas hominis,* a commensal trichomonad, a commercially available PCR assay is available targeting part of the 18 s ribosomal RNA (rRNA). Submission of samples should be diarrheic and free from litter as formed stool rarely tests positive even if a subclinical shedder (NC State University CVM, Submission of Samples for *T. foetus* PCR Testing [69]). The sample, roughly the size of a lima bean should be submitted in a sterile tube and the remainder of the volume filled with isopropyl alcohol, without the need for refrigeration. Unfortunately PCR cannot prove the absence of infection.

Chronic experimentally induced infection with *T. foetus* is limited to the colon, cecum and ileum [28]. The distribution of *T. foetus* organisms within the colon is not homogenous and histopathological diagnosis on

Table 4 Risk factors related to feline infections by *Tritrichomonas foetus*¶

Country	Age in month	Sex-male	Purebred	Housing	History of diarrhea in past 6 months	Food	Refs
Canada	<6 – 0.6 (0.1–3.4)	2.0 (0.5–7.9)	26.3 (3.8–1142.2)**	>5 cats per house – 4.6 (1.3–20.8)**	Another cat – 4.4 (1.3–16.2)** Self – 1.7 (0.4–6.4)	Fed a raw food diet – 5.4 (1.5–19.6)**	[61]
France	<12 – #2.5(0.6-10.2)+	NC	NC	NC		NC	[58]
Germany	≤12 – 0.9 (0.7-1.0)*	NC	Norwegian Forest – 25.9 (7.6-87.7)***	NC	Another cat – 3.2 (1.2–9.9)** Self – 3.2 (1.1- 8.7)*	NC	[35]
Norway	NC	NC		NC	NC ($P = 0.1$)		[62]
UK	6-12 (29.4%); >12 (15.2%)***		Pedigree (37.8%); Non-pedigree (6.0%)***				[66]
UK	≤12, #13.4(1.7-107.7)**	NC	# > 999.9 Siamese and Bengal #7.3 (2.1-25.9)**				[57]
USA	Infected mean 8 vs non- infected mean 64.8***		Abyssinians, Siamese and Bengal**				[54]
USA		#> 999.9**					[41]
USA	NC	NC			Self – 3.5 (1.1-11.3)*		[60]

¶Odds ratio is given; 95% confidence interval is in bracket. Blank cells: no data available.
#:Calculated by the authors of current manuscript according to [56]; P value from the original paper.
*$P < 0.05$; **$P < 0.01$; ***$P < 0.001$; +$P = 0.057$.
NC: No correlation was detected.

Table 5 Data included in metadata analysis of odds ratio of young cats with *Tritrichonomas foetus* infections

One year old or younger			Older than one year old			Reference
Positive	Negative	Total	Positive	Negative	Total	
13	35	48	1	36	37	[57]
17	76	93	3	44	47	[58]
65	563	628	33	730	763	[59]
5	14	19	6	26	32	[62]
100	313	413	92	515	607	[66]
9	3	12	1	22	23	[96]
209	1004	1213	136	1373	1509	

samples procured by necropsy, surgery or endoscopy in cats with naturally acquired infection had a sensitivity of 56% [42]. The probability of diagnosing *T. foetus* infection on histopathology is increased with the number of samples submitted. Thus examination of multiple samples will increase the likelihood of diagnosis with a minimum of 6 colon samples required to have a ≥95% confidence of detecting *T. foetus* on at least one sample [42]. A species (sequence) specific fluorescent antibody in situ hybridization (FISH) probe has been developed for the detection of *T. foetus* on formalin fixed samples allowing confirmation of location and molecular identification of a trichomonad [70]. A study examined an chromogenic in situ hybridization (CISH) technique using *T. foetus* and *P. hominis* probes on formalin archived small and large intestinal samples collected from young (4 weeks to 2 years of age) cats with diarrhea [71]. This technique is apparently more reliable than FISH technique as mammalian red blood cells, roughly the same size as trichomonads, auto-fluoresce. Four of the 102 samples were found to be positive, with three testing positive for the *T. foetus* probe and one with the *P. hominis* probe.

10. Treatment

The natural course of diarrhea in cats infected with *T. foetus* is waxing and waning, giving the false impression that therapy may be effective, but often relapsing after discontinuation of treatment [3]. Trichomonads rely on hydrogenosomal fermentation of pyruvate making them susceptibility to 5-nitroimidazole antibiotics, such as metronidazole, tinidazole and ronidazole [72]. Therapeutics reported in the literature include: paromomycin, fenbendazole, furazolidone, nitazoxanide, metronidazole, tinidazole and ronidazole [3,28]. One of the earliest reported descriptions of treatment was paromomycin, an aminoglycoside used to treat *Trichomonas vaginalis*, a human protozoal infection of the genital tract, at the same dose used to treat cryptosporidiosis in cats [3]. In the 25 cats studied, evaluated 3 days to 6 months after treatment, only three had normal stool without *T. foetus* isolated from their stool. Forty percent of the cats in the study continued to have diarrhea after treatment, of which 9 had positive fecal smears, and in the 12 cats that had normal stools, 22% of those cats tested ($n = 9$) had positive fecal smears. Three of the cats in the study were kittens and 2 of them suffered side-effects including acute renal failure, deafness and cataracts. These kittens were included in a case series of 4 kittens that suffered severe side-effects (acute renal failure, deafness and cataracts) after treatment with oral paromomycin [73]. Paromomycin has also been tested in vitro using a 24-h sensitivity assay and the results showed no effect at minimum lethal concentrations (MLC) ≤ 80 μg/mL [74]. Eleven of the original 25 cats were subsequently treated with fenbendazole and then 2-weeks later by furazolidone [3]. There was a decrease in the number of cats having diarrhea, although the stool was described as semi-formed in 9 of the cats with confirmed shedding trichomonads for the following 10-months. Furazolidone has shown equal 24-hour susceptibilities of *T. foetus* cultures to that of metronidazole and ronidazole at MLC of 0.625 to 2.5 μg/mL [74]. In experimentally infected cats, nitazoxanide, a nitrothiazole benzamide compound, with broad-spectrum antiprotozoal activity, decreased the number of trichomonads shed in the feces but failed to eliminate the *T. foetus* infection, although it did eliminate the cryptosporidial infection in those cats that were co-infected. Reported side-effects of nausea and foul-smelling dark diarrhea make it even less attractive as a therapeutic.

Nitroimidazoles (metronidazole, tinidazole and ronidazole) have been investigated both in vitro and in vivo in experimentally induced infections [74-76]. Metronidazole did not show any inhibitory effect in vitro at concentrations ≤10 μg/mL in contrast to tinidazole and ronidazole which had an inhibitory effect at MLC of ≥0.1 μg/mL [75]. Kather et al. demonstrated in vitro results that contradict these findings, as both metronidazole (1.25 to 2.5 μg/mL) and ronidazole (0.625 to 2.5 μg/mL) had a 24-h kill effect on *T. foetus* isolates, although ronidazole had lower 24-h MLC for some isolates [74]. Time-kill assays, which evaluate the degree of growth inhibition and survival during 24-h incubation demonstrated a significant difference in the survival kinetics of *T. foetus* in culture incubated with metronidazole as compared to ronidazole, with ronidazole being more effective [74]. Tinidazole has been investigated twice in vitro with reported MLC of ≥0.1 μg/mL and ≥10 μg/mL [75,76]. The disparity may be ascribable to different strains used in the two experiments.

The efficacy of metronidazole in vitro has not been translated to an in vivo efficacy, although transient improvement in clinical signs do occur independent of elimination of the *T. foetus* infection, the reasons proposed include alteration in bacterial microflora, elimination of *Giardia* co-infection or immunomodulatory effect [33,74]. Interestingly, treatment of infected cats with antibiotics that kill natural microbiota will increase shedding of *T. foetus*, as the organism is dependent on host bacteria for acquisition of micronutrients [75]. Tinidazole cleared experimentally induced *T. foetus* infection within 3-days, but the trichomonads were detected within 6 to 8 weeks after discontinuation of the treatment [76]. The poor in vivo efficacy may be related to its increased absorption and reduced concentration within the intestines. Ronidazole has been investigated in experimentally infected cats and shedding discontinued within 3-days of initiating therapy at 10 mg/kg, dosed orally every 12 h, although relapse was detected but the cultured organisms retrieved from the feces remained susceptible to ronidazole in vitro [75]. Relapses were reported in cats receiving a dose of 30 mg/kg twice daily but not in cats receiving 50 mg/kg twice daily. One reason for better efficacy of ronidazole as compared to other nitroimidazoles may be due to improved trapping of the activated compounds within the intestine [75].

Nitroimidazole resistant trichomonads are hydrogenosomal pyruvate:ferredoxin oxidoreductase deficient, and compensate by increased glycolysis and alternative cytosolic pathways. Ronidazole resistance is defined as aerobic MLC ≥100 µg/mL and is both inherent and acquired [77]. Resistant strains of *T. foetus* to ronidazole have been documented in cats with confirmed treatment failure after excluding the possibility of reinfection or urogenital nidus, and is related to the cross resistance of the organism to all nitroimidazole drugs [77].

Ronidazole is not registered for human or veterinary use and informed consent is necessary prior to use in cats and should only be prescribed in confirmed cases. The current recommended dose is 30 mg/kg, once daily for 14-days [75]. Relapse is common and cats with resolved clinical signs can continue to carry the organism and thus vigilant and prolonged post-treatment monitoring is indicated. No adverse effects were reported in the original study that examined ronidazole as a treatment for *T. foetus* at doses as high as 50 mg/kg, twice daily and hematology and biochemistry results remained within reference range and did not change as compared to pretreatment values [75]. Subsequent to this, four cases of neurological toxicity in cats treated with ronidazole in the range of 30 to 50 mg/kg were reported. The clinical signs included, having a blank stare, "slow motion" movements, agitation, facial tremors, trembling of the extremities, unable to jump or walk stairs and hyperesthesia which started three to nine days after initiating ronidazole, lasting one to four weeks in duration [78]. A lower dose of ronidazole, 10-30 mg/kg once daily, for 14 days, together with a probiotic (Pro-Kolin Enterogenic, Protexin, Probiotics International) was compared to a placebo control and ronidazole at the same dose, frequency and duration in age matched cats diagnosed with *T. foetus*-associated diarrhea [79]. No side-effects were noted with relapse reported in both groups but cats that received the probiotic with the ronidazole were less likely to relapse.

11. Conclusions

Feline trichomonosis is caused by *T. foetus*. The etiology was determined merely one and half a decades ago. The current manuscript comprehensively reviews the trichomonad biology and the disease itself. The authors hope this will provides individuals who are interesting in the topic with one source for updated information.

12. Abbreviations

bp: base pair; BL: bovine lymphosarcoma; BVEC: Bovine vaginal epithelial cells; CISH: Chromogenic in situ hybridization; CP: Cysteine protease; CVM: College of Veterinary Medicine; dpi: days post infection; EL: Elongation factor; FISH: Fluorescent antibody in situ hybridization; GI: Gastrointestinal; IPEC: Porcine intestinal epithelial cell; ITS: Internal transcribed spacer; LPG: Lipophosphoglycan; MDH: malate dehydrogenase; MDM: Modified Diamond's Medium; MLC: Minimum lethal concentration; NC: North Carolina; OR: Odds ratio; RAPD: Random amplified polymorphic DNA; RFLP: Restriction fragment length polymorphism; RUSVM: Ross University School of Veterinary Medicine.

13. Competing interests

The authors declare that they have no competing interests.

14. Authors' contributions

CY conceived the manuscript, and wrote all sections except the ones by LSK who was responsible for clinical signs associated with gastrointestinal tract infection, diagnosis and treatment. Both authors read and approved the final manuscript.

15. Authors' information

CY is an Associate Professor of Parasitology at Ross University School of Veterinary Medicine (RUSVM). CY has studied *T. foetus* for more than five years and published five refereed paper on the subject and 45 refereed manuscripts on other topics. CY had headed the Parasitology section of Wyoming State Veterinary Laboratory (WSVL) between 2008 and 2013, where about 8000 *T. foetus* testing was annually performed. LSK is an European Specialist in Internal Medicine and an Assistant Professor of Internal Medicine at RUSVM. LSK has 15 years of clinical experience working with companion animals including cats as a veterinarian and has frequently diagnosed and treated feline trichomonosis.

16. Acknowledgments

The authors are very grateful to Dr A Lee Willingham of RUSVM for his critical review of the manuscript. Drs. Esteban Soto and Edyta Bajak of RUSVM translated literature published in Spanish and Polish, respectively. The cost for publication is provided by an intramural grant of RUSVM One Health Center for Zoonoses and Tropical Veterinary Medicine.

Author details

[1]Department of Biomedical Sciences, Ross University School of Veterinary Medicine, P.O. Box 334, Basseterre, St. Kitts, West Indies. [2]Department of Clinical Sciences, Ross University School of Veterinary Medicine, P.O. Box 334, Basseterre, St. Kitts, West Indies. [3]One Health Center for Zoonoses and Tropical Veterinary Medicine, Ross University School of Veterinary Medicine, P.O. Box 334, Basseterre, St. Kitts, West Indies.

17. References

1. Yao C (2012) Opportunistic human infections caused by *Tritrichomonas* species: a mini-review. Clin Microbiol Newsl 34:127–131
2. Yao C (2013) Diagnosis of *Tritrichomonas foetus*-infected bulls, an ultimate approach to eradicate bovine trichomoniasis in US cattle? J Med Microbiol 62:1–9
3. Gookin JL, Breitschwerdt EB, Levy MG, Gager RB, Benrud JG (1999) Diarrhea associated with trichomonosis in cats. J Am Vet Med Assoc 215:1450–1454
4. Levy MG, Gookin JL, Poore M, Birkenheuer AJ, Dykstra MJ, Litaker RW (2003) *Tritrichomonas foetus* and not *Pentatrichomonas hominis* is the etiologic agent of feline trichomonal diarrhea. J Parasitol 89:99–104
5. Kessel JF (1928) Trichomoniasis in kittens. Trans R Soc Trop Med Hyg 22:61–80
6. Benchimol M (2004) Trichomonads under Microscopy. Microsc Microanal 10:528–550
7. Lipman NS, Lampen N, Nguyen HT (1999) Identification of pseudocysts of *Tritrichomonas muris* in Armenian hamsters and their transmission to mice. Lab Anim Sci 49:313–315
8. Mariante RM, Lopes LC, Benchimol M (2004) *Tritrichomonas foetus* pseudocysts adhere to vaginal epithelial cells in a contact-dependent manner. Parasitol Res 92:303–312
9. Pereira-Neves A, Ribeiro KC, Benchimol M (2003) Pseudocysts in trichomonads–new insights. Protist 154:313–329
10. Gruffydd-Jones T, Addie D, Belak S, Boucraut-Baralon C, Egberink H, Frymus T, Hartmann K, Hosie MJ, Lloret A, Lutz H, Marsilio F, Möstl K, Pennisi MG, Radford AD, Thiry E, Truyen U, Horzinek MC (2013) Tritrichomoniasis in cats: ABCD guidelines on prevention and management. J Feline Med Surg 15:647–649
11. Lappin MR (2005) Enteric protozoal diseases. Vet Clin North Am Small Anim Pract 35:81–88
12. Levy MG, Gookin JL, Poore MF, Litaker RW, Dykstra M (2001) Information on parasitic gastrointestinal tract infections in cats. J Am Vet Med Assoc 218:194–195
13. Manning K (2010) Update on the diagnosis and management of *Tritrichomonas foetus* infections in cats. Top Companion Anim Med 25:145–148
14. Payne PA, Artzer M (2009) The biology and control of Giardia spp and Tritrichomonas foetus. Vet Clin North Am Small Anim Pract 39:993–1007
15. Tolbert MK, Gookin J (2009) *Tritrichomonas foetus*: a new agent of feline diarrhea. Compend Contin Educ Vet 31:374–381
16. Reinmann K, Muller N, Kuhnert P, Campero CM, Leitsch D, Hess M, Henning K, Fort M, Muller J, Gottstein B, Frey CF (2012) *Tritrichomonas foetus* isolates from cats and cattle show minor genetic differences in unrelated loci ITS-2 and EF-1alpha. Vet Parasitol 185:138–144
17. Slapeta J, Craig S, McDonell D, Emery D (2010) *Tritrichomonas foetus* from domestic cats and cattle are genetically distinct. Exp Parasitol 126:209–213
18. Slapeta J, Muller N, Stack CM, Walker G, Lew-Tabor A, Tachezy J, Frey CF (2012) Comparative analysis of *Tritrichomonas foetus* (Riedmuller, 1928) cat genotype, *T. foetus* (Riedmuller, 1928) cattle genotype and *Tritrichomonas suis* (Davaine, 1875) at 10 DNA loci. Int J Parasitol 42:1143–1149
19. Sun Z, Stack C, Slapeta J (2012) Sequence differences in the diagnostic region of the cysteine protease 8 gene of *Tritrichomonas foetus* parasites of cats and cattle. Vet Parasitol 186:445–449
20. Morin-Adeline V, Lomas R, O'Meally D, Stack C, Conesa A, Sapeta J (2014) Comparative transcriptomics reveals striking similarities between the bovine and feline isolates of *Tritrichomonas foetus*: consequences for in silico drug-target identification. BMC Genomics 15:955
21. Walden HS, Dykstra C, Dillon A, Rodning S, Givens D, Bird R, Newton J, Lindsay D (2013) A new species of *Tritrichomonas* (Sarcomastigophora: Trichomonida) from the domestic cat (*Felis catus*). Parasitol Res 112:2227–2235
22. Felleisen RS (1998) Comparative genetic analysis of tritrichomonadid protozoa by the random amplified polymorphic DNA technique. Parasitol Res 84:153–156
23. Hampl V, Pavlicek A, Flegr J (2001) Construction and bootstrap analysis of DNA fingerprinting-based phylogenetic trees with the freeware program FreeTree: application to trichomonad parasites. Int J Syst Evol Microbiol 51:731–735
24. Tachezy J, Tachezy R, Hampl V, Sedinova M, Vanacova S, Vrlik M, Van Ranst M, Flegr J, Kuldaa J (2002) Cattle pathogen *Tritrichomonas foetus* (Riedmuller, 1928) and pig commensal *Tritrichomonas suis* (Gruby & Delafond, 1843) belong to the same species. J Eukaryot Microbiol 49:154–163
25. Kleina P, Bettim-Bandinelli J, Bonatto SL, Benchimol M, Bogo MR (2004) Molecular phylogeny of Trichomonadidae family inferred from ITS-1, 5.8S rRNA and ITS-2 sequences. Int J Parasitol 34:963–970
26. Walker RL, Hayes DC, Sawyer SJ, Nordhausen RW, Van Hoosear KA, BonDurant RH (2003) Comparison of the 5.8S rRNA gene and internal transcribed spacer regions of trichomonadid protozoa recovered from the bovine preputial cavity. J Vet Diagn Invest 15:14–20
27. Lun ZR, Chen XG, Zhu XQ, Li XR, Xie MQ (2005) Are *Tritrichomonas foetus* and *Tritrichomonas suis* synonyms? Trends Parasitol 21:122–125
28. Gookin JL, Levy MG, Law JM, Papich MG, Poore MF, Breitschwerdt EB (2001) Experimental infection of cats with *Tritrichomonas foetus*. Am J Vet Res 62:1690–1697
29. Hale S, Norris JM, Slapeta J (2009) Prolonged resilience of *Tritrichomonas foetus* in cat faeces at ambient temperature. Vet Parasitol 166:60–65
30. Van der Saag M, McDonell D, Slapeta J (2011) Cat genotype *Tritrichomonas foetus* survives passage through the alimentary tract of two common slug species. Vet Parasitol 177:262–266
31. Rosypal AC, Ripley A, Stockdale Walden HD, Blagburn BL, Grant DC, Lindsay DS (2012) Survival of a feline isolate of *Tritrichomonas foetus* in water, cat urine, cat food and cat litter. Vet Parasitol 185:279–281
32. Stockdale HD, Dillon AR, Newton JC, Bird RC, Bondurant RH, Deinnocentes P, Barney S, Bulter J, Land T, Spencer JA, Lindsay DS, Blagburn BL (2008) Experimental infection of cats (Felis catus) with *Tritrichomonas foetus* isolated from cattle. Vet Parasitol 154:156–161
33. Foster DM, Gookin JL, Poore MF, Stebbins ME, Levy MG (2004) Outcome of cats with diarrhea and *Tritrichomonas foetus* infection. J Am Vet Med Assoc 225:888–892
34. Xenoulis PG, Lopinski DJ, Read SA, Suchodolski JS, Steiner JM (2013) Intestinal *Tritrichomonas foetus* infection in cats: a retrospective study of 104 cases. J Feline Med Surg 15:1098–1103
35. Kuehner KA, Marks SL, Kass PH, Sauter-Louis C, Grahn RA, Barutzki D, Hartmann K (2011) *Tritrichomonas foetus* infection in purebred cats in Germany: prevalence of clinical signs and the role of co-infection with other enteroparasites. J Feline Med Surg 13:251–258
36. Mardell EJ, Sparkes AH (2006) Chronic diarrhoea associated with *Tritrichomonas foetus* infection in a British cat. Vet Rec 158:765–766
37. Stockdale H, Rodning S, Givens M, Carpenter D, Lenz S, Spencer J, Dykstra C, Lindsay D, Blagburn B (2007) Experimental infection of cattle with a feline isolate of *Tritrichomonas foetus*. J Parasitol 93:1429–1434
38. Holliday M, Deni D, Gunn-Moore DA (2009) *Tritrichomonas foetus* infection in cats with diarrhoea in a rescue colony in Italy. J Feline Med Surg 11:131–134
39. Stockdale HD, Givens MD, Dykstra CC, Blagburn BL (2009) *Tritrichomonas foetus* infections in surveyed pet cats. Vet Parasitol 160:13–17
40. Dahlgren SS, Gjerde B, Pettersen HY (2007) First record of natural *Tritrichomonas foetus* infection of the feline uterus. J Small Anim Pract 48:654–657
41. Gray SG, Hunter SA, Stone MR, Gookin JL (2010) Assessment of reproductive tract disease in cats at risk for *Tritrichomonas foetus* infection. Am J Vet Res 71:76–81
42. Yaeger MJ, Gookin JL (2005) Histologic features associated with *tritrichomonas foetus*-induced colitis in domestic cats. Vet Pathol 42:797–804
43. Burgess DE, Knoblock KF, Daugherty T, Robertson NP (1990) Cytotoxic and hemolytic effects of *Tritrichomonas foetus* on mammalian cells. Infect Immun 58:3627–3632
44. Corbeil LB, Hodgson JL, Jones DW, Corbeil RR, Widders PR, Stephens LR (1989) Adherence of *Tritrichomonas foetus* to bovine vaginal epithelial cells. Infect Immun 57:2158–2165
45. Singh BN, Lucas JJ, Beach DH, Shin ST, Gilbert RO (1999) Adhesion of *Tritrichomonas foetus* to bovine vaginal epithelial cells. Infect Immun 67:3847–3854
46. Singh BN, Lucas JJ, Hayes GR, Kumar I, Beach DH, Frajblat M, Gilbert RO, Sommer U, Costello CE (2004) *Tritrichomonas foetus* induces apoptotic cell death in bovine vaginal epithelial cells. Infect Immun 72:4151–4158
47. Tolbert MK, Stauffer SH, Gookin JL (2013) Feline *Tritrichomonas foetus* adhere to intestinal epithelium by receptor-ligand-dependent mechanisms. Vet Parasitol 192:75–82
48. Tolbert MK, Stauffer SH, Brand MD, Gookin JL (2014) Cysteine protease activity of feline *Tritrichomonas foetus* promotes adhesion-dependent cytotoxicity to intestinal epithelial cells. Infect Immun 82:2851–2859
49. Da Rocha-Azevedo B, De Melo-Braga MB, Silva-Filho FC E (2005) Intra-strain clonal phenotypic variation of *Tritrichomonas foetus* is related to the cytotoxicity exerted by the parasite to cultured cells. Parasitol Res 95:106–112

50. Kania SA, Reed SL, Thomford JW, BonDurant RH, Hirata K, Corbeil RR, North MJ, Corbeil LB (2001) Degradation of bovine complement C3 by trichomonad extracellular proteinase. Vet Immunol Immunopathol 78:83–96
51. Allenspach K (2011) Clinical immunology and immunopathology of the canine and feline intestine. Vet Clin North Am Small Anim Pract 41:345–360
52. Stokes C, Waly N (2006) Mucosal defence along the gastrointestinal tract of cats and dogs. Vet Res 37:281–293
53. Aydintug MK, Leid RW, Widders PR (1990) Antibody enhances killing of *Tritrichomonas foetus* by the alternative bovine complement pathway. Infect Immun 58:944–948
54. Queen EV, Marks SL, Farver TB (2012) Prevalence of selected bacterial and parasitic agents in feces from diarrheic and healthy control cats from Northern California. J Vet Intern Med 26:54–60
55. Polak KC, Levy JK, Crawford PC, Leutenegger CM, Moriello KA (2014) Infectious diseases in large-scale cat hoarding investigations. Vet J 201:189–195
56. Szumilas M (2010) Explaining Odds Ratios. J Can Acad Child Adolesc Psychiatry 19:227–229
57. Gunn-Moore DA, McCann TM, Reed N, Simpson KE, Tennant B (2007) Prevalence of *Tritrichomonas foetus* infection in cats with diarrhoea in the UK. J Feline Med Surg 9:214–218
58. Profizi C, Cian A, Meloni D, Hugonnard M, Lambert V, Groud K, Gagnon AC, Viscogliosi E, Zenner L (2013) Prevalence of *Tritrichomonas foetus* infections in French catteries. Vet Parasitol 196:50–55
59. Galián M, Heusinger A, Gentil M, Müller E (2011) *Tritrichomonas fetus* in cats. Argos - Informativo Veterinario 134:44-45.
60. Gookin JL, Stebbins ME, Hunt E, Burlone K, Fulton M, Hochel R, Talaat M, Poore M, Levy MG (2004) Prevalence of and risk factors for feline *Tritrichomonas foetus* and giardia infection. J Clin Microbiol 42:2707–2710
61. Hosein A, Kruth SA, Pearl DL, Richardson D, Maggs JC, Peach HA, Peregrine AS (2013) Isolation of *Tritrichomonas foetus* from cats sampled at a cat clinic, cat shows and a humane society in southern Ontario. J Feline Med Surg 15:706–711
62. Tysnes K, Gjerde B, Nodtvedt A, Skancke E (2011) A cross-sectional study of *Tritrichomonas foetus* infection among healthy cats at shows in Norway. Acta Vet Scand 53:39
63. Bissett SA, Gowan RA, O'Brien CR, Stone MR, Gookin JL (2008) Feline diarrhoea associated with *Tritrichomonas cf. foetus* and Giardia co-infection in an Australian cattery. Aust Vet J 86:440–443
64. Kingsbury DD, Marks SL, Cave NJ, Grahn RA (2010) Identification of *Tritrichomonas foetus* and *Giardia* spp. infection in pedigree show cats in New Zealand. N Z Vet J 58:6–10
65. Mancianti F, Nardoni S, Mugnaini L, Zambernardi L, Guerrini A, Gazzola V, Papini RA (2015) A retrospective molecular study of select intestinal protozoa in healthy pet cats from Italy. J Feline Med Surg 17:163–167
66. Paris J, Wills S, Balzer H-J, Shaw D, Gunn-Moore D (2014) Enteropathogen co-infection in UK cats with diarrhoea. BMC Vet Res 10:13
67. Colon Flush Technique [http://www.youtube.com/watch?v=JMfZ9M80V8E] Accessed 15 Jan 2015
68. *T. foetus vs. Giardia* [http://www.youtube.com/watch?v=aF06jlbcF8E] Accessed 15 Jan 2015
69. NC State University CVM, Submission of Samples for T. foetus PCR Testing [http://www.JodyGookin.com]. Accessed 15 Jan 2015
70. Gookin JL, Stone MR, Yaeger MJ, Meyerholz DK, Moisan P (2010) Fluorescence in situ hybridization for identification of *Tritrichomonas foetus* in formalin-fixed and paraffin-embedded histological specimens of intestinal trichomoniasis. Vet Parasitol 172:139–143
71. Mostegl MM, Wetscher A, Richter B, Nedorost N, Dinhopl N, Weissenbock H (2012) Detection of *Tritrichomonas foetus* and *Pentatrichomonas hominis* in intestinal tissue specimens of cats by chromogenic in situ hybridization. Vet Parasitol 183:209–214
72. Kulda J (1999) Trichomonads, hydrogenosomes and drug resistance. Int J Parasitol 29:199–212
73. Gookin JL, Riviere JE, Gilger BC, Papich MG (1999) Acute renal failure in four cats treated with paromomycin. J Am Vet Med Assoc 215:1821–1823. 1806
74. Kather EJ, Marks SL, Kass PH (2007) Determination of the in vitro susceptibility of feline *Tritrichomonas foetus* to 5 antimicrobial agents. J Vet Intern Med 21:966–970
75. Gookin JL, Copple CN, Papich MG, Poore MF, Stauffer SH, Birkenheuer AJ, Twedt DC, Levy MG (2006) Efficacy of ronidazole for treatment of feline *Tritrichomonas foetus* infection. J Vet Intern Med 20:536–543
76. Gookin JL, Stauffer SH, Coccaro MR, Poore MF, Levy MG, Papich MG (2007) Efficacy of tinidazole for treatment of cats experimentally infected with Tritrichomonas foetus. Am J Vet Res 68:1085–1088
77. Gookin JL, Stauffer SH, Dybas D, Cannon DH (2010) Documentation of in vivo and in vitro aerobic resistance of feline *Tritrichomonas foetus* isolates to ronidazole. J Vet Intern Med 24:1003–1007
78. Rosado TW, Specht A, Marks SL (2007) Neurotoxicosis in 4 cats receiving ronidazole. J Vet Intern Med 21:328–331
79. Lalor SL, Gunn-Moore DA (2012) Effects of concurrent ronidazole and probiotic therapy in cats with *Tritrichomonas foetus*-associated diarrhoea. J Feline Med Surg 14:650–658
80. Doi J, Hirota J, Morita A, Fukushima K, Kamijyo H, Ohta H, Yamasaki M, Takahashi T, Katakura K, Oku Y (2012) Intestinal *Tritrichomonas suis* (=*T. foetus*) infection in Japanese cats. J Vet Med Sci 74:413–417
81. Midlej V, Pereira-Neves A, Kist LW, Bogo MR, Benchimol M (2011) Ultrastructural features of *Tritrichomonas mobilensis* and comparison with *Tritrichomonas foetus*. Vet Parasitol 182:171–180
82. Bell ET, Gowan RA, Lingard AE, McCoy RJ, Slapeta J, Malik R (2010) Naturally occurring *Tritrichomonas foetus* infections in Australian cats: 38 cases. J Feline Med Surg 12:889–898
83. Bissett SA, Stone ML, Malik R, Norris JM, O'Brien C, Mansfield CS, Nicholls JM, Griffin A, Gookin JL (2009) Observed occurrence of *Tritrichomonas foetus* and other enteric parasites in Australian cattery and shelter cats. J Feline Med Surg 11:803–807
84. Steiner JM, Xenoulis PG, Read SA, Suchodolski JS, Globokar M, Huisinga E, Thuere S (2007) Identification of *Tritrichomonas foetus* DNA in feces from cats with diarrhea from Germany and Austria. J Vet Intern Med 21:649
85. Pham D (2009) Chronic intermittent diarrhea in a 14-month-old Abyssinian cat. Can Vet J 50:85–87
86. Galián M, Gentil M, Heusinger A, Müller E (2011) *Tritrichomonas foetus* as a cause of diarrhoea in cats. Tierärztliche Umschau Parasiten-Spezial 1:5-8
87. Castrén L, Vainio-Siukola K, Laaksonen I, Saari S (2011) *Tritrichomonas foetus* as a cause of feline chronic large bowel diarrhoea. Suomen Eläinlääkärilehti 117:371–378
88. Schrey C, Mundhenk L, Grubers A, Henning K, Frey C (2009) *Tritrichomonas foetus* as a cause of diarrhoea in three cats. Kleintierpraxis 54:93–96
89. Xenoulis PG, Saridomichelakis MN, Read SA, Suchodolski JS, Steiner JM (2010) Detection of *Tritrichomonas foetus* in cats in Greece. J Feline Med Surg 12:831–833
90. Mugnaini L, Papini R, Gorini G, Passantino A, Merildi V, Mancianti F (2012) Pattern and predictive factors of endoparasitism in cats in Central Italy. Rev Med Vet 163:89–94
91. van Doorn DC, de Bruin MJ, Jorritsma RA, Ploeger HW, Schoormans A (2009) Prevalence of *Tritrichomonas foetus* among Dutch cats. Tijdschr Diergeneeskd 134:698–700 (in Dutch)
92. Hensinger T (2009) *Trichomonas foetus*. A pathogen responsible for diarrhoea in cats. Weterynaria w Praktyce 6:80–81
93. Lim S, Park SI, Ahn KS, Oh DS, Ryu JS, Shin SS (2010) First report of feline intestinal trichomoniasis caused by *Tritrichomonas foetus* in Korea. Korean J Parasitol 48:247–251
94. Miro G, Hernandez L, Montoya A, Arranz-Solis D, Dado D, Rojo-Montejo S, Mendoza-Ibarra JA, Ortega-Mora LM, Pedraza-Diaz S (2011) First description of naturally acquired *Tritrichomonas foetus* infection in a Persian cattery in Spain. Parasitol Res 109:1151–1154
95. Forshell U, Osterman-Lind E (2010) Chronic diarrhoea caused by *Tritrichomonas foetus* in the cat. Svensk Veterinärtidning 62:19–21
96. Frey CF, Schild M, Hemphill A, Stunzi P, Muller N, Gottstein B, Burgener IA (2009) Intestinal *Tritrichomonas foetus* infection in cats in Switzerland detected by in vitro cultivation and PCR. Parasitol Res 104:783–788
97. Burgener IA, Frey CF, Kook PH, Gottstein B (2010) *Tritrichomonas foetus*: a new intestinal parasite in Swiss cats. Schweiz Arch Tierheilkd 151:383–389 (in German)
98. Gunn-Moore D, Tennant B (2007) *Tritrichomonas foetus* diarrhoea in cats. Vet Rec 160:850–851

A novel panel of monoclonal antibodies against Schmallenberg virus nucleoprotein and glycoprotein Gc allows specific orthobunyavirus detection and reveals antigenic differences

Kerstin Wernike[1†], Emiliana Brocchi[2†], Paolo Cordioli[2^], Yann Sénéchal[3], Christian Schelp[3], Anne Wegelt[1], Andrea Aebischer[1], Gleyder Roman-Sosa[1], Ilona Reimann[1] and Martin Beer[1*]

Abstract

A panel of monoclonal antibodies (mAbs) specific for the nucleocapsid (N) protein or the glycoprotein Gc of Schmallenberg virus (SBV), a novel member of the Simbu serogroup (genus *Orthobunyavirus*, family *Bunyaviridae*), was produced and used to analyze antigenic differences among members of this serogroup. Reactivity with various SBV-isolates and other Simbu serogroup viruses was assessed by an indirect immunofluorescence test and by immunoblotting. The Gc-specific mAbs detected different SBV isolates as well as two closely related members of the Simbu serogroup. In addition, one mAb showed a highly specific reactivity with the homologous SBV strain only. Based on their differing reactivity with different SBV-strains, these antibodies represent a valuable novel tool to rapidly determine the phenotype of new SBV isolates. In contrast, the N-specific mAbs showed a broad reactivity spectrum and detected not only all the tested SBV-isolates, but also several other viruses of the Simbu serogroup. One out of these mAbs even recognized all of the tested Simbu serogroup viruses in the indirect immunofluorescence assay. In order to further characterize the N-specific antibodies, PepScan analysis was performed and a specific epitope could be identified. In summary, the newly generated mAbs showed differing pan-Simbu virus-, pan-SBV- as well as SBV-isolate-specific reactivity patterns. Thus, they represent valuable tools for the development of novel antigen and antibody detection systems either specific for SBV or, in a broader approach, for the pan-Simbu serogroup diagnostics.

Introduction

In late 2011, a hitherto unknown teratogenic orthobunyavirus was discovered in Central Europe and named Schmallenberg virus (SBV) [1]. It causes severe congenital malformation, stillbirth or premature birth, when pregnant ruminants are infected during a critical period of gestation. SBV is a member of the genus *Orthobunyavirus* within the family *Bunyaviridae* [1]. Orthobunyaviruses are divided into 18 serogoups and among these SBV belongs to the Simbu serogroup [2,3]. The closest relatives of SBV are Sathuperi virus (SATV) and Douglas virus (DOUV) [2]. However, the Simbu serogroup also includes Akabane virus (AKAV) and Aino virus (AINOV), as well as Oropouche virus (OROV), which is the only member of the serogroup capable to infect humans.

Like in typical bunyaviruses, the SBV genome consists of three single-stranded RNA segments which encode six proteins. According to their size they are named large (L), medium (M) and small (S). The nucleocapsid (N) protein and a small non-structural protein (NSs) are encoded in overlapping open reading frames by the S segment, two glycoproteins (Gn and Gc), as well as a non-structural protein (NSm) are encoded by the M segment, and the RNA-dependent RNA polymerase which represents the central element of the orthobunyaviral replication complex [4] is encoded by the L segment [5,6].

* Correspondence: martin.beer@fli.bund.de
†Equal contributors
^Deceased
[1]Institute of Diagnostic Virology, Friedrich-Loeffler-Institut (FLI), Suedufer 10, 17493 Greifswald - Insel Riems, Germany
Full list of author information is available at the end of the article

The N-protein has a molecular weight of 25 kDa, oligomerizes as a tetramer [7], and is not only essential for viral genome encapsidation, but is also involved in viral RNA-transcription and replication [7,8]. Furthermore, it is the most conserved protein among orthobunyaviruses, and elicits a strong humoral immune response in infected animals [9-11]. The glycoproteins Gn and Gc with molecular masses of approximately 35 kDa and 110 kDa, respectively, represent type I integral transmembrane proteins which are further modified by N-linked glycosylation [8]. They form spikes on the virus particle and are essential for viral attachment and cell fusion. It has been described before for certain bunyaviruses, that Gn and Gc are targeted by neutralizing antibodies [5]. Similar roles are also assumed for the SBV Gn and Gc, but remain to be confirmed. In contrast to the nucleocapsid protein, the glycoproteins, especially Gc, show the most variable sequences among the protein-coding genes of SBV and related viruses [12-15].

Currently, molecular and serological detection systems for SBV primarily base on the N-protein [16,17]. In the present study, monoclonal antibodies (mAb) specific for N as well as for Gc were prepared and characterized. Special emphasis was set on the investigation of the suitability of the mAbs for application in SBV diagnostics and for the characterization of virus isolates.

Materials and methods

Virus purification

SBV, strain BH80/11, was propagated in Vero cell monolayers and harvested when the cytopathic effect (CPE) was maximal; supernatant fluid was clarified by centrifugation at 4000 rpm for 30 min, added to 8% of PEG 6000 in 0.5 M NaCl, and then placed overnight at 4 °C in agitation. The suspension was centrifuged at 5000 rpm for 30 min and the pellet was resuspended in phosphate-buffer saline solution, pH 7.4 (PBS) at a 20X concentration compared to the initial volume. Following further clarification by centrifugation (5000 rpm for 30 min), the viral suspension was purified by ultracentrifugation at 35 000 rpm for 2 h (rotor TST41 Kontron) through a 25% (w/w) sucrose cushion and the pellet was resuspended in PBS. The concentrated antigen was kept at −70 °C until use.

MAbs production

Two Balb/c mice were primed with intraperitoneal injections of 4×10^6 BHK-21 cells infected with SBV strain BH80/11 (dilutions in PBS). After one month, mice were boosted as follows: one using again the initial antigen preparation, and the second one using partially purified virus (500 µg of total protein containing approximately 50 µg of viral proteins).

Three days after the boost, mice were humanely sacrificed and hybridomas were generated by fusion of splenocytes with NSO myeloma cells following standard procedures [18]. Briefly, at least 10^8 spleen cells were recovered from each mouse and fused with NSO myeloma cells at a 10:1 ratio using PEG 4000. Fused cells diluted in Dulbecco's modified Eagle medium, supplemented with hypoxanthine/aminopterin/thymidine and 20% fetal calf serum, were distributed over five microplates (200 µL per well). Growing colonies were observed in all wells; in order to select hybridomas secreting monoclonal antibodies specific for SBV, the supernatants were screened by indirect immunofluorescence (IIF) test using SBV-infected Vero cells, grown into 96-well microplates and fixed by 80% acetone. Non-infected Vero cells served as negative controls.

The positive hybridoma cells were cloned by limiting dilution in order to obtain antibodies from one single cell. The supernatant from exhausted cultures was then used as source of mAb.

Indirect ELISA

ELISA was performed in 96-well Nunc Maxisorp ELISA plates. The plates were coated over night at 4 °C using 50 µL/well of partially purified SBV-antigen at a saturating concentration (produced as described above) diluted in ELISA coating buffer (0.05 M carbonate/bicarbonate buffer, pH 9.6). Plates were washed three times with 250 µL of washing buffer (PBS containing 0.05% Tween 20) and subsequently incubated with 50 µL/well of undiluted hybridoma culture supernatants for 1 h at 37 °C. After three washes, a peroxidase-conjugated goat anti-mouse immunoglobulin antibody (produced in-house) optimally diluted in PBS containing 0.05% Tween 20 and 1% yeast extract was incubated for 1 h at 37 °C. After a final washing cycle, 50 µL/well of substrate solution (0.5 mg/mL orthophenylenediamine and 0.02% H_2O_2 in 50 mM phosphate citrate buffer, pH 5) was added. The colorimetric reaction was stopped after 10 min using 2 N sulfuric acid and the absorbance values were read at 492 nm using an ELISA reader.

Virus-neutralization test (VNT)

Serial two-fold dilutions of each hybridoma supernatant (duplicate wells) in 25 µL of serum-free culture medium were incubated for 1 h at 37 °C with an equal volume of cell culture supernatant containing 100 tissue culture infectious dose 50 ($TCID_{50}$) of SBV. Subsequently, 50 µL of Vero cells at a dilution of 4×10^5 cells/mL in medium containing 10% fetal calf serum were added to each well. After incubation for 72–96 h at 37 °C with 5% CO_2, wells were scored for CPE and neutralizing titers were expressed as the reciprocal of the final mAb dilution required to neutralize 100% of the inoculated cultures.

Immunofluorescence test

The hybridoma supernatants were characterized by an IIF-test using SBV-infected BHK-21 cells, clone BRS5 (L194, Collection of Cell Lines in veterinary Medicine [CCLV]) as antigen matrix [17]. The BHK-21 cells were infected with one of the following SBV strains: BH80/11 (isolated from bovine blood in 2011 on KC cells [L1062 CCLV]), BH619/12 (isolated from sheep serum in 2012 on Vero cells [L0228 CCLV]), BH652/12 (isolated from bovine blood in 2012 on BHK cells [L0164 CCLV]), D512/12, D495/12-1, and D495/12-2 (all three isolated in 2012 and kindly provided by Andreas Moss, Lebensmittel- und Veterinärinstitut Oldenburg, Germany). In addition, the mAbs were tested against closely related Simbu serogroup viruses, namely Simbu virus (SIMV), DOUV, SATV, Sabo virus (SABOV), Shamonda virus (SHAV), AKAV, AINOV, Peaton virus (PEAV), and OROV. All Simbu serogroup viruses were kindly provided by Peter Kirkland (Elizabeth Macarthur Agricultural Institute, Australia) and Robert Tesh (University of Texas Medical Branch, USA).

In addition, the mAbs were tested in DNA-transfected BSR-T7/5 cells (L583 CCLV, [19]), transiently expressing SBV-N, all M-segment encoded proteins (Gn, Gc, M) and Gn or Gc separately. For the construction of the expression plasmids pCITE_N, pCITE_M, pCITE_Gn and pCITE_Gc, the open reading frame (ORF) of SBV-N and SBV-M and the genomic regions encoding Gn and Gc, respectively, were amplified by RT-PCR from supernatants of SBV-infected BHK-21 cells. RNA was isolated by using the QIAmp viral RNA Mini Kit (Qiagen) and amplified with the QIAGEN OneStep RT-PCR Kit (Qiagen). Primers used for S were as follows: SBV_N_F (5'CCAATCTAGACCGAT GTTGATACCGAATTGCTG 3'), SBV_N_R (3' GAG TGCGGCCGCTTTAGATGTTGATACCGAATTG 5'), for M: SBV_Gn_F (5' GAAAAACACGATGATAATACCATG CTTCTCAACATTGTCTTG 3'), SBV_Gc_R (3' GTGGT GCTCGAGTGCGGCCGCTCACTT AAATTT ATTTTC CATTT GG 5'), for Gn: SBV_Gn_F and SBV_Gn_R (3' GT GGTGCTCGAGTGCGGCCGCTT ACCTTGTTTTCG GCAATGCT TTATAG 5') and for Gc: SBV_Gc_F (5' GA AAAACA CGATGATAATACCATGGAAACTAG TATT AACTGCAAAAACA 3') and SBV_Gc_R. The RT-PCR fragments were cloned into plasmid pCITE-2a (Novagen). After XbaI/NcoI digestion, the PCR fragment of SBV-N was ligated into the NcoI/XbaI digested plasmid resulting in plasmid pCITE_N. Plasmid constructs pCITE_M, pCITE_Gn and pCITE_Gc were generated by restriction-free cloning [20]. For protein expression, plasmid-DNA was transfected into BSR-T7/5 cells which stably express the phage T7 RNA polymerase [19] using Lipofectamine 2000 (Invitrogen) according to manufacturer's protocols. At 24 h post transfection, the transfected cells were used for the investigation of the mAbs by IIF-staining.

SDS–PAGE and Western blot analysis

The reactivity of the hybridoma supernatants with the SBV-strains mentioned above as well as with SIMV, DOUV, SATV, SABOV, SHAV, AKAV, AINOV, and OROV was additionally analyzed by Western blot (WB). The viruses were propagated on BHK-cells (L0164 CCLV) and were deep frozen at −70 °C when a generalized cytopathic effect became evident after 24 – 48 h post infection. Uninfected BHK-cells were used as a negative control. The proteins were separated by sodium dodecyl sulfate polyacrylamide gel electrophoresis (SDS-PAGE) under reducing or non-reducing conditions and transferred onto a nitrocellulose membrane using a Trans-Blot SD Semi-Dry Transfer Cell device (Bio-Rad). The nitrocellulose membranes were blocked for 1 h using 5% non-fat dry milk diluted in PBS and subsequently incubated with the hybridoma supernatants (diluted 1:20 in PBS) overnight at 4 °C followed by a horseradish peroxidase-conjugated anti-mouse antibody (Dako, diluted 1:200 in PBS) for 1 h at room temperature. Proteins were visualized using the Super Signal West Pico Chemiluminescent substrat (Thermo Scientific).

PepScan analysis of anti-N monoclonal antibodies

A library of biotinylated overlapping peptides covering the entire N-protein sequence was synthesized (New England Peptide, USA). Biotinylated peptides were 16 amino acids (aa) long with an overlap of 13 aa. Synthesis was successful for all requested peptides except for peptides number B10 and D08 which were excluded from the analysis because they did not pass quality control (please see Additional file 1 for sequence information).

Biotinylated peptides were coated on 96-well streptavidin plates (IDEXX International, USA) and the N-specific mAbs were subsequently tested for binding activity on each peptide. In addition, binding activity of full-length recombinant N-protein (rN) was assessed as a control on the same plate. The rN-protein was cloned in pET28a and expressed in E. coli BL21 cells (Novagen, UK). Water soluble His-tagged protein was purified by affinity chromatography on Ni^{2+}-columns [21] and biotinylated subsequently (EZ-Link® Sulfo-NHS-LC-Biotinylation Kit, Thermo Scientific). The indirect ELISA was performed as follows: Streptavidin plates were washed three times with PBS containing 0.1% Tween-20. Peptides (5.0 to 7.5 mg/mL in DMSO) were diluted 1:400 in PBS pH 7.2 and coated using 100 μL/well during 1 h at room temperature. Plates were then washed three times using washing buffer (PBS containing 0.1% Tween-20). Subsequently, 100 μL of the diluted hybridoma supernatants were added to each well and incubated for 1 h at room temperature. After three additional washing steps, 100 μL/well of goat anti-mouse peroxidase-conjugated antibody (Bio-Rad) were added and incubated for 1 h at room temperature. Dilutions were both prepared in PBS containing 0.1% Tween-20 and 10% goat serum. Finally, the plates were washed three times with washing buffer and subsequently 3,3′,5,5′-tetramethylbenzidine (TMB substrate) was added to each well. The color development was stopped after 10 min and optical densities (OD) were measured at 450 nm using a spectrophotometer. When two contiguous peptides were recognized, it was assumed that the binding area was the common amino acid sequence of the two contiguous peptides.

The identified epitopes were highlighted in the three-dimensional structure of SBV-N [22] using the PyMOL software [23].

Results

MAb production

A panel of 47 hybridomas, generated by fusion processes from two immunized mice, was found to produce mAbs specifically reactive with homologous SBV in IIF and indirect ELISA tests.

In a preliminary characterization aimed at selection of mAbs for further studies, the 47 MAbs showed two different immunofluorescence patterns (described in the following paragraph), the majority reacted in western blot with either a band of approximately 25 kDa or a band of 110 kDa. The former did not show neutralizing activity, while most of the latter did neutralize SBV infectivity, suggesting a strong involvement of the target protein in virus neutralization mechanisms.

After preliminary characterization and diversification, a subset of 16 hybridomas was submitted to cloning procedures and the produced mAbs were used for the following more detailed investigations.

Evaluation of the 16 mAbs in VNT, IIF test and Western blot analysis

In the IIF tests, six mAbs reacted with transiently expressed SBV-N (pCITE_N transfected cells) and ten with SBV-M (pCITE_M transfected cells) (Table 1).

When analyzed in WB (non-reducing conditions), using the homologous strain BH80/11, four out of the six SBV-N-reactive mAbs bound a protein of the approximate molecular weight of the N-protein (25 kDa, Figure 1). The remaining two mAbs (3H9 and 3A11) did not recognize any denatured SBV antigen in cell lysates (Table 2). None of the six mAbs was reactive under reducing conditions (data not shown). The 10 mAbs which reacted with pCITE_M transfected cells detected a Gc-specific band of about 110 kDa in WB (Table 2 and Figure 1).

All mAbs showed a strong reactivity in BHK21-cells infected with the homologous SBV strain BH80/11. However, the individual mAbs showed different fluorescence staining patterns. By using the SBV-N-reactive mAbs a cytoplasmatic fluorescence and granular inclusions could be observed (see Figure 2A for an example). In contrast, a more diffuse, homogenous immunofluorescence around the nuclei of the infected cells was produced by SBV-M-reactive mAbs (Figure 2B).

Eventually, the target-specificity of the mAbs was determined by combining the results of WB analysis and IIF tests described above: 6 out of the 16 characterized mAbs were specific for the N-protein, and 10 specifically reacted with Gc. Investigation of the virus neutralizing capability by VNT showed that none of the six anti-N mAbs was able to neutralize virus infectivity, in contrast to seven out of 10 anti-Gc mAbs, which demonstrated neutralizing activity (Table 2).

Apart from the homologous strain BH80/11, five additional SBV isolates were used to investigate the reactivity of the mAbs. The results of both, WB analysis and IIF tests were in agreement for all isolates except for mAb 5 F8 (Tables 1 and 2). In IIF, this antibody detected 4 out of 6 SBV isolates, whereas in WB, it reacted only with the isolate BH80/11-4, which was used for the mAb production.

The reactivity of the mAbs with nine related Simbu viruses was subsequently also investigated. The N-specific mAbs were able to detect DOUV, SATV, and SHAV infected cells (see Figure 3 for an example) and four out of six mAbs reacted also with SIMV, SABOV, and AKAV infected cells in IIF tests. The mAb 1H4 even showed a pan-Simbu reactivity as it detected all of the tested Simbu serogroup viruses. Of the Gc-specific mAbs, one detected SATV and four recognized SATV as well as DOUV. However, the remaining 5 mAbs did not recognize any of the tested Simbu viruses (Table 1). In WB, all the SBV N-specific mAbs except 3H9 and 3A11 reacted with DOUV, SIMV, SATV, and SHAV, three of them also detected SABOV and AKAV, and mAb 1H4 showed reactivity with all tested Simbu viruses except AINOV. Among the Gc-specific mAbs, one showed positive signals with DOUV and another three were able to detect SATV (Table 2).

Epitope mapping and location on the three-dimensional structure of anti-N monoclonal antibodies

The anti-N mAbs showed the broadest reactivity spectrum against all the tested bunyaviruses, hence determining the relevant epitopes could be helpful to explain the observed patterns. For this purpose, a PepScan approach was applied, in which overlapping peptides that covered the complete sequence of the N-protein were synthesized and tested with the respective mAbs in an ELISA.

The mAbs 4E12 and 1H4 showed a strong and reproducible binding activity to some contiguous peptides allowing the localization of the target epitope (Figures 4 and 5). MAb 4E12 bound strongly to the peptides A07,

Table 1 Characterization of anti-SBV mAbs by immunofluorescence test

MAbs	indirect immunofluorescence test (IIFT)															IIFT pCITE clones		
	Schmallenberg virus						DOUV	SIMV	SATV	SHAV	SABOV	AKAV	AINOV	PEAV	OROV	Schmallenberg virus		
	BH80/11-4	BH619/12-3	BH652/12	D512/12	D495/12-1	D495/12-2										S	M	Gc
4E12	+	+	+	+	+	+	+	+	+	+	+	+	-	-	-	+		
1H4	+	+	+	+	+	+	+	+	+	+	+	+	+	+	+	+		
3H3	+	+	+	+	+	+	+	+	+	+	+	+	-	-	-	+	-	
3E3	+	+	+	+	+	+	+	+	+	+	+	+	-	-	-	+		
3H9	+	+	+	+	+	+	+	-	+	+	-	-	-	-	-	+	-	
3A11	+	+	+	+	+	+	+	-	+	+	-	-	-	-	-	+		
2G10	+	+	+	+	+	+	-	-	-	-	-	-	-	-	-	-	+	+
4D9	+	+	+	+	+	+	-	-	-	-	-	-	-	-	-	-	+	+
2H11	+	+	+	+	+	+	+	-	+	-	-	-	-	-	-	-	+	+
4E5	+	+	+	+	+	+	-	-	-	-	-	-	-	-	-	-	+	+
5 F8	+	+	+	+	-	-	-	-	-	-	-	-	-	-	-		+	+
1C11	+	+	+	+	+	+	+	-	+	-	-	-	-	-	-		+	+
1 F4	+	+	+	+	+	+	-	-	+	-	-	-	-	-	-		+	+
4B6	+	+	+	+	+	+	-	-	-	-	-	-	-	-	-	-	+	+
1C1	+	+	+	+	+	+	+	-	+	-	-	-	-	-	-	-	+	+
3A5	+	+	+	+	+	+	+	-	+	-	-	-	-	-	-	-	+	+

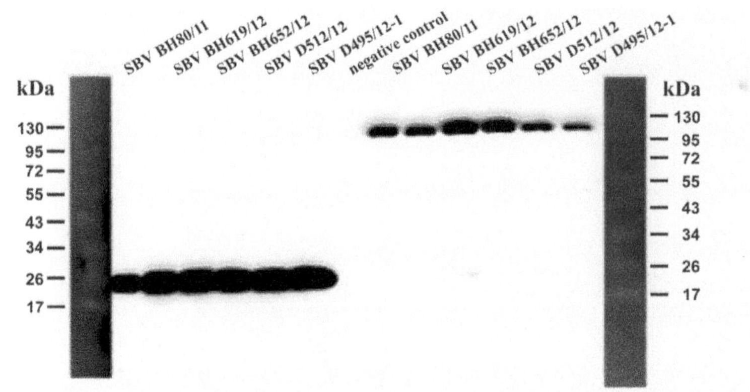

Figure 1 Western blot analysis of mAbs 4E12 and 1F4. The anti-N mAb 4E12 is shown in lanes 1 to 7, and mAb 1F4 (anti-Gc) in lanes 7 to 13.

A08 (OD > 5.0) and to a lower extent to A09 (OD 1.9). MAb 1H4 bound strongly to the peptide A08 (OD 3.9) and on a clearly lower level to A07 (OD 1.0). Since peptides A07 (aa 19–34), A08 (aa 22–37) and A09 (aa 25–40) are contiguous peptides within the N-protein of SBV strain BH80/11 (Figure 5) it could be assumed that this aa region represents the binding area of the mAbs 4E12 and 1H4 or is at least a part of it. However, for the remaining four N-specific mAbs, no binding activity could be detected in the peptide ELISA although all mAbs strongly bound to the full length N-protein (Figure 4). Two of these four mAbs showed also no reactivity in WB-analyses, indicating a conformation-dependent nature of their target epitopes.

The reactions of 3E3 and 4E12 with peptide F03 and of 3H9 with peptides F01 and G01 could not be confirmed and are possibly due to conjugate artifacts.

The epitope formed by peptides A07, A08, and A09 corresponds to amino acid positions 19 to 40 of SBV strain BH80/11 and could be localized at the external face of the N-protein tetramer in the crystal structure of SBV-N [22] (Figure 6).

Discussion

The Simbu serogroup of the genus *Orthobunyavirus* contains viruses of different medical and veterinary relevance and members of this group have been isolated worldwide [24]. OROV, the only virus in the serogroup that can infect humans, was responsible for outbreaks of acute febrile illness in South America [25,26]. AKAV, a serious threat to the livestock industry, caused epizootics of congenital defects in Asia, Australia, or in the Middle East [27-30]. An AKAV-infection during a critical period of gestation can lead to the birth of severely malformed offspring, premature birth or stillbirth. Identical symptoms are induced by an infection of pregnant ruminants with other members of the Simbu serogroup as e.g. AINOV or SBV [30-34]. SBV, a novel orthobunyavirus and the first European member of this serogroup, was discovered for the first time in late 2011. Since then, the virus caused a large epidemic in domestic and wild ruminants all over Europe [35-37]. To enable early detection of an SBV-spread into previously unaffected regions and to monitor emergence of other Simbu serogroup viruses, sensitive and specific diagnostic test systems are required.

The N-protein represents the most abundant protein in the virion as well as in virus-infected cells and is currently widely used for serological detection of SBV infections [16,17]. In addition, the N-protein encoding gene provides a reliable target of SBV molecular diagnostics tests. Furthermore, due to its high immunogenicity, N-specific antibodies are detectable early after infection as well as in convalescent animals providing a reliable basis for serological diagnosis [38,39]. However, due to the high sequence conservation of the N-gene, antibody cross-reactivity occurs among members of the same serogroup [17,40,41]. Accordingly, the N-specific mAbs produced in the present study recognized several viruses of the Simbu serogroup (Tables 1 and 2). Nevertheless, only the mAb 1H4 allowed detection of all the tested virus strains in the immunofluorescence test. This antibody therefore represents a promising candidate for the development of serological screening tests which cover the entire Simbu serogroup. The mAb could e.g. be applied in a blocking or competing ELISA format.

Table 2 Characterization of anti-SBV mAbs by ELISA, neutralization test, and western blot

MAbs	ELISA	VNT	Western blot (kDa)														
			Schmallenberg virus						DOUV	SIMV	SATV	SHAV	SABOV	AKAV	AINOV	OROV	
			BH80/11-4	BH619/12-3	BH652/12	D512/12	D495/12-1	D495/12-2									Specifity
4E12	+	<1/2	~25	~25	~25	~25	~25	~25	~25	~25	~25	~25	~25	~25	-	-	**nucleocapsid protein**
1H4	+	<1/2	~25	~25	~25	~25	~25	~25	~25	~25	~25	~25	~25	~25	-	~25	**nucleocapsid protein**
3H3	+	<1/2	~25	~25	~25	~25	~25	~25	~25	~25	~25	~25	~25	~25	-	-	**nucleocapsid protein**
3E3	+	<1/2	~25	~25	~25	~25	~25	~25	~25	~25	~25	~25	-	-	-	-	**nucleocapsid protein**
3H9	+	<1/2	-	-	-	-	-	-		-	-	-	-				**nucleocapsid protein**
3A11	+	<1/2	-	-	-	-	-	-		-	-	-	-				**nucleocapsid protein**
2G10	+	<1/2	~110	~110	~110	~110	~110	~110									**glycoprotein Gc**
4D9	+	pos	~110	~110	~110	~110	~110	~110									**glycoprotein Gc**
2H11	+	<1/2	~110	~110	~110	~110	~110	~110	~110	-	-	-	-				**glycoprotein Gc**
4E5	+	pos	~110	~110	~110	~110	~110	~110									**glycoprotein Gc**
5 F8	+	1/8	~110	-	-	-	-	-									**glycoprotein Gc**
1C11	+	1/16	~110	~110	~110	~110	~110	~110	-	-	~110	-	-				**glycoprotein Gc**
1 F4	+	1/4	~110	~110	~110	~110	~110	~110	-	-	-	-	-				**glycoprotein Gc**
4B6	+	1/8	~110	~110	~110	~110	~110	~110									**glycoprotein Gc**
1C1	+	1/16	~110	~110	~110	~110	~110	~110		-	~110	-	-				**glycoprotein Gc**
3A5	+	<1/2	~110	~110	~110	~110	~110	~110		-	~110	-	-				**glycoprotein Gc**

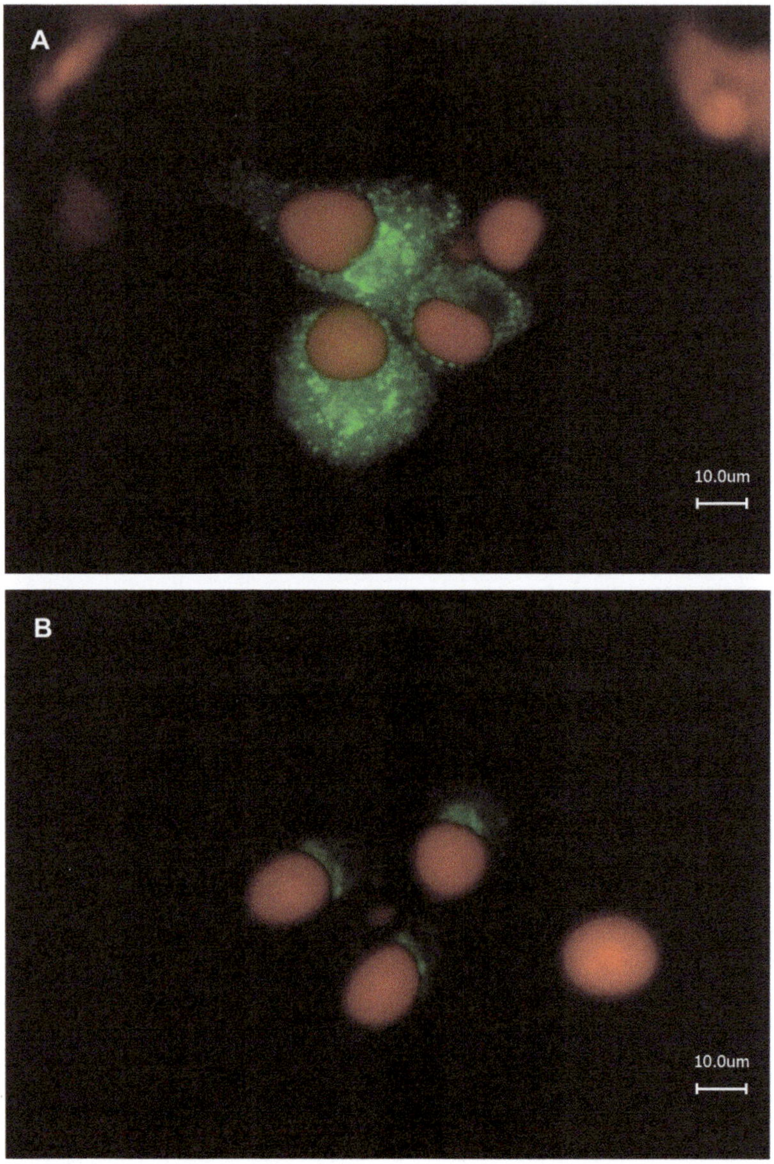

Figure 2 Indirect immunofluorescence test. MAbs 4E12 (anti-N, **A**) and 1F4 (anti-Gc, **B**) were analyzed in an indirect immunofluorescence test using BHK-21 cells infected with SBV strain BH80/11 as antigen matrix.

Using PepScan analysis, the epitope of mAb 1H4 and 4E12 could be localized to amino acid positions 19 to 40 of the SBV BH80/11-N-protein. These results are not in agreement with a previously with another mAb identified antigenic epitope located between aa 51 to 76 [41]. However, the respective experiments have been performed using a bacterially expressed full-length recombinant SBV-N-protein, whereas a peptide library was applied in the present study, which might explain the diverging results. Using 3D modelling, the epitope recognized by mAbs 1H4 and 4E12 could be located to the external surface of the tetramer formed by the N-protein in complex with the RNA molecule, rendering this domain accessible to the humoral immune system. However, even though these two mAbs bound to the same epitope in the PepScan analysis, they showed differences in their reactivity with Simbu serogroup viruses in IIF and WB. It can therefore be assumed that mAbs 1H4 and 4E12 bind to different key amino acid residues within overlapping linear epitopes.

For several of the mAbs used in this study a specific epitope could not be identified, indicating that the respective antibodies bind to discontinuous epitopes [42]. In such cases, the antibodies are not directed against a linear stretch of aa, but recognize a set of amino acid residues in the antigen that are brought together only by the folding of the molecule [42]. Since with the applied PepScan technology only linear epitopes can be mapped,

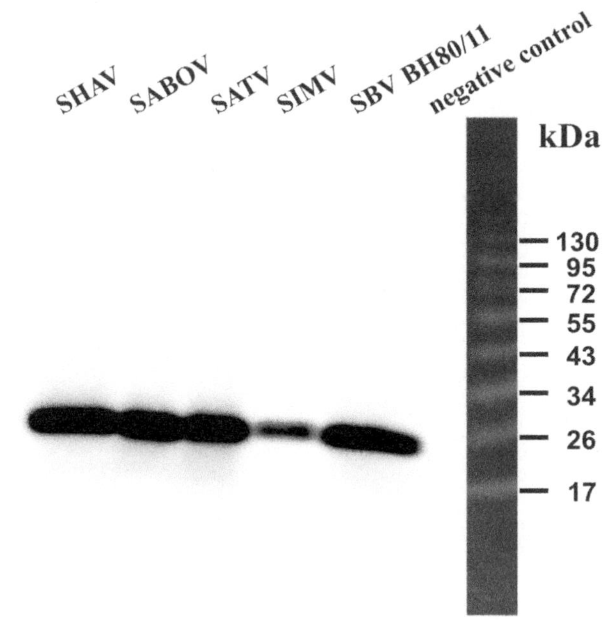

Figure 3 Western blot analysis of mAbs 4E12 with Simbu serogroup viruses. Mock-infected BHK-21 cells were used as negative control.

it is not suitable to investigate conformation-dependent epitopes. This might explain the failure to define epitopes for each of the antibodies.

Virus neutralization activity was observed for none of the generated anti-N mAbs, which is in agreement with previous studies. Although N represents the immunodominant protein in several members of the *Bunyaviridae* family, it has been shown before, that anti-N antibodies usually do not have neutralizing activity. In contrast, almost all neutralizing antibodies are directed against the glycoproteins [9,43-45]. This is in accordance with the results of the present study: 7 out of 10 mAbs specific for M-segment encoded proteins were positive in the VNT. Furthermore, all the isolated glycoprotein-specific antibodies were directed against Gc, suggesting that the virus particle-associated Gc is more immunogenic than Gn. It has already been shown before in immunization experiments, e.g. using the bunyavirus LaCrosse virus, that the Gc-protein can be the main target of the humoral immune response [9,46].

In contrast to the conserved S-segment, the M-segment is variable between different SBV strains and between different virus species of the Simbu serogroup. A region of especially high sequence variability was recently described within the gene encoding Gc [13,14]. Consequently, five out of the 10 Gc-specific mAbs exclusively detected SBV isolates in the present study. The remaining five mAbs additionally recognized DOUV and SATV, which are the most closely related viruses to SBV based on M-segment sequences [2]. However, cross-reactivity against other Simbu serogroup viruses was not observed.

Interestingly, two of the mAbs which detected SBV as well as DOUV and SATV (mAbs 1C1 and 1C11) are possibly directed against the same epitope within the Gc-glycoprotein. This was recently suggested based on their identical reactivity profile with an escape-mutant SBV (resistant to neutralization) which was generated by mAb 1C11 (Brocchi and Cordioli, personal communication). In addition, the mAb 1C11 (or alternatively 1C1) has already been successfully employed as competitor-conjugated mAb in a competitive ELISA which allows antibody detection in different species [47].

The mAb 2H11 did not bind as strong as the other Gc-mAbs to Gc-protein expressed in transfected cells, even though it recognized a product of the approximate molecular size of the mature Gc in western blot and reacted with virus-infected cells in the IIF test. Maybe, this antibody recognizes the SBV-Gc better in a conformation which relies

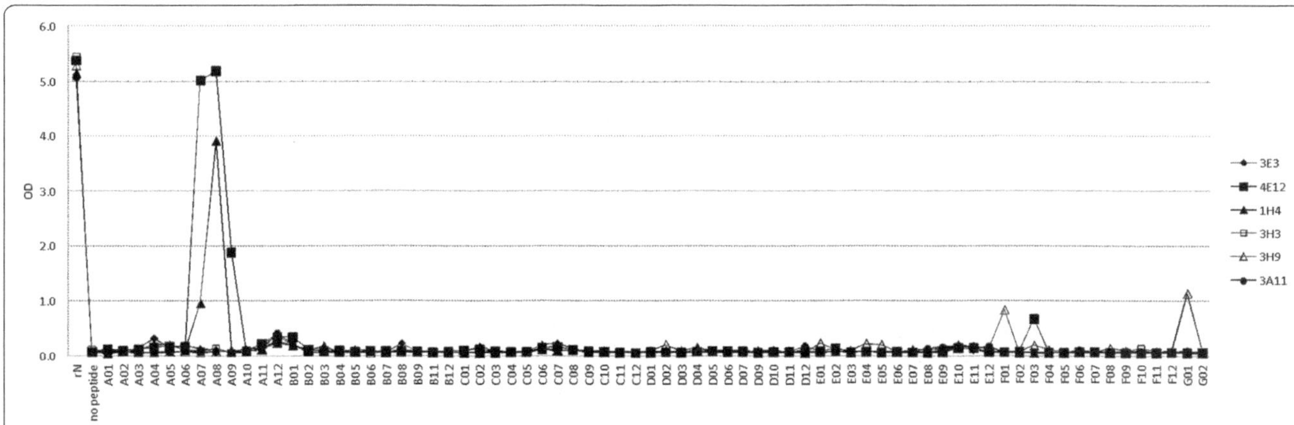

Figure 4 PepScan analysis of the anti-N antibodies. Binding of mAbs 3E3 clone 10 (filled diamond), 4E12 clone 9 (filled square), 1H4 clone 7 (filled triangle), 3H3 clone 2 (open square) 3H9 clone 4 (open triangle), and 3A11 clone 2 (filled circle) to full length N-protein (rNP) and to N-protein (Np) peptides.

```
Schmallenberg virus  MSSQFIFEDVPQRNAATFNPEVGYVAFIGKYGQQLNFGVARVFFLNQKKAKMVLHKTAQPSVDLTFGGVKFTVVNNHFPQYVSNPVPDNAITLHRMSGYL
Douglas virus        .....................................S..............................................................
Simbu virus          .AN...........LS..S..A.......R.......S.V....................N...........L...N....TA.......L....L....
Sathuperi virus      ....................................................................................................
Shamonda virus       ....................................................................................................
Sabo virus           .A.....D............DT......S....H...T...........................................IA.....T.L.........
Akabane virus        .AN....N............DA......S........T...................P........A..............TA...S.T.F....I....
Aino virus           .AN....Q......L.............A.H.A....DTV..............S.............I...L........TA.....T.L....L....
Peaton virus         .AN....Q......L.............A...A....DTV..............S.............I...L........TA.....T.L....L....
Oropouche virus      -M.E...N.....TTS..D..AA....EAR...V..A..V...........D..R..SR.M........Q.AM.......FQ.......GL....L....
Schmallenberg virus  ....................................................................................................

Schmallenberg virus  ARWIADTCKASVLKLAEASAQIVMPLAEVKGCTWADGYTMYLGFAPGAEMFLDAFDFYPLVIEMHRVLKDNMDVNFMKKVLRQRYGTMTAEEWMTQKITE
Douglas virus        ...V................................................................................................
Simbu virus          ...T.EQV.NNQV.....T.A.............N.................ET.E.F....D.......G......R.A.......LL..Q......V.
Sathuperi virus      ...V................................................................................................
Shamonda virus       ....................................................................................................
Sabo virus           ...V.EL.RGNQI.....ATL.............N.................ET.E......D.......G......R.........L.......T..EA
Akabane virus        ...V.EQ...NQI.F...A.T.............S...A.............ET.E......D....I..G......R.........QL......S.LDA
Aino virus           .K.V..Q..TNQI.....MEK.............TE.L..............ET.E......D.......G......R.........L...Q......DA
Peaton virus         .K.V..Q..TNQI.....MEK.............TE.L..............ET.E......D.......G......R.........L...Q......DA
Oropouche virus      ...AFTQMR-.PI.Q..FR.TV.V..........N..DA......A......QT.T.F............G................QK..Q..REE.VA
Schmallenberg virus  ....................................................................................................

Schmallenberg virus  IKAAFNSVGQLAWAKSGFSPAARTFLQQFGINI
Douglas virus        .................................
Simbu virus          V....DA...I............A.......TV
Sathuperi virus      .................................
Shamonda virus       .................................
Sabo virus           VR......A.IS...T.......A..AN...Q.
Akabane virus        V....G..A.IS...........A..A....Q.
Aino virus           VR....A....S...........A..A......
Peaton virus         VR....A....S..............A......
Oropouche virus      VR...EA..T....RT.......D..R....D.
Schmallenberg virus  .................................
```

4E12

1H4

Figure 5 Sequence alignment of N-protein of Simbu serogroup viruses. Amino acids that match those of SBV are indicated by dots. The linear epitopes identified by using pepscanning are highlighted, a strong ELISA reaction is represented in dark grey (mAb 4E12) or dark blue (mAb 1H4), whereas a weaker reaction is indicated in light grey (4E12) or light blue (1H4).

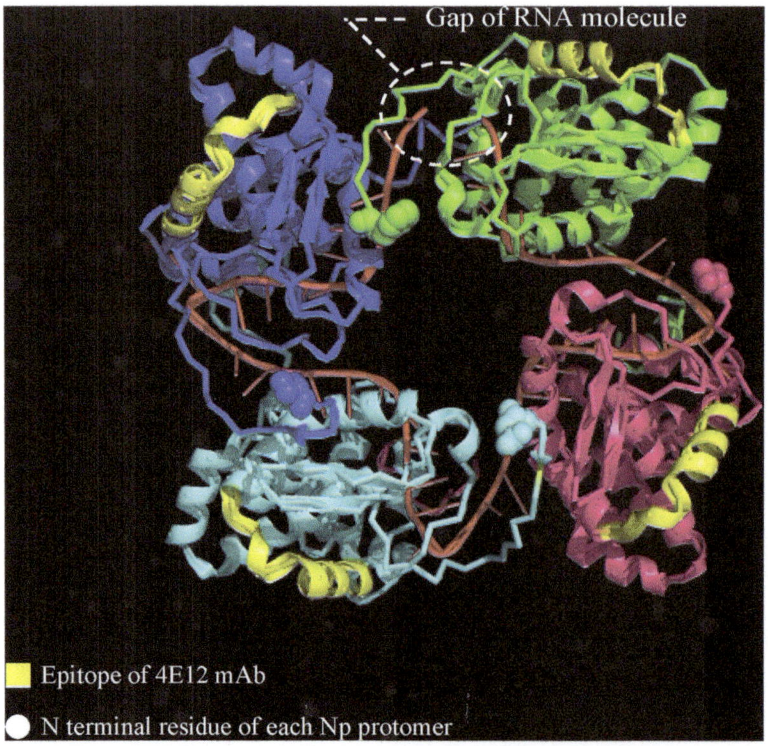

Figure 6 Location of the antigenic site of mAb 4E12 in the three-dimensional structure of SBV-N. The structure of SBV-N was obtained from [22]. This figure was prepared using the PyMOL program [23].

on the presence of the Gn-protein indicating that the mAb either reacts with the Gn-Gc complex and/or with the Gc alone once it is chaperoned by Gn. This hypothesis is supported by previous studies in Bunyamwera virus which demonstrated the importance of Gn in the transport of Gc to the Golgi and in Gc-Gn-heterodimerization [48,49].

Another intriguing finding of the present study was the highly specific binding pattern of the Gc-specific mAb 5F8 which reacted almost exclusively with the homologous SBV strain BH80/11. Similar observations have previously been described for AKAV- and AINOV-specific mAbs [50,51]. However, the respective virus strains were isolated during a period of more than 30 years (AKAV from 1959 to 1990, and AINOV between 1964 and 1995) on two different continents, which explains the observed antigenic differences. In contrast, the SBV strains used in the present study were collected only during 2011 or 2012 and in a spatially limited area. Nevertheless, different mAb-reactivity patterns were obtained for these isolates. Thus, the mAbs investigated in this study provide a valuable tool to rapidly determine the phenotype of SBV isolates and to characterize newly emerging virus strains. Furthermore, they represent attractive options for the development of novel immunodiagnostic assays which might allow differentiation of SBV and other Simbu serogroup viruses.

Additional file

Additional file 1: Sequences of peptides synthesized for SBV N-protein. A library of biotinylated overlapping peptides covering the entire N-protein sequence was synthesized, the peptides were 16 amino acids (aa) long with an overlap of 13 aa.

Competing interests

Yann Sénéchal and Christian Schelp are employees of IDEXX Switzerland, this does not alter the adherence to the journal policies on sharing data and reagents.

Authors' contributions

KW performed western blot and immunofluorescence analysis and drafted the manuscript. EB and PC produced the mAbs and performed the initial characterization. YS and CS conceived and performed PepScan analysis. AW and IR designed and tested the pCITE constructs. AA participated in the western blot analysis. GRS located the antigenic site in the three-dimensional structure of SBV-N. MB conceived the study, and participated in its design. All authors read and approved the final manuscript.

Acknowledgements

We thank Mr. Adrian Wyttenbach for excellent technical assistance with the pepscanning experiments. We are also very grateful to Peter Kirkland (Elizabeth Macarthur Agricultural Institute, Australia) and Robert Tesh (University of Texas Medical Branch, USA) for kindly providing Simbu serogroup viruses.

Author details

[1]Institute of Diagnostic Virology, Friedrich-Loeffler-Institut (FLI), Suedufer 10, 17493 Greifswald - Insel Riems, Germany. [2]Istituto Zooprofilattico Sperimentale della Lombardia e dell'Emilia Romagna, Via Bianchi 7, 25125 Brescia, Italy. [3]IDEXX Switzerland AG, Stationsstrasse 12, 3097 Liebefeld-Bern, Switzerland.

References

1. Hoffmann B, Scheuch M, Höper D, Jungblut R, Holsteg M, Schirrmeier H, Eschbaumer M, Goller KV, Wernike K, Fischer M, Breithaupt A, Mettenleiter TC, Beer M (2012) Novel orthobunyavirus in cattle, Europe, 2011. Emerg Infect Dis 18:469–72
2. Goller KV, Höper D, Schirrmeier H, Mettenleiter TC, Beer M (2012) Schmallenberg virus as possible ancestor of Shamonda virus. Emerg Infect Dis 18:1644–6
3. Yanase T, Kato T, Aizawa M, Shuto Y, Shirafuji H, Yamakawa M, Tsuda T (2012) Genetic reassortment between Sathuperi and Shamonda viruses of the genus Orthobunyavirus in nature: implications for their genetic relationship to Schmallenberg virus. Arch Virol 157:1611–6
4. Guu TS, Zheng W, Tao YJ (2012) Bunyavirus: structure and replication. Adv Exp Med Biol 726:245–66
5. Walter CT, Barr JN (2011) Recent advances in the molecular and cellular biology of bunyaviruses. J Gen Virol 92:2467–84
6. Chowdhary R, Street C, Travassos da Rosa A, Nunes MR, Tee KK, Hutchison SK, Vasconcelos PF, Tesh RB, Lipkin WI, Briese T (2012) Genetic characterization of the Wyeomyia group of orthobunyaviruses and their phylogenetic relationships. J Gen Virol 93:1023–34
7. Dong H, Li P, Elliott RM, Dong C (2013) Structure of Schmallenberg orthobunyavirus nucleoprotein suggests a novel mechanism of genome encapsidation. J Virol 87:5593–601
8. Elliott RM, Blakqori G (2011) Molecular Biology of Orthobunyaviruses. In: Plyusnin A, Elliott RM (ed) Bunyaviridae Molecular and Cellular Biology. Caister Academic Press, Norfolk, UK, pp 1–39
9. Gonzalez-Scarano F, Shope RE, Calisher CE, Nathanson N (1982) Characterization of monoclonal antibodies against the G1 and N proteins of LaCrosse and Tahyna, two California serogroup bunyaviruses. Virology 120:42–53
10. Meroc E, Poskin A, Van Loo H, Quinet C, Van Driessche E, Delooz L, Behaeghel I, Riocreux F, Hooyberghs J, De Regge N, Caij AB, Van den Berg T, Van der Stede Y (2013) Large-scale cross-sectional serological survey of Schmallenberg virus in Belgian cattle at the end of the first vector season. Transbound Emerg Dis 60:4–8
11. Wernike K, Silaghi C, Nieder M, Pfeffer M, Beer M (2014) Dynamics of Schmallenberg virus infection within a cattle herd in Germany, 2011. Epidemiol Infect 142:1501–4
12. Kobayashi T, Yanase T, Yamakawa M, Kato T, Yoshida K, Tsuda T (2007) Genetic diversity and reassortments among Akabane virus field isolates. Virus Res 130:162–71
13. Fischer M, Hoffmann B, Goller KV, Höper D, Wernike K, Beer M (2013) A mutation 'hot spot' in the Schmallenberg virus M segment. J Gen Virol 94:1161–7
14. Coupeau D, Claine F, Wiggers L, Kirschvink N, Muylkens B (2013) In vivo and in vitro identification of a hypervariable region in Schmallenberg virus. J Gen Virol 94:1168–74
15. Hulst M, Kortekaas J, Hakze-van der Honing R, Vastenhouw S, Cornellissen J, van Maanen K, Bossers A, Harders F, Stockhofe N, van der Poel W (2013) Genetic characterization of an atypical Schmallenberg virus isolated from the brain of a malformed lamb. Virus Genes 47:505–14
16. Bilk S, Schulze C, Fischer M, Beer M, Hlinak A, Hoffmann B (2012) Organ distribution of Schmallenberg virus RNA in malformed newborns. Vet Microbiol 159:236–8
17. Breard E, Lara E, Comtet L, Viarouge C, Doceul V, Desprat A, Vitour D, Pozzi N, Cay AB, De Regge N, Pourquier P, Schirrmeier H, Hoffmann B, Beer M, Sailleau C, Zientara S (2013) Validation of a commercially available indirect ELISA using a nucleocapside recombinant protein for detection of Schmallenberg virus antibodies. PLoS One 8:e53446
18. Galfrè G, Milstein C (1981) Preparation of monoclonal antibodies: strategies and procedures. Methods Enzymol 73:3–46
19. Buchholz UJ, Finke S, Conzelmann KK (1999) Generation of bovine respiratory syncytial virus (BRSV) from cDNA: BRSV NS2 is not essential for virus replication in tissue culture, and the human RSV leader region acts as a functional BRSV genome promoter. J Virol 73:251–9
20. Geiser M, Cebe R, Drewello D, Schmitz R (2001) Integration of PCR fragments at any specific site within cloning vectors without the use of restriction enzymes and DNA ligase. Biotechniques 31:88–90, 92
21. Block H, Maertens B, Spriestersbach A, Brinker N, Kubicek J, Fabis R, Labahn J, Schafer F (2009) Immobilized-metal affinity chromatography (IMAC): a review. Methods Enzymol 463:439–73
22. Dong H, Li P, Bottcher B, Elliott RM, Dong C (2013) Crystal structure of Schmallenberg orthobunyavirus nucleoprotein-RNA complex reveals a novel RNA sequestration mechanism. RNA 19:1129–36

23. DeLano WL (2002) The PyMOL user's Manual. DeLano Scientific, San Carlos, CA
24. Saeed MF, Li L, Wang H, Weaver SC, Barrett AD (2001) Phylogeny of the Simbu serogroup of the genus Bunyavirus. J Gen Virol 82:2173–81
25. Vasconcelos HB, Azevedo RS, Casseb SM, Nunes-Neto JP, Chiang JO, Cantuaria PC, Segura MN, Martins LC, Monteiro HA, Rodrigues SG, Nunes MR, Vasconcelos PF (2009) Oropouche fever epidemic in Northern Brazil: epidemiology and molecular characterization of isolates. J Clin Virol 44:129–33
26. Bastos Mde S, Figueiredo LT, Naveca FG, Monte RL, Lessa N, Pinto de Figueiredo RM, Gimaque JB, Pivoto Joao G, Ramasawmy R, Mourao MP (2012) Identification of Oropouche Orthobunyavirus in the cerebrospinal fluid of three patients in the Amazonas, Brazil. Am J Trop Med Hyg 86:732–5
27. Brenner J, Tsuda T, Yadin H, Chai D, Stram Y, Kato T (2004) Serological and clinical evidence of a teratogenic Simbu serogroup virus infection of cattle in Israel, 2001–2003. Vet Ital 40:119–23
28. Inaba Y, Kurogi H, Omori T (1975) Letter: Akabane disease: epizootic abortion, premature birth, stillbirth and congenital arthrogryposis-hydranencephaly in cattle, sheep and goats caused by Akabane virus. Aust Vet J 51:584–5
29. Kurogi H, Inaba Y, Goto Y, Miura Y, Takahashi H (1975) Serologic evidence for etiologic role of Akabane virus in epizootic abortion-arthrogryposis-hydranencephaly in cattle in Japan, 1972–1974. Arch Virol 47:71–83
30. Kirkland PD, Barry RD, Harper PA, Zelski RZ (1988) The development of Akabane virus-induced congenital abnormalities in cattle. Vet Rec 122:582–6
31. Noda Y, Uchinuno Y, Shirakawa H, Nagasue S, Nagano N, Ohe R, Narita M (1998) Aino virus antigen in brain lesions of a naturally aborted bovine fetus. Vet Pathol 35:409–11
32. Uchinuno Y, Noda Y, Ishibashi K, Nagasue S, Shirakawa H, Nagano M, Ohe R (1998) Isolation of Aino virus from an aborted bovine fetus. J Vet Med Sci 60:1139–40
33. Konno S, Moriwaki M, Nakagawa M (1982) Akabane disease in cattle: congenital abnormalities caused by viral infection. Spontaneous disease. Vet Pathol 19:246–66
34. Conraths FJ, Peters M, Beer M (2013) Schmallenberg virus, a novel orthobunyavirus infection in ruminants in Europe: potential global impact and preventive measures. N Z Vet J 61:63–7
35. EFSA. "Schmallenberg" virus: analysis of the epidemiological data (November 2012). EFSA Supporting Publications 2012 EN-360 http://www.efsa.europa.eu/en/supporting/doc/360e.pdf. Accessed 15/07/2013.
36. EFSA. "Schmallenberg" virus: analysis of the epidemiological data (May 2013). EFSA Supporting Publications 2013 EN-3429 http://www.efsa.europa.eu/de/supporting/doc/429e.pdf. Accessed 15/07/2013.
37. Wernike K, Conraths F, Zanella G, Granzow H, Gache K, Schirrmeier H, Valas S, Staubach C, Marianneau P, Kraatz F, Höreth-Böntgen D, Reimann I, Zientara S, Beer M (2014) Schmallenberg virus-two years of experiences. Prev Vet Med 116:423–34
38. Fafetine JM, Tijhaar E, Paweska JT, Neves LC, Hendriks J, Swanepoel R, Coetzer JA, Egberink HF, Rutten VP (2007) Cloning and expression of Rift Valley fever virus nucleocapsid (N) protein and evaluation of a N-protein based indirect ELISA for the detection of specific IgG and IgM antibodies in domestic ruminants. Vet Microbiol 121:29–38
39. Jansen van Vuren P, Potgieter AC, Paweska JT, van Dijk AA (2007) Preparation and evaluation of a recombinant Rift Valley fever virus N protein for the detection of IgG and IgM antibodies in humans and animals by indirect ELISA. J Virol Methods 140:106–14
40. Fischer M, Schirrmeier H, Wernike K, Wegelt A, Beer M, Hoffmann B (2013) Development of a pan-Simbu real-time reverse transcriptase PCR for the detection of Simbu serogroup viruses and comparison with SBV diagnostic PCR systems. Virol J 10:327
41. Zhang Y, Wu S, Wang J, Wernike K, Lv J, Feng C, Zhang J, Wang C, Deng J, Yuan X, Lin X (2013) Expression and purification of the nucleocapsid protein of Schmallenberg virus, and preparation and characterization of a monoclonal antibody against this protein. Protein Expr Purif 92:1–8
42. Van Regenmortel MH (1989) Structural and functional approaches to the study of protein antigenicity. Immunol Today 10:266–72
43. Yu L, Zhang L, Sun L, Lu J, Wu W, Li C, Zhang Q, Zhang F, Jin C, Wang X, Bi Z, Li D, Liang M (2012) Critical epitopes in the nucleocapsid protein of SFTS virus recognized by a panel of SFTS patients derived human monoclonal antibodies. PLoS One 7:e38291
44. Magurano F, Nicoletti L (1999) Humoral response in Toscana virus acute neurologic disease investigated by viral-protein-specific immunoassays. Clin Diagn Lab Immunol 6:55–60
45. Boshra H, Lorenzo G, Busquets N, Brun A (2011) Rift valley fever: recent insights into pathogenesis and prevention. J Virol 85:6098–105
46. Pekosz A, Griot C, Stillmock K, Nathanson N, Gonzalez-Scarano F (1995) Protection from La Crosse virus encephalitis with recombinant glycoproteins: role of neutralizing anti-G1 antibodies. J Virol 69:3475–81
47. Cordioli P, Lelli D, Moreno A, Pezzoni G, Gamba D, Canelli E, Brocchi E (2013) Competitive mAb-Based ELISA for the Detection of Antibodies Against Schmallenberg Virus. 16th International Symposium of the World Association of Veterinary Laboratory Diagnosticians, Berlin
48. Lappin DF, Nakitare GW, Palfreyman JW, Elliott RM (1994) Localization of Bunyamwera bunyavirus G1 glycoprotein to the Golgi requires association with G2 but not with NSm. J Gen Virol 75:3441–51
49. Shi X, Lappin DF, Elliott RM (2004) Mapping the Golgi targeting and retention signal of Bunyamwera virus glycoproteins. J Virol 78:10793–802
50. Yoshida K, Ohashi S, Kubo T, Tsuda T (2000) Comparison of intertypic antigenicity of Aino virus isolates by dot immunobinding assay using neutralizing monoclonal antibodies. J Clin Microbiol 38:4211–4
51. Akashi H, Inaba Y (1997) Antigenic diversity of Akabane virus detected by monoclonal antibodies. Virus Res 47:187–96

11

Field and experimental data indicate that the eastern cottontail (*Sylvilagus floridanus*) is susceptible to infection with European brown hare syndrome (EBHS) virus and not with rabbit haemorrhagic disease (RHD) virus

Antonio Lavazza[1,7*], Patrizia Cavadini[1,7], Ilaria Barbieri[1], Paolo Tizzani[2], Ana Pinheiro[3,8,9], Joana Abrantes[3,10], Pedro J Esteves[3,11], Guido Grilli[4], Emanuela Gioia[5], Mariagrazia Zanoni[1], Pier Giuseppe Meneguz[2], Jean-Sébastien Guitton[6], Stéphane Marchandeau[6], Mario Chiari[1] and Lorenzo Capucci[1,7]

Abstract

The eastern cottontail (*Sylvilagus floridanus*) is an American lagomorph. In 1966, it was introduced to Italy, where it is currently widespread. Its ecological niche is similar to those of native rabbits and hares and increasing overlap in distribution brings these species into ever closer contact. Therefore, cottontails are at risk of infection with the two lagoviruses endemically present in Italy: Rabbit Haemorrhagic Disease virus (RHDV) and European Brown Hare Syndrome Virus (EBHSV). To verify the susceptibility of *Sylvilagus* to these viruses, we analyzed 471 sera and 108 individuals from cottontail populations in 9 provinces of north-central Italy from 1999 to 2012. In total, 15–20% of the cottontails tested seropositive for EBHSV; most titres were low, but some were as high as 1/1280. All the cottontails virologically tested for RHDV and EBHSV were negative with the exception of one individual found dead with hares during a natural EBHS outbreak in December 2009. The cottontail and the hares showed typical EBHS lesions, and the EBHSV strain identified was the same in both species (99.9% identity). To experimentally confirm the diagnosis, we performed two trials in which we infected cottontails with both EBHSV and RHDV. One out of four cottontails infected with EBHSV died of an EBHS-like disease, and the three surviving animals developed high EBHSV antibody titres. In contrast, neither mortality nor seroconversion was detected after infection with RHDV. Taken together, these results suggest that *Sylvilagus* is susceptible to EBHSV infection, which occasionally evolves to EBHS-like disease; the eastern cottontail could therefore be considered a "spill over" or "dead end" host for EBHSV unless further evidence is found to confirm that it plays an active role in the epidemiology of EBHSV.

Introduction

The eastern cottontail (*Sylvilagus floridanus*) is a lagomorph belonging to the *Leporidae* family, which also includes hares (genus *Lepus*) and the European rabbit (genus *Oryctolagus*). The genus *Sylvilagus* separated from the genera *Lepus* and *Oryctolagus* around 12 million years ago [1-3]. The genetic distances among the three genera are almost the same. *Sylvilagus floridanus* originated in North America and was translocated to various European countries including France (1953), Spain (1980), Switzerland (1982) and Italy, where it was introduced to Piemonte, in Northern Italy, in 1966 and subsequently to many other regions (i.e., Lombardia, Veneto, Emilia-Romagna, Marche, Toscana) for hunting purposes. Currently, the eastern cottontail is widespread in the western part of the Po Valley, and the largest "Italian" population still lives in Piemonte, where it occupies an ecological niche typical of the brown hare (*Lepus europaeus*). The risks of crop damage and

* Correspondence: antonio.lavazza@izsler.it
[1]IZSLER, Istituto Zooprofilattico Sperimentale della Lombardia e dell'Emilia Romagna "Bruno Ubertini", Via Bianchi 7/9, 25124 Brescia, Italy
[7]OIE Reference Laboratory for Rabbit Haemorrhagic Disease at IZSLER Via Bianchi 7/9, 25124 Brescia, Italy
Full list of author information is available at the end of the article

possible competition for space and food with other lagomorphs as well as of introduction of highly virulent strains of *Francisella tularensis* have already been highlighted [4-6]. Indeed, due to its high reproductive performance, the cottontail has colonized the hare's historical range, and currently, interspecific competition may represent an important factor limiting hare populations [7]. In particular, the cottontail is blamed for having caused a drastic decline in hare populations in simplified agro-ecosystems, i.e. in areas with a low biodiversity and landscape heterogeneity, in which the two species are sympatric, competing for daytime refuges and feeding sites [8].

Rabbit haemorrhagic disease (RHD) and European brown hare syndrome (EBHS) are two highly contagious and acute fatal diseases caused by distinct but antigenically correlated caliciviruses [9]. RHD was first reported in 1984 in the People's Republic of China [10] and subsequently in many other countries throughout the world reviewed in [11]. EBHS was first described in Sweden in 1980 [12,13] and is present only in Europe. Both diseases were first reported in Italy in the late 1980s and have been considered endemic since then [14]. Based on both the results of experimental trials and epidemiological data, RHD and EBHS had been initially considered genus-specific, the former infecting only wild and domestic European rabbits (*Oryctolagus cuniculus*) [15] and the latter both brown hares (*Lepus europaeus*) [16] and mountain hares (*Lepus timidus*). A new RHDV-related pathogenic virus emerged in France in 2010; in the following few years, it spread to Italy, Spain, Portugal and Great Britain [17-20]. Among the specific characteristics of the new virus, which has been named RHDV2 [17], is its ability to infect and cause an EBHSV-like disease in Cape Hares (*Lepus capensis* subsp. *mediterraneus*) in Sardinia [21]. RHDV2 was also identified in an Italian hare (*Lepus corsicanus*) in a single case in Sicily [22]. These two events suggest a possible species jump of lagoviruses between lagomorph genera.

The main aim of the present study was to determine the role of *S. floridanus* as the host, vehicle or reservoir of lagoviruses in Italy. Gregg et al. [23] found that *S. floridanus* does not show clinical signs of RHD when challenged with RHDV, but their study does not give information on a possible subclinical infection. In order to study the susceptibility of *S. floridanus* to RHDV and EBHS, and therefore to better evaluate the role of this species in the epidemiology of pathogenic lagoviruses, we analyzed the results of serological and virological surveys conducted in north-central Italy over a 13-year period. To support field results, we additionally performed experimental trials to assess the reproducibility of both RHD and EBHS in seronegative cottontails. Taken together, the results obtained indicate that cottontails are susceptible to EBHSV but not to RHDV infection.

Materials and methods

Epidemiological surveys

During the first survey, we considered three different areas, Roleto, Sezzadio and Tollara, in the Province of Alessandria (lat. 44.916; long. 8.6148) in northwestern Italy (Figure 1). This was an active surveillance monitoring site and the areas were chosen according to the following criteria: i) typical habitat for *S. floridanus*; ii) high density of *S. floridanus* (>50 individuals/km^2); iii) simultaneous presence of brown hares; iv) prohibition of hunting. We shot approximately 15 individuals in each study area at bimonthly intervals between July 1999 and January 2000 and then again in May and August 2000. In total, we collected blood samples from 252 animals (122 males, 130 females).

The second survey consisted of passive monitoring and surveillance and was conducted from 2003 to 2012. We analyzed 219 blood samples and 108 carcasses from cottontails captured or found dead in 9 provinces of north-central Italy (Figure 1). The number of cottontail carcasses examined each year was highly variable and depended on local surveillance programs (3 on 2006, 23 on 2007, 12 on 2008, 2 on 2009, 50 on 2011 and 18 on 2012).

Clinical case

In late 2009, an EBHS outbreak occurred in a fenced-in area of approximately 1 km^2 at Cerro Maggiore (+45° 34′ 55.79″, +8° 58′ 31.52″) north of Milan (Figure 1), where a high density of hares (25 individuals/km^2) and cottontails (>50 individuals/km^2) was present. Over a ten-day period (24 December 2009 – 3 January 2010), several hares and some cottontails were found dead, but due to post mortem alterations and predator activity, the carcasses of only two hares and one cottontail were brought to the laboratory for examination. After necropsy, we examined the organs for EBHSV using conventional virological methods. One year later (January 2011), we revisited the same area to assess the serological status of surviving cottontails and hares by taking, respectively, 11 and 25 blood samples from their ear veins.

Serological analysis

To detect antibodies against RHD and EBHS, we analyzed the serum samples using two specific competitive ELISA (cELISA). These tests, one for each virus (RHDV and EBHS), were developed in-house at the OIE Reference Laboratory, and the procedures are extensively described in the "OIE Manual of Diagnostic Tests and Vaccines for Terrestrial Animals" [24]. The tests are based on competition for the antigen between anti-RHDV or anti-EBHS antibodies adsorbed to the solid phase and those possibly present in the serum sample added to the plate well. The antigen (RHDV or EBHSV) was used at a fixed and pre-

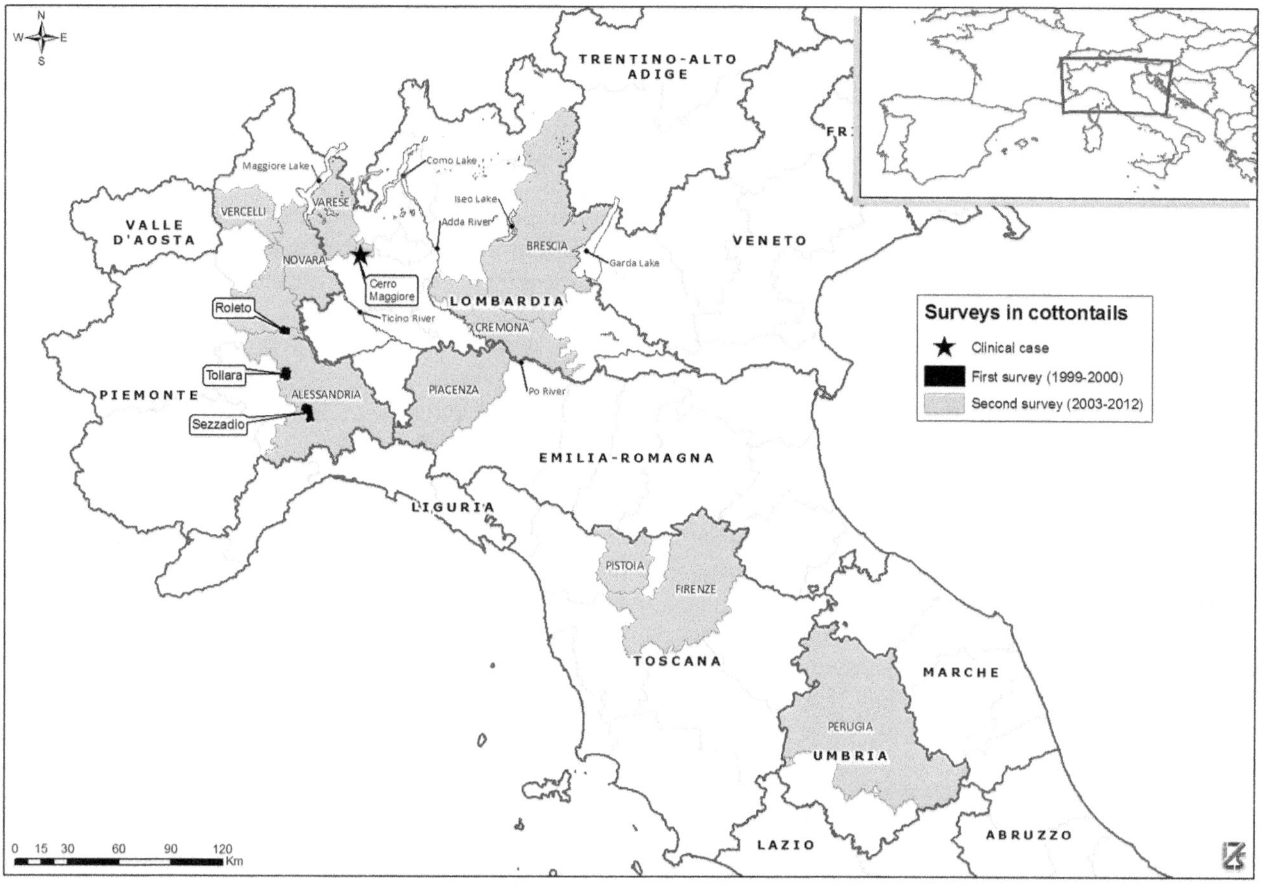

Figure 1 Maps showing sites in northern and central Italy where cottontails were sampled. The map shows the sites and areas of north-central Italy where cottontails were sampled during the two epidemiological surveys and where the clinical case of EBHS in cottontails was observed.

determined concentration [14,23-26]. Such ELISA have a high specificity because they primarily measure antibodies binding the antigenic determinants forming the viral surface. Regarding the data interpretation, because this was the first time a serological approach was applied with *S. floridanus*, we used the same cut-off value for rabbits and hares. The sera were classified as negative if the absorbance value of the first dilution (1/10) decreased by less than 20% of the reference value (i.e. the first dilution of the negative control serum) and positive if the absorbance value decreased by 30% or more. Sera with a decrease between 20% and 30% were considered equivocal. The titre of positive sera corresponded to a dilution yielding an absorbance value of approximately 50% of the value of the negative control serum. In order to detect anti-EBHSV and anti-RHDV IgM in the sera of experimentally infected animals, we used two similar sandwich ELISA developed using anti-isotype MAbs (IgM-ELISAs) after having ascertained that *S. floridanus* IgM were also recognized by the test [24].

Virological analysis

Carcasses and/or organs from the hares, rabbits and cottontails collected during the second survey, from a clinical case, and from experimental trials were submitted to necropsy and virological examination for EBHS and/or RHD. In particular, the liver and spleen were examined using methods commonly employed in routine laboratory diagnostics, i.e., sandwich ELISA and RT-PCR. These are also "in house" tests, fully described in the "OIE Manual of Diagnostic Tests and Vaccines for Terrestrial Animals" [24].

Genomic analysis

Total RNA was isolated from liver homogenates of one hare and one cottontail using the Trizol reagent (Invitrogen) according to the manufacturer's instructions. Reverse transcription (RT) was carried out with an oligo(dT) primer using the High Capacity cDNA Reverse Transcription Kit (Applied Biosystem) according to the protocol suggested by the supplier. The gene encoding the capsid protein VP60 was amplified by PCR in two overlapping regions (PCR1-959 bp: EBHS-F2 5'-CTGGAATATGAATG GTGAAACC-3', EBHS6-R 5'- GAGCGCTGCTCAACG TAGAA-3'; PCR2-915 bp: EBHS5-F 5'- CGACAGGAA GAGGATCGTCT-3', EBHSV-R7 5'-AAACCTGGGGCT GGACCAGC-3'). Cycle conditions were 5 min at 95 °C followed by 40 cycles of 30 s at 95 °C, 30 s at 58 °C, 1 min at 72 °C and a final extension of 7 min at 72 °C. The PCR products were purified from agarose gel and sequenced twice in both directions with the PCR primers by an automated fluorescence-based technique according to the manufacturer's instructions (ABI-PRISM 3130 Genetic Analyzer, Applied Biosystems); they were assembled with SeqMan Pro (DNASTAR, Lasergene 10).

The resultant sequences were put into the local alignment search tool (BLAST) in the GenBank library to confirm the specificity of a positive reaction and to estimate the degree of identity with the detected strain. The sequences obtained were aligned with the available GenBank sequences using ClustalW, as implemented in MEGA 5.1 [27].

Due to the phenotypic similarities existing between cottontails and brown hares, especially when they are young and sub-adult, and in consideration of the exceptionality of the case observed, it was decided to confirm the genetic identity of the studied animals as *Sylvilagus* sp.. Therefore a set of discriminating genetic markers was amplified by PCR. The following have been shown to have specific SNP for *Oryctolagus*, *Sylvilagus* and *Lepus* genera: CXCR4 [28], CCR5 [29], IGHG hinge region [30] and IGHG CH2 [31]. The mitochondrial Cytb was also analyzed. Total genomic DNA was extracted from frozen liver tissue using the EasySpin Genomic DNA Minipreps Tissue Kit (Citomed). PCR amplification of the set of nuclear and mitochondrial markers was conducted using primers designed on available sequences from *Oryctolagus cuniculus* or *Sylvilagus* sp. (GenBank Acession Numbers: CCR5: DQ142884; CXCR4: EU258276; IGHG: AY386696; CytB: HQ143462). The PCR primer pairs for each genetic marker, amplified fragment length and annealing temperatures are indicated in Table 1. The PCR reaction was performed with 0.5 μL of DNA in a final volume of 5 μL containing 2.5 μL of HotStarTaq DNA Polymerase Multiplex PCR Master Mix (Qiagen) and 2 pmol of each oligonucleotide. Cycle conditions were 15 min at 95 °C followed by 35 cycles of 30 s at 95 °C, 30 s at the annealing temperature and 45 s at 75 °C (see Table 1 for the annealing temperatures). A final extension was carried out for 20 min at 60 °C. After purification, PCR products were sequenced on an automatic sequencer (ABI PRISM 310 Genetic Analyzer, PE Applied Biosystems) using the same PCR primers.

The obtained sequences were aligned with published sequences available in GenBank using ClustalW [32] as implemented in the BioEdit software [33] and adjusted by visual inspection. For each genetic marker studied, the denomination and GenBank accession number of the nucleotide sequences are reported in Tables 1 and 2.

For each genetic marker, pairwise distances were calculated in MEGA5.1 [27] using the options p-distance and complete deletion of positions with gaps or missing data.

Experimental reproducibility of RHD and EBHS in cottontails

To assess the reproducibility of RHD and EBHS in cottontails, we used seven conventional rabbits (New Zealand hybrids) of approximately four months of age, two captive-reared sub-adult brown hares and ten cottontails, which were live-trapped and then brought to the animal facility of IZSLER in Brescia. All animals were housed individually in cages in three isolation units. The negative serological status of each animal was verified by a blood sample taken just prior to infection.

The RHDV used for infection was our laboratory's reference strain, RHDV-BS89. The experimental infection contained approximately 10^5 lethal doses (LD_{50})/mL [34], Mortarino, personal communication, 1990. The EBHS

Table 1 Primers used for PCR amplification and sequencing

Genetic marker	Primer	Primer sequence (5'-3')	Amplified fragment length	Annealing temperature (°C)
CCR5	CCR5F	TCTACCTGCTCAACCTGGCCA	574	58
	CCR5R	TGTTGGAGCTGCTGCAGTTA		
CXCR4	CXCR4F	CATCTTCTTGACTGGCATAG	804	49
	CXCR4RJ1	GCGTTAGCTGGAGTGAAAA		
IGHG hinge region	FG12	TCAGGCCCAGACTGTAGACC	680	60
	RE	ACGGTCCCCCAGGAGTTCA		
IGHGCH2	F3	GTGAGTCCCATTAGCCTCAC	830	60
	RG31	TTGGAAGGAATCAGGACAGC		
CytB	CytBF	TTCAAATCCTAACCGGCCTA	500	47.5
	CytBR	AACCTAGGGCGTCCTTAATT		

Table 2 Genetic distances between the studied individual and published Sylvilagus, Oryctolagus and Lepus nucleotide sequences

	Sylvilagus	Sample	*Oryctolagus*	Genbank accession numbers
CCR5				
Sylvilagus	----	----	----	DQ017768
Sample	0.009	----	----	KF620521
Oryctolagus	0.056	0.056	----	DQ142884
Lepus	0.047	0.045	0.059	DQ146763
CXCR4				
Sylvilagus	----	----	----	EU258272
Sample	0.001	----	----	KF620522
Oryctolagus	0.009	0.010	----	EU258276
Lepus	0.011	0.012	0.011	EU258265
IGHG hinge region				
Sylvilagus	----	----	----	DQ206979
Sample	0.015	----	----	KF620519
Oryctolagus	0.038	0.045	----	DQ206981
Lepus	0.068	0.075	0.060	DQ206976
IGHG CH2				
Sylvilagus	----	----	----	AJ295223
Sample	0.017	----	----	KF620520
Oryctolagus	0.048	0.036	----	AJ430862
Lepus	0.043	0.031	0.038	AJ295217
Cyt B				
Sylvilagus	----	----	----	HQ143462
Sample	0.002	----	----	KF620523
Oryctolagus	0.150	0.152	----	HQ596486
Lepus	0.144	0.146	0.144	AY745113

isolate (i.e., EBHS reference strain EBHSV-BS89, GenBank accession number X98002) derived from a severe outbreak of EBHS in naturally infected, captive hares. The inoculum corresponded to a 10% (w/v) liver suspension in PBS, and its infectivity and virulence have been assessed in previous experiments [16]. The inocula were diluted in sterile PBS (EBHSVBS89 = 1:2, and RHDVBS89 = 1:10) and filtered on a 0.2 μm Millipore filter before being used. To ensure that the recorded serological results were in fact due to RHDV replication, we inactivated a few mL of RHDV inoculum with 1% formaldehyde for 24 h at 25 °C.

In the first trial, two cottontails and three rabbits were infected with a 2 mL dose of RHDV-BS89 via the oronasal route, two cottontails and two rabbits were administered an inactivated inoculum by the same route, and the remaining two cottontails and two rabbits were maintained as uninfected controls. The animals were kept in three separate rooms, divided according to the type of treatment; they were assessed daily for mortality or the presence of clinical signs over a two-week period. Blood samples were taken at 14 and 28 days post infection (pi) for serological analysis of both specific anti-RHDV antibodies and IgM isotype antibodies. In the second experiment, four seronegative cottontails and two seronegative hares were infected via the oro-nasal route with 2 mL of EBHSV-BS89. The animals were kept in separate cages in the same room, checked daily for the presence of clinical signs and mortality for two weeks and serologically controlled for both specific anti-EBHSV antibodies and IgM isotype antibodies at eleven and 32 days pi.

Experiments were carried out in accordance with the European Communities Council Directive of 24 November 1986 (86/609/EEC) and with National laws and regulations regarding the care and use of animals. At the end of the experiments, the surviving animals were humanely euthanized.

Results

Epidemiological surveys

The results of the serological survey performed in 1999–2000 in three different areas of the province of Alessandria are reported in Figure 2. Overall, in serum samples from cottontails, seroprevalences of 17.9% and 33.7% were observed for EBHSV and RHDV antibodies, respectively. These values were reduced to 11.9% and 14.3%, respectively, when considering titres equal to or higher than 1/20. A number of cottontails sera exhibited high titres for EBHSV (i.e., up to 1/1280); in contrast, the highest RHDV titre was only 1/80 and was detected in only one serum sample. Twenty-nine sera were positive for both viruses (65% and 34% of EBHSV and RHDV positive sera, respectively). In 14 of them, the EBHSV titres were higher than the RHDV ones and in the remaining 15 samples, RHDV titres were slightly higher or the titres were similar (1/10-1/20) for the two viruses. In contrast, positive samples were not uniformly geographically distributed. In fact, all serum samples collected in one area (Roleto) were negative or <1/20 for both EBHSV and RHDV antibodies; indeed, no positive samples were found for RHDV during the visits in January and for EBHSV during two visits (September and January) (data not shown). In addition, we observed that the seroprevalence of EBHS in the two areas that had positive sera (i.e., Sezzadio and Tollara) increased with time (data not shown). In particular, at Tollara, all the sera sampled in July 1999 were negative, but the prevalence increased to 26.7% in September 1999 and to 33.3% in both November 1999 and January 2000, with titres as high as 1/40, 1/80 and 1/640, respectively.

During the period from 2003 to 2012, following the implementation of surveillance programs in north-central Italy, 219 blood samples were taken from cottontails in nine provinces. The results of the serological analysis for EBHSV antibodies are detailed in Table 3. The overall prevalence was 20.1%; in particular, 16.0% of animals tested had low titres (1/10–1/20); an almost equal percentage exhibited medium (1/40–1/160 = 2.2%) or high titres (1/320 to 1/640 = 1.9%), and the remaining samples (79.9%) were negative. During this second survey, we also received and examined 108 carcasses of cottontails, captured or found dead. After necropsy, regardless of the presence of specific lesions, the target organs (i.e., liver and spleen) were examined to detect lagoviruses (i.e., EBHSV and RHDV). All carcasses were negative for both lagoviruses.

Clinical case

At necropsy, the lesions detected in the two hares and the single cottontail found dead during the outbreak exhibited lesions typical of EBHS: congestion of tracheal mucosa, petechial lung haemorrhages, friable, fatty and discoloured liver with an accentuated lobular pattern, and congestion and enlargement of the spleen. All these animals tested virologically positive for EBHSV in the liver and spleen. The results of the serological assessment undertaken one year after the outbreak are reported in Figure 3. All analyzed hares were positive and showed an average antibody titre higher than that of cottontails. Of the eleven cottontails sampled, five (45.5%) had titres between 1/10 and 1/80 and six (54.5%) tested negative.

Because the necropsied animals (i.e., two hares and one cottontail) were naturally infected by EBHS, the identified strains from both species were amplified, sequenced and compared. The capsid protein (VP60) amplified by RT-PCR from the cottontail was completely sequenced (GenBank JX195102) and compared to the sequence of virus isolated from one hare found dead in the same area and period (GenBank KF591083). The nucleotide identity of the two strains was 99.9%, and the amino acid identity was 100%, indicating the presence of the same viral strain in the two species. The sequences obtained for all five amplified genetic markers were closer to published *Sylvilagus* sequences than to *Oryctolagus* or *Lepus* sequences. Analysis of the variable sites for each genetic marker revealed a few positions that differed between the published *Sylvilagus* sp. sequences and our sample; there was consistently more variation between *Sylvilagus* sp. and *Oryctolagus* or *Lepus* published sequences. Consistently, for all analysed genetic markers, the genetic distances were

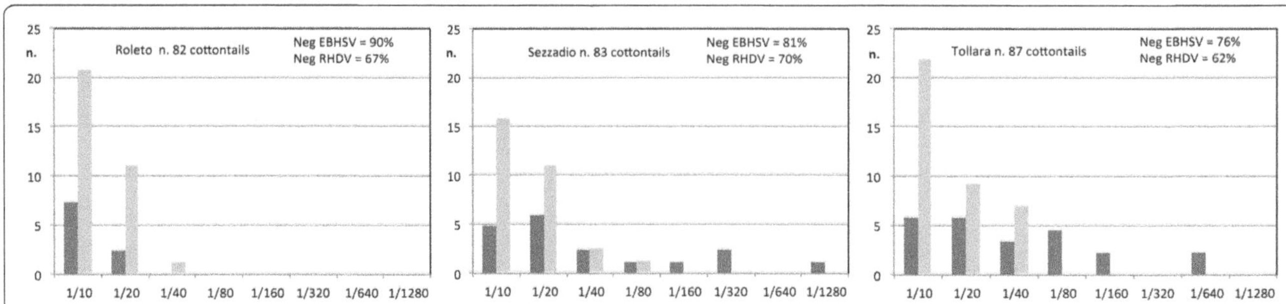

Figure 2 Results of serological analysis for RHD and EBHS antibodies in cottontails during the first survey. Results of serological analysis for RHD and EBHS in cottontail sera from three areas in the Alessandria province (black columns = AbRHDV; grey columns = AbEBHSV).

Table 3 Results of serological analysis for EBHS in cottontail sera during the second survey (2003–2010)

Year titre	2003	2004	2005	2006	2007	2008	2009	2010	2011	2012	TOTAL
Neg.	7	8	30	7	56	11	1	10	28	17	175
1/10	0	0	7	5	1	3	0	0	11	1	28
1/20	0	0	2	2	0	0	0	0	3	0	7
1/40	0	0	1	0	1	1	0	0	0	0	3
1/80	0	0	0	1	0	1	0	0	0	0	2
1/160	0	0	0	0	0	0	0	0	0	0	0
1/320	0	0	0	0	0	0	1	0	0	0	1
1/640	0	0	0	1	0	2	0	0	0	0	3
1/1280	0	0	0	0	0	0	0	0	0	0	0
Total	7	8	40	16	58	18	2	10	42	18	219

significantly lower for the *Sylvilagus* sample pair (0.001–0.017) than for *Oryctolagus* sample (0.010–0.152) or *Lepus* sample (0.012–0.146) pairs (Table 2). Thus, the genetic markers analysed confirm that the studied individual was a *Sylvilagus* and thus it had been correctly identified on the basis of its gross appearance.

Experimental reproducibility of EBHS and RHD in cottontails

The inoculation of RHDV caused an acute form of RHD in the three seronegative rabbits, which all died within 72 h pi and exhibited typical signs and lesions. RHDV positivity was confirmed by a sandwich ELISA test (data not shown). All remaining animals, i.e., all the cottontails and those rabbits inoculated with inactivated RHDV or kept as uninfected controls, remained healthy during the 14 days of observation. Their sera were collected at 14 and 28 days pi, and no antibodies, either IgM or total specific antibodies, were detected using RHDV ELISA (data not shown).

During the second trial, which involved inoculation with EBHSV, one cottontail out of four died at four days pi, and at necropsy it had typical gross lesions attributable to EBHS. The identification of EBHSV was confirmed by virological ELISA. In the sera of the two hares and three cottontails that survived, we detected seroconversion with IgM titres up to 1/40 000 and total specific antibodies up to 1/1280.

Discussion

Cottontails were first introduced in Italy in 1966 and then in France in 1972. Massive introductions were then made from the late 1970's to the late 1980's mainly in Italy and France but also in Switzerland, Spain and Luxemburg [35]. Following these introductions, cottontails established in Italy, where populations progressively increased from the late 1970s to the late 1980s. During the same period, two new diseases, RHD and EBHS, emerged within the European lagomorph species *O. cuniculus* and *L. europaeus* in China and northern Europe, respectively. RHD and EBHS are similar; they are acute and lethal forms of hepatitis caused by two distinct but related lagoviruses. RHDV infects wild and domestic rabbits whereas EBHSV infects hares, both in the wild and in captivity. They are responsible for high mortality rates and account for a strong economic burden on the rabbit and

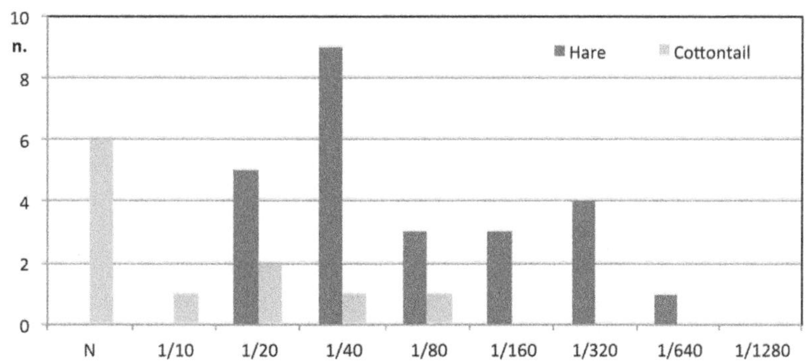

Figure 3 Results of serological analysis for EBHS in hare and cottontail sera after the clinical case. Results of serological analysis for EBHS in hare ($n = 25$) and cottontail ($n = 11$) sera after the outbreak in Cerro Maggiore in 2011 (black columns = hares; grey columns = cottontails).

hare industries and on game animal management.. Therefore, this study was designed to better investigate the role of cottontails (*S. floridanus*) in the epidemiology of lagoviruses and in particular, to ascertain whether this species could be infected by any of the known pathogenic lagoviruses, i.e., RHDV or EBHSV. Overall, the results of two consecutive epidemiological surveys, experimental trials and observations of a natural outbreak of EBHS in sympatric hares and cottontails are indicative of natural susceptibility among cottontails to EBHSV, albeit with only sporadic cases of clinical disease.

Our first approach was to evaluate the serological results obtained from cottontail sera using the same ELISA parameters (i.e., threshold values and titre computation) that are employed for serology of RHD in rabbits and EBHS in hares. A general analysis of the data indicates that these parameters could be considered acceptable for cottontail serology as well. In fact, in cottontails experimentally infected with EBHSV, serological titres reached high values within a few days and the kinetics were similar to those induced by EBHSV in hares. These results suggest that the initially chosen threshold ELISA values, identical to those established for hares, were appropriate for cottontails as well. Therefore, the serological results obtained from cottontails can be considered reliable.

The results of the first serological survey indicate that approximately 20% of the tested cottontails may have been naturally exposed to EBHSV; the high EBHSV titres found in some seropositive cottontails were comparable to those detected in the sera of RHD-convalescent rabbits [24,36] and EBHS-convalescent hares [14,37]. In addition, we observed that the seroprevalence of EBHSV in the areas of Sezzadio and Tollara, where high titres were found, increased with time, in agreement with the epidemiological characteristics of EBHS that indicate a strong seasonal peak in incidence in the autumn [14]. With regard to RHDV serology, the titres detected were always too low to be considered directly induced by RHDV or by a cross-reaction with EBHSV-induced antibodies. However, the prevalence of low titre RHDV-positive sera was higher than that for EBHSV. This result strongly suggests, as a possible explanation, the presence in cottontails of a non-pathogenic lagovirus genetically related to those found in rabbits [38].

The results of the second serological survey conducted across a ten-year period confirmed the presence of specific EBHSV antibodies among cottontail populations in north-central Italy. The prevalence found in cottontails was similar to that commonly detected in hares hunted in low-density hare populations in northern Italy [39,40].

The experimental trials confirmed that cottontails are not susceptible to experimental infection with RHDV, as previously observed [22], but clearly demonstrated that EBHSV can infect *S. floridanus* via the oro-nasal route that corresponds to the natural way of transmission. In addition, a detectable level of seroconversion was observed in the surviving animals (i.e., three cottontails and two hares), comparable with the levels detected in convalescent hares in natural outbreaks [14,37,39]. The fact that the two experimentally infected hares did not die of EBHS is not unexpected; the mortality rate observed in previous experiments was quite variable, ranging from zero to 50% [Lavazza and Capucci, personal data].

In late 2009, the occurrence of one natural case of EBHS in sympatric populations of hares and cottontails living in a fenced-in area strongly supported these results. Several hares and cottontails were found dead during the outbreak; two hares and one cottontail, delivered to the laboratory, tested positive for EBHSV, and the genomic comparison between the strains identified from both species revealed 100% VP60 amino acid identity, indicating the presence of the same EBHSV strain in the two species. In addition, a serological survey conducted in the same area one year later revealed that approximately half the *Sylvilagus* individuals had had contact with the virus, as indicated by low-medium antibody titres.

Considering the outcome of field surveys and experimental trials we may conclude that cottontails appear to be susceptible to EBHSV infection and are likely more resistant to the development of overt disease than hares. In fact, their susceptibility to EBHSV does not appear to be a problem for the conservation of this invasive species; no outbreaks were recorded in free-living populations other than the one in late 2009. However, by being infected with EBHSV, cottontails may play a certain role in the spread of the virus. We demonstrated that in nature cottontails become infected but only sporadically develop the disease. EBHSV circulates in cottontails but the serological results could also arise if the virus spreads through a sympatric hare population and the cottontails become simply affected as "spill-over" or "dead end" host. Since we do not have a reliable estimate of the prevalence nor do we know whether the infection is dose-dependent or to what extent the viral infectivity and spread in the field are amplified, we cannot confirm that cottontails play an active role in the epidemiology of EBHSV unless further evidence is found.

The susceptibility of *S. floridanus* to EBHSV broadens our perspective on its epidemiological role in lagovirus diseases. The fact that cottontails support EBHSV replication could influence the evolution and outcome of EBHS in hares at a local level and could act as an example of "parasite mediated competition" [41]. In fact, according to the proposed epidemiological model of spread of this disease [38], the ability of EBHSV to infect and/or kill hares in endemic areas is inversely proportional to their population densities. Therefore, since cottontails living in sympatry with hares are quite common in some European countries, the EBHS model should also consider the impact of this species. In particular, cottontails likely act as a carrier of EBHSV and may favour the introduction, persistence and spread of the virus and the occurrence of EBHS cases. This may be especially true in open hunting areas, characterized by simplified agro-ecosystems, which cannot sustain stable, high density hare populations even on a short time scale [7].

In conclusion, further studies are needed to verify the incidence of EBHS infections in sympatric populations of hares and cottontails and to better define, either experimentally or in natural outbreaks, the characteristics (i.e., morbidity, mortality rates, age of affected animals, gross lesions, seroconversion, etc.) of the disease in cottontails. In addition, it is necessary to search for lagovirus genome sequences in organs of healthy cottontails using sensitive molecular methods to ascertain whether they are hosts of non-pathogenic lagoviruses. Finally, considering the capacity of the recently identified RHDV2 to infect species other than the European rabbit, the possibility that RHDV2 can infect or cause disease in *S. floridanus* should be verified, either experimentally or through field observations.

The cottontail is widespread in northern Italy, and any eradication action, even if recommended by the Council of Europe (Recommendation no. R 85–14, 1985), should be considered unfeasible. Considering the adaptability of this species, a further expansion in Northern Italy is likely to occur in the coming years and its population density is likely to increase [42]. Given this context, the possible health interactions with native hares, especially in sympatric populations, must be carefully evaluated through the application of a continuous surveillance program.

Abbreviations

RHD: Rabbit haemorrhagic disease; EBHS: European brown hare syndrome; cELISA: Competitive ELISA; MAbs: Monoclonal antibodies; IgM-ELISAs: Anti-isotype MAbs sandwich ELISAs; LD_{50}: Lethal dose; pi: Post infection.

Competing interests

The authors declare that they have no competing interests.

Authors' contributions

AL, MC, PC, LC, SM, JSG, JA and PJE contributed to the general interpretation of the data and the writing of the manuscript. In addition, PT and PGM contributed to the execution of the first survey. EG, GG, MZ and MC collected samples and epidemiological data during the second survey and the clinical outbreak. AL and LC performed virological and serological analyses. LC carried out the immunoassay for virus typing. PC carried out the molecular phylogenetic studies of the viral isolates. AP, JA and PJE carried out the molecular genetic studies for the species confirmation of cottontails. MC, GG and MZ performed necropsies on the animals and pathological examinations. All authors read and approved the final manuscript.

Acknowledgements

The authors gratefully acknowledge Science Docs (Jennie S. Lavine) for the English language editing of this manuscript. We are also very grateful to Giuliana Botti, Debora Campagna, Gianni Bozzoni, and Cristina Palotta for their skilled technical assistance and to Mr. Giovanni Pozzi for his availability during the clinical outbreak.

Author details

[1]IZSLER, Istituto Zooprofilattico Sperimentale della Lombardia e dell'Emilia Romagna "Bruno Ubertini", Via Bianchi 7/9, 25124 Brescia, Italy. [2]Dipartimento di Produzioni Animali, Epidemiologia ed Ecologia, Università degli Studi di Torino, Via Nizza 52, 10126 Torino, Italy. [3]CIBIO-UP, Centro de Investigação em Biodiversidade e Recursos Genéticos Universidade do Porto, InBio, Laboratório Associado, Campus Agrário de Vairão, Vairão, Portugal. [4]Dipartimento di Scienze Veterinarie e Sanità Pubblica (DIVET), Università degli Studi di Milano, Via Celoria 10, 20133 Milan, Italy. [5]Veterinary Practitioner, Via Negri 26, 29122 Piacenza, Italy. [6]ONCFS, National Hunting and Wildlife Agency, Department of Studies and Research, CS 42355, 44323 Nantes, Cedex 3, France. [7]OIE Reference Laboratory for Rabbit Haemorrhagic Disease at IZSLER Via Bianchi 7/9, 25124 Brescia, Italy. [8]Departamento de Biologia, Faculdade de Ciencias, Universidade do Porto, Porto, Portugal. [9]SaBio - Instituto de Investigacion en Recursos Cinegeticos (CSIC-UCLM-JCCM), Ciudad Real, Spain. [10]INSERM, U892, Universite de Nantes, 44007 Nantes, France. [11]CESPU, Instituto de Investigação e Formação Avançada em Ciências e Tecnologias da Saúde, 4585-116 Gandra, Portugal.

References

1. Matthee CA, van Vuuren JB, Bell D, Robinson TJ (2004) A molecular supermatrix of the rabbits and hares (Leporidae) allows for the identification of five intercontinental exchanges during the Miocene. Syst Biol 53:433–447
2. van der Loo W, Abrantes J, Esteves PJ (2009) Sharing of endogenous lentiviral gene fragments among leporid lineages separated for more than 12 million years. J Virol 83:2386–2388
3. Pinheiro A, de Mera IGF, Alves PC, Gortázar C, de la Fuente J, Esteves PJ (2013) Sequencing of modern Lepus VDJ genes shows that the usage of VHn genes has been retained in both Oryctolagus and Lepus that diverged 12 million years ago. Immunogenetics 65:777–784
4. Arthur CP, Chapuis JL (1983) L'introduction de Sylvilagus floridanus en France: historique, dangers et expérimentation en cours. CR Soc Biogéogr 59:333–356 (in French)
5. Chapuis JL, Forgeard F, Didillon MC (1985) Étude de *Sylvilagus floridanus* en région méditerranéenne dans des conditions de semi-liberté. Régime alimentaire au cours d'un cycle annuel par l'analyse micrographique des fèces. Gibier Faune Savage 3:5–31 (in French)
6. Silvano F, Acquarone C, Cucco M (2000) Distribution of the eastern cottontail *Sylvilagus floridanus* in the province of Alessandria. Hystrix 2:75–78
7. Vidus Rosin A, Gilio N, Meriggi A (2008) Introduced lagomorphs as a threat to "native" lagomorphs: the case of the Eastern cottontail (*Sylvilagus floridanus*) in northern Italy. In: Alves PC, Ferrand N, Hacklander K (ed) Lagomorph biology, evolution, ecology and conservation. Springer, Eidenberg, pp 153–165
8. Vidus Rosin A, Montagna A, Meriggi A, Serrano Perez S (2009) Density and habitat requirements of sympatric hares and cottontails in northern Italy. Hystrix 20:101–110
9. Wirblich C, Meyers G, Ohlinger VF, Capucci L, Eskens U, Haas B, Thiel HJ (1994) European brown hare syndrome virus - relationship to rabbit hemorrhagic disease virus and other caliciviruses. J Virol 68:5164–5173
10. Liu SJ, Xue HP, Pu BQ, Quian NH (1984) A new viral disease in rabbits. Anim Hus Vet Med 16:253–255
11. Abrantes J, van der Loo W, Le Pendu J, Esteves PJ (2012) Rabbit haemorrhagic disease (RHD) and rabbit haemorrhagic disease virus (RHDV): a review. Vet Res 43:12
12. Gustaffson K, Svensson T, Uggla A (1989) Studies on an idiopathic syndrome in the brown hare (Lepus europaeus P.) and mountain hare (Lepus timidus L.) in Sweden, with special reference to hepatic lesions. Zentralbl Veterinarmed A 36:631–637
13. Gavier-Widén D, Mörner T (1991) Epidemiology and diagnosis of the European brown hare syndrome in Scandinavian countries: a review. Rev Sci Tech 10:453–458
14. Scicluna MT, Capucci L, Lavazza A (1994) European brown hare syndrome in northern Italy: results of a virological and serological survey. Rev Sci Tech 13:893–904
15. Lenghaus C, Westbury H, Collins B, Ratnamoban N, Morrissy C (1994) Overview of the RHD Project in Australia. In Rabbit Haemorrhagic Disease: Issues in Assessment for Biological Control. Edited by Williams R, Munro R. Camberra, Australia: Australian Government Printing Service, pp 104–129

16. Lavazza A, Scicluna MT, Capucci L (1996) Susceptibility of hares and rabbits to the European brown hare syndrome virus (EBHSV) and rabbit hemorrhagic disease virus (RHDV) under experimental conditions. Zentralbl Veterinarmed B 43:401–410
17. Le Gall-Reculé G, Lavazza A, Marchandeau S, Bertagnoli S, Zwingelstein F, Cavadini P, Martinelli N, Lombardi G, Guérin J, Lemaitre E, Decors A, Boucher S, Le Normand B, Capucci L (2013) Emergence of a new lagovirus related to rabbit haemorrhagic disease virus. Vet Res 44:81
18. Dalton KP, Nicieza I, Balseiro A, Muguerza MA, Rosell JM, Casais R, Álvarez ÁL, Parra F (2012) Variant rabbit hemorrhagic disease virus in young rabbits, Spain. Emerg Infect Dis 18:2009–2012
19. Abrantes J, Lopes AM, Dalton KP, Melo P, Correia JJ, Ramada M, Alves PC, Parra F, Esteves PJ (2013) New variant of rabbit hemorrhagic disease virus, Portugal, 2012–2013. Emerg Infect Dis 19:1900–1902
20. Westcott DG, Frossard J-P, Everest D, Dastjerdi A, Duff JP, Choudhury B (2014) Incursion of RHDV2-like variant in Great Britain. Vet Rec 174:333
21. Puggioni G, Cavadini P, Maestrale C, Scivoli R, Botti G, Ligios C, Le Gall-Reculé G, Lavazza A, Capucci L (2013) The new french 2010 variant of the rabbit hemorrhagic disease virus causes an RHD-like disease in the Sardinian cape hare (Lepus capensis mediterraneus). Vet Res 44:96
22. Camarda A, Pugliese N, Cavadini P, Circella E, Capucci L, Caroli A, Legretto M, Mallia E, Lavazza A (2014) Detection of the new emerging rabbit hemorrhagic disease type 2 virus (RHDV2) in Sicily from rabbit (Oryctolagus cuniculus) and Italian hare (Lepus corsicanus). Res Vet Sci 97:642–645
23. Gregg DA, House C, Meyer R, Berninger M (1991) Viral haemorrhagic disease of rabbits in Mexico: epidemiology and viral characterization. Rev Sci Tech 10:435–451
24. Capucci L, Lavazza A (2012) Rabbit Haemorrhagic Disease. In OIE Manual of Diagnostic Tests and Vaccines for Terrestrial Animals. 6th edition. Edited by the World Organisation For Animal Health (OIE). Paris, France: Biological Standards Commission, pp 941–955.
25. Capucci L, Scicluna MT, Lavazza A (1991) Diagnosis of viral haemorrhagic disease of rabbits and the European brown hare syndrome. Rev Sci Tech 10:347–370
26. Capucci L, Frigoli G, Ronsholt L, Lavazza A, Brocchi E, Rossi C (1995) Antigenicity of the rabbit hemorrhagic disease virus studied by its reactivity with monoclonal antibodies. Virus Res 37:221–238
27. Tamura K, Peterson D, Peterson N, Stecher G, Nei M, Kumar S (2011) MEGA 5: molecular evolutionary genetics analysis using maximum likelihood, evolutionary distance, and maximum parsimony methods. Mol Biol Evol 28:2731–1739
28. Abrantes J, Esteves PJ, Carmo CR, Müller A, Thompson G, van der Loo W (2008) Genetic characterization of the chemokine receptor CXCR4 gene in lagomorphs: comparison between the families Ochotonidae and Leporidae. Int J Immunogenet 35:111–117
29. Carmo CR, Esteves PJ, Ferrand N, van der Loo W (2006) Genetic variation at chemokine receptor CCR5 in leporids: alteration at the 2nd extracellular domain by gene conversion with CCR2 in Oryctolagus, but not in Sylvilagus and Lepus species. Immunogenetics 58:494–501
30. Esteves PJ, Carmo C, Godinho R, van der Loo W (2006) Genetic diversity at the hinge region of the unique immunoglobulin heavy gamma (IGHG) gene in leporids (Oryctolagus, Sylvilagus and Lepus). Int J Immunogenet 33:171–177
31. Esteves PJ, Alves PC, Ferrand N, van der Loo W (2002) Restriction fragment alleles of the rabbit IGHG genes with reference to the rabbit IGHGCH2 or e locus polymorphism. Anim Genet 33:309–311
32. Thompson JD, Higgins DG, Gibson TJ (1994) CLUSTAL W: improving the sensitivity of progressive multiple sequence alignment through sequence weighting, position-specific gap penalties and weight matrix choice. Nucleic Acids Res 22:4673–4680
33. Hall TA (1999) BioEdit: a user-friendly biological sequence alignment editor and analysis program for windows 95/98/NT. Nucleic Acids Symp Ser 41:95–98
34. Capucci L, Scicluna MT, Lavazza A, Brocchi E (1990) Purificazione e caratterizzazione dell'agente eziologico della malattia virale emorragica del coniglio. Sel Vet 31:301–312
35. Sasse C (1983) Ecological consequences of the introduction of the American cottontail, Sylvilagus floridanus, into Europe. Report Council of Europe SN-US, 83, Research Institute for Nature Management, Leersum, The Netherlands, p 33
36. Cooke BD, Robinson AJ, Merchant JC, Nardin A, Capucci L (2000) Use of ELISAs in field studies of rabbit haemorrhagic disease (RHD) in Australia. Epidemiol Infect 124:563–576
37. Drews B, Roellig K, Szentiks CA, Fickel J, Schroeder K, Duff P, Lavazza A, Hildebrandt TB, Goeritz F (2011) Epidemiology, control and management of an EBHS outbreak in captive hares. Vet Microbiol 154:37–48
38. Capucci L, Fusi P, Lavazza A, Pacciarini ML, Rossi C (1996) Detection and preliminary characterization of a new rabbit calicivirus related to rabbit haemorrhagic disease virus but non-pathogenic. J Virol 70:8614–8623
39. Lavazza A, Guberti V, Ferri M, Zanni ML, Poglayen G, Nardin A Capucci L (1999) Epidemiology of European brown hare syndrome (EBHS) in Modena province (North Italy). In Proceedings 4th International Congress of Veterinary Virology, ESVV: 24–27 August 1997; Edimburgh. European Society of Veterinary Virology, pp 34–37
40. Chiari M, Bonavetti E, Zanoni M, Lavazza A (2012) Application of a surveillance program in wild European brown hares (Lepus europeaus) in Brescia province, north Italy. In Proceedings of the 8th Italian Congress of Teriologia: 9–11 May 2012; Piacenza. Edited by Hystrix Italian Journal of Mammalogy; p 40
41. Tompkins DM, Parish DM, Hudson PJ (2002) Parasite-mediated competition among red-legged partridges and other lowland game birds. J Wildl Manag 66:445–450
42. Bertolino S, Ingegno B, Girardello M (2011) Modelling the habitat requirements of invasive Eastern Cottontail (*Sylvilagus floridanus*) introduced to Italy. Eur J Wildlife Res 57:264–267

Susceptibility to and transmission of H5N1 and H7N1 highly pathogenic avian influenza viruses in bank voles (*Myodes glareolus*)

Aurora Romero Tejeda[1†], Roberta Aiello[1*†], Angela Salomoni[1], Valeria Berton[1], Marta Vascellari[2] and Giovanni Cattoli[1]

Abstract

The study of influenza type A (IA) infections in wild mammals populations is a critical gap in our knowledge of how IA viruses evolve in novel hosts that could be in close contact with avian reservoir species and other wild animals. The aim of this study was to evaluate the susceptibility to infection, the nasal shedding and the transmissibility of the H7N1 and H5N1 highly pathogenic avian influenza (HPAI) viruses in the bank vole (*Myodes glareolus*), a wild rodent common throughout Europe and Asia. Two out of 24 H5N1-infected voles displayed evident respiratory distress, while H7N1-infected voles remained asymptomatic. Viable virus was isolated from nasal washes collected from animals infected with both HPAI viruses, and extra-pulmonary infection was confirmed in both experimental groups. Histopathological lesions were evident in the respiratory tract of infected animals, although immunohistochemistry positivity was only detected in lungs and trachea of two H7N1-infected voles. Both HPAI viruses were transmitted by direct contact, and seroconversion was confirmed in 50% and 12.5% of the asymptomatic sentinels in the H7N1 and H5N1 groups, respectively. Interestingly, viable virus was isolated from lungs and nasal washes collected from contact sentinels of both groups. The present study demonstrated that two non-rodent adapted HPAI viruses caused asymptomatic infection in bank voles, which shed high amounts of the viruses and were able to infect contact voles. Further investigations are needed to determine whether bank voles could be involved as silent hosts in the transmission of HPAI viruses to other mammals and domestic poultry.

Introduction

Influenza type A (IA) viruses are subtyped on the basis of two surface proteins, the haemagglutinin (HA) and the neuraminidase (NA), which govern the viral lifecycle at cellular entry and the release of progeny virions. To date, 16 HA and 9 NA subtypes have been described and isolated from wild water birds, the known primary natural reservoir of IA viruses [1]. However, the identification of two novel influenza A-like viruses, the H17N10 and the H18N11 strains isolated from a little yellow-shouldered bat from Guatemala [2] and from a flat-faced fruit bat from Peru [3], respectively, has prompted attention towards new mammalian species as possible hosts or reservoirs of unknown IA viruses.

Although transmission of IA viruses from avian to mammalian hosts is considered to be a rare event, due to the complexity of the transmission pathways and the different interfaces connecting both populations [4,5], species-adapted influenza lineages of avian origin are already circulating in swine, horses, dogs and humans [6,7], independently from the avian reservoir. The first evidence of natural infection with avian origin IA viruses in wild mammals was reported in harbour seals in 1979–1980 [8,9]. Since then, evidence of natural IA-related infections has been reported in several wild mammalian species such as mink [10], stone marten [11], raccoon [12], feral cat [13], feral dog [14], captive tiger and leopard [15], captive Owston's palm civet [16], and skunk [17]. Recently, the discovery that wild pikas can be naturally infected with HPAI H5N1 [18] and LPAI H9N2 [19] subtypes has extended the range of known terrestrial free-ranging

* Correspondence: raiello@izsvenezie.it
†Equal contributors
[1]Istituto Zooprofilattico Sperimentale delle Venezie (IZSVe), OIE/FAO and National Reference Laboratory for Newcastle Disease and Avian Influenza, OIE Collaborating Centre for Infectious Diseases at the Human-Animal Interface, Viale dell'Università 10, Legnaro, 35020 Padova, Italy
Full list of author information is available at the end of the article

mammals hosting IA viruses. Moreover, susceptibility to low pathogenic IA viruses has been demonstrated by experimental infection in live-trapped synanthropic species such as cottontail rabbits [20] and the striped skunk [21].

Although the susceptibility of some wild mammals to avian IA infections has been documented, the potential role of these species in the IA ecology and its relevance in public health have received limited attention [18,21-23]. Very little information is available on how wild birds can spread IA viruses to free-living wild mammals within their natural habitat [18], and whether virus adaptation to these hosts could represent an advantage for transmission to other species, such as terrestrial mammals, poultry and eventually humans [4,22]. In this regard, a small number of studies have identified the presence of mammalian wildlife (rodents and racoons) as a risk factor associated with the spread of IA viruses among commercial poultry and duck farms [24-26], and although an evident link between the presence of wild rodents and the occurrence of IA infections in poultry farms does not exist, rodent control is widely recommended as biosecurity measure to limit the spread of IA viruses within poultry flocks [27,28].

Synanthropic rodents are highly mobile in urban and rural areas, and may represent a risk for virus transmission within and among poultry farms [28]. In addition, they may be at a higher risk of co-infection with avian and mammalian IA strains, providing conditions for reassortment in nature [22]. Interestingly, seroconversion to IA has been demonstrated in wild-caught rodents during several low pathogenic avian influenza (LPAI) and HPAI outbreaks in poultry, although no virus isolation attempts from lungs or other collected organs have provided successful results [28-31]. Moreover, it has been demonstrated that LPAI viruses derived from wild birds are able to efficiently replicate in lungs of wild-caught house mice without prior adaptation, elucidating the possible role of this species in outbreak dynamics on poultry farms [28]. Remarkably, Achenbach et al. confirmed that recently-infected mallards had been able to transmit a LPAI H7N3 isolate to rats directly or through environmental contamination in an artificial barnyard [32].

In the present study, we evaluated the susceptibility to infection, the nasal shedding and the transmissibility of two HPAI isolates of H7N1 and H5N1 subtypes in the bank vole (*Myodes glareolus*), a wild rodent common throughout Europe and Asia, with the aim of elucidating the potential role of wild synanthropic populations of rodents in IA virus ecology.

Materials and methods

Viruses

The two HPAI isolates used for this study were H7N1 A/ostrich/Italy/2332/2000 (Os/H7N1) [GenBank: PB2:DQ991309, PB1:DQ991310, PA:DQ991311, HA:DQ991312, NP:DQ991313, NA:DQ991314, MA:DQ991315, NS: DQ991316], isolated during the Italian epidemic of 1999–2000 [33], and H5N1 A/turkey/Turkey/1/2005 (Tk/H5N1) [GenBank: PB2: EF619975, PB1: EF619976, PA: EF619979, HA: EF619980, NP: EF619977, NA: EF619973, MA: EF619978, NS: EF619974]. The two viruses were replicated in the allantoic cavity of 9- to 11-days old embryonated-specific pathogen-free (SPF) hen eggs according to OIE guidelines [34], and allantoic fluids were titrated to calculate the 50% Embryo Infectious Dose (EID_{50}) using the Reed and Muench formula [35].

Animals

Eighty five (male and female) bank voles (*Myodes glareolus*) of 4–6 weeks of age (13–16 g body weight) were obtained from a colony originally derived from the Istituto Superiore di Sanità (ISS, Rome, Italy). Prior to each experiment, all animals were left for acclimatization to the local environment for at least 1 week. Bank voles were housed in mouse cages with standard rodent feed and water *ad libitum*, and were weekly supplemented with grain seeds. Cages were prepared with a 3–4 cm bedding layer, and animals were provided with sufficient nesting material and environmental enrichments in order to express their species-specific behaviour (digging and burrowing). All in vivo experiments, approved by the IZSVe Ethics Committee (CE.IZSVE.24/2014) and authorized by the Italian Ministry of Health (Decree N.180/2011-B), were performed in containment facilities (BSL-3) and in accordance with the relevant legislation on the use of animals for scientific purposes [36].

Study design

Serology

Prior to challenge, blood was collected from all voles (tail vein) and sera were tested by means of a competitive commercial anti-nucleoprotein (NP) influenza ELISA (ID-screen®, IDVet, Montpellier, France) and through the Haemagglutination Inhibition (HI) test according to the WHO procedure used for mammal sera [37], using the challenge viruses as antigens (naïve sera from animals of each experimental group were tested only with the corresponding challenge virus). The same tests were used to evaluate the seroconversion on convalescent sera.

Nasal shedding experiment

Since no preliminary information existed regarding the infectivity of HPAI viruses in bank voles, the challenge dose of each selected virus was established as ten times the 50% Mouse Lethal Dose (MLD_{50}) as for previous experiments in BALB/c mice [38].

To evaluate the occurrence of nasal shedding, two groups of 12 male and female bank voles each (groups Os/H7N1 and Tk/H5N1) were inoculated intranasally, under light anesthesia (50 mg/kg ketamine and 4 mg/kg xylazine, intraperitoneally), with 50 µL of PBS-diluted allantoic fluid containing 10 times the MLD_{50} calculated in Balb/C mice, equivalent to $10^{3.75}$ and $10^{4.4}$ EID_{50}/0.1 mL of the H7N1 and H5N1 viruses, respectively. Three voles were used as negative controls and were mock-infected with 50 µL of sterile phosphate-buffered saline (PBS)-diluted allantoic fluid.

On a daily basis, challenged animals were monitored for the onset of clinical signs. Animals reaching the humane endpoint (weight loss greater than 20% and/or severe depression and respiratory distress) were euthanized. On days 3, 5, 7 and 9 post-infection (pi), three subjects were randomly selected and euthanized to collect organs. Brain, lungs and trachea tissues were collected from each animal along with a nasal wash (using 400 µL of sterile PBS). On day 3 post-inoculation, all control voles were also euthanized for collection of samples. Brain and nasal washes were tested by quantitative real time reverse transcriptase polymerase chain reaction (qRRT-PCR), while whole lungs and trachea were paraffin-embedded for histopathological and immunohistochemical (IHC) examination. Virus isolation in SPF embryonated hen eggs was attempted from all qRRT-PCR positive samples.

Pathogenicity and contact transmission experiment

Two groups of 24 female voles each were used for the transmission experiments; each group was randomly selected after weaning and reared together in a proper size cage (2065 cm^2 floor area). For each isolate, the experimental group included 12 infected voles (groups I-Os/H7N1 and I-Tk/H5N1) and 12 sentinels. The voles of each infected group were challenged by the intranasal route, as previously described, with 50 µL of PBS-diluted isolate. Twenty-four hours later, infected voles were moved into a clean cage hosting a group of 12 serologically naïve sentinels. Contemporaneously, 10 mock-infected voles were used as controls.

On a daily basis, all animals were observed for the onset of clinical signs and for mortality, and body weight was monitored on days 2, 4, 7 and 9 pi. Significance in body weight changes was calculated by the Student's *t*-test, and a *P* value less than 0.05 ($p < 0.05$) was considered statistically significant. On days 3 and 4 pi, post-contact (pc) and post-inoculation, two animals per group (infected, sentinels and control, respectively) were randomly selected and euthanized to collect nasal washes and different organs including lungs, trachea, brain, spleen, kidney and intestine. On day 30 pi/29 pc, all remaining voles were humanly euthanized, and convalescent sera were collected to determine seroconversion.

RRT-PCR and qRRT-PCR

Sample preparation. One hundred milligrams of tissues were homogenized in 200 µL of lysis buffer of the commercial kit Nucleospin RNA (Macherey Nagel, Düren, Germany), using the TissueLyser II (Qiagen, Germantown, USA) and following a homogenization program of 30 Hz for 3 min. The homogenates were clarified by centrifugation and tested by means of RRT-PCR.

RNA extraction. Viral RNA was extracted from 100 µL of clarified supernatant from tissue samples or from nasal washes, using the commercial kit Nucleospin RNA II and following the manufacturer's instructions. Viral RNA was eluted in 60 µL of RNAse-free water and stored at −80 °C after the addition of 1 µL of RNasin Plus RNase Inhibitor (Promega®, Madison, USA).

One-Step RRT-PCR and qRRT-PCR. The extracted RNA was amplified using the published primers and probe from Spackman et al. [39], targeting the conserved matrix (M) gene of the IA virus. Five microlitres of RNA were added to the reaction mixture, composed of 300 nM of forward and reverse primers (M25F and M124-R, respectively) and 100 nM of fluorescent label probe (M + 64). The amplification reaction was performed in a final volume of 25 µL using the commercial QuantiTect Multiplex RT-PCR kit (Qiagen, Hilden, Germany). The RRT-PCR was performed using the following protocol: 20 min at 50 °C and 15 min at 95 °C, followed by 40 cycles at 94 °C for 45 s and 60 °C for 45 s. According to the internal validation trails, the samples with a threshold cycle (Ct) higher than 35 were considered negative; however, all Ct values obtained for each sample were reported in the results.

The same one-step RRT-PCR protocol was used for the qRRT-PCR analysis. The synthetic RNA used as reference standard was created in vitro by means of the MegaScript® T7 kit (Invitrogen, CA, USA) from the H7N1 (A/Ostrich/Italy/2332/2000) and H5N1 (A/turkey/Turkey/1/2005) HPAI strains.

Virus isolation

Nasal washes (around 200 µL) were diluted in 400 µL of PBS containing antibiotics (10 000 IU/mL of penicillin, 10 mg/mL of streptomycin, 5000 UI/mL of nystatin and 250 mg/mL of gentamycin sulphate), while tissue samples (100 mg) were homogenized using sterile polypropylene micropestles (Sigma-Aldrich, Hamburg, Germany) in 700 µL of PBS containing antibiotics, and then clarified by centrifugation. Processed samples were propagated into the allantoic cavities of 9 to 11 days-old SPF embryonated hen eggs according to the OIE guidelines [34].

Histopathology and Immunohistochemistry

After 24 h, the lungs and trachea collected from the infected and mock-infected voles were fixed in 10% neutral phosphate-buffered formalin, paraffin-embedded, and stained with hematoxylin-and-eosin method for histopathological examination. The immunohistochemistry (IHC) was carried out by an automated immunostainer

(Autostainer™ Link 48 Dako, Italy). Briefly, the antigen retrieval was performed with Proteinase K (Dako, Italy) for 3 min at room temperature (RT). Endogenous peroxidases were neutralized by incubating the sections with the EnVision FLEX Peroxidase-Blocking Reagent (Dako, Italy) for 10 min at RT. Sections were incubated with a primary monoclonal antibody against IA virus nucleoprotein (Clone 1331, BIODESIGN International, USA), applied at 1:500 dilution for 10 min at RT. The EnVision FLEX/HRP (Dako, Carpinteria, CA, USA) and the EnVision FLEX Substrate Buffer EnVision FLEX DAB+ were used as the detection system and chromogen, respectively. Sections were then counterstained with the EnVision FLEX Hematoxylin (Dako, Italy). The specificity of the immunostaining was verified by incubating some sections with PBS instead of the specific primary antibody.

Results

Nasal shedding experiment

Serology

All voles sampled prior to infection tested negative for IA virus by means of a commercial ELISA and HI tests, while convalescent sera were not collected due to the short duration of this experiment (9 days).

Clinical signs and mortality

None of the twelve H7N1-infected voles showed any clinical sign throughout the experiment. Only one out of twelve H5N1-infected voles started to display the clinical signs of the disease (mild depression) on day 2 pi, being humanely euthanized on day 7 pi (severe depression and respiratory distress). All mock-infected voles remained asymptomatic throughout the duration of the experiment.

qRRT-PCR

Nasal shedding was detected in 1/3 voles of the Os/H7N1 group sampled on days 3 and 5 pi, showing 2.7 × and 7.9×10^7 viral copies/μL, respectively. On day 7 pi, 1/3 nasal washes recorded a viral load of 1.89×10^4 viral copies/μL (Figure 1). The nasal washes collected on day 9 pi, as well as all the brain samples collected from infected voles of this group at different points of infection, tested negative by qRRT-PCR. Results of nasal shedding of infected voles with both HPAI viruses at different time points of infection are reported in Table 1.

In H5N1-infected voles (Table 1), a peak of nasal shedding was recorded on day 3 pi, since 3/3 nasal washes tested positive with an average viral load of 1.27×10^9 copies/μL (Figure 1). On day 5 pi, one out of three nasal washes collected tested positive, recording a viral load of 9.4×10^4 viral copies/μL, while 2/3 nasal washes tested positive by qRRT-PCR on day 9 pi, with an average viral load of 7.62×10^5 viral copies/μL (Figure 1). Interestingly, the brain sample collected on day 7 pi from the only symptomatic H5N1-infected vole tested positive with a viral load of 7.17×10^4 copies/μL, while the remaining brain samples collected were negative.

All samples collected from the mock-infected voles were negative by means of qRRT-PCR.

Virus isolation

Viable virus was isolated from one qRRT-PCR positive nasal wash collected from one H7N1-infected vole on day 5 pi (Table 1), while no viable virus was recovered from any sample collected from H5N1-infected voles.

Histopathology and IHC

Histopathological examination of lungs collected from H7N1-infected animals revealed lesions in 3/12 voles, mainly characterized by multifocal purulent and catarrhal bronchitis in one vole on day 3 pi, and by multifocal pyogranulomatous bronchopneumonia in two animals on day 7 pi (Table 1). Only two voles presented multifocal alveolar haemorrhages and diffuse pulmonary congestion on days 5 and 9 pi, respectively. No histopathological findings were observed in the tracheas collected from the H7N1-infected animals. Positive IHC staining was observed in the trachea and in the lungs sampled on day 3 pi from two different infected voles belonging to this group (Figure 2).

In the lungs collected from Tk/H5N1-infected voles, multifocal pyogranulomatous bronchopneumonia with lymphohistiocytic infiltrate was evident in 2/2 voles on day 5 pi, and in 1/3 voles on days 7 and 9 pi, respectively. Only one animal showed multifocal interstitial pneumonia on day 5 pi. In addition, none of the tracheas collected at different points of infection showed any pathological lesion. Despite the evident histopathological lesions observed in the lungs of 5/12 Tk/H5N1-infected voles, no positive IHC staining was detected in the lungs and tracheas evaluated in this experimental group. None of the mock-infected voles showed any significant histopathological lesions nor positivity to IHC staining in the lungs and trachea.

Pathogenicity and by contact transmission experiment

Clinical signs and mortality

None of the voles belonging to group I-Os/H7N1 showed any clinical sign within 30 days of the observation period, although mild reduction in body weight compared to the control group was observed on day 9 pi (Figure 3A). However, the difference in body weight loss at different days pi between both groups was not statistically significant ($p >$ 0.05). Moreover, no clinical signs were observed in the sentinel group throughout the observation period.

One out of twelve H5N1-infected voles (group I-Tk/H5N1) showed depression, anorexia and severe respiratory signs on day 2 pi, and died during handling. No visual signs of disease were observed in the remaining infected

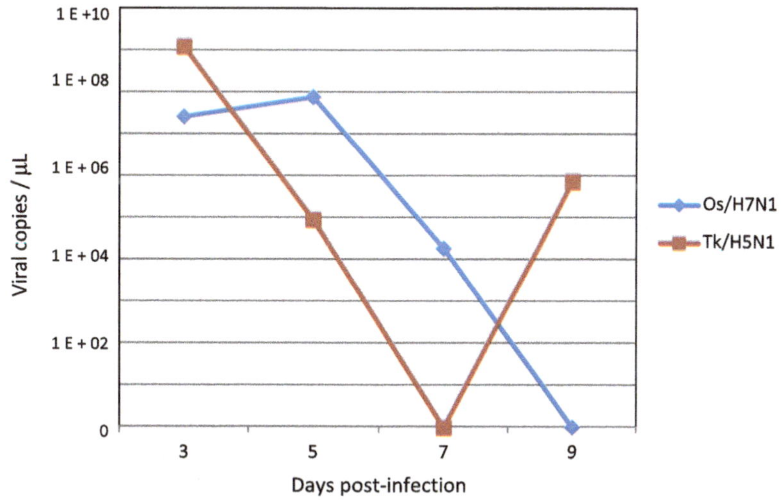

Figure 1 Nasal shedding of infected voles at different time points of infection. Mean of the viral shedding (viral copies/µL) recorded on nasal washes collected on days 3, 5, 7 and 9 pi from intranasally infected voles with $10^{3.75}$ EID_{50}/0.1 mL of the Os/H7N1 strain (group Os/H7N1) and $10^{4.4}$ EID_{50}/0.1 mL of the Tk/H5N1 strain (group Tk/H5N1).

voles and neither in all the contact sentinels; as well, the mean body weight recorded at different days pi showed no significant difference ($p > 0.05$) when compared to the control group (Figure 3B).

RRT-PCR

From the I-Os/H7N1 group, viral RNA was detected in all lungs collected on days 3 and 4 pi, and in 1/2 nasal washes collected on days 3 and 4 pi, respectively (Table 2). Moreover, viral RNA was detected in extra-respiratory organs such as the spleen (2/2), kidney (1/2) and brain (1/2) of infected and asymptomatic voles on day 3 pi. All samples collected from intestines tested negative by molecular test. From the contact sentinels of the Os/H7N1 group, all samples collected on day 3 pc tested negative, while one out of two lungs and one nasal

Table 1 Results of the nasal shedding experiment

Day pi	H7N1 A/ostrich/Italy/2332/2000 (Os/H7N1)				H5N1 A/turkey/Turkey/1/2005 (Tk/H5N1)				
	Nasal wash		Lungs/trachea		Nasal wash		Brain		Lungs
	qRRT-PCR (Ct/SQ)	VI	HP	IHC	qRRT-PCR (Ct/SQ)	VI	qRRT-PCR (Ct/SQ)	VI	HP
3	-	-	npl	+ trachea	+ (25.08/1.16 × 10^8)	-	-	/	npl
	-	/	npl	-	+ (21.14/3.70 × 10^9)	-	-	/	npl
	+ (24.0/2.7 × 10^7)	-	Multifocal purulent and catarrhal bronchitis	+ lungs	+ (29.4/2.60 × 10^6)	-	-	/	npl
5	+ (22.5/7.9 × 10^7)	+	npl	-	-	/	-	/	Multifocal of PBP with lymphohistiocytic infiltrate
	-	/	npl	-	-	/	-	/	Multifocal of PBP with lymphohistiocytic infiltrate
	-	/	Multifocal alveolar haemorrhages	-	+ (33.18/9.40 × 10^4)	-	-	/	Multifocal of interstitial pneumonia
7	-	/	npl	-	-	/	+(33.49/7.17 × 10^4)[a]	-	Multifocal PBP
	-	/	Multifocal PBP	-	-	/	-	/	npl
	+ (34.19/1.89 × 10^4)	-	Multifocal PBP	-	-	/	-	-	npl
9	-	/	Diffuse congestion	-	+ (34.68/2.50 × 10^4)	-	-	-	Multifocal PBP
	-	/	npl	-	+ (30.03/1.50 × 10^6)	-	-	/	npl
	-	/	npl	-	-	/	-	/	npl

Ct: quantification cycle; SQ: starting quantity (viral copies/µL); VI: virus isolation; HP: histopathological findings; IHC: immunohistochemical stain; –: negative; /: not performed; npl: no pathological lesions; PBP: pyogranulomatous bronchopneumonia, [a]bank vole with clinical signs.
This Table shows the qRRT-PCR and virus isolation results of the nasal washes and brains collected from the voles intranasally infected with both HPAI strains at different time points of infection. The results of the histopathological findings and IHC examination of the lungs and trachea collected from the infected voles are also reported.

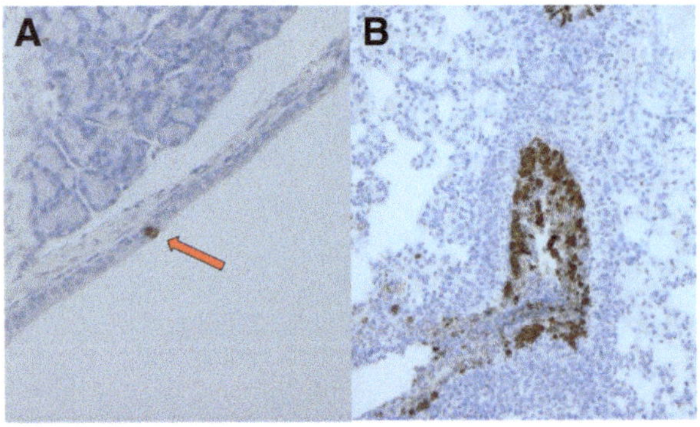

Figure 2 Immunohistochemical detection of HPAI viruses in paraffin-embedded tissue sections from infected voles. Positive staining by IHC in trachea **(A)** (red arrow) and lungs **(B)** collected on day 3 pi from two voles intranasally infected with $10^{3.75}$ EID_{50}/0.1 mL of the Os/H7N1 virus.

wash collected on day 4 pc tested positive by RRT-PCR (Table 2).

All lungs and nasal washes collected from H5N1-infected voles (group I-Tk/H5N1) were positive on days 3 and 4 pi. Moreover, one brain sample was positive in 1/2 voles on day 4 pi. Interestingly, the lungs, nasal wash and spleen collected from the only symptomatic H5N1-infected vole were positive by RRT-PCR on day 2 pi. From the contact sentinels of this group, the lungs collected from one animal on day 4 pc tested positive.

Virus isolation

Viable virus was isolated from all lungs collected on days 3 and 4 pi from infected voles of the group I-Os/H7N1 (Table 2). When virus isolation was attempted from other RRT-PCR positive organs, viable virus was isolated only from spleen on day 3 pi. Moreover, viable virus was isolated from the RRT-PCR positive lungs collected from the sentinel on day 4 pc.

As for the I-Tk/H5N1 group, viable virus was isolated from 5/5 RRT-PCR positive lungs collected from 2 infected voles on days 3 and 4 pi, respectively, and from the symptomatic vole that had died on day 2 pi (Table 2). All nasal washes collected on day 3 pi tested positive by VI. No virus isolation attempts were successful from other RRT-PCR positive extra-pulmonary organs, such as the brain and spleen collected from the infected group. Interestingly, viable virus was isolated from one RRT-PCR positive lung collected on day 4 pc from one in contact sentinel.

Serology

Six out of eight H7N1-infected voles (75%) tested positive by either competitive ELISA and HI tests on day 30 pi (Table 3). The HI titres ranged from 1:10 to 1:40. Four out of eight contact sentinels (50%) from the Os/H7N1 group were positive by ELISA and confirmed by HI test, with titres comparable to those of the infected voles (ranging from 1:10 to 1:40).

Regarding the I-Tk/H5N1 group, 7/7 infected voles (100%) seroconverted by both ELISA and HI tests, with HI titres ranging from 1:10 to 1:20. Only one out of eight (12.5%) contact sentinels tested positive by means of ELISA, but that individual was negative by HI.

Discussion

The aim of this study was to investigate the susceptibility of the bank vole to infection with two HPAI strains, the H5N1 A/turkey/Turkey/1/2005 (Tk/H5N1) and the H7N1 A/ostrich/Italy/2332/2000 (Os/H7N1) isolates, and to establish whether those avian viruses are transmitted by infected animals to naïve co-housed sentinel voles.

In the nasal shedding experiment, no clinical signs were observed in any of the H7N1-infected voles, while only one vole infected with the H5N1 virus displayed severe clinical signs. Voles infected with both HPAI viruses demonstrated evident nasal shedding; however, the number of voles shedding virus (particularly on day 3 pi) was higher in the group of voles infected with the Tk/H5N1 virus in comparison to the animals infected with the Os/H7N1 strain (100% of shedders vs. 33%, respectively). Interestingly, Tk/H5N1-infected voles shed the virus for a longer period than those infected with Os/H7N1, since positivity in nasal washes was recorded until day 9 pi in this group (66.6% vs. 0% of shedders). Quantitatively, voles infected with the Tk/H5N1 virus shed a higher amount of viruses than voles infected with the Os/H7N1 strain, especially on days 3 and 9 pi (1.27×0^9 vs. 2.7×10^7 and 7.6×10^5 vs. 0 viral copies/μL, respectively). Infected voles showed a similar shedding pattern to those reported in BALB/c mice infected with the same infectious doses of both HPAI isolates [38], although a different clinical outcome and mortality rate were observed in infected animals (100% mortality within 7 days pi of BALB/c mice infected with both strains vs. 0 and 8.3% of mortality in infected voles with Os/H7N1 and Tk/H5N1 strains, respectively). Viable virus was isolated from one nasal wash collected on day 5 pi from one Os/H7N1-infected vole, demonstrating that these animals are able to shed viable infectious particles to the environment. In contrast, no viable virus was recovered in the nasal washes collected from the Tk/H5N1-infected voles, despite their positivity by means of RRT-PCR. Due to the scarcity of original sample material, it was not possible to replicate the isolation attempts, which may explain the low virus isolation rate observed. However, the viable H5N1 virus was isolated in nasal washes collected in the pathogenicity and transmission experiment.

The histopathological examination of the respiratory tract of asymptomatic voles infected with both HPAI

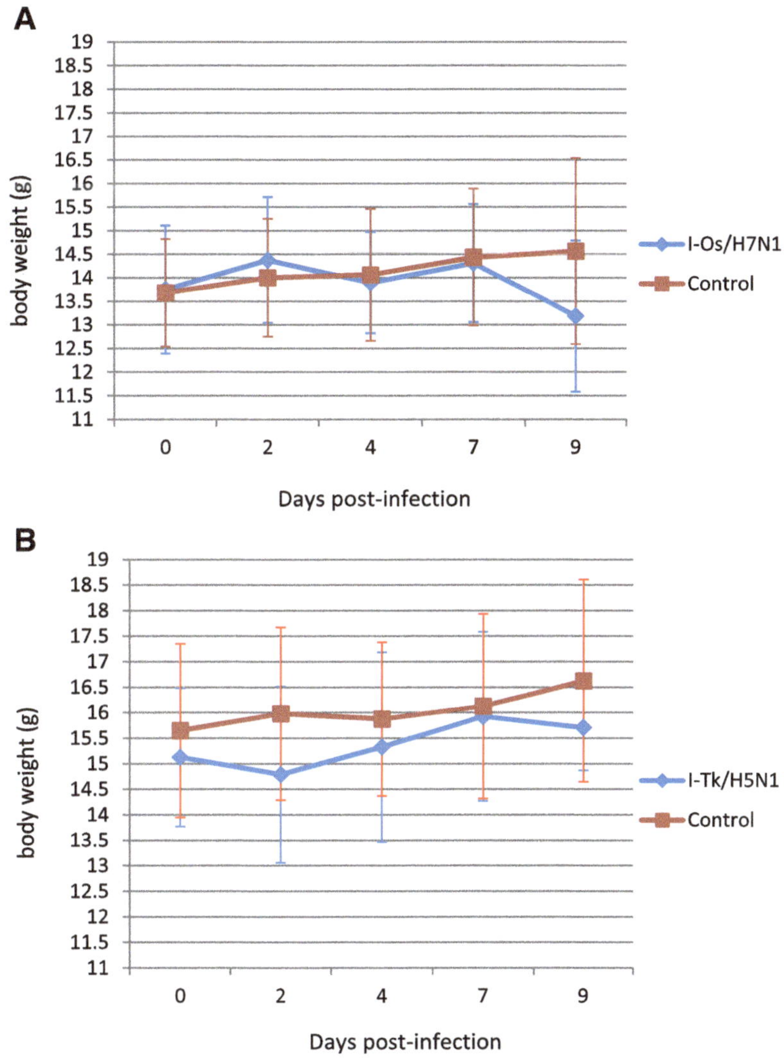

Figure 3 Mean body weight changes of control voles and voles infected with HPAI viruses. Body weight of bank voles intranasally inoculated with **(A)** $10^{3.75}$ EID_{50}/0.1 mL of Os/H7N1 virus and **(B)** $10^{4.4}$ EID_{50}/0.1 mL of Tk/H5N1 virus (group I-Tk/H5N1). Data shown are the mean ± SD (error bars) of body weight changes of inoculated voles in comparison to the control group. No significant difference ($p > 0.05$) was noticed between the body weight recorded at different points in all experimental groups.

strains demonstrated the presence of lesions due to the influenza infection, mainly characterized by multifocal pyogranulomatous bronchopneumonia, in 25% (3/12) and 41% (5/12) of infected voles with Os/H7N1 and Tk/H5N1 viruses, respectively. However, IHC positivity was only detected in trachea and lungs of two Os/H7N1-infected voles on day 3 pi, confirming the occurrence of viral replication in the upper and lower respiratory tract for this strain. Although no IHC positivity was observed in any organ collected from Tk/H5N1-infected animals, the positivity obtained by RRT-PCR on nasal washes in this same group suggests that further studies of the upper respiratory tract of voles (especially nasal mucosa and turbinates) are needed.

As observed in the nasal shedding experiment, all voles infected with the Os/H7N1 virus in the transmission experiment did not show any clinical sign, while only one vole infected with Tk/H5N1 displayed several respiratory signs and died on day 2 pi. Moreover, both infected groups showed no significant difference in body weight variations compared to the control group at different time points of infection. Despite the asymptomatic infection, the two selected HPAI viruses spread systemically in bank voles, since viral RNA from both of them was detected in extra-pulmonary organs, such as brain, kidney and spleen. Interestingly, as observed in the nasal shedding experiment, viral RNA was found in the nasal washes collected in a higher number of animals infected with the Tk/H5N1

Table 2 Results of the pathogenicity and by contact transmission experiment

Virus	Sample	Day pi/pc	Infected			Sentinels		
			RRT-PCR	Ct ± SD	VI	RRT-PCR	Ct	VI
Os/H7N1	Lungs	3	+2/2	26.22 ± 1.1	+2/2	-	-	nt
		4	+2/2	22.33 ± 0.08	+2/2	+1/2	28.24	+1/1
	Nasal wash	3	+1/2	32.13	-	-	-	nt
		4	+1/2	30.57	-	+1/2	35	-
	Brain	3	+1/2	30.01	-	-	-	nt
		4	-	-	nt	-	-	nt
	Spleen	3	+2/2	28 ± 3.5	+1/2	-	-	nt
		4	-	-	nt	-	-	nt
	Kidney	3	+1/2	29.6	-	-	-	nt
Tk/H5N1	Lungs	2[a]	+1/1	20.22	+1/1	nt	nt	nt
		3	+2/2	22.19 ± 2	+2/2	-	-	nt
		4	+2/2	27.3 ± 3.4	+2/2	+1/2	24.03	+1/1
	Nasal wash	2[a]	+1/1	26.95	-	nt	nt	nt
		3	+2/2	29 ± 2.1	+2/2	-	-	nt
		4	+2/2	34.7 ± 0.1	-	-	-	nt
	Brain	2[a]	-	-	nt	nt	nt	nt
		3	-	-	nt	-	-	nt
		4	+1/2	33.48	-	-	-	nt
	Spleen	2[a]	+1/1	33.12	-	nt	nt	nt
		3	-	-	nt	-	-	nt
		4	-	-	nt	-	-	nt

pi: post-infection; pc: post-contact; Ct: quantification cycle; SD: standard deviation; VI: virus isolation; [a]dead vole with clinical signs on day 2 pi; –: all samples tested negative; nt: not tested.

RRT-PCR (mean of Ct values ± SD) and virus isolation results of the different organs and nasal washes collected from infected voles and in contact sentinels on days 3 and 4 pi/pc.

virus than in those infected with the Os/H7N1 strain. Although the oral-fecal route of transmission could not be ruled out in this experiment, these findings suggest that the respiratory route may be the predominant mode of transmission of both HPAI viruses in this species. In fact, the viable virus was isolated from the lungs and nasal washes of infected voles, while no evidence of positivity and/or viral replication was observed in any of the intestines collected. However, further experiments using the oral route of inoculation will be necessary to clarify whether influenza viruses are able to replicate in the gastrointestinal tract of voles, and if infected animals are able to shed viruses to the environment by means of the feaces.

Importantly, voles infected with both HPAI viruses were able to infect in contact voles. No clinical signs of disease were observed in any of the sentinels, although virological (lungs and nasal washes) positivity was confirmed on day 4 pc in 2 and 1 sentinels from the Os/H7N1 and Tk/H5N1 groups, respectively. Although both the selected HPAI strains harboured the PB2 E627K mutation; which is correlated with higher pathogenicity, adaptation and transmission in mammals [40,41]; the Os/H7N1 virus displayed a higher rate of transmission than the Tk/H5N1

Table 3 Results of seroconversion of the pathogenicity and contact transmission experiment

Virus	Inoculated				Sentinels			
	Clinical signs	Mortality	Seroconversion		Clinical signs	Mortality	Seroconversion	
			ELISA	HI			ELISA	HI
Os/H7N1	Not observed	0% (0/8)	75% (6/8)	75% (6/8)[a]	Not observed	0% (0/8)	50% (4/8)	50% (4/8)[b]
Tk/H5N1	Severe respiratory signs (1/8)	12.5% (1/8)	100% (7/7)	100% (7/7)[c]	Not observed	0% (0/8)	12.5% (1/8)	0% (0/8)

[a]HI titers: 1:10 ($n = 1$), 1:20 ($n = 3$), 1:40 ($n = 2$); [b]HI titers: 1:10 ($n = 1$), 1:20 ($n = 1$), 1:40, ($n = 2$); [c]1:10 ($n = 3$), 1:20 ($n = 4$).

Clinical signs, mortality and seroconversion by means of ELISA and HI tests of inoculated and in contact sentinel voles on days 30 pi and 29 pc, respectively.

virus, since seroconversion was confirmed in 50% (4/8) and 12.5% (1/8) of sentinels at the end of the experiment, respectively.

Although our experimental design did not include the sampling of nasal washes on day 1 pi, it was demonstrated that both LPAI and HPAI viruses replicate in the upper respiratory tract (in particular, in the nasal turbinates) of mice [28,42,43] and other mammals [21,44] as early as day 1 pi. Moreover, we also excluded the possibility that the natural infection of sentinels was due to residual inoculums in the nasal cavity of the inoculated voles, since sentinels were put in contact with the infected animals after the recommended period of 6 h post inoculation to avoid any contamination [45].

The present study demonstrated that the bank vole is susceptible to infection with highly pathogenic H5N1 and H7N1 viruses of avian origin without prior adaptation, shedding viable virus in the environment, and transmitting the virus to contact voles. Interestingly, infection with the same HPAI strains demonstrated high pathogenicity and 100% of mortality in BALB/c mice [38], while infected voles were more resistant to the clinical condition and displayed zero or very low mortality rate. These important findings may suggest that wild rodents could play a role as silent hosts in IA virus epidemiology, contributing to the spread of HPAI virus infections during an outbreak. If this occurs under natural conditions, the circulation of IA viruses in these rodents may provide opportunities for the acquisition of mammalian adaptive mutations, which could minimize the barriers to interspecies transmission of these viruses. However, the study of synanthropic wild mammals, and in particular wild rodents, is a critical and important gap in our knowledge of how IA viruses may evolve in new hosts [22], considering that these species share the same ecological habitats as waterfowl and live commensally around domestic poultry farms [32], thus running the risk of being exposed to IA viruses.

Bank voles are geographically distributed in central Europe, in the South to Northern Spain and Italy, the Balkans, Western and Northern Turkey, as well as in Britain and Ireland [46], sharing a wide variety of habitats (woodland, river and stream banks, scrub and parkland) with the wild reservoirs of all avian IA strains and other terrestrial mammals. Importantly, voles are well identified as natural hosts for viruses of zoonotic interest, such as hantavirus Puumala virus [47], flavivirus tick borne encephalitis virus [48], orthopoxvirus cowpox virus [49], and parechovirus Ljungan virus [50]. The transmission of most of these viruses from rodents to humans is believed to occur through inhalation of aerosols contaminated by viruses shed in excreta, saliva and urine of infected animals; and several outdoor activities, such as camping and cleaning rodent infestations are considered important risk factors associated with their transmission [51]. In addition, multiple infections in voles with zoonotic pathogens such as *Borrelia* and *Bartonella* [52], as well as the presence of other pathogens as *Leptospira*, *Babesia* and *Anaplasma* have been reported [53]. All these findings demonstrate that voles are potentially susceptible to be infected by several pathogens with zoonotic potential, which could be transmitted directly or indirectly to other wild rodents and mammals.

Further investigations are needed to address the virological presence and the natural seroprevalence of IA viruses in free-living bank voles and other wild rodents, in the hope that a more conclusive epidemiologic scenario of IA infections in these synanthropic species may be provided, especially when avian and wild mammalians populations overlap in nature [22]. In addition, it would be important to understand whether the infection with IA viruses in synanthropic mammalian species may have a substantial impact on the public health, and if these species could be involved in the IA transmission to other synantropic populations of rodents, domestic poultry and mammals.

Two non-rodent adapted HPAI viruses caused asymptomatic infection in bank voles, which shed viable infectious particles capable of infecting in-contact sentinels. Infection of BALB/c mice with the same strains in previous experiments caused 100% mortality and severe clinical signs, thus suggesting that voles are more resistant to the disease caused by HPAI viruses, but still potentially capable of transmitting the virus. Additional studies are needed to elucidate the potential role of wild rodents in the epidemiology of HPAI infections.

Abbreviations

IA: Influenza type A; HPAI: Highly pathogenic avian influenza; LPAI: Low pathogenic avian influenza; HA: Haemagglutinin; NA: Neuraminidase; NP: Nucleoprotein; SPF: Specific pathogen-free; EID_{50}: 50 percent Embryo Infectious Dose; MLD_{50}: 50 percent Mouse Lethal Dose; PBS: Phosphate-buffered saline; HI: Haemagglutination inhibition test; pi: Post-infection; pc: Post-contact; RRT-PCR: Real time reverse transcription polymerase chain reaction; qRRT-PCR: Quantitative RRT-PCR; Ct: Quantification cycle; HP: Histopathological; IHC: Immunohistochemical stain; VI: Virus isolation; PBP: Pyogranulomatous bronchopneumonia.

Competing interests

The authors declare that they have no competing interests.

Authors' contributions

ART participated in the design of the study, carried out the in vivo tests and drafted the manuscript. RA participated in the design of the study and carried out the in vivo tests. AS carried out the molecular studies. VB carried out the virological analysis. MV carried out the histopathological and immunohistochemical assays. GC conceived the study, participated in the design of the study and coordinated all the activities of the project. All authors read and approved the final manuscript.

Acknowledgements

This work has been financially supported by the Italian Ministry of Health RC 06/2010. Authors wish to thank Dr Franco Mutinelli for providing the animals used in this study, and Dr Michele Di Bari for his invaluable technical support for in vivo studies. Authors also thank Dr Claudia Zanardello for her scientific contribution to this article and Francesca Ellero for her useful linguistic support.

Author details
[1]Istituto Zooprofilattico Sperimentale delle Venezie (IZSVe), OIE/FAO and National Reference Laboratory for Newcastle Disease and Avian Influenza, OIE Collaborating Centre for Infectious Diseases at the Human-Animal Interface, Viale dell'Università 10, Legnaro, 35020 Padova, Italy.
[2]Histopathology Laboratory, IZSVe, Viale dell'Università 10, Legnaro, 35020 Padova, Italy.

References

1. Webster RG, Bean WJ, Gorman OT, Chambers TM, Kawaoka Y (1992) Evolution and ecology of influenza A viruses. Microbiol Rev 56:152–179
2. Tong S, Li Y, Rivailler P, Conrardy C, Castillo DA, Chen LM, Recuenco S, Ellison JA, Davis CT, York IA, Turmelle AS, Moran D, Rogers S, Shi M, Tao Y, Weil MR, Tang K, Rowe LA, Sammons S, Xu X, Frace M, Lindblade KA, Cox NJ, Anderson LJ, Rupprecht CE, Donis RO (2012) A distinct lineage of influenza A virus from bats. Proc Natl Acad Sci U S A 109:4269–4274
3. Tong S, Zhu X, Li Y, Shi M, Zhang J, Bourgeois M, Yang H, Chen X, Recuenco S, Gomez J, Chen LM, Johnson A, Tao Y, Dreyfus C, Yu W, McBride R, Carney PJ, Gilbert AT, Chang J, Guo Z, Davis CT, Paulson JC, Stevens J, Rupprecht CE, Holmes EC, Wilson IA, Donis RO (2013) New world bats harbor diverse influenza A viruses. PLoS Pathog 9:e1003657
4. Reperant LA, Kuiken T, Osterhaus AD (2012) Adaptive pathways of zoonotic influenza viruses: from exposure to establishment in humans. Vaccine 30:4419–4434
5. Dórea FC, Cole DJ, Stallknecht DE (2013) Quantitative exposure assessment of waterfowl hunters to avian influenza viruses. Epidemiol Infect 141:1039–1049
6. Harder TC, Siebert U, Wohlsein P, Vahlenkamp T (2013) Influenza A virus infections in marine mammals and terrestrial carnivores. Berl Munch Tierarztl Wochenschr 126:500–508
7. Reperant LA, Rimmelzwaan GF, Kuiken T (2009) Avian influenza viruses in mammals. Rev Sci Tech 28:137–159
8. Geraci JR, St Aubin DJ, Barker IK, Webster RG, Hinshaw VS, Bean WJ, Ruhnke HL, Prescott JH, Early G, Baker AS, Madoff S, Schooley RT (1982) Mass mortality of harbor seals: pneumonia associated with influenza A virus. Science 215:1129–1131
9. Webster RG, Hinshaw VS, Bean WJ, Van Wyke KL, Geraci JR, St Aubin DJ, Petursson G (1981) Characterization of an influenza A virus from seals. Virology 113:712–724
10. Yoon KJ, Schwartz K, Sun D, Zhang J, Hildebrandt H (2012) Naturally occurring Influenza A virus subtype H1N2 infection in a Midwest United States mink (*Mustela vison*) ranch. J Vet Diagn Invest 24:388–391
11. Klopfleisch R, Wolf PU, Wolf C, Harder T, Starick E, Niebuhr M, Mettenleiter TC, Teifke JP (2007) Encephalitis in a stone marten (*Martes foina*) after natural infection with highly pathogenic avian influenza virus subtype H5N1. J Comp Pathol 137:155–159
12. Horimoto T, Maeda K, Murakami S, Kiso M, Iwatsuki-Horimoto K, Sashika M, Ito T, Suzuki K, Yokoyama M, Kawaoka Y (2011) Highly pathogenic avian influenza virus infection in feral raccoons. Japan. Emerg Infect Dis 17:714–717
13. Gordy JT, Jones CA, Rue J, Crawford PC, Levy JK, Stallknecht DE, Tripp RA, Tompkins SM (2012) Surveillance of feral cats for influenza A virus in north central Florida. Influenza Other Respir Viruses 6:341–347
14. Su S, Zhou P, Fu X, Wang L, Hong M, Lu G, Sun L, Qi W, Ning Z, Jia K, Yuan Z, Wang H, Ke C, Wu J, Zhang G, Gray GC, Li S (2014) Virological and epidemiological evidence of avian influenza virus infections among feral dogs in live poultry markets, china: a threat to human health? Clin Infect Dis 58:1644–1646
15. Keawcharoen J, Oraveerakul K, Kuiken T, Fouchier RA, Amonsin A, Payungporn S, Noppornpanth S, Wattanodorn S, Theambooniers A, Tantilertcharoen R, Pattanarangsan R, Arya N, Ratanakorn P, Osterhaus DM, Poovorawan Y (2004) Avian influenza H5N1 in tigers and leopards. Emerg Infect Dis 10:2189–2191
16. Roberton SI, Bell DJ, Smith GJ, Nicholls JM, Chan KH, Nguyen DT, Tran PQ, Streicher U, Poon LL, Chen H, Horby P, Guardo M, Guan Y, Peiris JS (2006) Avian influenza H5N1 in viverrids: implications for wildlife health and conservation. Proc Biol Sci 273:1729–1732
17. Britton AP, Sojonky KR, Scouras AP, Bidulka JJ (2010) Pandemic (H1N1) 2009 in skunks, Canada. Emerg Infect Dis 16:1043–1045
18. Zhou J, Sun W, Wang J, Guo J, Yin W, Wu N, Li L, Yan Y, Liao M, Huang Y, Luo K, Jiang X, Chen H (2009) Characterization of the H5N1 highly pathogenic avian influenza virus derived from wild pikas in China. J Virol 83:8957–8964
19. Yu Z, Cheng K, Sun W, Xin Y, Cai J, Ma R, Zhao Q, Li L, Huang J, Sang X, Li X, Zhang K, Wang T, Qin C, Qian J, Gao Y, Xia X (2014) Lowly pathogenic avian influenza (H9N2) infection in Plateau pika (Ochotona curzoniae), Qinghai Lake, China. Vet Microbiol 173:132–135
20. Root JJ, Shriner SA, Bentler KT, Gidlewski T, Mooers NL, Spraker TR, VanDalen KK, Sullivan HJ, Franklin AB (2014) Shedding of a low pathogenic avian influenza virus in a common synanthropic mammal–the cottontail rabbit. PLoS One 9:e102513
21. Root JJ, Shriner SA, Bentler KT, Gidlewski T, Mooers NL, Ellis JW, Spraker TR, VanDalen KK, Sullivan HJ, Franklin AB (2014) Extended viral shedding of a low pathogenic avian influenza virus by striped skunks (*Mephitis mephitis*). PLoS One 9:e70639
22. Runstadler J, Hill N, Hussein IT, Puryear W, Keogh M (2013) Connecting the study of wild influenza with the potential for pandemic disease. Infect Genet Evol 17:162–187
23. Vandalen KK, Shriner SA, Sullivan HJ, Rooot JJ, Franklin AB (2009) Monitoring exposure to avian influenza viruses in wild mammals. Mammal Rev 39:167–177
24. Duvauchelle A, Huneau-Salaün A, Balaine L, Rose N, Michel V (2013) Risk factors for the introduction of avian influenza virus in breeder duck flocks during the first 24 weeks of laying. Avian Pathol 42:447–456
25. Wakawa AM, Abdu PA, Oladele SB, Sa'idu L, Mohammed SB (2012) Risk factors for the occurrence and spread of Higlhy Pathogenic Avian Influenza H5N1 in commercial poultry farms in Kano, Nigeria. Sokoto J of Vet Sci 10:40–51
26. McQuiston JH, Garber LP, Porter-Spalding BA, Hahn JW, Pierson FW, Wainwright SH, Senne DA, Brignole TJ, Akey BL, Holt TJ (2005) Evaluation of risk factors for the spread of low pathogenicity H7N2 avian influenza virus among commercial poultry farms. J Am Vet Med Assoc 226:767–772
27. Koch G, Elbers ARW (2005) Outdoor ranging of poultry: a major risk factor for the introduction and development of High-Pathogenicity Avian Influenza. NJAS 54:179–194
28. Shriner SA, Vandalen KK, Mooers NL, Ellis JW, Sullivan HJ, Root JJ, Pelzel AM, Franklin AB (2012) Low-pathogenic avian influenza viruses in wild house mice. PLoS One 7:e39206
29. Nettles VF, Wood JM, Webster RG (1985) Wildlife surveillance associated with an outbreak of lethal H5N2 avian influenza in domestic poultry. Avian Dis 29:733–741
30. Shortridge KF, Gao P, Guan Y, Ito T, Kawaoka Y, Markwell D, Takada A, Webster RG (2000) Interspecies transmission of influenza viruses: H5N1 virus and a Hong Kong SAR perspective. Vet Microbiol 74:141–147
31. Henzler DJ, Kradel DC, Davison S, Ziegler AF, Singletary D, DeBok P, Castro AE, Lu H, Eckroade R, Swayne D, Lagoda W, Schmucker B, Nesselrodt A (2003) Epidemiology, production losses, and control measures associated with an outbreak of avian influenza subtype H7N2 in Pennsylvania (1996–98). Avian Dis 47:1022–1036
32. Achenbach JE, Bowen RA (2011) Transmission of avian influenza A viruses among species in an artificial barnyard. PLoS One 6:e17643
33. Capua I, Mutinelli F, Bozza MA, Terregino C, Cattoli G (2000) Highly pathogenic avian influenza (H7N1) in ostriches (*Struthio camelus*). Avian Pathol 29:643–646
34. OIE Manual of Diagnostic Tests and Vaccines for Terrestrial Animals 2014. http://www.oie.int/fileadmin/Home/eng/Health_standards/tahm/2.03.04_AI.pdf. Accessed 15 December 2014.
35. Reed LJ, Muench H (1938) A simple method of estimating fifty per cent endpoints. Am J of Hyg 27:493–497
36. Directive 2010/63/EU of the European Parliament and of the Council of 22 September 2010 on the protection of animals used for the scientific purposes. http://eur-lex.europa.eu/legal-content/EN/TXT/?qid=1414768135290&uri=CELEX:32010L0063. Accessed 15 December 2014.
37. WHO Manual on Animal Influenza Diagnosis and Surveillance. http://www.who.int/csr/resources/publications/influenza/en/whocdscsrncs20025rev.pdf Accessed 15 December 2014.
38. Rigoni M, Toffan A, Viale E, Mancin M, Cilloni F, Bertoli E, Salomoni A, Marciano S, Milani A, Zecchin B, Capua I, Cattoli G (2010) The mouse model

is suitable for the study of viral factors governing transmission and pathogenesis of highly pathogenic avian influenza (HPAI) viruses in mammals. Vet Res 41:66

39. Spackman E, Senne DA, Myers TJ, Bulaga LL, Garber LP, Perdue ML, Lohman K, Daum LT, Suarez DL (2002) Development of a real-time reverse transcriptase PCR assay for type A influenza virus and the avian H5 and H7 hemagglutinin subtypes. J Clin Microbiol 40:3256–3260
40. Zhang H, Li X, Guo J, Li L, Chang C, Li Y, Bian C, Xu K, Chen H, Sun B (2014) The PB2 E627K mutation contributes to the high polymerase activity and enhanced replication of H7N9 influenza virus. J Gen Virol 95:779–786
41. de Jong RM, Stockhofe-Zurwieden N, Verheij ES, de Boer-Luijtze EA, Ruiter SJ, de Leeuw OS, Cornelissen LA (2013) Rapid emergence of a virulent PB2 E627K variant during adaptation of highly pathogenic avian influenza H7N7 virus to mice. Virol J 10:276–286
42. Whiteley A, Major D, Legastelois I, Campitelli L, Donatelli I, Thompson CI, Zambon MC, Wood JM, Barclay WS (2007) Generation of candidate human influenza vaccine strains in cell culture - rehearsing the European response to an H7N1 pandemic threat. Influenza Other Respir Viruses 1:157–166
43. Cox RJ, Major D, Hauge S, Madhun AS, Brokstad KA, Kuhne M, Smith J, Vogel FR, Zambon M, Haaheim LR, Wood J (2009) A cell-based H7N1 split influenza virion vaccine confers protection in mouse and ferret challenge models. Influenza Other Respir Viruses 3:107–117
44. Hinshaw VS, Webster RG, Easterday BC, Bean WJ, Jr (1981) Replication of avian influenza A viruses in mammals. Infect Immun 34:354–361
45. Edenborough KM, Gilbertson BP, Brown LE (2012) A mouse model for the study of contact-dependent transmission of influenza A virus and the factors that govern transmissibility. J Virol 86:12544–12551
46. Wilson DE and Reeder DM (2005) Mammal Species of the World (MSW3), 3rd Edition. http://www.vertebrates.si.edu/msw/mswcfapp/msw/taxon_browser.cfm?msw_id=4452. Accessed 15 December 2014.
47. Tersago K, Crespin L, Verhagen R, Leirs H (2012) Impact of Puumala virus infection on maturation and survival in bank voles: a capture/mark/recapture analysis. J Wildl Dis 48:148–156
48. Knap N, Korva M, Dolinšek V, Sekirnik M, Trilar T, Avšič-Županc T (2012) Patterns of tick/borne encephalitis virus infection in rodents in Slovenia. Vector Borne Zoonotic Dis 12:236–242
49. Chantrey J, Meyer H, Baxby D, Begon M, Bown KJ, Hazel SM, Jones T, Montgomery WI, Bennett M (1999) Cowpox: reservoir hosts and geographic range. Epidemiol Infect 122:455–460
50. Hauffe HC, Niklasson B, Olsson T, Bianchi A, Rizzoli A, Klitz W (2010) Ljungan virus detected in bank voles (*Myodes glareolus*) and yellow-necked mice (*Apodemus flavicollis*) from Northern Italy. J Wildl Dis 46:262–266
51. Winter CH, Brockmann SO, Piechotowski I, Alpers K, Van der Heiden M, Koch J, Stark K, Pfaff G (2009) Survey and case–control study during epidemics of Puumala virus infection. Epidemiol Infect 137:1479–1485.
52. Buffet JP, Marsot M, Vaumourin E, Gasqui P, Masséglia S, Marcheteau E, Huet D, Chapuis JL, Pisanu B, Ferquel E, Halos L, Vourc'h G, Vayssier-Taussat M (2012) Co-infection of *Borrelia afzelii* and *Bartonella spp.* in bank voles from a suburban forest. Comp Immunol Microbiol Infect Dis 35:583–589
53. Kallio ER, Begon M, Birtles RJ, Bown KJ, Koskela E, Mappes T, Watts PC (2014) First report of Anaplasma phagocytophilum and Babesia microti in rodents in Finland. Vector Borne Zoonotic Dis 14:389–393

13

Evaluation of the capability of the PCV2 genome to encode miRNAs: lack of viral miRNA expression in an experimental infection

Fernando Núñez-Hernández[1], Lester J Pérez[2], Gonzalo Vera[3], Sarai Córdoba[3], Joaquim Segalés[1,4], Armand Sánchez[3,5] and José I Núñez[1*]

Abstract

Porcine circovirus type 2 (PCV2) is a ssDNA virus causing PCV2-systemic disease (PCV2-SD), one of the most important diseases in swine. MicroRNAs (miRNAs) are a new class of small non-coding RNAs that regulate gene expression post-transcriptionally. Viral miRNAs have recently been described and the number of viral miRNAs has been increasing in the past few years. In this study, small RNA libraries were constructed from two tissues of subclinically PCV2 infected pigs to explore if PCV2 can encode viral miRNAs. The deep sequencing data revealed that PCV2 does not express miRNAs in an in vivo subclinical infection.

Introduction, methods, and results

Porcine circovirus type 2-systemic disease (PCV2-SD) is a devastating disease that causes important economic losses [1]. The disease is essentially caused by PCV2, a single stranded DNA, non enveloped virus belonging to the *Circoviridae* family [2]. The PCV2 genome encodes four ORFs. ORF1 encodes for two proteins (Rep and Rep') which are involved in replication. ORF2 encodes for the Cap protein, which constitutes the unique structural protein. The two proteins coded by ORF3 and ORF4 have been related with cellular apoptosis while the function of both still needs further research [3].

MicroRNAs (miRNAs) comprise a class of small non-coding RNAs that post-transcriptionally regulate the expression of many genes by mRNA degradation or translation inhibition [4]. miRNAs are involved in the modulation of gene expression and replication of many viruses and play a pivotal role in host-virus interactions. In addition, many viruses encode miRNAs that can play a role in the infection process. To date, 308 hairpin precursors and 502 mature miRNAs have been discovered in several viruses as shown in the miRBase [5], most of them encoded by herpesviruses, which is the virus family with the highest miRNAs encoding capacity [6,7]. Other viruses belonging to the families *Polyomaviridae, Adenoviridae, Papillomaviridae, Baculoviridae* and *Ascoviridae* encode miRNAs in low numbers [8-12]. Recently, a Human Torque Teno virus, a small, ssDNA virus from the *Anelloviridae* family, that encodes a miRNA involved in interferon modulation has been described [13]. All of them share in common to be DNA viruses, with an essential nuclear phase in their replication cycle, necessary for initial miRNA biogenesis. miRNAs encoded by RNA viruses is a matter of controversy [14-16].

In the present study, the expression of miRNAs in subclinically PCV2 infected pigs was analysed using high throughput sequencing. Firstly, in silico prediction was carried out in order to check if the PCV2 genome encodes possible miRNA precursors. The Vmir prediction algorithm [17] was used to predict the possible presence of hairpin structures in the PCV2 genome compatible with the existence of miRNAs. Computational prediction of viral miRNAs indicated that 41 miRNA candidates could be identified, 16 of them with a score among 100-150 and two with a score >150 (Figure 1). In order to explore whether these candidates were present in the virus, next-generation sequencing (NGS) of small RNAs was carried out from tonsil and mediastinal lymph node of animals subclinically infected with PCV2.

* Correspondence: ignacio.nunez@cresa.uab.es
[1]Centre de Recerca en Sanitat Animal (CReSA), UAB-IRTA, Campus de la Universitat Autònoma de Barcelona, Bellaterra, Cerdanyola del Vallès, Spain
Full list of author information is available at the end of the article

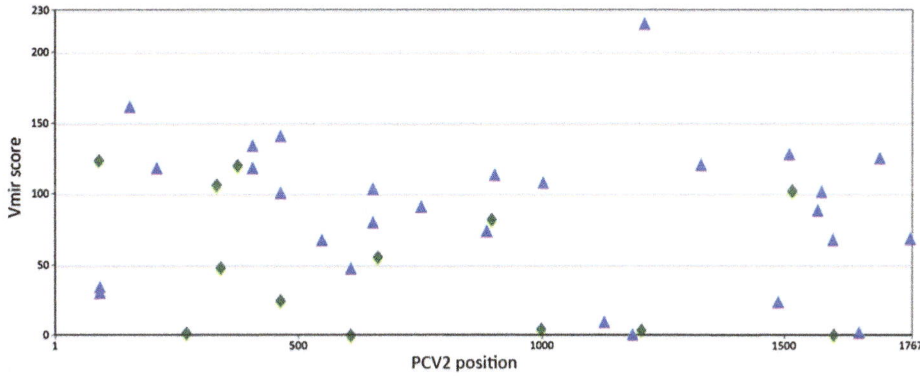

Figure 1 Hairpin structures predicted for PCV2 genome of Sp-10-7-54-13 isolate (accession number GU049342) by using Vmir with default parameters. Green diamonds and blue triangles indicate stem-loop structures in direct or reverse orientation, respectively.

We have reported previously modification of the expression pattern of host miRNAs due to the PCV2 infection [18]. For both purposes, four animals were inoculated with $7 \times 10^{4.8}$$TCID_{50}$ of PCV2 isolate Sp-10-7-54-13 [19] and two animals were inoculated with PBS. Animal experiments were carried out at the CReSA facilities, all procedures were performed under the supervision of the Ethical and Animal Welfare Committee of the UAB in compliance with national guidelines and EU regulations. At 21 days post-inoculation samples were taken and total RNA extractions were carried out in order to construct small RNA libraries as described in [20] with some modifications. A total of 12 small RNA libraries were constructed in a two-step ligation procedure with the 3′ and 5′ adaptors from IDT technologies. Amplification by RT-PCR was carried out with fusion primers containing sequences complementary to the 3′ and 5′ adaptors used for miRNA library construction and sequences complementary to the A and B adaptors used for high-throughput (HT) sequencing with the GS FLX 454 device (Roche) at CRAG (Centre de Recerca Agrogenòmica, Universitat Autònoma de Barcelona, Spain). From the total reads obtained (1 106 437), primer sequences were trimmed and only those insert sequences between 15 and 29 nucleotides and with total number of sequences ≥3 were kept for further analysis. This procedure resulted in a total of 796 710 reads.

The analysis of the reads that aligned to the *Sus scrofa* genome are reported elsewhere because these sequences constitute porcine miRNAs [18]. For viral miRNA discovery, sequences were blasted to the PCV2 isolate Sp-10-7-54-13 genome (NCBI Reference Sequence: GU049342) considering only sequences with 100% of alignment and identity (perfect match). In order to search potential viral miRNAs, a blast against the viral genome was done with an increased number of mismatches in the extremes due to miRNA variability (isomiRs) [21,22]. The presence of isomiRs entails differences in length and point mutations in both extremes, with the 3′-terminus having a higher proportion of such mutations. In some cases, a blast was done allowing internal variations with a <100% of alignment in order to consider the variability of the viral genome [23]. Also, sequences were blasted to the output of Vmir hairpin PCV2 structures.

No hits were found in the viral PCV2 genome sequence (GU049342) with a 100% homology. One candidate of 18 nt with 58 copies was identified when allowing <100% of alignment and identity in the ORF2, positions 1189 to 1206. In accordance with the Vmir prediction, these positions were included in the pre-miRNA candidate MD18, (the hairpin with the highest score), presenting one internal mismatch, and 94.4% sequence identity. The secondary structure and the minimum free energy of the pre-miRNA candidate was analysed with MFold software [24] (Figure 2). As this candidate presented a point mutation, and due to the described variability of the virus, the corresponding viral DNA fragment from the mediastinal lymph node of an infected animal was amplified and Sanger sequenced. Because the exact candidate sequence was not found in the viral sequence (94.4% sequence identity), it was not considered a miRNA encoded by the virus. The miRNA candidate sequence was compared to the porcine genome Sscrofa10.2 (GCA_000003025.4) using blast and showed 100% sequence identity with the ssc-miR-29a hairpin precursor located in chromosome 18. Also, the 18 nt miRNA candidate sequence was compared to the miRBase (v.21) showing 100% sequence identity with miR-29a-5p. The alignment of this region was carried out including all PCV2 sequences available in the databases (Figure 3). miR-29a-5p has been described in many species like human, bovine, mouse, but it has not been described in pigs, where the precursor miR-29 has been included in miRBase along with the mature ssc-miR-29a-3p. From the total reads obtained in this study, 1276 sequences of 22 nt, comprising the 18 nt of the candidate, blasted to the miR-29a-5p. From all of the above data,

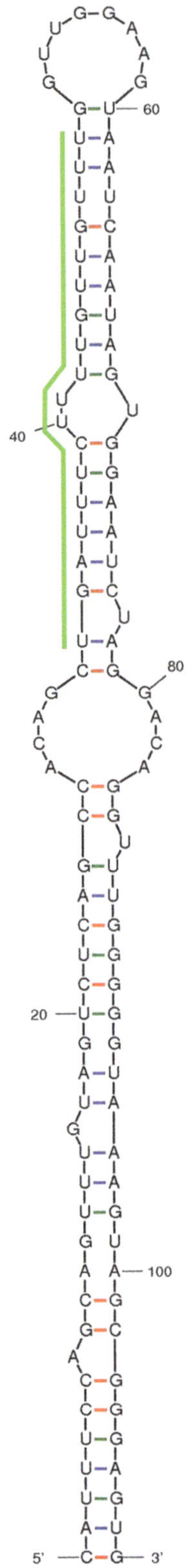

Figure 2 Folding structure using MFold of pre-miRNA candidate predicted by Vmir. The minimum free energy (ΔG) calculated was -26.60 Kcal/mol. Position of the miRNA candidate sequence detected by next-generation sequencing is indicated into the pre-miRNA structure with a green line.

miR-29a-5p can be considered as a miRNA encoded by the porcine genome and the 18 nt candidate as one of the miR-29a-5p isomiRs.

Discussion

This is the first study that tries to identify if PCV2 can encode miRNAs. PCV2 is a ssDNA virus with a nuclear phase in its replicating cycle [25]. This step is considered essential for the production of viral miRNAs, considering that the first steps in miRNA maturation take place in the cellular nucleus [26]. Nevertheless, high throughput sequencing has failed to identify any miRNA encoded by the viral genome in the natural host after an experimental infection. Thus, PCV2 may increase the list of DNA viruses not encoding miRNAs, as Cowpox virus [7]. Notwithstanding, the capacity of PCV2 to encode miRNAs has to be evaluated in cell culture, in a different clinical form or at a different time points.

Only one miRNA candidate was initially identified, but the posterior analysis indicated that it was a host miRNA, miR-29a-5p. The homology of the viral sequence with miR-29a-5p, with only one internal mismatch, led us to analyze with more detail if miR-29a-5p can regulate the expression of the Cap protein. A miR-29a-5p target prediction was evaluated using Miranda software [27] in order to explore if the Cap gen constitutes a target. As expected, a predicted target was identified in ORF2, with a low free energy of -21.65 Kcal/mol and a high complementarity score of 187. The alignment of the region with all PCV2 isolates available in the database indicated that A, C and T, but not G, has been found at position 1202 respecting Sp-10-7-54-13. All substitutions lead to a non synonymous change. The lack of the presence of G at position 1202 could be due to restriction in the protein conformation or due to the pressure exerted by miR-29a-5p in order to avoid regulation by this miRNA. If this is a consequence of viral evolution as [28] proposed, it needs further investigation. How viruses can evolve to avoid the inhibition by host miRNAs is a critical question. Some authors indicate that this evolution allows viruses to replicate without being targeted by host miRNAs by encoded viral miRNAs or modifying the expression of host miRNAs [29]. On the other hand, the secondary structure of MD18 could avoid the regulation by miR-29a-5p due to the inaccessibility of the target sequence as has been proposed for HIV [16].

In a previous study [18], in subclinically infected pigs, we demostrated that PCV2 can alter the miRNA expression pattern of the host. If PCV2 can express miRNAs in vitro has to be determined, but in its natural host, in a subclinical infection, NGS failed to indentify viral miRNAs. The exploration of the possible capacity of PCV2 to encode miRNAs could contribute to the understanding of

miRNA/PCV2 strains	Nucleotide Sequence	aa	No of isolates
	1188 1202 1209	173	
mir-29a-5p	ACTGATTTCTTTTGGTGTTCAG[a]		
PCV2 Sp-10-7-54-13	G T TG	N	977
PCV2 A/2002	G C TG	S	6
PCV2 Henan-1	G A TG	I	1
(-)[b]	G TG	T	0

Figure 3 Alignment of miR-29a-5p with positions 1188-1209 of the Sp-10-7-54-13 sequence and all PCV2 available sequences in the EMBL database. A representative of each sequence is included in the alignment. The number of isolates with the same sequence is shown. The derived amino acid (aa position 173) from nucleotide change at position 1202 is indicated. [a]U has been replaced by T to facilitate the understanding of the figure. [b]No viral sequence was found in the database with this sequence.

the pathogenesis of PCV2, especially for the candidate with highest score identified by the in silico prediction. In addition, further studies on the similarity of this candidate with miR-29a-5p, and its significance, could shed light on how miRNAs affect viral evolution [30].

Competing interests
The authors declare that they have no competing interests.

Authors' contributions
JIN and AS conceived, designed and coordinated this study. FNH, and LJP performed the experiments. JIN and FNH analyzed data. JS, and SC, contributed reagents/material/analysis tools. JIN and FNH wrote the paper. GV performed the bioinformatics analysis. JS critically read the manuscript. All authors read and approved the final manuscript.

Acknowledgements
The authors thank all the personnel of the animal facilities at CReSA. This work was supported by the projects AGL2007-66371-C02 and AGL2010-22358-C02 from MINECO (Spanish government). FN-H is the recipient of a PhD fellowship FI-DGR (AGAUR) from Generalitat de Catalunya. The authors thank Dr. Kevin Dalton for editing the manuscript.

Author details
[1]Centre de Recerca en Sanitat Animal (CReSA), UAB-IRTA, Campus de la Universitat Autònoma de Barcelona, Bellaterra, Cerdanyola del Vallès, Spain. [2]Centro Nacional de Sanidad Agropecuaria (CENSA), La Habana, Cuba. [3]Departament de Genètica Animal, Centre de Recerca en AgriGenòmica (CRAG), CSIC-IRTA-UAB-UB, Universitat Autònoma de Barcelona, Barcelona, Bellaterra, Spain. [4]Departament de Sanitat i Anatomia Animals, Universitat Autònoma de Barcelona, Barcelona, Bellaterra, Spain. [5]Departament de Ciència Animal i dels Aliments, Universitat Autònoma de Barcelona (UAB), Barcelona, Bellaterra, Spain.

References
1. Segalés J (2012) Porcine circovirus type 2 (PCV2) infections: clinical signs, pathology and laboratory diagnosis. Virus Res 164:10–19
2. Segalés J, Allan GM, Domingo M (2005) Porcine circovirus diseases. Anim Health Res Rev 6:119–142
3. Gao Z, Dong Q, Jiang Y, Opriessnig T, Wang J, Quan Y, Yang Z (2014) ORF4-protein deficient PCV2 mutants enhance virus-induced apoptosis and show differential expression of mRNAs in vitro. Virus Res 183:56–62
4. Bartel DP (2004) MicroRNAs: genomics, biogenesis, mechanism, and function. Cell 116:281–297
5. miRBase: the microRNA database [http://www.mirbase.org]
6. Grundhoff A, Sullivan CS (2011) Virus-encoded microRNAs. Virology 411:325–343
7. Skalsky RL, Cullen BR (2010) Viruses, microRNAs, and host interactions. Annu Rev Microbiol 64:123–141
8. Sullivan CS, Grundhoff AT, Tevethia S, Pipas JM, Ganem D (2005) SV40-encoded microRNAs regulate viral gene expression and reduce susceptibility to cytotoxic T cells. Nature 435:682–686
9. Sano M, Kato Y, Taira K (2006) Sequence-specific interference by small RNAs derived from adenovirus VAI RNA. FEBS Lett 580:1553–1564
10. Qian K, Pietila T, Ronty M, Michon F, Frilander MJ, Ritari J, Tarkkanen J, Paulin L, Auvinen P, Auvinen E (2013) Identification and validation of human papillomavirus encoded microRNAs. PLoS One 8:e70202
11. Hussain M, Taft RJ, Asgari S (2008) An insect virus-encoded microRNA regulates viral replication. J Virol 82:9164–9170
12. Singh J, Singh CP, Bhavani A, Nagaraju J (2010) Discovering microRNAs from Bombyx mori nucleopolyhedrosis virus. Virology 407:120–128
13. Kincaid RP, Burke JM, Cox JC, de Villiers EM, Sullivan CS (2013) A human torque teno virus encodes a microRNA that inhibits interferon signaling. PLoS Pathog 9:e1003818
14. Ouellet DL, Plante I, Landry P, Barat C, Janelle ME, Flamand L, Tremblay MJ, Provost P (2008) Identification of functional microRNAs released through asymmetrical processing of HIV-1 TAR element. Nucleic Acids Res 36:2353–2365
15. Schopman NC, Willemsen M, Liu YP, Bradley T, van Kampen A, Baas F, Berkhout B, Haasnoot J (2012) Deep sequencing of virus-infected cells reveals HIV-encoded small RNAs. Nucleic Acids Res 40:414–427
16. Whisnant AW, Bogerd HP, Flores O, Ho P, Powers JG, Sharova N, Stevenson M, Chen CH, Cullen BR (2013) In-depth analysis of the interaction of HIV-1 with cellular microRNA biogenesis and effector mechanisms. MBio 4:e000193
17. Grundhoff A (2011) Computational prediction of viral miRNAs. Methods Mol Biol 721:143–152
18. Nunez-Hernandez F, Perez LJ, Munoz M, Vera G, Tomas A, Egea R, Cordoba S, Segales J, Sanchez A, Nuñez JI (2015) Identification of microRNAs in PCV2 subclinically infected pigs by high throughput sequencing. Vet Res 46:18
19. Fort M, Sibila M, Nofrarias M, Perez-Martin E, Olvera A, Mateu E, Segalés J (2010) Porcine circovirus type 2 (PCV2) Cap and Rep proteins are involved in the development of cell-mediated immunity upon PCV2 infection. Vet Immunol Immunopathol 137:226–234
20. Timoneda O, Nunez-Hernandez F, Balcells I, Munoz M, Castello A, Vera G, Perez LJ, Egea R, Mir G, Cordoba S, Rosell R, Segalés J, Tomas A, Sanchez A, Nunez JI (2014) The role of viral and host microRNAs in the Aujeszky's disease virus during the infection process. PLoS One 9, e86965
21. Ebhardt HA, Tsang HH, Dai DC, Liu Y, Bostan B, Fahlman RP (2009) Meta-analysis of small RNA-sequencing errors reveals ubiquitous post-transcriptional RNA modifications. Nucleic Acids Res 37:2461–2470
22. Morin RD, O'Connor MD, Griffith M, Kuchenbauer F, Delaney A, Prabhu AL, Zhao Y, McDonald H, Zeng T, Hirst M, Eaves CJ, Marra MA (2008) Application of massively parallel sequencing to microRNA profiling and discovery in human embryonic stem cells. Genome Res 18:610–621
23. Firth C, Charleston MA, Duffy S, Shapiro B, Holmes EC (2009) Insights into the evolutionary history of an emerging livestock pathogen: porcine circovirus 2. J Virol 83:12813–12821
24. Zuker M (2003) Mfold web server for nucleic acid folding and hybridization prediction. Nucleic Acids Res 31:3406–3415
25. Tischer I, Peters D, Pociuli S (1995) Occurrence and role of an early antigen and evidence for transforming ability of porcine circovirus. Arch Virol 140:1799–1816
26. Cullen BR (2010) Five questions about viruses and microRNAs. PLoS Pathog 6:e1000787

27. Enright AJ, John B, Gaul U, Tuschl T, Sander C, Marks DS (2003) MicroRNA targets in Drosophila. Genome Biol 5:R1
28. Bogerd HP, Skalsky RL, Kennedy EM, Furuse Y, Whisnant AW, Flores O, Schultz KL, Putnam N, Barrows NJ, Sherry B, Scholle F, Garcia-Blanco MA, Griffin DE, Cullen BR (2014) Replication of many human viruses is refractory to inhibition by endogenous cellular microRNAs. J Virol 88:8065–8076
29. Cullen BR (2013) How do viruses avoid inhibition by endogenous cellular microRNAs? PLoS Pathog 9:e1003694
30. Guo YE, Steitz JA (2014) Virus meets host microRNA: the destroyer, the booster, the hijacker. Mol Cell Biol 34:3780–3787

14

Evaluation of porcine epidemic diarrhea virus transmission and the immune response in growing pigs

Kimberly Crawford[1], Kelly Lager[1*], Laura Miller[1], Tanja Opriessnig[2,3], Priscilla Gerber[2,3] and Richard Hesse[4]

Abstract

Clinical disease associated with porcine epidemic diarrhea virus (PEDV) infection in naïve pigs is well chronicled; however, information on endemic PEDV infection is limited. To characterize chronic PEDV infection, the duration of infectious virus shedding and development of protective immunity was determined. On Day 0 (D0), a growing pig was challenged with PEDV and 13 contacts were commingled. On D7, 9 contact pigs (principal virus group (PG)), were selected, moved to a separate room and commingled with one sentinel pig (S1). This process was repeated weekly with S2, S3 and S4. The PG was PEDV-positive by PCR from D3-11, with some pigs intermittently positive to D42. Pigs S1 and S2 were PEDV-positive within 24 hours of commingling. Antibodies were detected in all PG by D21 and by 7 days post-contact in S1 and S2. Pigs S3 and S4 were PCR and antibody negative following commingling. To evaluate protective immunity, 5 naïve pigs (N) and the PG were challenged (N/C, PG/C) with homologous virus on D49. All N/C pigs were PEDV PCR-positive by D52 with detection out to D62 in 3/5 N/C pigs. All PG/C pigs were PEDV PCR-negative post-challenge. By D63, all N/C seroconverted. Although PEDV RNA was demonstrated in pigs after primary infection until D42, infectious PEDV capable of horizontal transmission to naïve pigs was only shed 14–16 days after infection to age-matched pigs. Homologous re-challenge 49 days post initial PEDV exposure did not result in re-infection of the pigs. This demonstrates potential for an effective PEDV vaccine.

Introduction

Porcine epidemic diarrhea virus (PEDV) was discovered in 1976 in the feces of young pigs with diarrhea, and subsequently demonstrated to induce diarrhea in pigs [1]. Retrospectively, this virus was determined to be the cause of an enteric disease in feeder/fattening pigs that was first described in England in 1971, and characterized by severe watery diarrhea with low mortality [2]. Although endemic PEDV infections have persisted in Europe until the present, the economic impact of the virus is considered to be minor [3]. PEDV was first detected in Asia in 1982 when the virus was isolated in Japan [4]. Within a few years it was recognized in other Southeast Asian countries. In contrast to Europe, the clinical impact of PEDV in Asia was much higher leading to the commercialization of both killed and attenuated vaccines in the late 1990s [5]. Vaccine use may have led to a reduction in prevalence of the disease; however, in 2010 severe PEDV outbreaks with high morbidity and mortality in suckling piglets were reported in China and were subsequently attributed to vaccine failure against new viral PEDV strains [5-7].

PEDV is a member of the *Coronaviridae* family and is an enveloped, single-stranded, positive-sense RNA virus with a 28 kb genome encoding non-structural proteins and four major structural proteins including spike, envelope, membrane, and nucleocapsid proteins [8]. The main method of PEDV transmission is fecal-oral; however the ability of the virus to aerosolize and be transported over large distances by air is being considered as an additional important route of virus transmission [9].

PEDV was first identified in the United States in April 2013 in sporadic outbreaks of severe diarrhea in young piglets with high mortality [10]. Within one year the disease spread to 31 states and associated with a 5-7% loss in pig production nationwide [11]. The first isolates identified in the United States had over 99% nucleotide identity to a Chinese isolate from the Anhui

* Correspondence: Kelly.lager@ars.usda.gov
[1]National Animal Disease Center, United States Department of Agriculture-Agricultural Research Services, Ames, IA, USA
Full list of author information is available at the end of the article

province suggesting a Chinese origin of infection, but the primary mode of entry into the United States is still under investigation [12,13]. In January 2014, a variant strain of PEDV with genetic evidence of a Chinese origin was identified in the U.S [14]. Although there is physical evidence for contaminated feed as a mode of transmission in a series of Canadian PEDV cases, such evidence does not exist for the initial introduction of PEDV in North America [15]. Swine are susceptible to PEDV infection at all stages of production with mild diarrhea and vomiting in adults, and severe diarrhea in neonatal pigs causing up to 100% mortality in this age group [3].

Although the clinical disease during an acute outbreak in a breeding herd is well chronicled, little information is available on endemic PEDV infection. The goals of this study were to assess PEDV transmission among pigs, evaluate the duration of shedding of infectious virus, and demonstrate protective immunity of nursery-aged pigs.

Materials and methods

Experimental design

Twenty-three, 4-week-old barrows from a PEDV-negative commercial source in Iowa, USA, were randomly assigned a livestock ear tag with a unique number placed in the left ear (Allflex USA, Dallas, TX, USA). A summary of the experimental design and the animal movement can be found in Figure 1. All animals were housed at the National Animal Disease Center, USDA-ARS campus in accordance with Institutional Animal Care and Use Committee protocols (protocol ACUP 2707) following the *"Guide for the Care and Use of Agricultural Animals in Research and Teaching"*. One ABSL2 isolation barn was dedicated to housing non-exposed animals (Barn 1) until moved to isolation Barn 2 for PEDV exposure. On Day (D) 0, a pig was selected from Barn 1 and placed into a room in Barn 2 at which time it was inoculated orally with PEDV and was designated as the "seeder" pig.

On D1 and 2, 1 and 12 naïve contacts, respectively, were commingled with the seeder pig. On D7, 9 pigs were randomly selected from the 13 contact pigs and moved into a new isolation room to serve as the principal virus reservoir group (PG). The seeder pig and 4 remaining contact pigs were designated as the Stationary Virus group (SG) and remained in the same room in Barn 2 throughout the duration of the study. On D7, one naïve sentinel age-matched pig (S1) was commingled with the PG. Seventy-two hours post-contact (D10), S1 was moved to a separate isolation room until necropsy. On D14 the PG pigs were moved into a clean isolation room and pig S2 was commingled until D17 at which time S2 was moved into a clean isolation room until necropsy. This process was repeated on D21 and 28 with pigs S3 and S4. On D49, the five remaining naïve age-matched sentinels (N) in Barn 1 were moved to a clean room in Barn 2. The N and PG were all challenged with PEDV virus and designated as N/C and PG/C, respectively. On D30 (21-days-post contact with PG), S1 was humanely euthanized and necropsied. All other pigs (SG, PG/C, N/C, and S2, S3, S4 pigs) were euthanized on D78. Gross examination was performed on all organ systems and blood was collected for serum.

Disinfection and maintenance of rooms

Rooms were cleaned daily by removing organic matter with tap water using a high-pressure hose. To prevent cross contamination between groups, room-specific boots, coveralls, and latex gloves were required for each room.

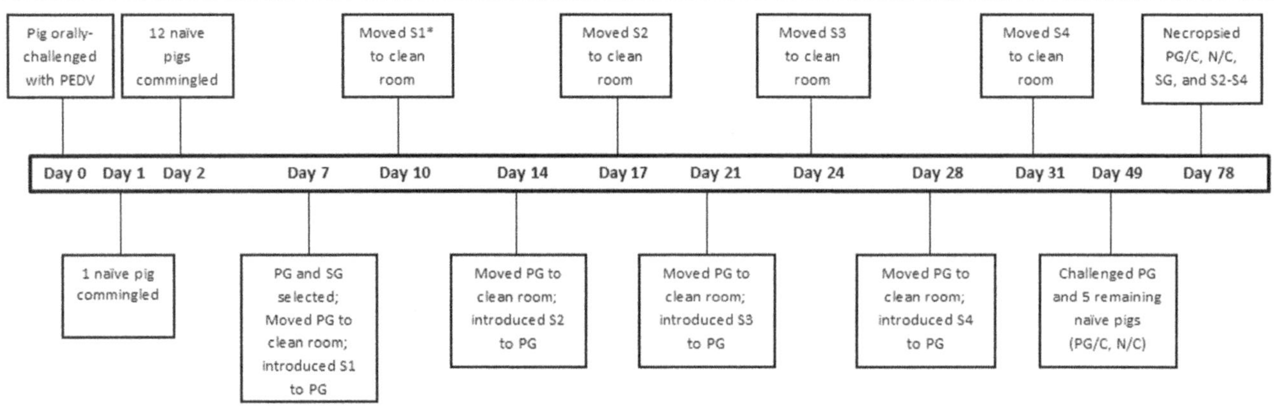

Figure 1 Experimental timeline of events. Experiment timeline from study initiation (Day 0) to termination (Day 78). On Day 0, the seeder pig was orally challenged with PEDV. On Days 1 and 2, 1 and 12 contact pigs, respectively were placed with the seeder pig. On Day 7, the Principle Group (PG) consisting of 9 contact pigs, and the Stationary Group (SG) consisting of 4 contact pigs and the seeder pig were selected. On Days 7, 14, 21, and 28, pigs S1, S2, S3, and S4, were commingled with the PG, respectively. On Days 10, 17, 24, and 31, the respective sentinel pig was removed and placed in a separate room. S1 was euthanized and necropsied on Day 30. All other study animals were euthanized and necropsied on Day 78. At Day 49 naïve pigs (N) and PG received PEDV challenge (PG/C: principal virus reservoir group post-challenge. N/C: naïve pigs post-challenge).

Due to animal movement requirements, several rooms in Barn 2 were used multiple times throughout the study; after each group or pig relocation, each room was cleaned and disinfected with a commercial multi-purpose disinfectant (Virkon® S, DuPont, Neogen, Lexington, KY, USA) following this protocol. Pigs and all disposable items were removed from the isolation room leaving an essentially bare concrete room with minimal corners, crevices, etc. If decking or penning was in the room, these items were disassembled as much as possible to allow powerwashing of all surfaces. The room was cleaned with low and high pressure water followed by a soaking with a disinfectant foam. The room was allowed to dry overnight. The second day the air filters were changed and the room was washed and soaked again with disinfectant foam followed by drying overnight. On the following day the room is considered acceptable for pig use. Movement between rooms was in the following order, SG, PG, S1, S2, S3, S4, and after challenge, SG, S2, S3, S4, PG/C and N/C. After moving through each room in sequence, a complete body shower was taken before exiting the barn. No respiratory masks were worn between rooms.

Clinical observations

All pigs were observed daily for general changes in health including diarrhea, rough hair coat, inappetence, and lethargy.

Sample collection

Rectal swabs were collected daily from all pigs in Barn 2 using a sterile polyester-tipped applicator (Puritan Medical Products, Guilford, ME) immersed in a 5 mL polystyrene round-bottom tube (BD Falcon, Franklin Lakes, NJ, USA) filled with 2 mL of minimal essential media (MEM). A summary of daily rectal swab collections by group can be found in Tables 1 and 2. The fecal swab samples were frozen at −80 °C until use. Blood was collected from all pigs in Barn 2 on D5, 7, 14, 21, 28, 35, 42, 49, 56, 63, 70, and 77 via jugular venipuncture using a 10 mL syringe with an 18 g X 1 ½" needle (BD Falcon, Franklin Lakes, NJ, USA) then transferred into an 8.5 mL plastic serum separator tube (BD Vacutainer®, 8.5 mL draw; Becton and Dickinson Company, Franklin Lakes, NJ). Blood was centrifuged at 1000 × *g* for 10 min. Following centrifugation, the serum portion of the blood was poured off into 2 mL cryogenic vials (Corning, Corning, NY) and stored at −80 °C until future use.

Inoculum

The PEDV isolate, US/Colorado/2013 (CO-13 PEDV) was supplied by the National Veterinary Services Laboratory, USDA-APHIS, Ames, Iowa (Lot 025 PDV 1303). The virus was propagated on African green monkey kidney (Vero) cells (ATCC, CCL-81) as follows. Vero cells were maintained in MEM supplemented with 10% fetal bovine serum as previously described [16]. Confluent monolayers were infected by decanting the MEM/serum media from a 25 cm^2 cell culture flask (BD Falcon, Franklin Lakes, NJ, USA), and washing three times with serum-free MEM and 2.5 μg/mL tosyl phenylalanyl chloromethyl ketone (TPCK) trypsin. Cells were inoculated with virus at an MOI of 0.1 in MEM-TPCK and incubated at 38.7 °C. Once cytopathic effect was evident on the cell monolayer, the flask was frozen and thawed twice, decanted into a 15 mL conical centrifuge tube (BD Falcon, Franklin Lakes, NJ, USA) and centrifuged at 1000 × *g* for 10 min. The supernatant was removed, aliquoted, and stored at −80 °C and used for inoculating the seeder pig (CO-13 PEDV stock #1; $1 \times 10^{5.8}$ $CCID_{50}$/mL). A larger stock of virus was prepared in a similar fashion and used to inoculate N/C and PG/C pigs at D49 (CO-13 PEDV stock #2; $1 \times 10^{6.0}$ $CCID_{50}$/mL).

Pigs were physically restrained and the virus inoculum was given orally using a 10 mL syringe (BD Falcon, Franklin Lakes, NJ, USA). The seeder pig was inoculated with a 6 mL volume of stock #1 virus at D0 providing an estimated challenge of $1 \times 10^{6.6}$ $CCID_{50}$ virus. At D49 the N/C and PG/C pigs were given a similar challenge (4 mL volume of stock #2 virus). Aliquots of each challenge virus were frozen at −80 °C for subsequent back-titration which revealed a titer of $1 \times 10^{5.3}$ $CCID_{50}$/mL and $1 \times 10^{4.5}$ $CCID_{50}$/mL for stock virus #1 and #2, respectively.

RNA extraction and real-time PCR

Each rectal swab sample was thawed and vortexed for 10 s and allowed to sit for 2–5 min to facilitate settling of the fecal debris. Approximately 200 μL of the sample was added to 500 μL of Lysis Binding Solution and mixed using the Thermomixer™ C (Eppendorf, AG, Hamburg, Germany) at 1400 rpm for 5 min at room temperature. The sample was then centrifuged at 13 000 × *g* for 3 min. Clarified lysates were obtained and nucleic acid extractions were performed using the MagMax Pathogen RNA/DNA kit (Life Technologies, Carlsbad, CA, USA) according to the manufacturer's protocol AM1836-feces (Life Technologies, Carlsbad, CA, USA). The extraction was carried out on the MagMax Express 24 (Life Technologies, Carlsbad, CA, USA). Following extraction, 5 μL of the nucleic acid templates were added to 20 μL of the Ambion® Path ID Multiplex One-Step RT-PCR reaction master mix (Life Technologies, Carlsbad, CA, USA). The PEDV N and S-gene real time RT-PCR reactions were based on recommendation by the University of Minnesota Veterinary Diagnostic Laboratory [17] and were ran in standard mode on a 7500 Fast Real-Time PCR System (Life Technologies, Carlsbad, CA, USA). The thermal cycler protocol started with 10 min at 45 °C, followed by 10 min at 95 °C. The final cycle consisted of 15 s at 95 °C

Table 1 Fecal swab PCR results for Stationary Group, Principal Group, and Sentinels from Day 2-42*

	2	3	4	5	6	7	8	9	10	11	12	13	14	15	16	17	18	19	20	21	22	23	24	25	26	27	28	29	30	31	32	33	34	35	40	41	42
SG-1	+	+	+	+	+	+	+	+	+	+	+	+	+	+	-	-	-	-	+	-	-	+	+	+	+	-	+	-	+	+	+	+	+	+	-	+	+
SG-2	+	+	+	+	+	+	+	+	+	+	+	-	-	+	-	-	-	-	-	-	-	-	-	-	-	-	-	-	-	-	-	-	+	-	-	-	-
SG-3	-	+	+	+	+	+	+	+	+	+	+	+	+	+	+	-	+	+	+	+	+	+	+	+	-	-	-	-	-	-	-	-	+	-	+	-	-
SG-4	-	+	+	+	+	+	+	+	+	+	+	+	+	+	+	-	-	-	-	-	-	-	-	-	-	-	-	-	-	-	-	-	+	-	-	-	-
SG-5	-	+	+	+	+	+	+	+	+	+	+	+	-	-	-	-	-	-	+	-	-	-	-	-	+	-	-	-	-	-	-	-	+	-	-	-	-
PG-1	-	+	+	+	+	+	+	+	+	+	+	+	+	+	+	+	-	+	+	+	+	+	+	+	-	-	-	-	-	-	-	-	-	-	-	-	-
PG-2	-	+	+	+	+	+	+	+	+	+	+	-	+	+	+	+	+	-	-	-	-	-	-	-	-	-	-	-	-	-	-	-	-	-	-	-	-
PG-3	-	+	+	+	+	+	+	+	+	+	+	+	+	+	+	+	+	+	+	+	+	+	+	+	+	+	-	-	-	-	-	-	-	-	-	-	-
PG-4	-	+	+	+	+	+	+	+	+	+	+	+	+	+	+	+	-	-	-	-	-	-	-	-	-	-	-	-	-	-	-	-	-	-	-	-	-
PG-5	-	+	+	+	+	+	+	+	+	+	+	+	+	+	+	+	-	-	+	-	-	-	-	-	-	-	-	-	-	-	-	-	-	+	-	-	-
PG-6	-	+	+	+	+	+	+	+	+	+	+	+	+	+	+	+	-	-	-	-	-	-	-	-	-	-	-	-	-	-	-	-	-	-	-	-	-
PG-7	-	+	+	+	+	+	+	+	+	+	+	+	+	+	+	+	+	+	+	+	+	-	-	-	-	-	+	+	+	-	-	-	-	-	-	+	+
PG-8	-	+	+	+	+	+	+	+	+	+	+	+	-	-	+	+	-	+	+	+	+	+	-	-	-	-	-	-	-	-	-	-	-	-	-	-	-
PG-9	-	+	+	+	+	+	+	+	+	+	+	+	-	-	+	+	+	+	+	-	-	-	-	-	-	-	-	-	-	-	-	-	-	-	-	-	-
S1						-	+	+	+	+	+	+	+	+	+	+	+	+	+	+	+	+	+	+	+	+	+	+	-								
S2													-	+	+	+	+	+	+	+	+	+	+	+	+	-	-	-	-	+	+	+	+	-	-	-	+
S3																				-	-	-	-	-	-	-	-	-	-	-	-	-	-	-	-	-	-
S4																											-	-	-	-	-	-	-	-	-	-	-

Table 2 Fecal swab PCR results for Stationary Group, Principal Group, Sentinels, and Naïve/Challenged group From Day 47–77**

	47	48	49	50	51	52	53	54	55	56	57	58	59	60	61	62	63	64	65	66	67	68	69	70	71	72	73	74	75	76	77
SG-1	-	-	-	-	-	-	-	-	-	-	-	-	-	-	-	-	-														
SG-2	-	-	-	-	-	-	-	-	-	-	-	-	-	-	-	-	-														
SG-3	-	-	-	-	-	-	-	-	-	-	-	-	-	-	-	-	-														
SG-4	-	-	-	-	-	-	-	-	-	-	-	-	-	-	-	-	-														
SG-5	-	-	-	-	-	-	-	-	-	-	-	-	-	-	-	-	-														
PG-1	-	-	-	-	-	-	-	-	-	-	-	-	-	-	-	-	-														
PG-2	-	-	-	-	-	-	-	-	-	-	-	-	-	-	-	-	-														
PG-3	-	-	-	-	-	-	-	-	-	-	-	-	-	-	-	-	-														
PG-4	-	-	-	-	-	-	-	-	-	-	-	-	-	-	-	-	-														
PG-5	-	-	-	-	-	-	-	-	-	-	-	-	-	-	-	-	-														
PG-6	-	-	-	-	-	-	-	-	-	-	-	-	-	-	-	-	-														
PG-7	-	-	-	-	-	-	-	-	-	-	-	-	-	-	-	-	-														
PG-8	-	-	-	-	-	-	-	-	-	-	-	-	-	-	-	-	-														
PG-9	-	-	-	-	-	-	-	-	-	-	-	-	-	-	-	-	-														
S2	-	-	-	+	-	-	-	-	-	-	-	-	-	-	-	-	-														
S3	-	-	-	-	-	-	-	-	-	-	-	-	-	-	-	-	-														
S4	-	-	-	-	-	-	-	-	-	-	-	-	-	-	-	-	-														
N/C1	-	-	-	-	+	+	+	+	+	+	+	+	+	-	-	-	-	-	-	-	-	-	-	-	-	-	-	-	-	-	-
N/C2	-	-	-	-	+	+	+	+	+	+	+	+	+	+	+	+	-	-	-	-	-	-	-	-	-	-	-	-	-	-	-
N/C3	-	-	-	-	+	+	+	+	+	+	+	+	+	+	+	+	-	-	-	-	-	-	-	-	-	-	-	-	-	-	-
N/C4	-	-	-	-	+	+	+	+	+	+	+	+	+	+	+	+	-	-	-	-	-	-	-	-	-	-	-	-	-	-	-
N/C5	-	-	-	-	+	+	+	+	+	+	+	+	+	-	-	-	-	-	-	-	-	-	-	-	-	-	-	-	-	-	-

*On Day 0, the seeder pig (SG-1) was orally challenged with PEDV. On Days 1 and 2, 1 and 12 contact pigs, respectively were placed with the seeder pig. On Day 7, the Principal Group (PG) consisting of 9 contact pigs, and the Stationary Group (SG) consisting of 4 contact pigs and the seeder pig were selected. On Days 7, 14, 21, and 28, Sentinel pigs S1, S2, S3, and S4, were commingled with the PG, respectively. On Days 10, 17, 24, and 31, the respective sentinel pig was removed and placed in a separate room. S1 was euthanized and necropsied on Day 30. All other study animals were euthanized and necropsied on Day 78. Samples not collected D36-39. **PG and N/C pigs were orally challenged with CO-13 PEDV on D49. Cycle Threshold of ≤ 35 = positive result (+); Cycle Threshold of ≥ 36 = negative result (–), empty box = sample not collected.

and then 45 s at 60 °C. The final cycle was run for 40 cycles using the FAM detector for PEDV. Positive and negative controls were included on each run. A cycle threshold (Ct) of less than 35 cycles was considered a positive result.

PEDV Spike 1 protein ELISA

The ELISA test was performed using a previously published method [18]. Briefly, each well of a 96-well microtiter plate (Nalgene Nunc International, Penfield, NY) was coated with 0.44 ng of S1 protein, incubated overnight, and blocked with 1% bovine serum. The 1/100 diluted samples of serum in PBS with 10% goat serum were reacted at 37 °C for 30 min, washed, and incubated with 20 000-fold diluted peroxidase-conjugated goat anti-porcine IgG. Using tetramethylbenzidine-hydrogen peroxide as the substrate, the reaction was visualized for 10 min at room temperature and terminated with 2.5 M sulfuric acid prior to OD measurement at 450 nm. Positive, negative, and blank samples were tested in duplicate on each plate.

Results

Clinical assessment

A watery, grey diarrhea was noted in the seeder pig 48 hours-post-inoculation with the cell culture-derived challenge material and lasted for approximately 5 days. Approximately 48–72 hours post-exposure with the seeder pig, the contact pigs showed intermittent signs of mild-moderate diarrhea lasting for approximately 7 days. No other clinical signs of diarrhea were appreciated in the contact pigs throughout the remainder of the study. S1, S3, and S4 showed no signs of diarrhea, while S2 had diarrhea for approximately 1 day 24 hours-post-contact with the PG. Post-challenge, the N/C group showed clinical signs of mild diarrhea beginning approximately 48 hours-post-inoculation that lasted for approximately 5 days with intermittent diarrhea in a few pigs for 3 weeks post-challenge. In contrast, no clinical signs were noted in the PG/C pigs post-challenge. The rectal swab fluids were not tested for other enteric pathogens.

PEDV RNA detection

On D0 all fecal swabs were negative for PEDV RNA. The seeder pig (SG-1) and contact pigs were PCR positive within 24 hours of inoculation (seeder pig) or contact (13 contact pigs). PCR results for D2-42 fecal swabs are summarized in Table 1. The seeder pig was positive from D1-15, and then intermittently thereafter through D42. The 4 contact pigs that were combined with the seeder pig to form the SG group were all positive from D3-12 and then intermittently through D35. PEDV RNA was detected in all PG pigs from D3-11, and at least 1/9 PG pigs was PCR positive from D3-30. From D30-34, 0/9 PG pigs were PCR positive. Fecal swabs were not collected from the PG pigs from D36-39 but on D35 and 42, 1/9 PG pigs showed a positive result. Each sentinel pig was negative for PEDV RNA at the time of contact with PG. PEDV RNA was detected in pigs S1 and S2 within 1 day of contact with the PG. S1 was positive until necropsy at 21 days post contact. S2 was positive for 11 days post contact and then intermittently afterwards through D34 (20 days post contact). PEDV RNA was not detected in any sample obtained from pigs S3 (commingled with PG on D21) and S4 (commingled with PG on D28).

After re-challenge at D49, all PG/C pigs were PCR negative for the remainder of the study (Table 2). Within three days post challenge (D52), 5/5 N/C pigs were PCR positive and remained so until D59, while 3/5 remained positive until D62.

PEDV antibody detection

In the PG group, 2/9, 8/9, and 9/9 pigs were positive for PEDV-antibodies by D7, 14, and 21, respectively. In the N/C group, 2/5 pigs were ELISA positive by D56 (7 days post challenge) and all pigs were positive from D63 to D78. S1 and S2 seroconverted by 7 days post-contact and S3 and S4 remained seronegative throughout the remainder of the study. Average ELISA OD readings for the PG, SG, and N/C groups are depicted in Figure 2.

Discussion

The rapid dissemination of PEDV across the US in months demonstrated the vulnerability of a concentrated, interwoven swine production system to a highly transmissible novel enteric pathogen. This unprecedented spread was dependent on many factors including the duration and magnitude of virus shedding from infected to naïve pigs. The goal of this study was to better understand the role of pig-to-pig transmission in the US PEDV epidemic by developing a model to characterize the host response to infection with PEDV.

In 4-week-old contact pigs, mild-to-moderate diarrhea was observed for approximately one week post exposure to a PEDV experimentally-infected seeder pig. No other clinical disease was observed in the contact pigs. Within 24 hours-post-inoculation or post-exposure, all rectal swabs were PCR positive demonstrating the rapidity of transmission and the potential for pigs to shed infectious virus. In the pigs "naturally" infected by contact, 13/13 pigs were PCR positive for 9 days and most pigs were positive for 2-weeks-post exposure during which time one or more of the pigs shed an infectious dose of virus to pigs S1 and S2. Like the 13 naturally exposed pigs, S1 and S2 became PCR positive within 24 hours of contact, and seroconverted within 2 weeks post-exposure. The speed by which all pigs became PEDV RNA positive and the potential for pigs to shed infectious virus up to 2-weeks-post infection to age-matched pigs, suggests the basic reproduction number or R_0 should be high for this virus.

As would be expected for a virus with a high R_0 value, the transmissibility of the virus would be enhanced by

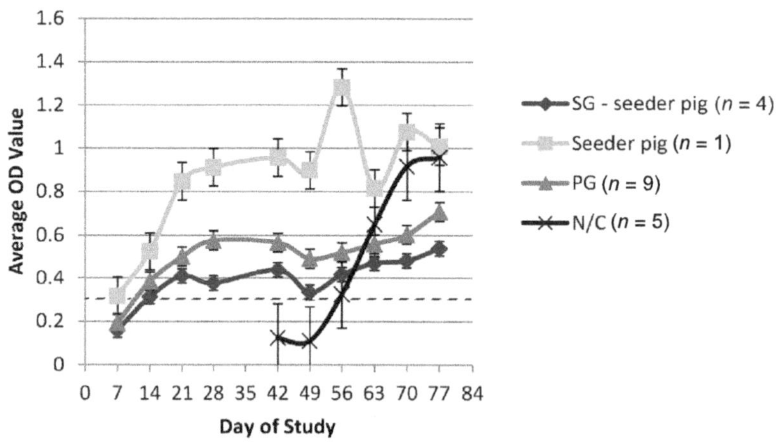

Figure 2 Average Optical Density (OD) of IgG antibody to PEDV. Average (OD) of IgG Antibody to PEDV over time in the Stationary Group without seeder pig included (SG - seeder), Seeder pig, Principal Group (PG), and Naïve/Challenge (N/C) group. On D 49, PG and N/C pigs orally challenged with PEDV strain USA/Colorado/2013. Dashed line represents cut-off optical density value of 0.3.

large numbers of naïve animals concentrated in small areas. In the case of PEDV, an enteric virus that can be shed in feces in large quantities, it is not a surprise that the virus would heavily contaminate transportation systems that would facilitate its spread throughout the US. Moreover, potential spread of the virus through contaminated feed and by air would allow this virus to circumvent most bio-security practices. Collectively, these factors combined to make a "perfect storm" for spread of PEDV in the US.

Based on negative PCR results and lack of specific antibody, pigs S3 and S4 were determined to have remained PEDV negative despite contact with PG pigs that were intermittently PCR positive. The negative status of S3 and S4 indicates the PG pigs did not shed infectious virus in sufficient quantity to infect age-matched pigs (aged 7 and 8 weeks, respectively). It is not known if younger, presumably more susceptible pigs might have become infected under similar conditions. Likewise, we do not know if the infectious character of the virus being shed changes with time, i.e., the rectal swabs are PCR positive but may not contain infectious virus. For this experiment, the PCR results were defined as positive or negative based on a Ct cutoff of 35, as recommended by the University of Minnesota Veterinary Diagnostic Laboratory. Whether or not this positive/negative cutoff correlates to infectious/non-infectious virus is not known.

Protective immunity to homologous challenge was observed in the PG pigs based on the absence of clinical disease following challenge, and the pigs remained PCR negative from D49 through 63. In contrast, following challenge at D49, the 11-week-old N/C pigs developed an intermittent mild diarrhea beginning 2–3 days post-challenge that lasted for several days. Within 48-hours post-challenge, 4/5 pigs were PEDV PCR positive and all 5 were positive from D52-59. The number of positive pigs reduced to 3/5 positive from D60-62.

Field reports describe age differences in clinical PEDV disease ranging from essentially 100% mortality in neonatal pigs to a moderate to mild diarrhea in older pigs and adults that may include vomiting. The minimal infectious dose, and the minimal lethal dose for different ages of swine are not known. Moreover, there could be considerable differences in the pathogenicity of different PEDV isolates, and innate resistance between genetic lines of swine. For the purposes of this paper, we chose to give a uniform dose to the younger (4 weeks-of-age) and older (11 weeks-of-age) pigs realizing that the older pigs might be less affected due to a relatively smaller dose, and the possibility that there may be inherent resistance to infection as pigs mature. Characterizing the relationship between age, challenge dose, and clinical disease is beyond the scope of this study. Although both age groups did become infected following challenge, back titrations of challenge virus suggests the younger pigs received a larger challenge dose than the older pigs (about 6 $\log_{10}$ vs. 5.1 $\log_{10}$) which limits any interpretation of the potential relationship between age, challenge dose and disease.

In this study, the 4-week-old pigs were more clinically affected when compared to 11-week-old pigs. None of the pigs in this study became clinically dehydrated or succumbed to the infection, and other than showing signs of diarrhea, it would have been difficult to discern any apparent illness if the pigs were housed on slatted floors. We presume this difference is mostly age-related as younger pigs are more susceptible to disease. However, the younger pigs became infected by contact with a seeder pig while the older pigs received a known oronasal challenge of cell culture propagated virus, and it is not known how these different routes of exposure might affect the pig. Although the study was not designed to compare the clinical effect of cell-culture propagated virus challenge vs. natural infection, it is interesting to compare the ELISA OD values for the one seeder and 5 N/C pigs that received an oronasal challenge to the 13 naturally infected pigs (Figure 2). The mean OD of the 6 inoculated pigs was higher than the naturally exposed pigs at each post-inoculation time point (7, 14, 21, and 28 days-post-inoculation). The importance of this trend and whether or not it would be reproducible in subsequent studies is not known. In addition, for the 13 contact pigs, the mean OD value was greater at each post-exposure time point for the PG group when compared to the 4 contact pigs in the SG group. This apparent trend could reflect exposure, albeit a short exposure, to "fresh" virus being shed by S1 and S2 when they were commingled with the PG for 3 days at D7 and 14, respectively. Perhaps this potential exposure affected the development of the humoral antibody response. Under the conditions of this study, an anamnestic humoral immune response was not observed following challenge of the 9 PG pigs. Lack of immunological memory was also observed in a report using the Belgian isolate, CV-777 [19]. Given that the N/C pigs replicated challenge virus and developed specific antibody, we are confident the PG pigs received an infectious homologous challenge and had no detectable replication of homologous challenge virus or rise in humoral antibody titer.

The infection of contact pigs exposed to the seeder pig, and the infection of S1 and S2 pigs demonstrated pig-to-pig transmission of infectious virus. In the case of the seeder and contact pigs, transmission happened quickly since all of the contact pigs were rectal swab positive within 24 h of contact to either the seeder pig, or the seeder pig and first contact pig. These results are similar to a recent report using a different US PEDV strain [20]. Similarly, S1 and S2 pigs were rectal swab positive within

24 h of contact with the PG group. Collectively, these results indicate pigs can rapidly become infected and shed infectious virus for at least 2 weeks. However, this study does not provide insight into the relationship between samples that are deemed positive by PCR and the presence of infectious virus in rectal swab fluids. In the case of the seeder pig infecting the 13 contact pigs, the seeder pig was positive from D1-15 and clearly shed infectious virus on D1 since the first contact pig was PCR positive by D2. Whether the 12 remaining contact pigs became infected by exposure to virus from the seeder pig or the first contact pig is unknown, but all were positive 24 h later on D3. All 9 PG pigs were PCR positive on D7 when S1 was commingled and at least one of these pigs shed infectious virus since S1 was PCR positive by the next day. When S2 was commingled on D14, 7/9 PG pigs were PCR positive and at least one was shedding infectious virus since S2 was positive on D15. At D21 and 28, 4 and 1 of 9 PG pigs were PCR positive, respectively, but none of the pigs shed an infectious dose based on lack of demonstrable infection in S3 and S4. The Negative/Positive status of the rectal swab was based on using the Ct value of 35; negative (>35) or positive (<35). This cutoff value was determined by the original designers at the University of Minnesota Veterinary Diagnostic Laboratory and is routinely used by other diagnostic laboratories performing either the original real-time PCR assay, or a modification of the assay (D. Madson, personal communication). Additional studies are warranted to understand the relationship between Ct value and the presence of infectious virus.

There is justifiable concern by the swine industry on how robust this virus is and what efforts are necessary to eliminate environmental contamination. In this study, there were movements of pigs into rooms that had previously housed PEDV-infected pigs. We did not conduct any environmental sampling of the rooms for PEDV contamination prior to use, thus we do not know what potential contamination might have existed in the room from preceding pigs. Each room was cleaned following the removal of previous pigs according to our standard protocol for cleaning the ABSL-2 isolation rooms. During the acute phase of the experiment it was not possible to assess if infectious virus may have been present in the room upon entry of the pigs because the pigs were already positive. Later in the experiment, we did not find evidence for pigs becoming infected upon movement into a room, i.e., S3 and S4 did not become infected when moved from the PG into separate isolation rooms. In addition, these rooms have been used subsequently for non-PEDV pig studies and no PEDV contamination was detected. Based on these experiences, we believe our routine cleaning protocol was adequate to inactivate PEDV contaminated surfaces.

In general, results from this study agree with recent observations by others that have experimentally infected 3- and 4-week-old pigs with US PEDV isolates resulting in the production of mild to moderate clinical disease [20]. Conversely, prior to this study, the longest duration of fecal shedding of PEDV was reported out to 24 days post-inoculation [20]. We detected intermittent viral shedding by PCR in several pigs up to D42 even though clinical signs diminished approximately 7 days post exposure. To our understanding, this is the longest length of PEDV shedding reported in pigs to date. Asymptomatic shedding of PEDV in pigs introduces a higher level of difficulty in the management of the disease throughout the swine industry.

In summary, this study and the work of others demonstrates how easily pigs become infected with PEDV, and may help explain the rapid transmission of virus recently observed in the US. In addition, pigs shed infectious virus for 2 weeks which would help explain how easily the virus was transmitted among farms. The apparent sterile immunity following primary infection suggests there may be value in a consistent feedback program, and it demonstrates potential for a vaccine to help manage the disease.

Competing interests
The authors declare that they have no competing interests.

Authors' contributions
KC and KL designed and performed the animal experiment and wrote the manuscript. RH, LM, TO, and PG contributed to the interpretation of results and helped draft the manuscript. All authors read and approved the final manuscript.

Acknowledgements
The authors would like to thank Sarah Anderson and Deborah Adolphson for their excellence in technical assistance. Mention of trade names or commercial products in this publication is solely for the purpose of providing specific information and does not imply recommendation or endorsement by the U.S. Department of Agriculture. USDA is an equal opportunity provider and employer.

Author details
[1]National Animal Disease Center, United States Department of Agriculture-Agricultural Research Services, Ames, IA, USA. [2]Veterinary Diagnostic and Production Animal Medicine, Iowa State University College of Veterinary Medicine, Ames, IA, USA. [3]The Roslin Institute, University of Edinburgh, Midlothian, UK. [4]Diagnostic Medicine/Pathobiology, College of Veterinary Medicine, Kansas State University, Manhattan, KS, USA.

References
1. Pensaert MB, De Bouck P (1978) A new coronavirus-like particle associated with diarrhea in swine. Arch Virol 58:243–247
2. Wood E (1977) An apparently new syndrome of porcine epidemic diarrhoea. Vet Rec 100:243–244
3. Saif L, Pensaert MB, Sestak K, Yeo SG, Jung K (2012) From Coronaviruses. In Disease of Swine. 10th edition. Edited by Zimmerman JJ, Karriker LA, Ramirez A, Schwartz KJ, Stevenson GW. Ames, Iowa, USA; Wiley-Blackwell. pp 501–524
4. Takahashi K, Okada K, Ohshima K (1983) An outbreak of swine diarrhea of a new-type associated with corona-virus like particles in Japan. Nihon Juigaku Zasshi 45:829–832
5. Wang XM, Niu BB, Yan H, Gao DS, Yang X, Chen L, Chang HT, Zhao J, Wang CQ (2013) Genetic properties of endemic Chinese porcine epidemic diarrhea virus strains isolated since 2010. Arch Virol 158:2487–2494

6. Sun RQ, Cai RJ, Chen YQ, Liang PS, Chen DK, Song CX (2012) Outbreak of porcine epidemic diarrhea in suckling piglets, China. Emerg Infect Dis 18:161–163
7. Li R, Qiao S, Yang Y, Su Y, Zhao P, Zhou E, Zhang G (2014) Phylogenetic analysis of porcine epidemic diarrhea virus (PEDV) field strains in central China based on the ORF3 gene and the main neutralization epitopes. Arch Virol 159:1057–1065
8. Song D, Park B (2012) Porcine epidemic diarrhoea virus: a comprehensive review of molecular epidemiology, diagnosis, and vaccines. Virus Genes 44:167–175
9. Alonso C, Goede DP, Morrison RB, Davies PR, Rovira A, Marthaler DG, Torremorell M (2014) Evidence of infectivity of airborne porcine epidemic diarrhea virus and detection of airborne viral RNA at long distances from infected herds. Vet Res 45:73
10. Stevenson GW, Hoang H, Schwartz KJ, Burrough ER, Sun D, Madson D, Cooper VL, Pillatzki A, Gauger P, Schmitt BJ, Koster LG, Killian ML, Yoon KJ (2013) Emergence of porcine epidemic diarrhea virus in the United States: clinical signs, lesions, and viral genomic sequences. J Vet Diagn Invest 25:649–654
11. Novel Swine Enteric Corona Virus Disease Testing Summary Report. [www.aasv.org/pedv/SECoV_weekly_report_140425.pdf]
12. Huang YW, Dickerman AW, Piñeyro P, Li L, Fang L, Kiehne R, Opriessnig T, Meng XJ (2013) Origin, evolution, and genotyping of emergent porcine epidemic diarrhea virus strains in the United States. MBio 4:e00737–e00813
13. Chen Q, Li G, Stasko J, Thomas JT, Stensland WR, Pillatzki AE, Gauger PC, Schwartz KJ, Madson D, Yoon KJ, Stevenson GW, Burrough ER, Harmon KM, Main RG, Zhang J (2014) Isolation and characterization of porcine epidemic diarrhea viruses associated with the 2013 disease outbreak among swine in the United States. J Clin Microbiol 52:234–243
14. Wang L, Byrum B, Zhang Y (2014) New variant of porcine epidemic diarrhea virus, United States, 2014. Emerg Infect Dis 20:917–919
15. Pasick J, Berhane Y, Ojkic D, Maxie G, Embury-Hyatt C, Swekla K, Handel K, Fairles J, Alexanderson S (2014) Investigation into the role of potentially contaminated feed as a source of the first-detected outbreaks of porcine epidemic diarrhea in Canada. Transbound Emerg Dis 61:387–410
16. Hoffman M, Wyler R (1988) Propagation of the virus of porcine epidemic diarrhea in cell culture. J Clin Microbiol 26:2235–2239
17. University of Minnesota Diagnostic Laboratory PEDV Rapid Diagnostic Test [http://www.cvm.umn.edu/sdec/prod/groups/cvm/@pub/@cvm/@sdec/documents/content/cvm_content_446628.pdf]
18. Gerber PF, Gong Q, Huang YW, Wang C, Holtkamp D, Opriessnig T (2014) Detection of antibodies against porcine epidemic diarrhea virus in serum and colostrum by indirect ELISA. Vet J 202:33–36
19. De Arriba ML, Carvajal A, Pozo J, Rubio P (2002) Mucosal and systemic isotype-specific antibody responses and protection in conventional pigs exposed to virulent or attenuated porcine epidemic diarrhoea virus. Vet Immunol Immunopathol 85:85–97
20. Madson D, Magstadt D, Arruda P, Hoang H, Sun D, Bower L, Bhandari M, Burrough E, Gauger P, Pillatzki A, Stevenson G, Wilberts B, Brodie J, Harmon K, Wang C, Main R, Zhang J, Yoon KJ (2014) Pathogenesis of porcine epidemic diarrhea virus isolate (US/Iowa/18984/2013) in 3-week-old weaned pigs. Vet Microbiol 174:60–68

Magnitude and kinetics of multifunctional CD4$^+$ and CD8β$^+$ T cells in pigs infected with swine influenza A virus

Stephanie C Talker[1†], Hanna C Koinig[1,2†], Maria Stadler[1], Robert Graage[2,5], Eva Klingler[2], Andrea Ladinig[2], Kerstin H Mair[1], Sabine E Hammer[1], Herbert Weissenböck[3], Ralf Dürrwald[4], Mathias Ritzmann[2,6], Armin Saalmüller[1] and Wilhelm Gerner[1*]

Abstract

Although swine are natural hosts for influenza A viruses, the porcine T-cell response to swine influenza A virus (FLUAVsw) infection has been poorly characterized so far. We have studied Ki-67 expression and FLUAVsw-specific production of IFN-γ, TNF-α and IL-2 in CD4$^+$ and CD8β$^+$ T cells isolated from piglets that had been intratracheally infected with a H1N2 FLUAVsw isolate. IFN-γ$^+$TNF-α$^+$IL-2$^+$ multifunctional CD4$^+$ T cells were present in the blood of all infected animals at one or two weeks after primary infection and their frequency increased in four out of six animals after homologous secondary infection. These cells produced higher amounts of IFN-γ, TNF-α and IL-2 than did CD4$^+$ T cells that only produced a single cytokine. The vast majority of cytokine-producing CD4$^+$ T cells expressed CD8α, a marker associated with activation and memory formation in porcine CD4$^+$ T cells. Analysis of CD27 expression suggested that FLUAVsw-specific CD4$^+$ T cells included both central memory and effector memory populations. Three out of six animals showed a strong increase of Ki-67$^+$perforin$^+$ CD8β$^+$ T cells in blood one week post infection. Blood-derived FLUAVsw-specific CD8β$^+$ T cells could be identified after an in vitro expansion phase and were multifunctional in terms of CD107a expression and co-production of IFN-γ and TNF-α. These data show that multifunctional T cells are generated in response to FLUAVsw infection of pigs, supporting the idea that T cells contribute to the efficient control of infection.

Introduction

Pigs are natural hosts for influenza A viruses and infections of humans with swine influenza A viruses (FLUAVsw) have been reported [1]. Moreover, the pig is considered as a "mixing vessel" i.e. a species where reassortments between avian and mammalian influenza virus strains can occur which may lead to the emergence of novel pandemic strains in humans. For example, in the 2009 pandemic H1N1 virus, genes closely related to swine North American and Eurasian H1N1 viruses were identified [2]. The 2009 pandemic H1N1 virus was frequently transmitted from farmers to pigs during the last years, thereby reflecting the zoonotic potential of this virus. As a consequence, this transmission established a new lineage of pandemic viruses (pandemic H1N2) in pigs via reassortment with circulating swine influenza viruses [3].

These observations, but also economic and animal welfare issues of FLUAVsw infections in pig production units, justify investigations on pig-FLUAVsw host-pathogen interactions. Of note, FLUAVsw infections are usually rapidly controlled by the porcine immune system and an elimination of replicating virus from the respiratory tract within one week has been reported [4]. Neutralizing antibodies appear in serum within seven days post inoculation [4]. It is assumed that these antibodies play a major role in control of infection, although a production of IgA antibodies by B cells in the nasal mucosa has also been reported [5].

The rapid control of FLUAVsw infections suggests that also cell-mediated immune responses contribute to viral

* Correspondence: wilhelm.gerner@vetmeduni.ac.at
†Equal contributors
[1]Institute of Immunology, Department of Pathobiology, University of Veterinary Medicine, Vienna, Austria
Full list of author information is available at the end of the article

clearance. However, while abundant knowledge exists on the role of influenza virus-specific $CD4^+$ and $CD8^+$ T cells in mice and humans [6], their role has not been studied in great detail in pigs. A FLUAVsw-specific proliferation of lymphocytes isolated from blood has been reported following infection of pigs with H3N2 and H1N1 FLUAVsw strains [7-9]. One study demonstrated the proliferation of blood-derived $CD4^+$ and $CD8^+$ T cells following vaccination with a human pandemic H1N1 vaccine [10]. Also, the presence of H1N1-specific IFN-γ producing T cells in tracheobronchial lymph nodes, spleen and nasal mucosa has been described [5]. More recently, increased frequencies of cytolytic T cells (CTLs), $CD4^+CD8\alpha^+$ T cells and regulatory T cells have been reported in lung tissue and bronchoalveolar lavage fluid of H1N1-infected pigs six days post infection [11].

However, none of these studies investigated the phenotype and functional properties of FLUAVsw-specific T cells in detail. Taking into account the rapid clearance of FLUAVsw infections, we hypothesized that highly differentiated $CD4^+$ and $CD8\beta^+$ T cells with multiple effector functions are involved in protective immune responses. Accordingly, we performed a detailed phenotypic and functional analysis of FLUAVsw-specific T cells occurring in blood of pigs experimentally infected with a FLUAVsw H1N2 isolate.

Materials and methods

Animals and virus

Nine three-week-old crossbred piglets ([Landrace × Large White] × Pietrain) were derived from a conventional breeding farm in Lower Austria and were kept in a biosafety level 2 facility at the University of Veterinary Medicine Vienna. Sows at the farm were free of FLUAVsw-specific antibodies. This was tested by a commercial ELISA (Ingezim Influenza A, 1.0.FLU.K3, Ingenasa, Madrid, Spain) at regular intervals. All piglets were vaccinated against *Mycoplasma hyopneumoniae* (MycoFLEX®, Boehringer Ingelheim, Ingelheim, Germany) and against porcine circovirus type 2 (CircoFLEX®, Boehringer Ingelheim) at three weeks of age. After arrival, the piglets were divided into a control group (three animals) and an infection group (six animals). Seronegativity for antibodies against Influenza A was confirmed by the Ingezim Influenza A, 1.0.FLU.K3 ELISA (Ingenasa) one day before FLUAVsw infection (four weeks of age). Piglets were infected twice at an interval of four weeks. Each time, 10 mL of virus suspension containing the FLUAVsw isolate A/swine/Kitzen/IDT6142/2007 (H1N2) with $10^{7.25}$ $TCID_{50}$/mL was administered intratracheally by the use of a laryngoscope to anesthetized piglets (Narketan®: Ketaminhydrochlorid 10 mg/kg body weight (BW), Vetoquinol, Lure, France; Stresnil®: Azaperon 1.2 mg/kg BW, Janssen Pharmaceutical, Beerse, Belgium). Control animals underwent the same procedure, but received phosphate buffered saline (PBS) instead. Daily, clinical examinations were carried out and recorded in a clinical score. Additionally, rectal temperature and body weight were measured daily and weekly, respectively. Euthanasia of pigs was performed either two or five weeks following the second infection. Piglets were anesthetized (Narketan®, Stresnil®), before T61® (T61®: Embutramid, Mebezoniumiodid, Tetracainhydrochlorid, 1 mL/10 kg BW, MSD, Whitehouse Station, NJ, USA) was administered. At necropsy, gross lung lesions were documented and samples from all seven lung lobes were fixed in 10% neutral buffered formalin. The samples were processed for 3 μm thick paraffin sections and stained with hematoxylin and eosin. The slides were examined for presence and quantity of the following parameters: (1) septal infiltration with mononuclear cells, (2) lobular atelectasis and interstitial fibrosis with metaplasia of alveolar epithelium, (3) interstitial formation of lymphoid follicles and/or bronchus-associated lymphoid tissue (BALT) hyperplasia.

The animal experiment was approved by the institutional ethics committee, the Advisory Committee for Animal Experiments (§12 of Law for Animal Experiments, Tierversuchsgesetz – TVG) and the Federal Ministry for Science and Research (reference number BMWF-68.205/0180-II/3b/2011).

FLUAVsw/Kitzen/IDT6142/2007 (H1N2) was originally isolated from an influenza outbreak in a pig herd in Saxony, Germany. It was isolated on primary porcine thymus cells and thereafter passaged on embryonated hen eggs (three passages) and on MDBK cells. The forth passage on MDBK cells was used for the experiments. The virulence of this passage of this strain had been proved by intratracheal and aerosol infection trials in pigs at IDT Biologika GmbH during the development of a swine influenza vaccine (EMEA/V/C/153) prior to the experiments reported here. The strain is able to induce dyspnea and fever in pigs at infection doses of $10^{8.55}$ $TCID_{50}$ MDBK at intratracheal infection. The sequences of hemagglutinin and neuraminidase are available from NCBI GenBank, accession numbers GQ161145 and GQ161146, respectively. This virus belongs to the human-like H1N2 swine influenza A viruses (huH1N2) which contain the hemagglutinin of H1N1 influenza A viruses which circulated in the human population in the 1970s/1980s and the neuraminidase of swine human-like H3N2 influenza A viruses isolated in the UK in the early 1990s [12].

Sample collection and isolation of peripheral blood mononuclear cells (PBMCs)

Blood samples were taken weekly by puncturing the anterior *vena cava* or the jugular vein. Leukograms (total white blood cell counts and differentials) were generated by using the hematology system ADVIA2120i (Siemens Healthcare Diagnostics, Eschborn, Germany). Serum samples were frozen at −20 °C for subsequent detection of neutralizing antibodies. PBMCs were isolated from heparinized blood by density gradient centrifugation with lymphocyte separation medium (PAA Laboratories, Pasching, Austria) as described elsewhere [13]. Isolated PBMCs were either directly used for ex vivo multicolor flow cytometry (FCM) and IFN-γ ELISpot assays or were cryopreserved for later in vitro experiments.

Serum neutralization test

Neutralizing antibodies were analyzed via serum neutralization tests as previously described [12]. Briefly, a serial dilution of sera was prepared and mixed with one of four different virus strains: A/sw/Bakum/1832/2000 (huH1N2), A/sw/Haselünne/IDT2617/2003 (avH1N1), A/sw/Bakum/IDT1769/2003 (huH3N2) and A/Jena/VI5256/2009 (panH1N1). Each strain was adjusted to 100 $TCID_{50}$. After incubation for 1 h at 37 °C, the virus-incubated sera were added to MDBK cell monolayers in microtiterplates. The medium of MDBK cell cultures was supplemented with porcine trypsin (γ-irradiated, final concentration 4 BAEE units/mL medium; Sigma-Aldrich, Schnelldorf, Germany) at the time of infection and again after 24 h. After 48 h of incubation at 37 °C, cells were fixed with acetone and investigated by indirect immunofluorescence, followed by ND_{50} calculation.

Phenotypic analysis of PBMCs performed ex vivo

For phenotypic analysis of $CD4^+$ and $CD8\beta^+$ T cells, freshly isolated PBMCs were suspended in PBS (without Ca^{2+}/Mg^{2+}, PAA) and 10% (v/v) porcine plasma (in-house preparation) and adjusted to 1×10^6 cells per sample. Monoclonal antibodies (mAbs) and secondary reagents used for cell surface staining are listed in Table 1. For detection of intracellular perforin and Ki-67, cells were fixed and permeabilized by in-house prepared fixation and permeabilization buffers containing saponin, as described previously [14]. Staining was performed in 96-well microtiterplates and cells were incubated for 20 min at 4 °C in the fridge. Free binding sites of secondary antibodies were blocked with whole mouse IgG molecules (2 μg per sample, Jackson ImmunoResearch, West Grove, PA, USA) during an additional incubation step prior to fixation and permeabilization.

ELISpot assays for IFN-γ production

96-well MultiScreen IP plates (Millipore, Billerica, MA, USA) were coated with mouse anti-swine IFN-γ mAb (clone pIFN-γ, Mabtech, Nacka Strand, Sweden) overnight at 4 °C (100 μL/well; 10 μg/mL in PBS), washed with PBS and subsequently blocked with cell culture medium (RPMI 1640 with stable glutamine supplemented with 10% [v/v] fetal calf serum, 100 IU/mL penicillin and 0.1 mg/mL streptomycin, all from PAA) for one hour at 37 °C. Per well, 3×10^5 freshly isolated PBMCs were incubated with the FLUAVsw infection strain (multiplicity of infection, MOI 0.1) or mock for 24 h at 37 °C. Samples incubated in cell culture medium served as additional negative control. Thereafter, plates were washed and incubated with biotin-labeled mouse anti-IFN-γ mAbs (clone PAN, Mabtech, 100 μL/well; 0.5 μg/mL in PBS) for one hour at room temperature. This was followed by incubation with streptavidin-alkaline phosphatase (1:2000 in PBS supplemented with 0.01% Tween20 and 0.1% BSA, Roche, Mannheim, Germany) for one hour at room temperature and subsequent addition of 5-bromo-4-chloro-3-indolyl phosphate/nitro blue tetrazolium substrate (100 μL/well, Sigma-Aldrich) according to manufacturer's instructions. After intense washing and drying of plates, spots were analyzed with an AID ELISpot reader (AID, Straßberg, Germany).

Intracellular cytokine staining

For intracellular staining of IFN-γ, TNF-α and IL-2 in $CD4^+$ and $CD8\beta^+$ T cells, PBMCs were defrosted and rested at 37 °C for eight hours (5×10^5 cells per well in 150 μL cell culture medium). Thereafter, FLUAVsw (infection strain, MOI = 0.1) was added to microcultures and left overnight for 18 h at 37 °C in a total volume of 200 μL. During the last four hours, Brefeldin A (BD GolgiPlug™, BD Biosciences, San Jose, CA, USA) was present in microcultures at a final concentration of 1 μg/mL. Mock- and medium-incubated cultures served as controls. For subsequent FCM staining in microtiterplates, cells were washed in PBS (without Ca^{2+}/Mg^{2+}) containing 3% (v/v) fetal calf serum and incubated with antibodies and secondary reagents listed in Table 1. Free binding sites of secondary antibodies were blocked with whole mouse IgG molecules (details see above) and Near-IR LIVE/DEAD stain kit (Life Technologies, Carlsbad, CA, USA) was used according to manufacturer's instructions. For fixation and permeabilization of cells, BD Cytofix/Cytoperm and BD Perm/Wash (both BD Biosciences) were used according to manufacturer's instructions.

In vitro expansion and functional analysis of $CD8\beta^+$ T cells

Defrosted PBMCs were labeled with CellTrace™ Violet Cell Proliferation Kit (Life Technologies) as described elsewhere [15]. Per well, 5×10^5 violet-stained PBMCs were plated together with FLUAVsw (infection strain, MOI 0.1) and were incubated at 37 °C for five days. At the fifth day, cells were restimulated for a second time with FLUAVsw (MOI 0.1) for another 18 h. Four hours

Table 1 Antibody panels

Antigen	Clone	Isotype	Fluorochrome	Labeling strategy	Source of primary Ab
Ex vivo Ki-67/CD4⁺ T cells					
CD3	PPT3	IgG1	PE	secondary antibody[a]	in house
CD4	74-12-4	IgG2b	Alexa488	secondary antibody[b]	in house
CD8α	11/295/33	IgG2a	PE-Cy7	secondary antibody[c]	in house
CD27	b30c7	IgG1	Alexa647	directly conjugated[d]	in house
CD45RC	3a56	IgG1	PerCP-Cy5.5	directly conjugated[e]	in house
SLA-DR	MSA3	IgG2a	Qdot605	directly conjugated	in house[f]
Ki-67	B56	IgG1	V450	directly conjugated	BD Biosciences
Ex vivo Ki-67/CD8β⁺ T cells					
CD3	PPT3	IgG1	PE	secondary antibody[a]	in house
CD8β	PG164A	IgG2a	Alexa488	Zenon labeling kit[g]	VMRD
CD27	b30c7	IgG1	Alexa647	directly conjugated[d]	in house
SLA-DR	MSA3	IgG2a	Qdot605	directly conjugated	in house[f]
Perforin	δ-G9	IgG2b	PerCP-eFluor710	directly conjugated	eBioscience
Ki-67	B56	IgG1	V450	directly conjugated	BD Biosciences
Triple cytokine staining/CD4⁺ T cells					
CD4	74-12-4	IgG2b	Alexa488	secondary antibody[b]	in house
CD8α	11/295/33	IgG2a	PE-Cy7	secondary antibody[c]	in house
CD27	b30c7	IgG1	BV421	biotin-streptavidin[h]	in house
IFN-γ	P2G10	IgG1	PE	directly conjugated	BD Biosciences
TNF-α	MAb11	IgG1	BV605	directly conjugated	BioLegend
IL-2	A150D3F1	IgG2a	APC	directly conjugated[i]	Life Technologies
Triple cytokine staining/CD8β⁺ T cells					
CD3	BB23-8E6-8C8	IgG2a	PE-Cy7	directly conjugated	BD Biosciences
CD8β	PG164A	IgG2a	Alexa488	Zenon labeling kit[g]	VMRD
CD27	b30c7	IgG1	BV421	biotin-streptavidin[h]	in house
IFN-γ	P2G10	IgG1	PE	directly conjugated	BD Biosciences
TNF-α	MAb11	IgG1	BV605	directly conjugated	BioLegend
IL-2	A150D3F1	IgG2a	APC	directly conjugated[i]	Life Technologies
In vitro expanded CD8β⁺ T cells					
CD4	74-12-4	IgG2b	PerCP-Cy5.5	directly conjugated	BD Biosciences
CD8β	PG164A	IgG2a	Alexa488	secondary antibody[j]	VMRD
CD107a	4E9/11	IgG1	Alexa647	directly conjugated	AbD Serotec
Pan-γδ	PPT16	IgG2b	PE-Cy7	biotin-streptavidin[k]	in house
IFN-γ	P2G10	IgG1	PE	directly conjugated	BD Biosciences
TNF-α	MAb11	IgG1	BV605	directly conjugated	BioLegend

[a]Goat anti-Mouse IgG1-PE, Southern Biotech.
[b]Goat anti-Mouse IgG2b-Alexa488, Life Technologies.
[c]Goat anti-Mouse IgG2a-PE-Cy7, Southern Biotech.
[d]Alexa Fluor-647 Protein Labeling Kit, Life Technologies.
[e]Lightning-Link™ PerCP-Cy5.5 Tandem Conjugation Kit, Innova Biosciences.
[f]Custom conjugation by Life Technologies.
[g]IgG2a-Alexa488 Zenon labeling kit, Life Technologies.
[h]Streptavidin-BV421, BioLegend.
[i]Lightning-Link™ APC Conjugation Kit, Innova Biosciences.
[j]Goat anti-Mouse IgG2a-Alexa488, Life Technologies.
[k]Streptavidin-PE-Cy7, eBioscience.

prior to harvesting of cells, anti-CD107a mAb was added, together with Brefeldin A (GolgiPlug™, BD Biosciences; final concentration 1 μg/mL) and Monensin (GolgiStop™, BD Biosciences; final concentration 1 μg/mL). Cell surface labeling and intracellular cytokine staining was performed with reagents listed in Table 1, under the conditions described above.

FCM analysis

FCM measurements were performed using a FACSCanto™ II flow cytometer (BD Biosciences) equipped with three lasers (405, 488 and 633 nm) and a High Throughput Sampler. Compensation was calculated automatically with single-stain samples. For analysis of ex vivo Ki-67 expression, at least 1×10^5 lymphocytes were collected. Between 5×10^5 and 1×10^6 lymphocytes were recorded for detection of intracellular cytokines. Gating strategies for identification of lymphocytes, doublet discrimination and exclusion of dead cells are shown in Additional file 1. Data was processed by FACSDiva software (Version 6.1.3; BD Biosciences) or FlowJo software (Version 7.6.5; Tree Star, Ashland, OR, USA) and transferred to Microsoft Excel (Office 2010; Microsoft, Redmond, WA, USA) for further calculations and preparation of graphs.

Swine leukocyte antigen haplotyping

Pigs were genotyped for their swine leukocyte antigen (SLA) class I and II haplotypes by running low-resolution PCR screening assays (PCR-SSP) on PBMC-derived genomic DNA as previously described [16].

Results

Clinical signs and pathological findings following FLUAVsw infection

Typically, influenza infection of pigs leads to a rapid onset of respiratory signs accompanied by fever and lethargy. To verify successful influenza infection and to evaluate protection from reinfection, animals were monitored daily for clinical signs of disease, including inspection, lung auscultation and measurement of rectal temperature. A clinical score was used to specify quality and severity of the observed signs. PBS-treated control animals (animal #1 to #3) did not show any signs of illness throughout the entire study (Figure 1A, first column and data not shown). All infected animals showed lethargy, fever (>40 °C, Additional file 2) and respiratory signs, including nasal discharge, coughing, dyspnea and abnormal lung auscultation, starting one day post intratracheal administration of virus. Exemplary scores for dyspnea and lung auscultation of all infected animals (#4 to #9) are displayed in Figure 1A. Severity and quality of these lower respiratory tract signs were similar among individuals, with the exception of animal #7, showing severe dyspnea and pleural friction rub in lung auscultation for several days following infection. All animals recovered within 7 to 9 days and did neither show clinical signs nor fever after the second infection. At necropsy, six (#4, #6, #8) and nine (#5, #7, #9) weeks post primary infection, the lungs of animals #4, #7, #8 and #9 showed localized lobular atelectasis with fibrous retraction at the edges of the cranial and middle lobes. Enlarged bronchial or mediastinal lymph nodes were found in animals #5, #6, #7, #8 and #9. Animal #7 additionally showed severe adhesive pleuritis and pericarditis. Animals #5 and #6 were without macroscopic changes. Compared to control animals, histopathology revealed increased peribronchial and interstitial infiltration of mononuclear cells in animals #4, #5, #8 and #9. Retracted lobules showed atelectasis with interstitial fibrosis, metaplasia of alveolar epithelium as well as hyperplastic bronchiolar epithelium (Additional file 3). In animal #7, in addition to increased mononuclear interstitial infiltration and BALT hyperplasia, histopathology showed multifocal purulent bronchopneumonia.

H1N2-neutralizing antibodies

Neutralizing antibodies are considered as a hallmark for strain-specific immunity following influenza infection. We analyzed H1N2-neutralizing antibodies in sera of infected and non-infected animals on a weekly basis. As displayed in Figure 1B, neutralizing antibodies were present in all infected animals (#4 to #9) one week after primary infection. Slightly higher titers were measured two weeks after primary infection. A boost of neutralizing antibodies following the second infection could be observed in animals #5, #6, #8 and #9. In all animals, neutralizing antibodies were detectable until euthanasia, 6 and 9 weeks after primary infection. Control animals (#1 to #3) were negative for neutralizing antibodies against H1N2 and all animals were negative for neutralizing antibodies against selected H1N1, H3N2 and panH1N1 strains throughout the study (data not shown).

Ex vivo Ki-67 expression

Ki-67 expression analysis has been used in human immunological studies to detect and quantify the expansion phase of T cells responding to vaccination against smallpox [17], yellow fever [17,18], but also infection with hantavirus [19] and H1N1 influenza A virus [20]. Similarly, we hypothesized that infection of pigs with FLUAVsw may lead to increased frequencies of blood-derived Ki-67$^+$ T-cell subsets in the time course following infection. Weekly, freshly isolated PBMCs were stained for Ki-67 expression in combination with different T-cell lineage and differentiation markers and analyzed by FCM. Peripheral blood TCR-$\gamma\delta^+$ T cells,

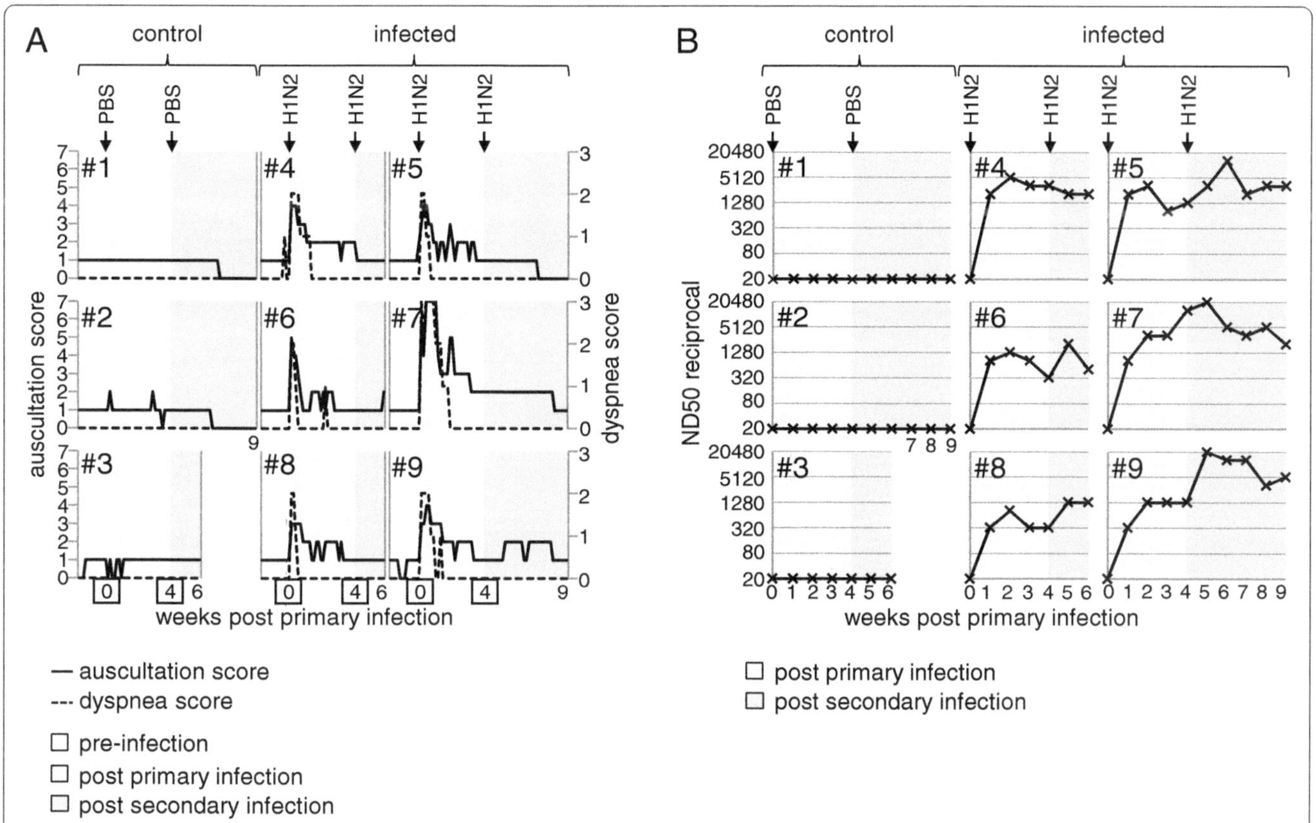

Figure 1 Clinical score and H1N2-neutralizing antibody titers. (A) From one week prior to the first infection until the end of the study either six or nine weeks post primary infection, piglets were daily monitored for clinical signs of disease. Auscultation score (solid line; 0 = physiologic, 1 = low-grade intensified vesicular, 2 = middle-grade intensified vesicular, 3 = high-grade intensified vesicular, 4 = bronchial, 5 = wheezing, 6 = rales, 7 = friction rub) and dyspnea score (dashed line; 0 = no dyspnea, 1 = dyspnea on exertion, 2 = dyspnea at rest, 3 = severe dyspnea) are shown for the three PBS-treated control animals (#1 to #3) and the six FLUAVsw-infected animals (#4 to #9). **(B)** Weekly collected serum samples were tested for H1N2-neutralizing antibodies by serum neutralization tests. Titers are expressed as the reciprocal neutralizing dose 50 (ND50). Data of PBS-treated (#1 to #3) and FLUAVsw-infected (#4 to #9) animals is shown in the time course following infections. (A and B) The background color in each diagram indicates different time spans: pre-infection (white), post primary infection (light grey) and post secondary infection (dark grey).

analyzed for CD2, CD8α, and CD27 expression, did not show any phenotypic changes or any increase in the absolute number of Ki-67 expressing cells following infection (data not shown). CD8β^{+} T cells, which represent porcine cytolytic T cells [21], were analyzed for the expression of perforin and CD27. By gating on CD27$^{dim/-}$perforin^{+} and CD27^{high}perforin^{-} Ki-67^{+}CD8β^{+} T cells, we distinguished perforin^{-} and perforin^{+} CD8β^{+} T cells (Figure 2A) and calculated absolute numbers in the time course following infection (Figure 2B). In three animals (#6, #8 and #9) we could detect a marked increase of Ki-67^{+}CD8β^{+} T cells one week after primary infection followed by a continuous decline in weeks 2 and 3. The expansion and contraction was mainly attributable to perforin^{+}Ki-67^{+}CD8β^{+} T cells. This might indicate an infection-related expansion of CD8β^{+} T cells in at least three (#6, #8 and #9) out of six animals. However, following the second infection, no increase of Ki-67^{+}CD8β^{+} T cells could be detected in these three animals, and only a slight increase was found in animals #4 and #7.

In parallel, we analyzed CD4^{+} T cells for FLUAVsw infection-related changes in Ki-67 expression. Expression of CD8α and CD27 were co-analyzed on Ki-67^{+}CD4^{+} T cells (Figure 2C). CD8α is expressed on activated and memory CD4^{+} T cells in swine [22,23] and down-regulation of CD27 has recently been described as a means to identify effector memory cells within porcine CD4^{+}CD8α^{+} T cells [24]. By respective gates, Ki-67^{+}CD4^{+} T cells were separated into naïve CD8α^{-} cells and antigen-experienced CD8α^{+} cells and, again, absolute numbers were calculated in the time course following infection (Figures 2C and D). In animals #6, #7 and #8, we observed a slight increase of Ki-67^{+}CD4^{+} T cells, one or two weeks after primary infection, with the majority of proliferating cells expressing the activation marker CD8α. Following the second infection, an increase of Ki-67^{+}CD4^{+} T cells could be detected in animals #4, #6 and #7. However, overall, no substantial increase, as seen for CD8β^{+} T cells in animals #6, #8 and #9, was found for the CD4^{+} T-cell population.

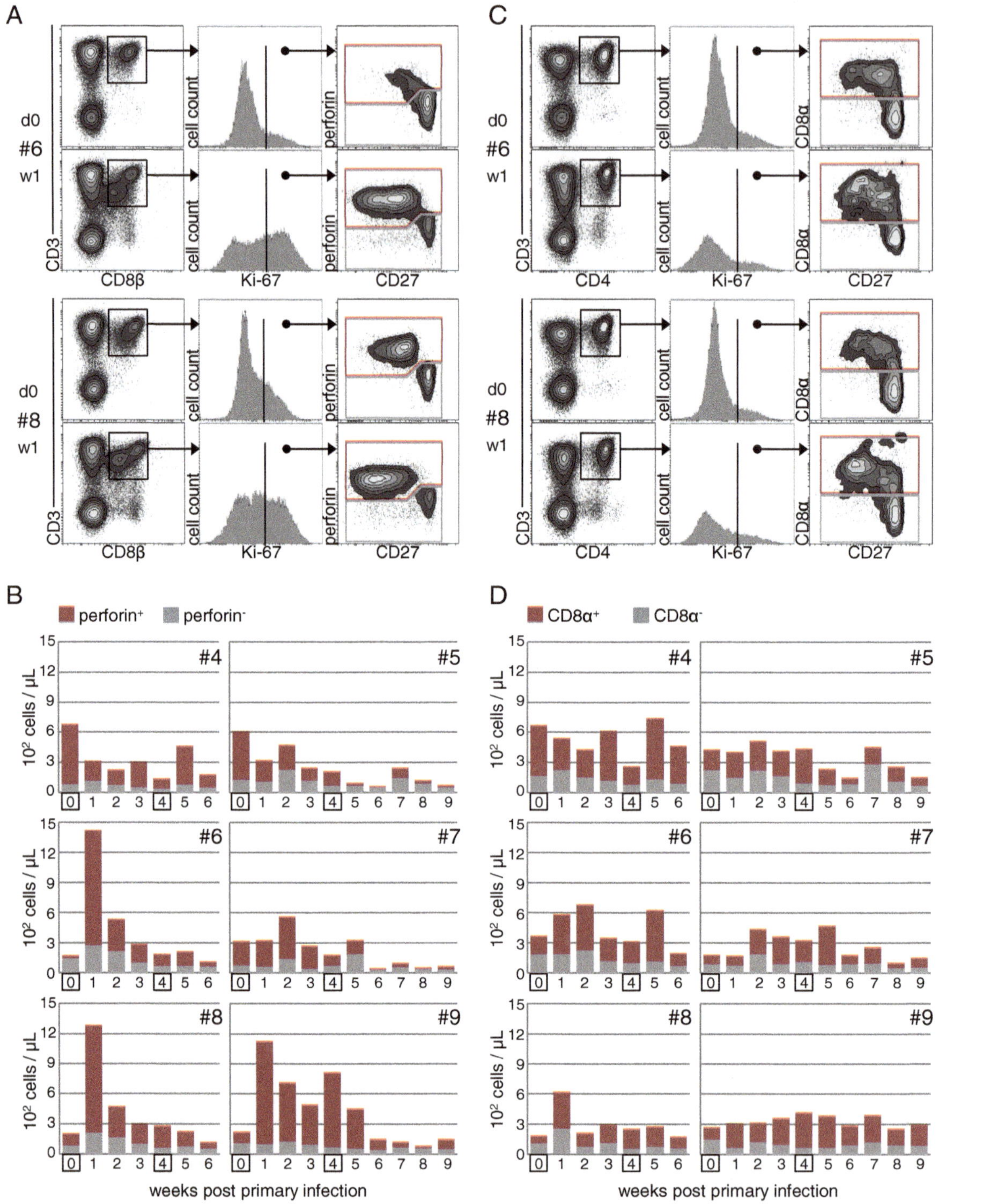

Figure 2 Kinetics of Ki-67$^+$CD8β$^+$ and Ki-67$^+$CD4$^+$ T cells in peripheral blood of FLUAVsw-infected pigs. Freshly isolated PBMCs were stained and analyzed for CD4, CD8α, CD8β, CD27, Ki-67 and perforin expression by FCM. **(A)** CD3$^+$CD8β$^+$ T cells were gated for Ki-67 expression and Ki-67$^+$ cells were further analyzed for expression of CD27 and perforin. Perforin$^+$ (red gate) and perforin$^-$ (grey gate) Ki-67$^+$CD3$^+$CD8β$^+$ T cells were further subgated for quantitative analysis over the time course following infection. **(C)** CD3$^+$CD4$^+$ T cells were gated for Ki-67 expression and Ki-67$^+$ cells were further analyzed for CD8α and CD27 expression. CD8α$^+$ (red gate) and CD8α$^-$ (grey gate) Ki-67$^+$CD3$^+$CD4$^+$ T cells were subgated for quantitative analysis over the time course following infection. **(A and C)** Exemplary raw data of animals #6 and #8, prior to infection and one week post infection, is shown. **(B and D)** Absolute numbers of Ki-67-expressing subsets within CD8β$^+$ T cells (B) and CD4$^+$ T cells (D) of six infected animals in the time course following infection. For calculation of absolute numbers, total lymphocyte counts were multiplied by percent values obtained by gating on the respective T-cell subpopulation.

IFN-γ ELISpot

Ex vivo Ki-67 expression kinetics of PBMCs pointed towards increased proliferative activity of T cells following FLUAVsw infection, but the specificity of this response remains uncertain. As a first approach to identify FLUAVsw-specific lymphocyte responses within PBMCs, we measured IFN-γ production in ELISpot assays following in vitro restimulation with homologous virus. As displayed in Figure 3, background levels of around 40 IFN-γ producing cells per 3×10^5 PBMCs were found in microcultures stimulated with mock supernatants or cell culture medium at all investigated time points (dark grey and light grey lines). Similar levels were found in virus-stimulated microcultures with PBMCs from non-infected control animals. Within PBMCs of all six infected animals, FLUAVsw-specific IFN-γ-producing cells could be detected already one week after primary infection (Figure 3, red lines). The magnitude of the IFN-γ response differed between individuals, with animal #9 having up to four times as many IFN-γ producing cells per 3×10^5 PBMCs as compared with the other animals. This difference was especially pronounced in week 1 after primary infection and in week 5, when animal #9 showed a clear booster response following the second infection. Booster responses were also found in PBMCs of animals #6 and #8. For an immediate comparison of the IFN-γ response in ELISpot assays and the neutralizing antibody titers, the trajectory curves of Figure 1B have been plotted into Figure 3. Overall, some synchronicity between the frequency of IFN-γ producing cells and antibody titers could be observed (animals #4, #6, #8 and #9), although there were opposing courses at certain periods or time points.

IFN-γ, TNF-α and IL-2 production by CD4⁺ T cells

As IFN-γ ELISpots indicated the presence of FLUAVsw-specific lymphocytes within PBMCs of infected animals, the next step was to assign a phenotype to these responding cells. On top, we aimed to identify potential multifunctional FLUAVsw-specific T cells, as the simultaneous production of different cytokines or effector molecules on the single T-cell level is proposed to be a hallmark of protective immune responses [25]. Accordingly, we performed intracellular cytokine staining for IFN-γ, TNF-α and IL-2 in $CD4^+$ and $CD8\beta^+$ T cells

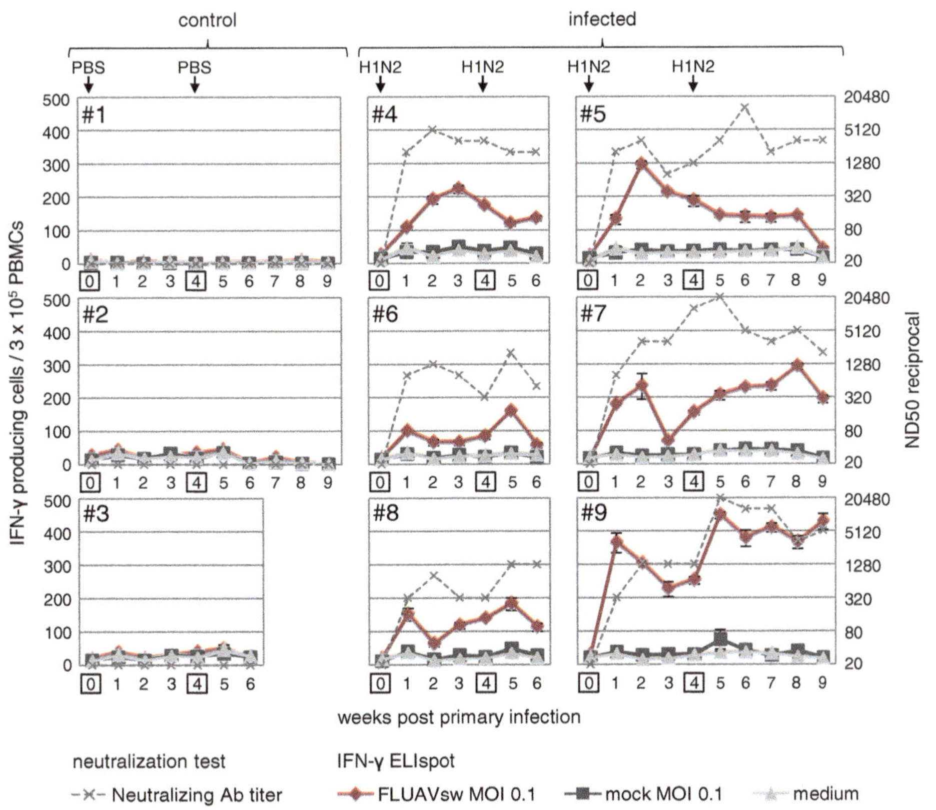

Figure 3 Kinetics of FLUAVsw-specific IFN-γ-producing T cells identified by ELISpot and H1N2-neutralizing antibody titers. For IFN-γ ELISpot, freshly isolated PBMCs were in vitro restimulated for 24 h with FLUAVsw (infection strain; MOI = 0.1). Mock- and medium-incubated cultures served as negative controls. Frequency of IFN-γ-producing cells within 3×10^5 PBMCs is displayed for FLUAVsw- (red line), mock- (dark grey line) and medium-incubated (light grey line) cultures. Neutralizing antibody titers are displayed in dashed grey lines according to the secondary y-axis (for details see caption of Figure 1B). Data of PBS-treated (#1 to #3) and FLUAVsw infected (#4 to #9) animals is shown in the time course following infections.

following FLUAVsw in vitro restimulation of PBMCs. As displayed in Figure 4A and Additional file 4, within $CD4^+$ T cells, double-cytokine-producing cells were virtually absent prior to infection, but could be identified from week 2 after primary infection onwards. Boolean gating was used to quantify single-, double- and triple-cytokine-producing $CD4^+$ T cells in the time course following infection, as displayed in Figure 4B. A detailed analysis of the frequency of $CD4^+$ T cells producing a particular single cytokine or cytokine combination is shown in Additional file 5. Overall, FLUAVsw-specific $cytokine^+CD4^+$ T cells were found to be increased from one (#7, #8) or two (all other animals) weeks after primary infection. Double- and triple-cytokine-producing cells started to be detectable at two weeks after primary infection. In animal #9, we observed a massive increase in the frequency of $cytokine^+$ $CD4^+$ T cells at one week post secondary infection (i.e. five weeks after primary infection). This increase was attributable mainly to IFN-γ single-producing and IFN-γ/TNF-α double-producing $CD4^+$ T cells (Additional file 5). Apart from animal #9, an increase of $cytokine^+CD4^+$ T cells following the second infection could be detected in animals #6, #7 and #8. Single-cytokine-producing $CD4^+$ T cells produced mainly IFN-γ or TNF-α. Double-cytokine-producing $CD4^+$ T cells predominantly produced IFN-γ in combination with TNF-α (Additional file 5).

Studies in humans and mice have shown that multiple-cytokine-producing T cells produce more cytokines on a per-cell basis compared to single-cytokine producers [26-28]. By comparing the median fluorescence intensity (MFI) obtained by FCM for the investigated cytokines (IFN-γ, TNF-α, IL-2) among single-, double- and triple-cytokine-producing $CD4^+$ T cells isolated from week 2 after primary infection onwards, we found higher quantities of IFN-γ and TNF-α in triple- and double-producers (Figures 5A and B and Additional file 6). IL-2 was slightly increased in triple-producers, compared with single- and double-producers. Overall, these findings might support the hypothesis that multiple-cytokine-producing FLUAVsw-specific T cells have a beneficial role in clearance of the infection.

Previous work of our group suggested that porcine $CD4^+CD8\alpha^+$ T cells can be differentiated upon their expression of CD27, with $CD27^+$ and $CD27^-$ cells resembling central memory (T_{CM}) and effector memory T helper cells (T_{EM}), respectively [24]. Therefore, we investigated the seven different cytokine-producing subsets identified by boolean gating for expression of CD8α and CD27. As shown in Figure 5C and Additional file 7, the vast majority of $cytokine^+CD4^+$ T cells expressed CD8α (with some notable exceptions of TNF-α and IL-2 single-producing cells), thereby displaying the phenotype of activated or antigen-experienced porcine $CD4^+$ T cells. However, within these $CD4^+CD8\alpha^+$ T cells, the CD27 expression profile did not allow for a clear assignment of responding cells to the $CD27^-$ T_{EM} or the $CD27^+$ T_{CM} subset, as all seven cytokine-producing subsets were distributed among both populations (Figure 5C and Additional file 7). In summary, these data indicate that $CD4^+$ T cells are involved in the immune response to influenza infection in pigs and that a considerable proportion of responding cells is multifunctional in terms of IFN-γ, TNF-α and IL-2 production.

Proliferation, degranulation and cytokine production by $CD8\beta^+$ T cells

Having observed typical clinical signs of FLUAVsw infection, indicative of active viral replication in the upper and lower respiratory tract, we expected to see a FLUAVsw-specific activation of MHC-I-restricted $CD8\beta^+$ T cells in infected pigs. As shown above, analysis of ex vivo Ki-67 expression in peripheral blood $CD8\beta^+$ T cells revealed expression dynamics reminiscent of an expansion and contraction phase of effector $CD8\beta^+$ T cells in at least three out of six animals. Using the overnight restimulation protocol established for the intracellular cytokine staining of $CD4^+$ T cells (Figure 4), we detected very low frequencies of FLUAVsw-specific cytokine-producing $CD8\beta^+$ T cells (Additional file 8). With the aim to increase the frequency of FLUAVsw-specific $CD8\beta^+$ T cells by in vitro expansion, we developed an alternative stimulation protocol, consisting of a 6-day culture of PBMCs, with a first FLUAVsw restimulation on day 0 and a second FLUAVsw restimulation on day 5 of culture. This prolonged incubation time enabled us to additionally investigate proliferation in mock- and FLUAVsw-stimulated cultures by the use of violet proliferation dye. Moreover, as hardly any $IL\text{-}2^+CD8\beta^+$ T cells could be detected by the overnight restimulation (Additional file 8), we decided to omit IL-2 and to analyze surface CD107a expression, indicative of degranulation, instead. PBMCs isolated at two weeks after primary infection, six weeks after primary infection (i.e. two weeks after secondary infection) and – where available – nine weeks after primary infection (i.e. five weeks after secondary infection) were analyzed. For each time point, intracellular IFN-γ and TNF-α, surface CD107a expression and violet proliferation were analyzed. Exemplary contour plots displaying all possible IFN-γ/TNF-α/CD107a/proliferation-marker combinations of gated $CD8\beta^+$ T cells are shown for one control animal (#3) and one infected animal (#8) at six weeks after primary infection (Figure 6A). $CD8\beta^+$ T cells of non-infected control animals showed some proliferation and degranulation, but hardly any cytokine production in response to FLUAVsw or mock stimulation. Within $CD8\beta^+$ T cells of infected animals, cytokine production was detected only in cells that had proliferated and all $cytokine^+$ cells also stained positive for the degranulation marker

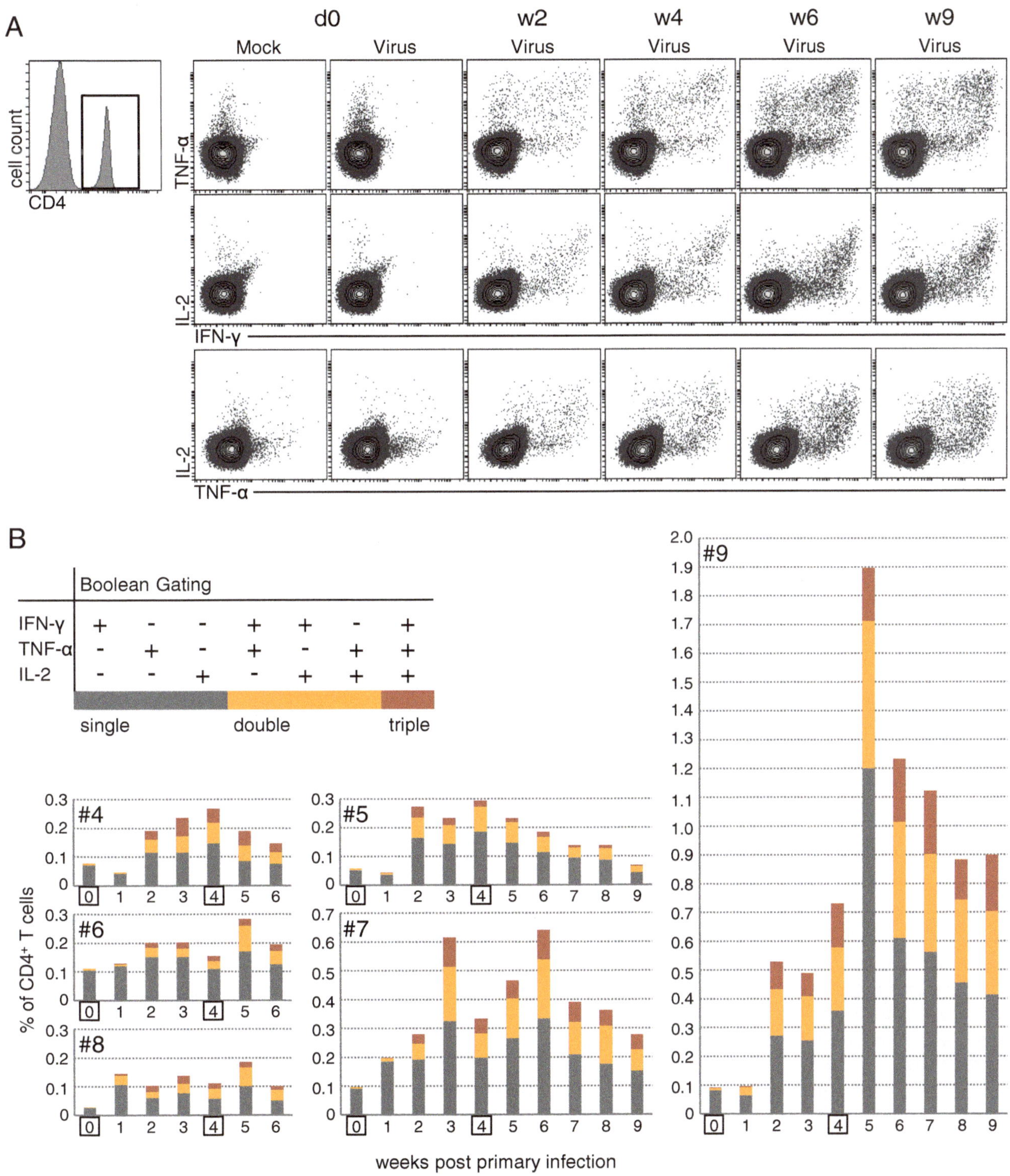

Figure 4 Kinetics of FLUAVsw-specific IFN-γ-/TNF-α-/IL-2-producing CD4⁺ T cells. Intracellular cytokine staining of defrosted PBMCs was performed following overnight in vitro restimulation with FLUAVsw (infection strain, MOI = 0.1; 18 h). Mock-incubated cultures served as negative controls. **(A)** CD4⁺ T cells were gated and analyzed for production of IFN-γ, TNF-α and IL-2. Contour plots show combinations of cytokines for selected time points following FLUAVsw infection. Exemplary data of animal #9 is shown. **(B)** Boolean gating was applied in order to identify single-, double-, and triple-cytokine-producing CD4⁺ T cells. Single- (dark grey), double- (orange) and triple- (red) cytokine-producing cells are shown as percent of total CD4⁺ T cells for all six infected animals in the time course following FLUAVsw infection.

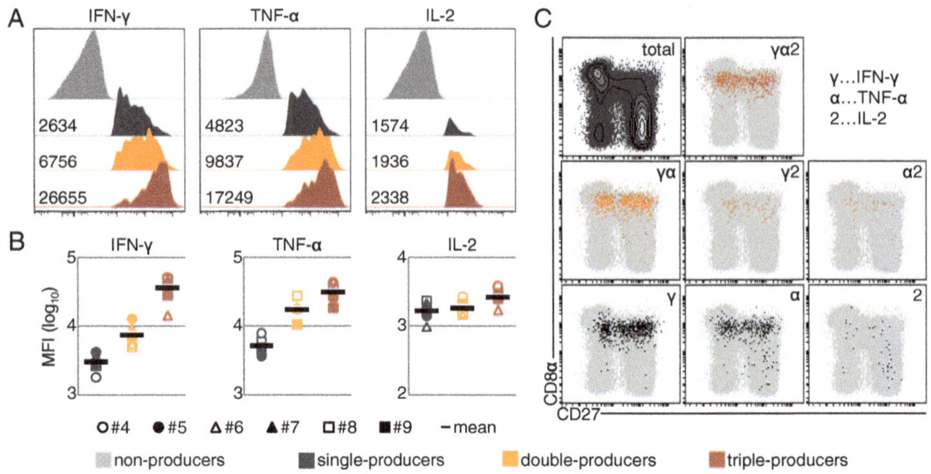

Figure 5 IFN-γ/TNF-α/IL-2 expression levels and CD8α/CD27 expression of cytokine-producing CD4⁺ T cells. (A + B) Fluorescence intensity of IFN-γ, TNF-α and IL-2 expression within single- (dark grey), double- (orange) and triple- (red) cytokine-producing $CD4^+$ T cells. **(A)** Histograms show exemplary data of animal #9 at six weeks post primary infection. Numbers indicate median fluorescence intensity (MFI) for each subset and the respective cytokine. **(B)** MFI of IFN-γ, TNF-α and IL-2 expression within single- (dark grey), double- (orange) and triple- (red) cytokine-producing $CD4^+$ T cells isolated at six weeks post primary infection. Data of all six infected animals is shown by individual symbols. The mean is indicated by the black bar. **(C)** CD8α and CD27 expression on total $CD4^+$ T cells (contour plot in the upper left and light grey dots in dot plots) and $CD4^+$ T cells producing a single cytokine (dark grey dots, bottom), two cytokines (orange dots, middle) or three cytokines (red dots, top). Representative raw data of animal #9, six weeks post primary infection, is shown.

CD107a (Figure 6A). Importantly, IFN-γ/TNF-α double positive $CD8\beta^+$ T cells were absent in mock-stimulated cultures, but clearly detectable upon FLUAVsw restimulation (Figure 6A, arrows). Having measured four different functions of $CD8\beta^+$ T cells simultaneously, we applied boolean gating to identify and quantify all subsets, differing in the type and number of functions. From 11 possible multifunctional subsets (i.e. ≥2 functions), three subsets dominated strongly: proliferating $CD107^+$ cells, (two functions), proliferating $CD107^+IFN\text{-}\gamma^+$ cells (three functions) and proliferating $CD107^+IFN\text{-}\gamma^+TNF\text{-}\alpha^+$ cells (four functions; Additional file 9). Therefore, the subsets were clustered according to the number of functions they exerted (Figure 6B). Results are displayed as percent of multifunctional cells within total $CD8\beta^+$ T cells. Animals #6 and #8 showed the highest frequency of FLUAVsw-specific multifunctional cells within $CD8\beta^+$ T cells, isolated at six weeks after primary infection, i.e. two weeks after secondary infection. A lower frequency was detected in animals #7 and #9 and no clear increase could be detected from the earliest to later time points. Hardly any virus-specific response could be detected in $CD8\beta^+$ T cells of animals #4 and #5, similar to the non-infected control animals (#1, #3). Notably, the lacking FLUAVsw-specific $CD8\beta^+$-T-cell response of animals #4 and #5 matched the results of the Ki-67 expression analysis (Figure 2B), as no expansion of Ki-67-expressing $CD8\beta^+$ T cells could be detected in these two animals. In summary, these data indicate the presence of FLUAVsw-specific multifunctional $CD8\beta^+$ T cells within PBMCs of four out of six animals.

SLA haplotyping

T-cell responses are influenced by the binding properties of particular major histocompatibility complex molecules that mediate the presentation of peptides to the T-cell receptor. To identify potential associations between the T-cell response and the SLA haplotype, a low-resolution SLA typing of the nine pigs included in the present study was performed and revealed a total of nine class I and eight class II haplotypes (Table 2). The most common class I haplotypes were Lr-01.0 (#4, #6, #7, #9) and Lr-24.0 (#3, #5, #6, #7), followed by Lr-25.0 (#1, #4) and Lr-59.0 (#2, #3). Unique class I haplotypes were Lr-45.0 (#1), Lr-08.0 (#2), Lr-18.0 (#5), Lr-40.0 (#8) and Lr-46.0 (#8). Within class II, the most frequent haplotype was Lr-0.15b (#2, #3, #4, #5, #6, #7), followed by Lr-0.09 (#3, #5, #6, #7) and Lr-0.25 (#1, #2, #4). Unique class II haplotypes were found in pig #1 (Lr-0.22), pig #8 (Lr-0.10/Lr-0.23) and pig #9 (Lr-0.33/Lr-0.35).

Discussion

In the present study, we aimed to investigate the kinetics and functional properties of FLUAVsw-specific $CD4^+$ and $CD8\beta^+$ T cells in the blood of FLUAVsw-infected pigs. We also decided to perform a homologous reinfection four weeks after the primary infection in order to monitor a potential expansion or change in functional attributes of FLUAVsw-specific memory T cells under such conditions. A FLUAVsw H1N2 isolate from Germany was used for infection and in vitro restimulation. H1N2 virus strains are constantly circulating in European pig

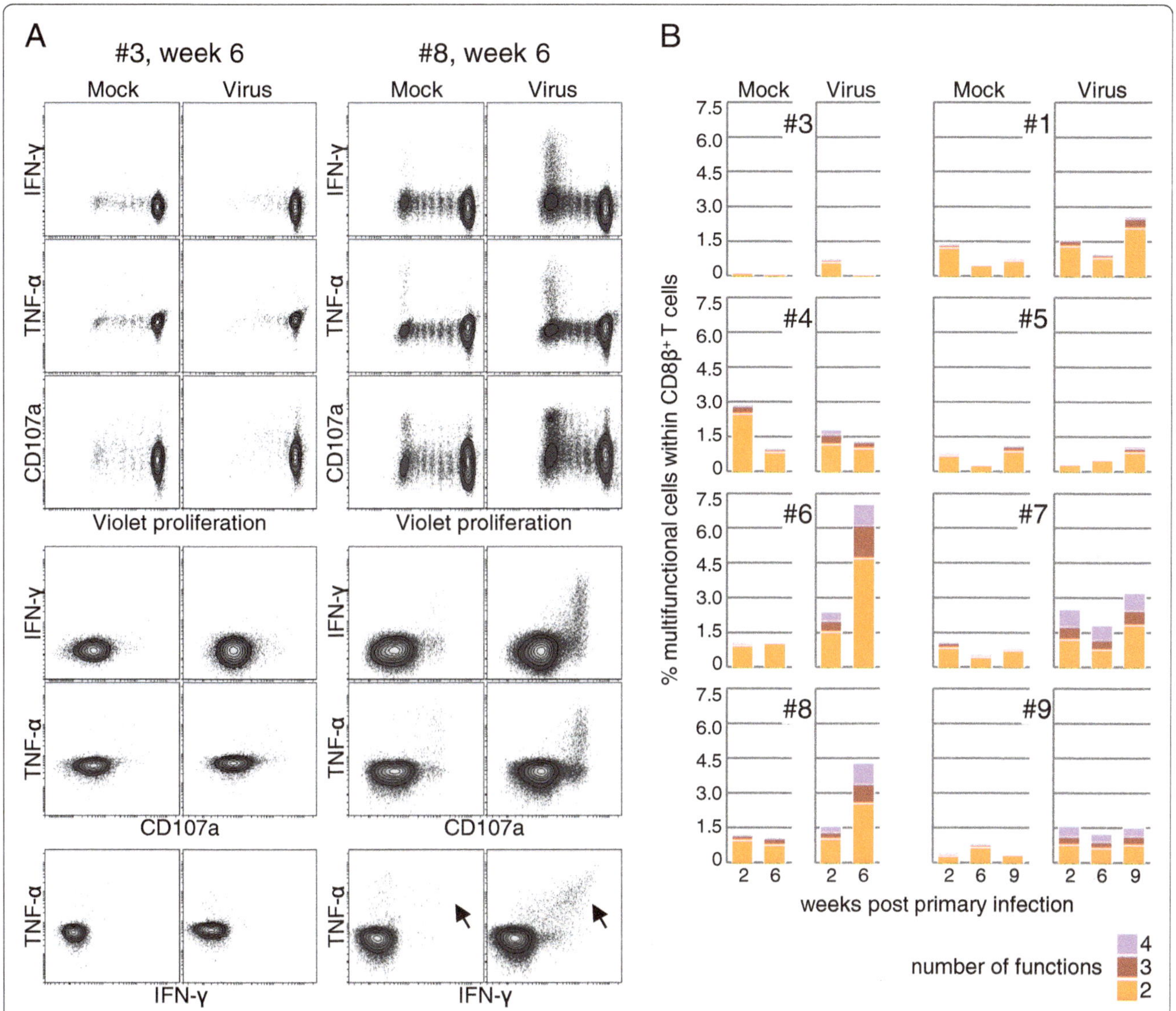

Figure 6 Proliferation, degranulation and cytokine production by FLUAVsw-specific CD8β⁺ T cells. Violet-labeled PBMCs isolated at 2, 6 and 9 weeks post primary infection were restimulated twice with FLUAVsw (infection strain, MOI = 0.1; day 0 and day 5 of culture) and analyzed by FCM on day 6 of culture. **(A)** CD8β⁺ T cells were gated (not shown) and analyzed for violet proliferation, surface CD107a expression and intracellular accumulation of IFN-γ and TNF-α. Contour plots show all possible marker combinations. Exemplary raw data of one non-infected control animal (#3) and one infected animal (#8) is shown for week 6 post primary infection. **(B)** Boolean gating was applied in order to identify multifunctional CD8β⁺ T cells, and resulting CD8β⁺ T-cell subsets were grouped by number of functions. Displayed is the frequency of CD8β⁺ T cells carrying out two or more functions within total CD8β⁺ T cells. Data of six FLUAVsw-infected animals (#4-9) and two non-infected control animals (#1, #3) is shown.

herds since the 1990s [4]; therefore our infection model should at least partially reflect field conditions.

To verify successful experimental infection with the intratracheally administered H1N2 isolate, clinical signs and post-mortem histopathological changes were examined. All infected animals developed clinical signs with fever, lethargy and lower-respiratory-tract signs, which have been described as the typical outcome of acute influenza infection [4,29]. Within one week, all animals recovered, which is consistent with the reported clearance of influenza virus from the porcine lung within seven days [4]. Clinical signs were absent from all animals upon reinfection with the same strain four weeks later. This is in accordance with previous studies, where pigs underwent a homologous reinfection [5,7,30,31]. Macroscopic lesions were either mild, and confined to localized lobular retractions at the edges of the cranial lobes, or were even absent. Microscopically, we observed mild to moderate infiltration of the lung tissue with mononuclear cells and lobular atelectasis with fibrous retraction as well as metaplastic and hyperplastic changes of the airway epithelium. These lesions were considered as

Table 2 Swine leukocyte antigen (SLA) haplotypes of pigs used in this study

		SLA allele specificity				SLA allele specificity		
Pig #	SLA class I haplotype	SLA-1	SLA-3	SLA-2	SLA class II haplotype	SLA-DRB1	SLA-DQB1	SLA-DQA
1	Lr-25.0	11XX	03XX	07XX	Lr-0.22	06XX	02XX(0204)	02XX
	Lr-45.0	08XX + cs02	07XX	w08XX + 10XX	Lr-0.25	13XX	09XX	04XX
2	Lr-08.0	04XX	03XX	07XX	Lr-0.15b	04XX	02XX	02XX
	Lr-59.0	11XX(1103)	05XX	jh02	Lr-0.25	13XX	09XX	04XX
3	Lr-24.0	blank	04XX/hb06	02XX	Lr-0.09	02XX	04XX	03XX
	Lr-59.0	11XX(1103)	05XX	jh02	Lr-0.15b	04XX	02XX	02XX
4	Lr-01.0	01XX	01XX	01XX	Lr-0.15b	04XX	02XX	02XX
	Lr-25.0	11XX	03XX	07XX	Lr-0.25	13XX	09XX	04XX
5	Lr-18.0	04XX	03XX	01XX	Lr-0.09	02XX	04XX	03XX
	Lr-24.0	blank	04XX/hb06	02XX	Lr-0.15b	04XX	02XX	02XX
6	Lr-01.0	01XX	01XX	01XX	Lr-0.09	02XX	04XX	03XX
	Lr-24.0	blank	04XX/hb06	02XX	Lr-0.15b	04XX	02XX	02XX
7	Lr-01.0	01XX	01XX	01XX	Lr-0.09	02XX	04XX	03XX
	Lr-24.0	blank	04XX/hb06	02XX	Lr-0.15b	04XX	02XX	02XX
8	Lr-40.0	16XX	05XX	10XX	Lr-0.10	04XX	08XX	03XX
	Lr-46.0	12XX	04XX/hb06	06XX	Lr-0.23	10XX/er01	06XX/zs12	01XX
9	Lr-01.0	01XX	01XX	01XX	Lr-0.33	11XX	02XX	02XX
	Lr-01.0	01XX	01XX	01XX	Lr-0.35	01XX	04XX	02XX

signs of late-stage influenza infection. The microscopic lesions observed in animal #7 resembled alterations present in intercurrent bacterial infections (such as *Mycoplasma* spp., *Pasteurella multocida* or *Haemophilus parasuis*) and were not representative for the infection group.

H1N2-neutralizing antibodies were detected at considerable levels already one week after infection, confirming the postulated relevance of the humoral response in the clearance of FLUAVsw infections. With the exception of animal #9, a clear boost in antibody titers was not observed, which is consistent with a study reporting the lack of a HI-titer increase after homologous reinfection [5].

As a first attempt to analyze the role of T cells in the control of FLUAVsw infection, we looked for expansion of CD4 and CD8β effector T cells via analysis of Ki-67 expression. In parallel, we followed the frequency of FLUAVsw-specific multiple-cytokine-producing T cells. The analysis of Ki-67$^+$ T cells has been successfully used in immunological studies addressing T-cell expansion in response to influenza A virus infections within PBMCs isolated from humans [20] and nonhuman primates [32]. In our study, we could identify a clear expansion of CD8β$^+$Ki-67$^+$perforin$^+$ T cells at one week after primary infection in three out of six animals. This heterogeneity is somewhat similar to results obtained by a study of human T cells [20], where, seven days after infection, a strong variation in the frequency of CD4$^+$CD38$^+$Ki-67$^+$ and CD8$^+$CD38$^+$Ki-67$^+$ T cells was observed between different individuals. In contrast, a more homogenous response in regard to expansion of blood-derived CD8$^+$CD38$^+$Ki-67$^+$ T cells has been reported for H1N1-infected rhesus macaques [32]. The reasons for the lack of a CD8β$^+$-T-cell expansion in the blood of at least two infected pigs (#4, #5) are speculative. Interestingly, these two animals also lacked a response of CD8β$^+$ T cells in the in vitro restimulation experiments addressing FLUAVsw-specific proliferation, cytokine production and CD107a expression (Figure 6B). These findings may suggest that a CTL response was only weakly triggered in these two animals. Clearly, a parallel analysis of the T-cell response present in the lung will lead to a more comprehensive overview of the cell-mediated response and its variation among individual pigs.

The lack of a substantial FLUAVsw infection-related expansion of CD4$^+$ T cells (in all animals) might be also due to a masking by T-cell responses to other environmental antigens encountered following weaning, and by T-cell responses to the vaccines (porcine circovirus type 2, *Mycoplasma hyopneumoniae*, see chapter 2.1) administered at three weeks of age. Indeed, in a previous study from our group we could show that, following weaning at three weeks of age, a considerable increase of CD4$^+$ T cells with an activated and/or memory phenotype occurs in blood [23].

These observations also provide some evidence that, despite the relatively young age of the piglets in this study at the time of the first infection (i.e. four weeks), CD4$^+$ T cells were already capable to respond to the FLUAVsw infection. Similarly, the observed expansion of CD8β$^+$ T cells in the blood of three animals following FLUAVsw infection might indicate that also this T-cell subset was already in a maturation stage enabling a reaction to this viral infection.

Multifunctional T cells have been proposed as a hallmark of protective immunity [18,26,27,33,34]. Performing triple-cytokine staining of in vitro restimulated PBMCs, we found that a considerable proportion of FLUAVsw-specific CD4$^+$ T cells can be activated to produce two or three of the cytokines IFN-γ, TNF-α and IL-2 simultaneously. Triple-cytokine-producing CD4$^+$ T cells were detectable in the blood of all infected pigs from two weeks post primary infection onwards. This rather late appearance in regard to the clearance of clinical signs questions their immediate role in the primary immune response against FLUAVsw, but may indicate relevance in the formation of memory T cells. Also, an increase of single-, double- and triple-cytokine-producing CD4$^+$ T cells was observed in four (#6, #7, #8, #9) out of six animals after the secondary infection, supporting the assumption that multifunctional CD4$^+$ T cells are a part of the FLUAVsw-specific memory-T-cell pool.

CD4$^+$ multifunctional T cells produced more IFN-γ, TNF-α and IL-2 on a per-cell level, and triple producers outranked double-producers, especially in the production of IFN-γ (Figures 5A and B and Additional file 6). This confirms an observation already made for murine [26,28] and human T cells [27,34,35]. For CD8β$^+$ T cells, IL-2 production was undetectable in the overnight restimulated cultures (Additional file 8). Interestingly, recent work from our laboratory showed that, even after polyclonal stimulation, CD8β$^+$ T cells isolated from porcine blood produce hardly any IL-2, whereas such T cells can be readily identified in bronchial lymph nodes [36]. This might indicate a rapid homing of IL-2-producing CD8β$^+$ T cells into lymphatic organs. Of note, human influenza-specific CD8$^+$ T cells were shown to produce IL-2 upon influenza A virus restimulation, but protection from severe illness was found to correlate only with preexisting IFN-γ$^+$CD8$^+$ T cells and no correlation was found for IL-2-producing CD8$^+$ T-cell subsets [37].

Generally, cytokine production of CD4$^+$ T cells was mostly associated with CD8α expression, which is described as a marker to distinguish naïve from antigen-experienced CD4$^+$ T cells in swine [22,23]. Cytokine combinations including IFN-γ appeared to be even more restricted to CD8α expression, which is in accordance with the description of IFN-γ being a signature cytokine of late-differentiated human T cells [38]. For CD27 expression, which was proposed to distinguish between effector and central memory CD4$^+$ T cells in swine [24], we could not find any cytokine-related patterns. Both, the putative CD8α$^+$CD27$^+$ central memory subset and the putative CD8α$^+$CD27$^-$ effector memory subset contained FLUAVsw-specific cytokine-producing T cells, indicating that both T-cell subsets contribute to the FLUAVsw-specific memory-T-cell pool in pigs.

A reliable frequency of FLUAVsw-specific CD8β$^+$ T cells could only be identified after a six-day in vitro expansion. These responding CD8β$^+$ T cells consisted mainly of IFN-γ/TNF-α-double-producing cells (Figure 6A, arrows). A dominant co-production of IFN-γ and TNF-α was also shown for human CD8$^+$ T cells responding to influenza peptide restimulation [39]. This co-production of the antiviral cytokines IFN-γ and TNF-α is described as the predominant functional signature of effector CD8$^+$ T cells in humans [38].

Similar to the variable frequencies of FLUAVsw-specific cytokine-producing CD4$^+$ T cells, we found considerable variation in magnitude and kinetics of FLUAVsw-specific cytokine-producing CD8β$^+$ T cells among individual pigs (Figure 6B). Strong variations of the CD8$^+$-T-cell response were also described for outbred mice following bacterial or viral infection [40]. In humans, a recent study of CD8$^+$-T-cell immunity across ethnicities highlighted the influence of different human leukocyte antigen class 1 haplotypes on the resulting individual differences in magnitude and quality of influenza-specific CD8$^+$ memory T cells [39]. Interestingly, the low-resolution swine leukocyte antigen (SLA) typing of the pigs used in our study revealed that pig #9, which showed a strong expansion of Ki-67$^+$CD8β$^+$ T cells and the highest frequencies of FLUAVsw-specific cytokine-producing CD4$^+$ T cells, had a homozygous SLA class I haplotype and was also homozygous for the SLA-DQA locus (Table 2). However, the SLA class I haplotype of animal #9 was also present in the CD8β$^+$-T-cell-non-responding pig #4, indicating that further factors or minor differences in the SLA class I haplotypes, only identifiable by high-resolution SLA typing, are responsible for the observed differences in the CD8β$^+$-T-cell response.

In conclusion, our data demonstrate the generation of FLUAVsw-specific CD4$^+$ and CD8β$^+$ T cells in the immune response to influenza A virus infection in the pig. The observed multifunctional profile of FLUAVsw-specific T cells suggests a function in protective immunity, similar to the relevance of multifunctional T cells in the control of viral infections in humans [25]. Clearly, this has to be addressed in heterologous reinfection studies, which will provide important insights into T-cell-mediated cross-protection. Of note, the T-cell responses described in this study were analyzed in blood, i.e. on a systemic level. In future studies it is necessary to analyze FLUAVsw-specific T cells also on the local level in the lung, as FLUAVsw infections do not cause viremia [4] and therefore represent a local infection. Work on this is in progress in our laboratory, indicating a strong enrichment of FLUAVsw-specific CD8β$^+$ T cells in the porcine lung (S.C. Talker and W. Gerner, unpublished data). Such an in-depth characterization of the porcine T-cell response to influenza infection will contribute to the development of improved vaccines for pig husbandry. These novel vaccines should also reduce viral transmission between swine and humans, a risk factor associated with the emergence of – potentially pandemic – reassortant influenza strains.

Additional files

Additional file 1: FCM gating strategy used for freshly isolated PBMCs (A) and for defrosted, in vitro restimulated PBMCs (B). (A + B) Lymphocytes were gated according to FSC-A/SSC-A characteristics. Consecutive FSC-H/FSC-W and SSC-H/SSC-W plots were used to gate on singlets. (B) For analyses with defrosted and in vitro restimulated PBMCs, dead cells were excluded by the use of the LIVE/DEAD stain Near-IR.

Additional file 2: Rectal temperatures in the time course. Rectal temperatures were recorded daily from one week prior to infection until the end of the study, i.e. 6 weeks or 9 weeks post primary infection. Mean values and standard deviations for the PBS-treated control pigs (grey line) and the H1N2-infected pigs (red line) are shown in the time course. Asterisks at one and two days post primary infection indicate significant differences between the infected and the control group ($p \leq 0.001$, unpaired *t*-test, SPSS Inc./ IBM, Chicago, IL, USA, Version 19).

Additional file 3: Representative macroscopic and histologic lesions in a FLUAVsw-infected pig (#4) in comparison to a control animal (#2). The control animal shows no macroscopic alterations at the edges of the right cranial and middle lung lobes (A). Histologically, the lung tissue of the control animal shows thin alveolar walls and no inflammatory cells in the alveolar spaces and alveolar septa (C). The bronchioles are lined by a cuboidal epithelium and there are few mononuclear cells in the surrounding interstitium (E). In the infected animal there are several consolidated and retracted lobules at the ventral edge of the cranial and middle lobe (B). Microscopically, there is diffuse infiltration with mononuclear cells, fibrosis and metaplastic transformation of alveolar epithelia to cuboidal formations (D). Bronchiolar epithelia are markedly hyperplastic with pseudostratified columnar appearance and the surrounding interstitium is infiltrated with numerous mononuclear cells (F). Bars: 150 μm (C,D); 80 μm (E,F).

Additional file 4: Kinetics of FLUAVsw-specific IFN-γ-/TNF-α-/IL-2-producing CD4$^+$ T cells. Intracellular cytokine staining of defrosted PBMCs was performed following overnight in vitro restimulation with FLUAVsw (infection strain, MOI = 0.1; 18 h). Mock-incubated cultures served as negative controls. CD4$^+$ T cells were gated and analyzed for production of IFN-γ, TNF-α and IL-2. Contour plots show combinations of cytokines for selected time points following FLUAVsw infection. (A) Exemplary data of animal #7 (intermediate response) and (B) animal #8 (low response) is shown.

Additional file 5: Kinetics of FLUAVsw-specific CD4$^+$ T-cell subsets producing different cytokines. Intracellular cytokine staining of defrosted PBMCs was performed following overnight in vitro restimulation with FLUAVsw (infection strain, MOI = 0.1; 18 h). Mock-incubated cultures served as negative controls. CD4$^+$ T cells were gated and analyzed for production of IFN-γ, TNF-α and IL-2 as in Figure 4. Boolean gating was applied in order to identify all seven subsets of cytokine-producing CD4$^+$ T cells. The frequency of the seven different cytokine-producing T-cell subsets are shown in stacked bar charts as percent of total CD4$^+$ T cells for all six infected animals in the time course following FLUAVsw infection.

Additional file 6: IFN-γ/TNF-α/IL-2 expression levels of cytokine-producing CD4$^+$ T cells. (A + B) Fluorescence intensity of IFN-γ, TNF-α and IL-2 expression within single- (dark grey), double- (orange) and triple- (red) cytokine-producing CD4$^+$ T cells. Histograms show data of cells isolated from animal #7 (A; intermediate response) and animal #8 (B; low response) at six weeks post primary infection. Numbers indicate median fluorescence intensity (MFI) for each subset and the respective cytokine. (C) MFI of IFN-γ, TNF-α and IL-2 expression within single- (dark grey), double- (orange) and triple- (red) cytokine-producing CD4$^+$ T cells isolated at two to six weeks post primary infection. Data of all six infected animals is shown by individual symbols. The mean is indicated by the black bar.

Additional file 7: CD8α/CD27 expression of cytokine-producing CD4$^+$ T cells. CD8α and CD27 expression on total CD4$^+$ T cells (contour plot in the upper left and light grey dots in dot plots) and CD4$^+$ T cells producing a single cytokine (dark grey dots, bottom), two cytokines (orange dots, middle) or three cytokines (red dots, top). Data of CD4$^+$ T cells from animal #7 (A; intermediate response) and animal #8 (B; low response) at six weeks post primary infection is shown.

Additional file 8: Production of IFN-γ, TNF-α and IL-2 by FLUAVsw-specific CD8β$^+$ T cells. Intracellular cytokine staining of defrosted PBMCs was performed following overnight in vitro restimulation with FLUAVsw (infection strain, MOI = 0.1; 18 h). Mock-incubated cultures served as negative controls. CD3$^+$CD8β$^+$ T cells were gated and analyzed for production of IFN-γ, TNF-α and IL-2. Contour plots show combinations of cytokines for selected time points following FLUAVsw infection. Exemplary data obtained with CD8β$^+$ T cells of animal #6 is shown.

Additional file 9: Multifunctional FLUAVsw-specific CD8β$^+$ T cells identified by proliferation, CD107a expression and cytokine production. Violet-labeled PBMCs isolated at 2, 6 and 9 weeks post primary infection were restimulated twice with FLUAVsw (infection strain, MOI = 0.1; day 0 and day 5 of culture). On day 6 of culture, PBMCs were analyzed by FCM for proliferation, CD107a expression and production of IFN-γ and TNF-α. Boolean gating was applied in order to identify multifunctional subsets of CD8β$^+$ T cells. All 11 multifunctional subsets (i.e. ≥ 2 functions) are shown in the left panel as stacked bar charts in % of total CD8β$^+$ T cells. In the right panel, the subsets are grouped according to the number of functions they exert (as shown in Figure 6B). Data of six FLUAVsw-infected animals (#4-9) and two non-infected control animals (#1, #3) is shown.

Competing interests
The authors declare that they have no competing interests.

Authors' contributions
SCT performed laboratory work and wrote the manuscript together with WG. HCK organized and conducted the animal experiment. MS and KHM assisted in laboratory work. RG, EK, AL, and MR were involved in organization and conduction of the animal experiment. SEH performed SLA haplotyping. HW performed the pathological examinations. RD performed serum neutralization tests. AS assisted in project design and drafting of the manuscript. WG designed and supervised the overall project. All authors read and approved the final manuscript.

Acknowledgments
This work was supported by a "start-up project" (PP35010261) of the University of Veterinary Medicine Vienna granted to WG. SCT was supported by a "vetmeduni success" stipend of the University of Veterinary Medicine Vienna. The authors thank Sandra Groiss for her excellent technical assistance in running the PCR assays for the pig SLA haplotyping.

Author details
[1]Institute of Immunology, Department of Pathobiology, University of Veterinary Medicine, Vienna, Austria. [2]University Clinic for Swine, Department for Farm Animals and Veterinary Public Health, University of Veterinary Medicine, Vienna, Austria. [3]Institute of Pathology and Forensic Veterinary Medicine, Department of Pathobiology, University of Veterinary Medicine, Vienna, Austria. [4]Viral Vaccines, Business Unit Animal Health, IDT Biologika GmbH, Dessau-Rosslau, Germany. [5]Present address: Institute of Veterinary Pathology, Vetsuisse-Faculty, University of Zurich, Zurich, Switzerland. [6]Present address: Clinic for Swine, Ludwig-Maximilians-University, Munich, Germany.

References

1. Myers KP, Olsen CW, Gray GC (2007) Cases of swine influenza in humans: a review of the literature. Clin Infect Dis 44:1084–1088
2. Neumann G, Noda T, Kawaoka Y (2009) Emergence and pandemic potential of swine-origin H1N1 influenza virus. Nature 459:931–939
3. Lange J, Groth M, Schlegel M, Krumbholz A, Wieczorek K, Ulrich R, Köppen S, Schulz K, Appl D, Selbitz H-J, Sauerbrei A, Platzer M, Zell R, Dürrwald R (2013) Reassortants of the pandemic (H1N1) 2009 virus and establishment of a novel porcine H1N2 influenza virus, lineage in Germany. Vet Microbiol 167:345–356
4. Van Reeth K, Brown IH, Olsen CW (2012) Influenza Virus. In: Zimmerman JJ, Karriker LA, Ramirez A, Schwartz KJ, Stevenson GW (ed) Diseases of Swine, 10th edition. Wiley-Blackwell, Hoboken, pp 557–571
5. Larsen DL, Karasin A, Zuckermann F, Olsen CW (2000) Systemic and mucosal immune responses to H1N1 influenza virus infection in pigs. Vet Microbiol 74:117–131
6. La Gruta NL, Turner SJ (2014) T cell mediated immunity to influenza: mechanisms of viral control. Trends Immunol 35:396–402
7. Heinen PP, van Nieuwstadt AP, de Boer-Luijtze EA, Bianchi ATJ (2001) Analysis of the quality of protection induced by a porcine influenza A vaccine to challenge with an H3N2 virus. Vet Immunol Immunopathol 82:39–56
8. Heinen PP, de Boer-Luijtze EA, Bianchi ATJ (2001) Respiratory and systemic humoral and cellular immune responses of pigs to a heterosubtypic influenza A virus infection. J Gen Virol 82:2697–2707
9. Pomorska-Mól M, Markowska-Daniel I, Kwit K, Czyzewska E, Dors A, Rachubik J, Pejsak Z (2014) Immune and inflammatory response in pigs during acute influenza caused by H1N1 swine influenza virus. Arch Virol 159:2605–2614
10. Lefevre EA, Carr BV, Inman CF, Prentice H, Brown IH, Brookes SM, Garcon F, Hill ML, Iqbal M, Elderfield RA, Barclay WS, Gubbins S, Bailey M, Charleston B, COSI (2012) Immune responses in pigs vaccinated with adjuvanted and non-adjuvanted A(H1N1)pdm/09 influenza vaccines used in human immunization programmes. PLoS One 7:e32400
11. Khatri M, Dwivedi V, Krakowka S, Manickam C, Ali A, Wang L, Qin Z, Renukaradhya GJ, Lee CW (2010) Swine influenza H1N1 virus induces acute inflammatory immune responses in pig lungs: a potential animal model for human H1N1 influenza virus. J Virol 84:11210–11218
12. Zell R, Bergmann S, Krumbholz A, Wutzler P, Dürrwald R (2008) Ongoing evolution of swine influenza viruses: a novel reassortant. Arch Virol 153:2085–2092
13. Saalmüller A, Jonjic S, Bühring HJ, Reddehase MJ, Koszinowski UH (1987) Monoclonal antibodies reactive with swine lymphocytes. II. Detection of an antigen on resting T cells down-regulated after activation. J Immunol 138:1852–1857
14. Gerner W, Käser T, Pintaric M, Groiss S, Saalmüller A (2008) Detection of intracellular antigens in porcine PBMC by flow cytometry: a comparison of fixation and permeabilisation reagents. Vet Immunol Immunopathol 121:251–259
15. Reutner K, Leitner J, Essler SE, Witter K, Patzl M, Steinberger P, Saalmüller A, Gerner W (2012) Porcine CD27: identification, expression and functional aspects in lymphocyte subsets in swine. Dev Comp Immunol 38:321–331
16. Essler SE, Ertl W, Deutsch J, Rütgen BC, Groiss S, Stadler M, Wysoudil B, Gerner W, Ho CS, Saalmüller A (2013) Molecular characterization of swine leukocyte antigen gene diversity in purebred pietrain pigs. Anim Genet 44:202–205
17. Miller JD, van der Most RG, Akondy RS, Glidewell JT, Albott S, Masopust D, Murali-Krishna K, Mahar PL, Edupuganti S, Lalor S, Germon S, Del Rio C, Mulligan MJ, Staprans SI, Altman JD, Feinberg MB, Ahmed R (2008) Human effector and memory $CD8^+$ T cell responses to smallpox and yellow fever vaccines. Immunity 28:710–722
18. Akondy RS, Monson ND, Miller JD, Edupuganti S, Teuwen D, Wu H, Quyyumi F, Garg S, Altman JD, Del Rio C, Keyserling HL, Ploss A, Rice CM, Orenstein WA, Mulligan MJ, Ahmed R (2009) The yellow fever virus vaccine induces a broad and polyfunctional human memory $CD8^+$ T cell response. J Immunol 183:7919–7930
19. Lindgren T, Ahlm C, Mohamed N, Evander M, Ljunggren HG, Björkström NK (2011) Longitudinal analysis of the human T cell response during acute hantavirus infection. J Virol 85:10252–10260
20. Wilkinson TM, Li CKF, Chui CSC, Huang AKY, Perkins M, Liebner JC, Lambkin-Williams R, Gilbert A, Oxford J, Nicholas B, Staples KJ, Dong T, Douek DC, McMichael AJ, Xu XN (2012) Preexisting influenza-specific $CD4^+$ T cells correlate with disease protection against influenza challenge in humans. Nat Med 18:274–280
21. Gerner W, Käser T, Saalmüller A (2009) Porcine T lymphocytes and NK cells – an update. Dev Comp Immunol 33:310–320
22. Saalmüller A, Werner T, Fachinger V (2002) T-helper cells from naive to committed. Vet Immunol Immunopathol 87:137–145
23. Talker SC, Käser T, Reutner K, Sedlak C, Mair KH, Koinig H, Graage R, Viehmann M, Klingler E, Ladinig A, Ritzmann M, Saalmüller A, Gerner W (2013) Phenotypic maturation of porcine NK- and T-cell subsets. Dev Comp Immunol 40:51–68
24. Reutner K, Leitner J, Müllebner A, Ladinig A, Essler SE, Duvigneau JC, Ritzmann M, Steinberger P, Saalmüller A, Gerner W (2013) CD27 expression discriminates porcine T helper cells with functionally distinct properties. Vet Res 44:18
25. Seder RA, Darrah PA, Roederer M (2008) T-cell quality in memory and protection: implications for vaccine design. Nat Rev Immunol 8:247–258
26. Darrah PA, Patel DT, De Luca PM, Lindsay RWB, Davey DF, Flynn BJ, Hoff ST, Andersen P, Reed SG, Morris SL, Roederer M, Seder RA (2007) Multifunctional T_H1 cells define a correlate of vaccine-mediated protection against Leishmania major. Nat Med 13:843–850
27. Kannanganat S, Ibegbu C, Chennareddi L, Robinson HL, Amara RR (2007) Multiple-cytokine-producing antiviral CD4 T cells are functionally superior to single-cytokine-producing cells. J Virol 81:8468–8476
28. Lindenstrøm T, Agger EM, Korsholm KS, Darrah PA, Aagaard C, Seder RA, Rosenkrands I, Andersen P (2009) Tuberculosis subunit vaccination provides long-term protective immunity characterized by multifunctional CD4 memory T cells. J Immunol 182:8047–8055
29. Pomorska-Mól M, Kwit K, Markowska-Daniel I, Kowalski C, Pejsak Z (2014) Local and systemic immune response in pigs during subclinical and clinical swine influenza infection. Res Vet Sci 97:412–421
30. Van Reeth K, Gregory V, Hay A, Pensaert M (2003) Protection against a European H1N2 swine influenza virus in pigs previously infected with H1N1 and/or H3N2 subtypes. Vaccine 21:1375–1381
31. De Vleeschauwer AR, Van Poucke SG, Karasin AI, Olsen CW, Van Reeth K (2011) Cross-protection between antigenically distinct H1N1 swine influenza viruses from Europe and North America. Influenza Other Respir Viruses 5:115–122
32. Weinfurter JT, Brunner K, Capuano SV, III, Li C, Broman KW, Kawaoka Y, Friedrich TC (2011) Cross-reactive T cells are involved in rapid clearance of 2009 pandemic H1N1 influenza virus in nonhuman primates. PLoS Pathog 7:e1002381
33. Betts MR, Nason MC, West SM, De Rosa SC, Migueles SA, Abraham J, Lederman MM, Benito JM, Goepfert PA, Connors M, Roederer M, Koup RA (2006) HIV nonprogressors preferentially maintain highly functional HIV-specific $CD8^+$ T cells. Blood 107:4781–4789
34. Precopio ML, Betts MR, Parrino J, Price DA, Gostick E, Ambrozak DR, Asher TE, Douek DC, Harari A, Pantaleo G, Bailer R, Graham BS, Roederer M, Koup RA (2007) Immunization with vaccinia virus induces polyfunctional and phenotypically distinctive $CD8^+$ T cell responses. J Exp Med 204:1405–1416
35. Duvall MG, Precopio ML, Ambrozak DA, Jaye A, McMichael AJ, Whittle HC, Roederer M, Rowland-Jones SL, Koup RA (2008) Polyfunctional T cell responses are a hallmark of HIV-2 infection. Eur J Immunol 38:350–363
36. Gerner W, Talker SC, Koinig H, Sedlak C, Mair KH, Saalmüller A (2015) Phenotypic and functional differentiation of porcine αβ T cells: current knowledge and available tools. Mol Immunol 66:3–13
37. Sridhar S, Begom S, Bermingham A, Hoschler K, Adamson W, Carman W, Bean T, Barclay W, Deeks JJ, Lalvani A (2013) Cellular immune correlates of protection against symptomatic pandemic influenza. Nat Med 19:1305–1312
38. Mahnke YD, Brodie TM, Sallusto F, Roederer M, Lugli E (2013) The who's who of T-cell differentiation: human memory T-cell subsets. Eur J Immunol 43:2797–2809
39. Quinones-Parra S, Grant E, Loh L, Nguyen THO, Campbell KA, Tong SYC, Miller A, Doherty PC, Vijaykrishna D, Rossjohn J, Gras S, Kedzierska K (2014) Preexisting $CD8^+$ T-cell immunity to the H7N9 influenza A virus varies across ethnicities. Proc Natl Acad Sci U S A 111:1049–1054
40. Rai D, Pham NL, Harty JT, Badovinac VP (2009) Tracking the total CD8 T cell response to infection reveals substantial discordance in magnitude and kinetics between inbred and outbred hosts. J Immunol 183:7672–7681

The innate immune response of equine bronchial epithelial cells is altered by training

Linda Frellstedt[1,2*], Philippe Gosset[3,4,5,6,7], Gwenola Kervoaze[3,4,5,6,7], Aymeric Hans[8], Christophe Desmet[9], Dimitri Pirottin[9], Fabrice Bureau[9], Pierre Lekeux[1] and Tatiana Art[1]

Abstract

Respiratory diseases, including inflammatory airway disease (IAD), viral and bacterial infections, are common problems in exercising horses. The airway epithelium constitutes a major physical barrier against airborne infections and plays an essential role in the lung innate immune response mainly through toll-like receptor (TLR) activation. The aim of this study was to develop a model for the culture of equine bronchial epithelial cells (EBEC) in vitro and to explore EBEC innate immune responses in trained horses. Bronchial epithelial biopsies were taken from 6 adult horses during lower airway endoscopy. EBEC were grown in vitro by an explant method. The innate immune response of EBEC was evaluated in vitro by treatment with TLR ligands. TLR3 is the most strongly expressed TLR at the mRNA level in EBEC and stimulation of EBEC with Poly(I:C), an analog of viral dsRNA, triggers a strong secretion of IFN-β, TNF-α, IL-6 and CXCL8. We further evaluated the EBEC innate immune response in horses that underwent a 4-month-training program. While training had no effect on TLR mRNA expression in EBEC as well as in bronchial biopsies, it increased the production of IFN-β after stimulation with a TLR3 ligand and decreased the secretion of TNF-α and IL-6 after stimulation with a TLR2 and TLR3 ligand. These findings may be implicated in the increased risk for viral and bacterial infections observed in sport horses. Altogether, we report a successful model for the culture of EBEC that can be applied to the investigation of pathophysiologic conditions in longitudinal studies.

Introduction

Respiratory diseases represent the second most common disorder requiring veterinary medical attention in adult horses [1]. They are also the second most common ailment in young racehorses [2,3] and result in huge economic losses to the racing industry. Both viral and bacterial infections as well as inflammatory conditions, such as Inflammatory Airway Disease (IAD), are mainly responsible for those respiratory diseases. Young horses are more susceptible to viral infection than older horses [4] and exercise potentiates this risk for viral infection [4,5]. Bacterial infections can occur as a primary disease or secondary to viral infections. IAD is a frequent problem in young sports horses, especially racehorses. Its prevalence varies from 7 to 70% depending on the geographic region and the horse population studied [6-9]. It is most frequently observed in 2 year olds [2,7,10-12] and has been associated with viral and/or bacterial infections [7,10-12]. The underlying pathophysiology of these respiratory diseases, especially the involvement of innate and adaptive immune mechanisms, is currently not well understood. However, intensive training has been reported to alter the innate immune response in the lung and the systemic circulation [13]. We have recently demonstrated that TLR3 mRNA expression as well as TNF-α and IFN-β production were down-regulated in equine pulmonary alveolar macrophages (PAM) from trained horses. On the contrary, TLR4 mRNA expression and cytokine secretion were amplified in blood monocytes.

The lung innate immune defense against pathogens also implicates the airway epithelium which strongly interacts with other resident cells and leukocytes. Indeed, the airway epithelium plays an essential role [14,15] firstly as a physical barrier between the external environment and the host [15,16] and secondly by modulating the inflammatory reaction and the response to pathogens [17]. The ciliated airway epithelium prevents colonization by inhaled bacteria through their physical removal by ciliary clearance and cough, through the presence of antimicrobial proteins in the mucus and through the recruitment of

* Correspondence: linda.frellstedt@ulg.ac.be
[1]Center of Equine Sports Medicine, University of Liege, Liege, Belgium
[2]CIRALE, École Nationale Vétérinaire de Maisons-Alfort, Goustranville, France
Full list of author information is available at the end of the article

phagocytic cells [15,17]. In immune cells, a variety of pathogen recognition receptors (PRR), located on the surface or in intracellular compartments, interact with pathogen-associated molecular patterns (PAMP) and control the host defense mechanisms. Toll-like receptors (TLR) represent important signaling PRR that recognize PAMP [18,19]. TLR2 heterodimerizes with TLR1 or TLR6; TLR1/2 and TLR2/6 recognize molecular pattern specific for gram-positive bacteria. TLR3 mediates the response to double-stranded RNA, a marker of viral infection. TLR4 recognizes bacterial lipopolysaccharide (LPS) specific for gram-negative bacteria. TLR5 responds to flagellin which can be found on flagellated bacteria. TLR7/8 recognizes viral single-stranded RNA. Finally, TLR9 mediates the response to unmethylated DNA (CpG) which can be part of bacteria or viruses [18,19]. Once TLR are stimulated by PAMP, a downstream cascade is activated which results in the production of interferons (IFN), pro-inflammatory cytokines, chemokines, and cytotoxic activities [18,19]. Type I interferons are central to the early antiviral response of virus-infected cells [15] and interfere with viral replication, protein synthesis as well as early cell apoptosis. Activation of TLR is essential for an immediate protection against viral and bacterial infection. Epithelial cells express a large array of TLR and their activation leads to the secretion of a variety of cytokines (IFN, IL-6, TNF-α) and chemokines (CXCL8) [16]. CXCL8 is an essential chemotactic factor for neutrophils and its production is associated with viral, bacterial and fungal infections [16]. The mucosal response, including the innate response, aims to clear the sensed pathogens and to control secondary effects associated with neutrophils and their products [14]. Altogether, this underlines that TLR activation in the airway epithelium is important in order to tightly control the intensity and duration of this response in favor of preventing respiratory lesions [14].

In the interest of defining the physiopathologic role of bronchial epithelial cells in respiratory diseases in horses, ex vivo approaches are needed as previously reported in humans [20]. Few reports describe the use of bronchial epithelial cell culture in horses [21-27] and even fewer have used this technique for the study of equine diseases [21,22,27]. In order to perform this kind of study, we developed a method of culture for equine bronchial epithelial cells (EBEC) using bronchial biopsies collected from living animals. This method offers the possibility to perform repeated sampling. After the development phase of this protocol, we were able to obtain EBEC responsive to TLR ligands similarly to the airway epithelium, at least when considering the innate immune response. Based on this method, we analyzed the impact of intense training and acute exercise on the expression and function of TLR in EBEC to identify their role in equine respiratory diseases. Our results demonstrate that the expression of these receptors was not modified although the production of some cytokines in response to TLR ligands was altered. Using this new culture method, we were able to demonstrate some alteration in the function of EBEC in horses submitted to intense training.

Materials and methods

Horses

Six healthy Standardbred horses (3 mares and 3 geldings, 3 to 6 years old, 495.3 ± 55.2 kg) were used for the first part of the study to develop optimal EBEC culture conditions and EBEC responsiveness in vitro. All horses were determined to be healthy by physical examination, complete blood cell count, serum biochemistry, endoscopic evaluation of the respiratory tract and examination of the tracheal and bronchoalveolar lavage fluid (cytology, bacteriology and virology). We also investigated whether lower airway inflammation would be induced by the biopsy sampling procedure. Daily physical examinations were performed as well as lower airway endoscopy including tracheal washes and broncho-alveolar lavages on day 0 (prior to biopsy sampling) as well as 2 and 8 days after biopsy sampling. All vital parameters remained normal in all horses. None of the horses developed a cough or abnormal mucus secretion. The cytology results of the tracheal washes and broncho-alveolar lavages remained normal in all horses (data not shown). During lower airway endoscopy, we did not observe any local inflammation (reddening, swelling) at the biopsy sites; whereas a fast healing process was detected. On day 8, it was often not possible to identify the biopsy site anymore.

Once the EBEC culture conditions had been defined, eight healthy untrained (UT) Standardbred horses (5 mares and 3 geldings, 2.5 ± 0.5 years, 450 ± 45 kg) were enrolled for the second part of our study. All horses were determined to be healthy by physical examination, complete blood cell count, serum biochemistry, endoscopic evaluation of the respiratory tract and examination of the tracheal and bronchoalveolar lavage fluid (cytology, bacteriology and virology). The horses had been vaccinated (equine herpesvirus 1 and 4, equine influenza, tetanus) and dewormed and were kept in a grass pasture prior to starting the study. During the training period, the horses were stabled individually in well-ventilated stalls on wood shavings. They were fed grass silage and grain. In addition, they had daily access to a large paddock for a minimum of 4 h.

Our protocols were approved by the Animal Ethics Committee of the National Veterinary School of Alfort (agreement number: 13/12/11-9) and the Animal Ethics Committee of the University of Liege (agreement number: 13–1510).

Training protocol

Prior to the start of the study, the horses were kept in a grass pasture for 3 months (untrained = UT). This period allowed the horses to get accustomed to the environment. The horses started with 8 weeks of moderate training (MT), meaning they were exercised on a sand track three times a week. Each training session consisted of a six minute warm-up at 5.5 m/s, then trotting at progressively increasing speeds (7.0 to 9.7 m/s) for 20 min, followed by a recovery period of 3 min at 5.5 m/s. This was followed by the intensive training (IT) period of 8 weeks. They were exercised five times a week. Three sessions per week were performed as during the moderate training period at gradually increasing speeds up to their individual maximum speeds for 20 min. Two sessions per week consisted of interval ("sprint") training at maximal speeds. During these sessions, the horses underwent a warm-up of 15 min at 5.5 m/s, followed by 7 min at 7.0 m/s, then during a period of 10 min the horses maintained speeds of 9.7 to 11.0 m/s with the intercalated intervals (3 × 90 s) at maximal speeds (11.0 to 13.4 m/s), finishing with a recovery period of 3 min at 5.5 m/s. Heart rates, distance and speed were monitored continuously during each training session using a GPS on-board system (Equine CS600X Trotting, Polar Electro France SAS).

Standardized exercise test (SET)

The horses underwent a SET on a treadmill until fatigue prior to and at the end of the training period. The SET was performed as previously published [9]. A fourth step was performed at 11.0 m/s until fatigue.

Reagents

All reagents were purchased from Life Technologies, Paisley, UK unless otherwise stated.

Sample collection

The horses were sedated with detomidine (0.002 mg/kg) and butorphanol (0.005 mg/kg). Lower airway endoscopy was performed (Karl Storz, Utrecht, Netherlands). Bronchial biopsies (2 × 2 mm) were collected between the 1st and 3rd generation bronchi with biopsy forceps (Pentax, Aartselaar, Belgium). The bronchial biopsies were placed in cold DMEM/F-12 medium (Lonza, Verviers, Belgium) supplemented with penicillin (100 IU/mL), streptomycin (100 µg/mL) and amphotericin (0.25 µg/mL). The samples were kept at 4 °C and processed for cell culture within 2 h of collection. Concurrently, bronchial biopsies were placed in RNAlater® and stored at −20 °C until analysis for TLR and cytokine mRNA expression.

In the second part of the study, bronchial biopsies were collected at rest (48 h prior to the SET) between the 1st and 3rd generation bronchi of the left lung and post-exercise (24 h after the SET) between the 1st and 3rd bronchi of the right lung from horses in the untrained and trained condition.

Cell culture

In preliminary experiments, we tested a number of different culture conditions in order to identify optimal culture conditions for EBEC. Tissue culture plates were coated with human placental collagen type I, human placental collagen type IV (Sigma-Aldrich, St. Louis, MO, USA), calf skin collagen G (Biochrom, Merck Millipore, Darmstadt, Germany) as well as a mix of human fibronectin with bovine serum albumin (BSA) (Merck Millipore, Darmstadt, Germany) and collagens. We also used different culture media: BEGM (Promocell, Heidelberg, Germany), LHC-8 medium, DMEM/F-12 with 2% ultroser, a mix of LHC-8 and DMEM/F-12, a mix of BEGM and DMEM/F-12, with and without growth factors (epithelial growth factor, bovine pituitary extract).

After collection, the bronchial biopsies were washed three times in DMEM/F-12 medium. The biopsies were then placed on coated tissue culture plates (6-well plates, NUNC, Thermo Fisher Scientific, Erembodegem-Aalst, Belgium) in a minimal volume of medium supplemented with penicillin (100 IU/mL), streptomycin (100 µg/mL) and amphotericin (0.25 µg/mL) and placed in the incubator at 37 °C with 5% CO_2 for 24–48 h in order to favor the adherence of the biopsy. For the second part of the study, bronchial biopsies were placed on collagen IV coated plates in DMEM/F-12 medium supplemented with 2% ultroser (Pall Life Science, Cergy-Saint-Christophe, France), penicillin (100 IU/mL), streptomycin (100 µg/mL) and amphotericin (0.25 µg/mL). The medium was changed every 2 to 3 days until the cell cultures reached confluency (three to four weeks). The epithelial cell cultures were assessed daily under the light microscope for confirmation of their growth pattern (polygonal shape), and to rule out possible contamination with fibroblasts. We obtained 5×10^5 to 1×10^6 cells from a single explant. Once cultures were confluent, the EBEC were detached with trypsin, placed into DMEM/F-12 medium with 10% fetal bovine serum (FBS; Fisher Scientific, Aalst, Belgium), penicillin (100 IU/mL), streptomycin (100 µg/mL) and amphotericin (0.25 µg/mL). The cells were centrifuged, placed in DMEM/F-12 medium with 2% ultroser and then transferred into 24-well tissue culture plates (1×10^5 cells per well) for cell proliferation and subsequent stimulation with TLR ligands. One aliquot of 1×10^5 EBEC was used for flow cytometry systematically at each passage of cells from each horse. Once confluency was reached again (five to seven days), EBEC were stimulated with TLR2/6, TLR3, TLR4, TLR7/8 and TLR9 ligands (FSL- 100 ng/mL; Poly(I;C)- 50 µg/mL (CAYLA, Toulouse, France); LPS- 100 ng/mL (Sigma-Aldrich, Saint-Louis, MO, USA); Gardiquimod- 1 µg/mL (CAYLA, Toulouse, France);

CpG- 1 μg/mL (composition: 5′-tccatgacgttcctgatgct-3′, class B CpG, Hycult Biotech, Uden, Netherlands), respectively. Systematically, EBEC from one well of non-stimulated cells were used for flow cytometry and EBEC from a second well of non-stimulated and stimulated cells were placed in Trizol® for the assessment of TLR mRNA expression. Only cells from the first passage, that were confirmed to be epithelial cells of excellent purity (at least 95% cytokeratin positive and negative for vimentin), were used for the evaluation of TLR mRNA expression, TLR stimulation and the recovery of supernatants for cytokine secretion.

Primary fibroblasts were grown from deeper bronchial biopsy tissue. They had an accelerated growth rate and reached confluency within 7–10 days.

Light microscopy

The primary EBEC and fibroblast cultures were monitored daily under a phase contrast inverted microscope (Olympus, Tokyo, Japan). The morphology of the EBEC was documented and fibroblast contamination of the EBEC cultures was ruled out.

Flow cytometry

To confirm the EBEC epithelial character, EBEC were assessed systematically during their transfer (first passage) and at the time of stimulation with TLR ligands. EBEC were labeled with anti-cytokeratin antibodies (mouse anti-human cytokeratin, clone MNF116, Dako, Hamburg, Germany). Anti-vimentin antibodies (mouse anti-bovine vimentin, clone Vim3B4, Dako, Hamburg, Germany) were used to confirm the absence of fibroblast contamination. Donkey anti-mouse IgG labeled with Alexa Fluor® 488 dye were used as secondary antibodies.

Once confluent, EBEC were detached from tissue culture plates with trypsin, placed in DMEM/F-12 medium with 10% FBS and cytocentrifuged. The cells were fixed in 1% formaldehyde, washed twice in 0.1% saponin to allow for cell permeabilization and then incubated with anti-cytokeratin or anti-vimentin antibodies for 30 min at 4 °C. The cells were again washed in 0.1% saponin and were incubated with the secondary antibodies for 30 min at 4 °C. Then they were washed twice in PBS and placed in 0.25% formaldehyde solution and analyzed within 24 h. Flow cytometry analysis was performed on a BD Flowcytometer (BD FACSCanto II, BD Biosciences, Erembodegem, Belgium). In all conditions, negative controls were prepared by omitting primary antibodies. The primary fibroblasts were stained with the same antibodies in order to confirm their mesenchymal origin.

Cytokine measurement by ELISA

Cell culture supernatants were assayed for TNF-α (R&D Systems, Abingdon, UK), IFN-β, IL-6 (USCN Life Science Inc., Wuhan, China) and CXCL8 (Kingfisher Biotech Inc., Breda, Netherlands) concentrations with commercially available equine ELISA kits.

Muscle tissue

Microbiopsies of the gluteus medius muscle were obtained as previously described [28]. This tissue served as calibrator/control tissue for the TLR expression as previously described [28] since muscle tissue is known to have the lowest TLR expression within the body tissues [29].

RNA isolation, cDNA synthesis and real-time PCR

RNA was isolated from bronchial biopsies, muscle biopsies and cultured EBEC with Trizol® reagent as described by the manufacturer. Contaminating DNA was eliminated using the Turbo DNA-free kit™. Concentration and quality of RNA were assessed by UV spectrophotometry (Nanodrop® ND2000, Thermo Fisher Scientific, Aalst, Belgium) and a 2100 Bioanalyzer (Agilent Technologies, Waldbronn, Germany). UV spectrophotometry allowed the determination of the ratio of absorbance at 260 nm and 280 nm. This ratio is used to assess the purity of RNA. A ratio of 1.8-2.0 was accepted as indication of "good quality" RNA. The quality of the RNA was further assessed by a 2100 Bioanalyzer. Only RNA samples with an RNA integrity number (RIN) ≥ 9 and a 28S:18S ratio of $> 2:1$ qualified as "good quality" RNA and were used for real-time PCR. cDNA were generated as previously described [28]. Gene expression of TLR1-9, fibroblast growth factor-1 (FGF-1), fibroblast specific protein-1 (FSP-1), E-cadherin, keratin19, IFN-β, TNF-α, IL-6 and CXCL8 was quantified by real-time PCR using Absolute Blue qPCR SYBR Green Mix (Fisher Scientific, Aalst, Belgium) on an Applied Biosystems 7900 HT thermocycler (Applied Biosystems, Carlsbad, CA, USA). Equine gene specific primers were designed from available published sequences [13,26,30,31] or designed in silico (Table 1). Specificity of PCR was confirmed by melting curve analysis, agarose gel electrophoresis and the absence of signals in RT minus RT reactions. All primers designed for this study were located in single exons except the primer for CXCL8 (2 separate exons). The absence of signals in RT minus RT reactions and the fact that all primers, except for one, were located in single exons confirm the absence of DNA contamination. Real-time quantitative PCR data for TLR1-9, FGF-1, FSP-1, E-cadherin, keratin19, IFN-β, TNF-α, IL-6 and CXCL8 were normalized to the geometric mean of three housekeeping genes (PGK1 (phosphoglycerokinase 1), PPIA (cyclophilin A), RPLO (ribosomal protein L0)) using qbase + software (Biogazelle, Zwijnaarde, Belgium). Muscle tissue was used as a calibrator for the characterization of TLR mRNA expression in bronchial

Table 1 Primer sequences used for real-time PCR analysis of mRNA expression of target and housekeeping genes

Name	Primer sequences forward/reverse (5′ to 3′)	Product (bp)	Exon	Reference
PGK1	CGTCAAAGACCTGATGTCCA	98	1	In silico designed
	TCTTGGCATGCTCATCAAAC			
PPIA	TGGGGAGAAATTTGATGATGA	116	1	In silico designed
	TGGCAGTGCAGATGAAGAAC			
RPLO	CCAAGGTTGAAGCAAAGGAA	99	1	[13]
	AAAGCTGGCTGAATTGGTTG			
FGF-1	AGAAGAATGGGAGCTGCAAA	138	1	In silico designed
	GGACTCCTTCAGGCTCCTCT			
FSP-1	GCCCTGGATGTGATGGTATC	93	1	In silico designed
	CAGCAGCTCCTTTAGCTCTGA			
E-cadherin	ATCCGCAGCCTCATATCATC	125	1	In silico designed
	CCCACCTGGGTCATTGTACT			
Keratin19	GAAGGAGACCATGCAGAACC	120	1	In silico designed
	CCCTGCTTCAGGTACCAGTC			
IFN-beta	CCCCGAGGACACAATGAACT	81	1	In silico designed
	ACCAATGCAGCATCCTCCTT			
TNF-alpha	AAGGACATCATGAGCACTGAA	80	1	In silico designed
	GGGCCCCCTGCCTTCT			
IL-6	CCTGGTGATGGCTACTGCTT	102	1	In silico designed
	TGCTGTTTGGTTTTGTCTGC			
CXCL8	TTGGCCGTCTTCCTGCTTT	101	2 Intron (959 bp)	In silico designed
	GGTTTGGAGTGCGTCTTGATG			

biopsies and EBEC. The dCT results were compared to the calibrator samples to derive the relative quantities.

Statistical analysis

TNF-α, IFN-β, IL-6 and CXCL8 concentrations as well as relative gene expression data were analyzed by a global linear mixed model (SAS, Cary, NC, USA). A general linear mixed model was used for data analysis because it combines a random effect (horses) and fixed effects (training, strenuous exercise, treatment with TLR ligands). The mixed model allows considering the random nature of the horses sample and accordingly, correcting for potential individual differences, while modeling the other (fixed) effects of interest in our study. In such a multifactorial and unbalanced design, results were reported as least square means (LSmeans) ± associated SE instead of simple means in order to correct each factor for possible contamination due to the other factors of the model. Differences were considered to be significant when p value was less than 0.05.

Results

Growth and characterization of EBEC in vitro

Homogenous cell populations consisting of non-ciliated EBEC were cultured successfully using an explant method. Our preliminary tests showed that the EBEC grew better on collagen IV coated plates in DMEM/F-12 medium with 2% ultroser (Table 2). The supplementation with growth factors had no effect on the growth of EBEC in our model. The cells had a polygonal shape which is typical for the morphology of epithelial cells (Figure 1A). The epithelial cell character was confirmed by positive staining for cytokeratin (Figure 1D) during each step of the EBEC culture (passage of EBEC and at time of stimulation) and during each phase of the study (untrained and trained horses). Fibroblast contamination represents a common problem in epithelial cell culture. Our data revealed that EBEC are negative for vimentin in comparison with cultures of fibroblasts (Figure 1D). Fibroblasts strongly expressed mRNA encoding for FGF-1 and FSP-1, whereas these mRNA were expressed about 100–1000 times less in EBEC (Figure 1B). In contrast, EBEC strongly expressed E-cadherin and keratin19 (Figure 1C). The EBEC phenotype was further confirmed by TLR mRNA expression, particularly of TLR3 (as discussed in the following paragraph). Figure 2 shows that EBEC have a similar pattern of TLR mRNA expression as the bronchial epithelial biopsy tissue itself. Furthermore, we show that the TLR mRNA expression was neither altered by our culture technique (Figure 2) nor by training of the horses (Figure 3B).

Table 2 Comparison of different cell culture conditions for the in vitro culture of EBEC

Matrix coating medium	Collagen I	Collagen IV	Collagen I + collagen IV	Collagen G	Fibronectin + BSA + collagen I	Fibronectin + BSA + collagen IV
BEGM	(+)	(+)	(+)	(+)	-	-
LHC-8	+(+)	++	+	+	-	-
DMEM/F12 + 2% Ultroser	+(+)	+++	++	+(+)	-	-
DMEM/F12 + 10% FBS	-	-	-	-	-	-
50% BEGM +50% DMEM/F12	+	+	+	+	-	-
50% LHC-8 + 50% DMEM/F12	+	(+)	+	(+)	-	-

No growth - ; limited growth for 10 days only (+) ; growth during 10 days only + ; growth during the entire culture period ++/+++.

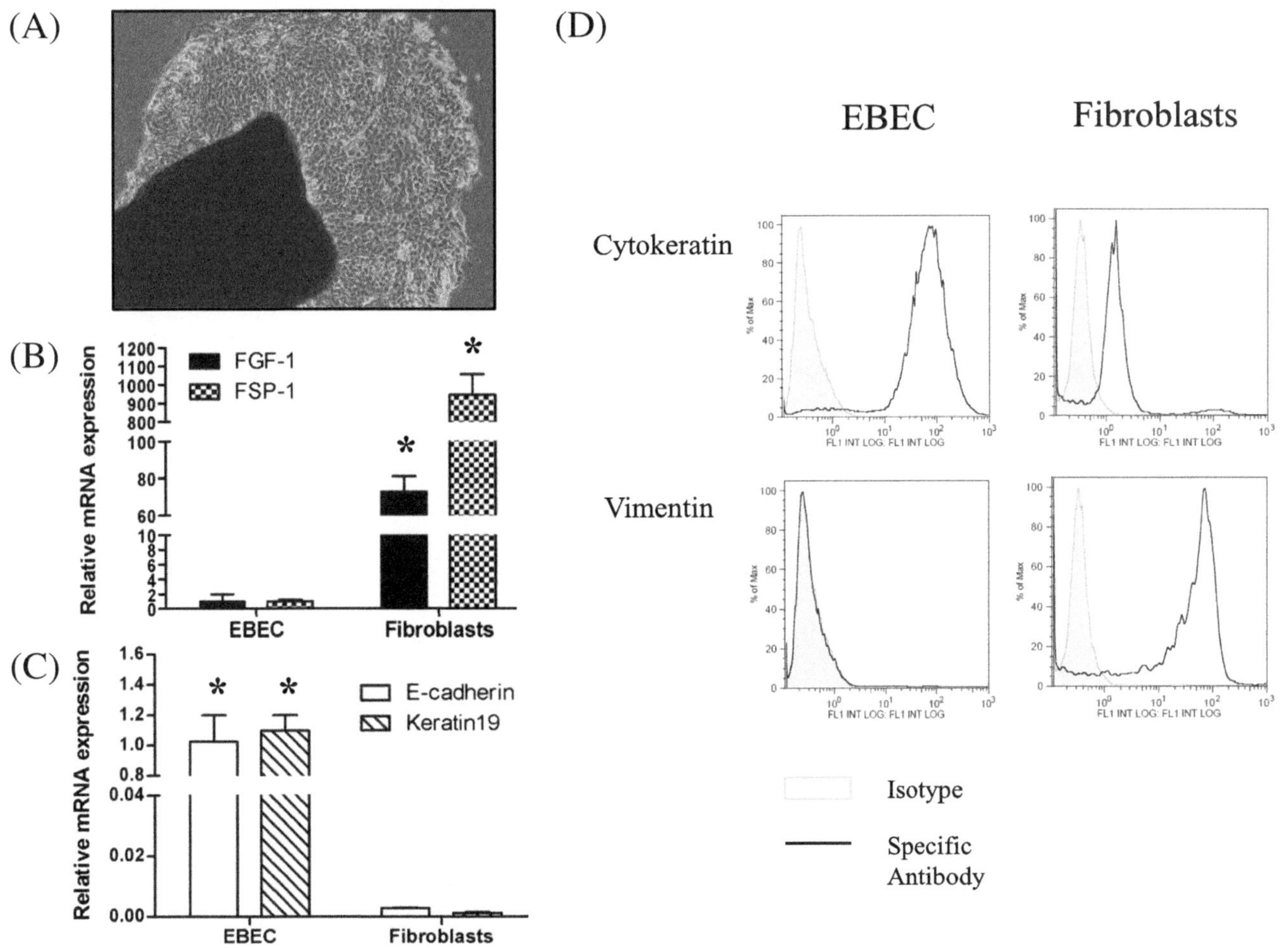

Figure 1 Characterization of equine bronchial epithelial cells (EBEC). (A) Morphological appearance of EBEC cultures 7 days after plating (phase contrast microscopy; objective magnification: x4). The biopsy is situated on the left bottom corner of the image. The biopsy is surrounded by growing EBEC. Note the polygonal shape of EBEC. **(B)** Relative mRNA expression of Fibroblast growth factor-1 (FGF-1) and Fibroblast specific protein-1 (FSP-1) in EBEC and fibroblasts. Significant differences ($P < 0.05$) in mRNA expression are identified with * for differences between EBEC and fibroblasts. **(C)** Relative mRNA expression of E-cadherin and Keratin19 in EBEC and fibroblasts. Significant differences ($P < 0.05$) in mRNA expression are identified with * for differences between EBEC and fibroblasts. **(D)** Flow cytometry analysis of in vitro cultured EBEC and fibroblasts for the epithelial cell marker cytokeratin and the mesenchymal cell marker vimentin. **(C-D)** EBEC were assessed at their first passage (4–6 weeks of culture). Fibroblasts were assessed at their first passage (7–10 days of culture). The phenotype and purity of EBEC were maintained during the study.

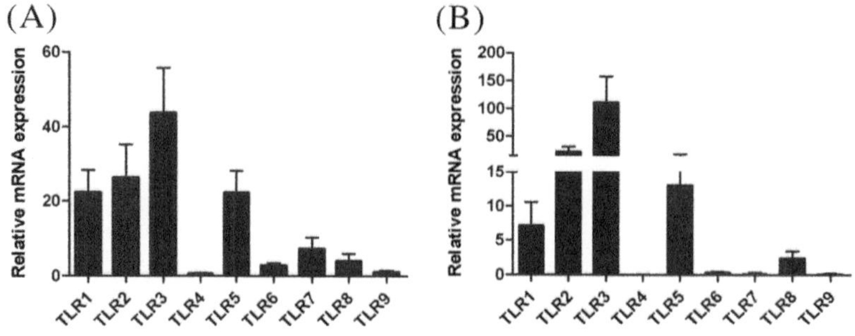

Figure 2 Relative mRNA expression of TLR1-9 in bronchial biopsies (A) and EBEC (B). Muscle tissue is used as a calibrator for TLR mRNA expression (muscle tissue = 1). Note that the profile of mRNA expression of TLR1-9 in bronchial biopsies and EBEC is similar, although the magnitude of TLR mRNA expression is amplified after in vitro culture of 4–6 weeks duration (first passage).

Our results indicate that our EBEC cultures had excellent purity, and that their phenotype was maintained during the study.

TLR expression in bronchial biopsies and in cultures of EBEC

To estimate the relevance of our culture model, we compared the expression of TLR in bronchial biopsies and EBEC. As previously described in EBEC [32,33], TLR3 was the most strongly expressed TLR at the mRNA level in bronchial biopsies (Figure 2A) as well as in EBEC cultured in vitro (Figure 2B), followed by TLR2, TLR5 and TLR1. However, the magnitude of TLR mRNA expression was amplified during in vitro culture. In both types of samples, the expression of TLR4, TLR6, TLR7 and TLR9 was low and nearly undetectable. Thus, we conclude that the pattern of TLR mRNA expression was similar between bronchial biopsies and EBEC.

Cytokine mRNA expression in EBEC stimulated in vitro with TLR ligands

To analyze the responsiveness of EBEC, we evaluated the cytokine production after stimulation with TLR ligands. The IFN-β mRNA expression was significantly increased only by treatment with Poly(I:C), a TLR3 ligand, after 3 ($P < 0.0001$) and 6 ($P < 0.005$) hours of incubation (Figure 4A). Treatment of EBEC with FSL ($P < 0.0003$), LPS ($P < 0.035$) and Poly(I:C) ($P < 0.0004$) induced a significant increase in mRNA expression of TNF-α (Figure 4B) after 3 hours of incubation. The mRNA expression of IL-6 (Figure 4C) and CXCL8 (Figure 4D) was significantly upregulated after 3 and 6 h of incubation

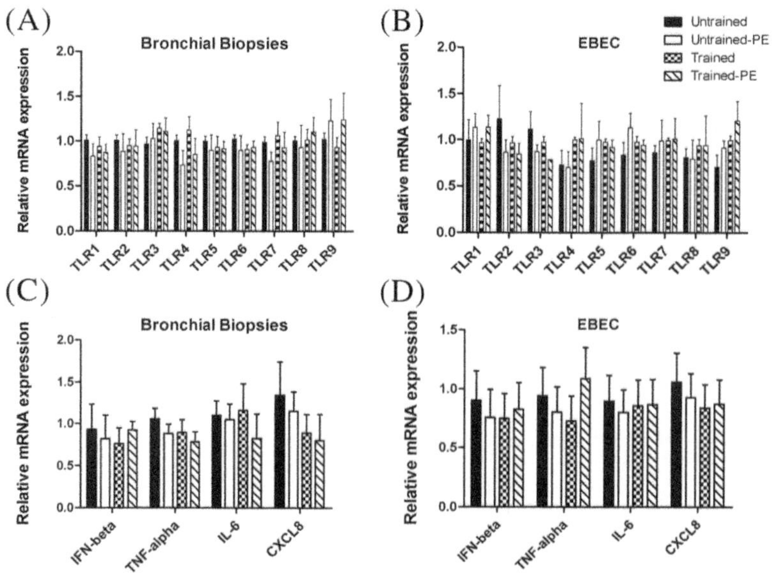

Figure 3 Relative mRNA expression of TLR1-9 and four cytokines in bronchial biopsies and cultured EBEC from untrained and trained horses. The relative mRNA expression of TLR1-9 **(A,B)** and four cytokines (IFN-β, TNF-α, IL-6, CXCL8) **(C,D)** was evaluated directly in bronchial biopsies **(A,C)** and in non-stimulated cultures of EBEC **(B,D)** obtained from biopsies collected from untrained and trained horses, at rest as well as after an acute exercise (PE = post-exercise). No significant differences were observed.

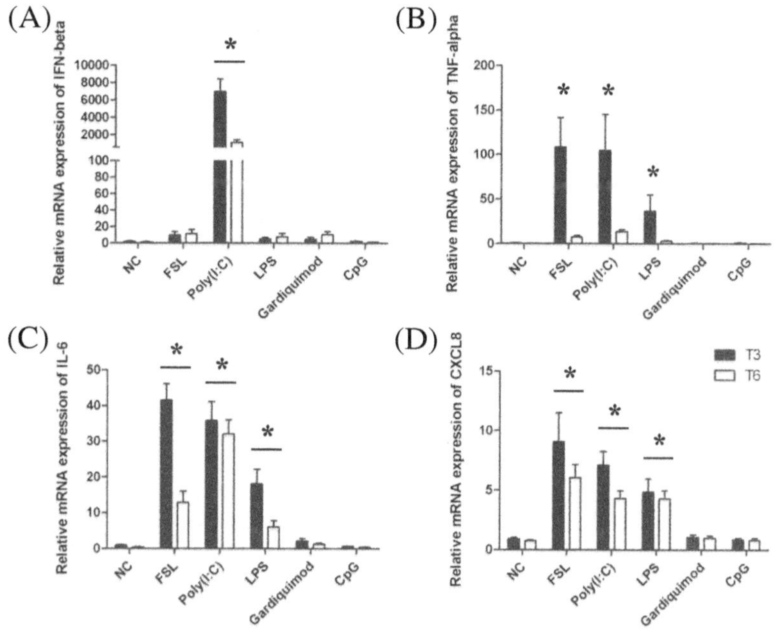

Figure 4 Relative mRNA expression of IFN-β, TNF-α, IL-6 and CXCL8 after stimulation of EBEC with TLR ligands. EBEC were stimulated with FSL, Poly(I:C), LPS, Gardiquimod and CpG. The mRNA expression of IFN-β **(A)**, TNF-α **(B)**, IL-6 **(C)** and CXCL8 **(D)** was evaluated after 3 and 6 h of incubation. Significant differences ($P < 0.05$) in mRNA expression are identified with * for differences between non-stimulated cells (NC) and cells stimulated with TLR ligands.

when the EBEC had been treated with FSL ($P < 0.006$; $P < 0.0001$), Poly(I:C) ($P < 0.0001$; $P < 0.0006$) and LPS ($P < 0.02$; $P < 0.0013$). Treatment of EBEC with Gardiquimod and CpG did not induce the mRNA expression of these cytokines (Figures 4A-D). While Gardiquimod and CpG represent appropriate TLR7/8 and TLR9 ligands, we conclude that the low expression of TLR7/8 and TLR9 in EBEC accounts for the non-responsiveness of EBEC to these ligands.

Cytokine production in EBEC stimulated in vitro with TLR ligands

Because the mRNA expression of cytokines is sometimes not correlated with the protein secretion in certain cells, we decided to examine the cytokine production in EBEC. Since the peak in cytokine mRNA expression was observed after 3 h of incubation, the cytokine production was measured after 6 h of stimulation. As previously reported [34], non-stimulated EBEC produced almost non-detectable levels of IFN-β, TNF-α and IL-6 but had an important baseline secretion of CXCL8 (Figures 5A-D). Only stimulation with Poly(I:C) significantly increased the production of IFN-β ($P < 0.0001$) (Figure 5A) and IL-6 ($P < 0.0001$) (Figure 5C). TNF-α secretion (Figure 5B) was significantly induced by treatment with FSL ($P < 0.0003$) and Poly(I:C) ($P < 0.0001$). CXCL8 secretion was significantly amplified by stimulation of EBEC with FSL ($P < 0.0001$), Poly(I:C) ($P < 0.0005$) and LPS ($P < 0.0005$) (Figure 5D). Treatment with Gardiquimod and CpG had no or limited effects on cytokine secretion (Figures 5A-D).

Since EBEC express low or undetectable levels of TLR7/8 and TLR9 and they did not respond to stimulation with a TLR7/8-ligand (Gardiquimod) or TLR9-ligand (CpG), for the second part of the study we focused on TLR2/6, TLR3, TLR4 in order to account for the most common respiratory pathogens in horses [13].

Training has no effect on TLR or cytokine mRNA expression in bronchial biopsies and non-stimulated EBEC

The TLR mRNA expression was examined directly in bronchial biopsy tissue and in non-stimulated EBEC cultured in vitro. Training or acute strenuous exercise had no effect on the TLR mRNA expression in either of them (Figure 3A and B). We also evaluated cytokine mRNA expression directly in bronchial biopsies and in non-stimulated EBEC in order to assess if training or acute exercise had an immediate effect on the baseline cytokine mRNA expression. No significant differences were observed after training or acute strenuous exercise regarding the mRNA expression of IFN-β, TNF-α, IL-6 or CXCL8 (Figure 3C and D).

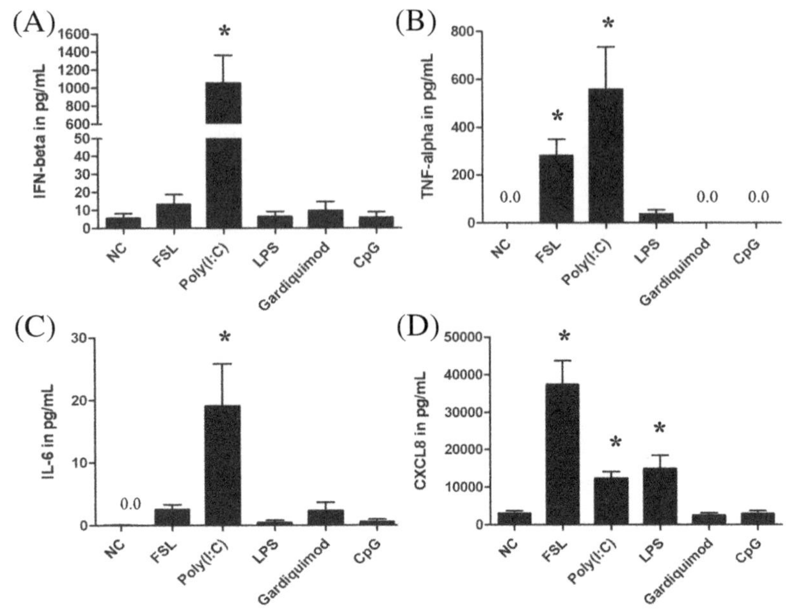

Figure 5 Production of IFN-β, TNF-α, IL-6 and CXCL8 after stimulation of EBEC with TLR ligands. EBEC were stimulated with FSL, Poly(I:C), LPS, Gardiquimod and CpG. The protein secretion of IFN-β **(A)**, TNF-α **(B)**, IL-6 **(C)** and CXCL8 **(D)** after 6 h incubation of EBEC in medium alone (NC) and after treatment with TLR ligands (FSL, Poly(I:C), LPS, Gardiquimod, CpG). Significant differences ($P < 0.05$) are identified with * for differences between non-treated cells (NC) and cells treated with TLR ligands.

Training alters the cytokine response to TLR ligands in EBEC

In order to assess the effect of training and/or acute exercise on the innate immune response, the cultured EBEC were treated with TLR2/6, TLR3 and TLR4 agonists. EBEC collected after an acute exercise responded to TLR ligands in a similar manner as the controls (Figures 6A-D). In contrast, the EBEC obtained from trained horses showed an increased secretion of IFN-β ($P < 0.0003$) (Figure 6A) and a lower production of TNF-α and IL-6 after treatment with FSL ($P < 0.05$; $P < 0.05$) and Poly(I:C) ($P < 0.0003$; $P < 0.01$) (Figure 6B and C). The TNF-α secretion of FSL- and Poly(I:C)-stimulated EBEC from trained horses after an acute exercise was restored to a level similar to untrained horses, whereas the IL-6 production was still strongly decreased (Figure 6C). The response to LPS for IL-6 and CXCL8 was not modified. Training and acute exercise had no effect on the CXCL8 secretion induced by TLR ligands (Figure 6D).

Discussion

We report the successful culture of EBEC in vitro from bronchial biopsies obtained in live horses. Our model allows us to culture EBEC from small biopsies obtained from the bronchial epithelium. EBEC do not cause any lower airway inflammation and do not present a risk for the horses. The in vitro cultured EBEC are responsive to TLR activation, therefore, they facilitate the investigation of pathophysiologic conditions in longitudinal studies as described in this work.

Previously, other authors have reported the successful culture of airway epithelial cells in horses [21-26]. The use of FBS in their culture medium was described and appeared to favor tight junction formation in their studies [25]. As shown by others [35-39], we found that FBS increased the contamination of EBEC cultures with fibroblasts, accelerated fibroblast growth and indirectly limited EBEC growth. Specific epithelial cell culture media are commonly used in human and veterinary research and were tested in our study. These defined media as well as specific growth factors did not support the growth of EBEC in our conditions. We hypothesize that the growth of EBEC from bronchial biopsies is even more fragile and sensitive than primary cell culture of airway epithelial cells recovered by digestion of bronchial epithelial tissue in which case large quantities of cells are made available. We show that DMEM/F-12 medium supplemented with a serum substitute (Ultroser G®) appeared to be the most appropriate medium for the culture of EBEC as we previously described in human BEC [20]. In this condition, we detected no detectable contamination by fibroblasts in our cultures. Moreover, the phenotype and cell purity were maintained during the culture as confirmed in a previous report using the same methodology in clinical immunology [20].

As expected, TLR3 was the most importantly expressed TLR at the mRNA level in EBEC, followed by TLR2,

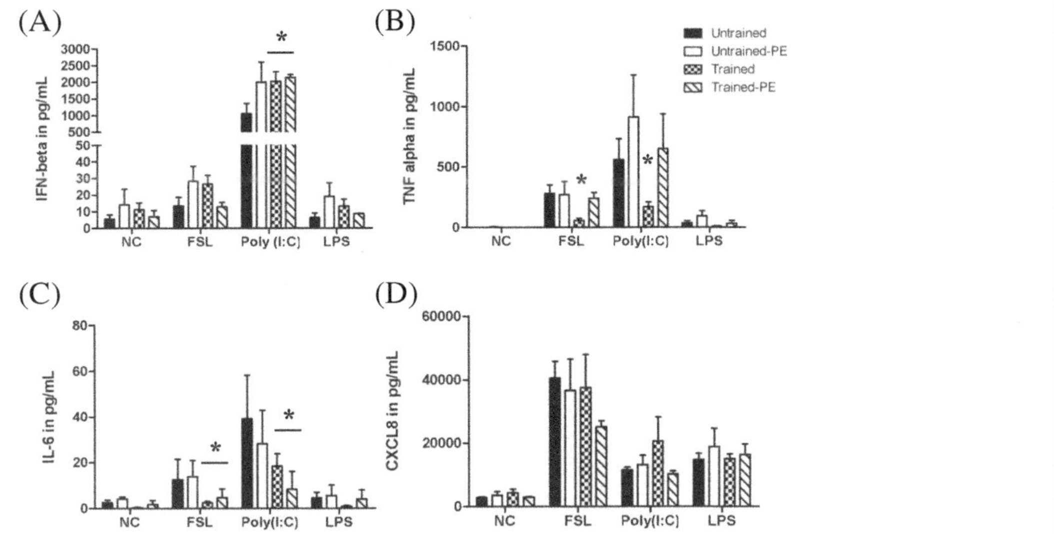

Figure 6 Ex vivo production of IFN-β, TNF-α, IL-6 and CXCL8 in EBEC from untrained and trained horses. EBEC were obtained from biopsies collected from untrained and trained horses, at rest as well as after an acute exercise (PE = post-effort). EBEC were cultured in vitro and stimulated with FSL, Poly(I:C) and LPS. We report the secretion of IFN-β **(A)**, TNF-α **(B)**, IL-6 **(C)** and CXCL8 **(D)** after 6 h of incubation in EBEC in medium alone (NC) and activated cells. Significant differences ($P < 0.05$) are identified with * for differences from EBEC in untrained horses.

TLR5 and TLR1. TLR4 and TLR6-9 were expressed at very low levels. TLR1-6 proved to be functional in our study with Poly(I:C) being the most efficient stimuli as a TLR3 agonist. These findings were in agreement with other studies [32,33,40]. Previously, Quintana et al. [26] described a model for the culture of equine respiratory epithelial cells and examined the expression of TLR1-4 and TLR6-10 mRNA. They reported decreased mRNA expression of TLR8-10 after 4 weeks of in vitro culture. In our model, the profile of TLR mRNA expression remained similar in EBEC when compared to bronchial biopsies although the magnitude of TLR mRNA expression was amplified during in vitro culture. Nonetheless, TLR3 was still the most importantly expressed TLR (also with the highest responsiveness) after several weeks of culture. The stimulation of TLR3 activates the transcription factors NF-κB and interferon regulatory factor 3 (IRF3) which significantly increase IFN-β, TNF-α, IL-6 and CXCL8 production confirming the importance of EBEC in the antiviral defense mechanisms of the lung [41]. Type-I IFN will inhibit viral replication, whereas the proinflammatory cytokines (TNF-α, IL-6) and chemokines (CXCL8) play important roles in immune cell recruitment. The mRNA expression of TLR4 appears to be lower in EBEC compared to its expression in human bronchial epithelial cells (HBEC) [32,33,40]. This could represent a protective mechanism in EBEC since horses are continuously exposed to large quantities of dust and organic particulates (shavings, straw, hay) that contain endotoxin [21]. Nevertheless, LPS stimulation induced the secretion of IL-6 and at a lower level TNF-α underlining the functionality of TLR4. Furthermore, Ainsworth et al. reported an upregulation of TLR4 in bronchial epithelial cells of horses with recurrent airway obstruction (RAO) which renders them more sensitive to such endotoxin exposure. We also report that TLR7-9 are not functional in EBEC as confirmed by the treatment with TLR7-9 agonists. This was in agreement with previous publications in HBEC [33,34].

The effect of training and acute exercise on TLR-associated airway epithelial cell function has not been reported previously. Several researchers have examined the effect of exercising in a cold environment on the airway epithelium. Bronchial epithelial cell damage, apoptosis, loss of ciliated epithelial cells and airway remodeling have been described in sled dogs [42] and horses [43]. In this study, neither training nor acute strenuous exercise had an effect on the mRNA expression at baseline of TLR or cytokines in bronchial biopsy tissue and EBEC. Our data underline that even though some damage can be observed in airway epithelium after exercise, this was not associated with airway inflammation and modulation of TLR mRNA expression. Only the exposure to TLR agonists, which mimicked experimental bacterial/viral infection, revealed altered EBEC function in cells from trained horses. Intense training but not acute exercise impaired the secretion of TNF-α and IL-6 only in response to FSL and Poly(I:C). FSL mimics infection with gram + bacteria, whereas Poly (I:C) mimics viral infection, thereby representing the most common equine pulmonary pathogens. The down-regulated production of pro-inflammatory cytokines could be caused by secretion of anti-inflammatory cytokines as suggested by others [44]. We did not evaluate anti-inflammatory cytokines (IL-10, IL-1ra, TGF-β) in this study, and therefore cannot argue their importance here. The decreased TNF-α secretion might also suggest a defect in cell recruitment by EBEC in trained horses. TNF-α is one of the first cytokines produced after stimulation with TLR ligands, exposure to pathogens or other irritants. It then stimulates the secretion of other cytokines and chemokines (CCL2, CCL3) that result in the recruitment of monocytes and their differentiation into dendritic cells and tissue macrophages. This alteration in cell recruitment might play an important role in limiting the lung defense mechanism and therefore, represent an essential mechanism in organ-specific regulation of immunity [45,46]. In contrast, IFN-β production by EBEC was increased after training. We recently described decreased TLR3 mRNA expression and decreased IFN-β production in equine PAM after training [13]. The increased IFN-β secretion by EBEC might reflect a compensatory mechanism for the low pulmonary IFN-β levels in trained horses. Altogether, the decreased type I IFN and cytokine secretion in the lung from trained horses might favor the development of viral infection and thereby, might increase secondary bacterial infection in the lung. As already mentioned in our previous work [13], our data show that the type and the intensity of the exercise (acute exercise/training) as well as the environmental conditions play an important role in the innate immune defense.

In conclusion, we report a successful model for the culture of EBEC in vitro that can be applied to the investigation of pathophysiologic conditions in longitudinal studies. These EBEC present a profile of expression and function of TLR similar to what we can find in bronchial biopsies and in other cell culture models. Training altered the IFN-β, TNF-α and IL-6 secretion in response to TLR2 and TLR3 ligands in EBEC and, therefore, may have important effects on immune cell recruitment in exercising horses. Altogether, this mechanism may be implicated in the increased risk for viral and bacterial infections observed in sport horses.

Abbreviations
BSA: Bovine serum albumin; CpG: Unmethylated CpG dinucleotides; EBEC: Equine bronchial epithelial cells; FBS: Fetal bovine serum; FGF-1: Fibroblast growth factor-1; FSL: Synthetic diacylated lipoprotein; FSP-1: Fibroblast specific protein-1; HBEC: Human bronchial epithelial cells; IAD: Inflammatory airway disease; IFN: Interferon; IT: Intensive training; LPS: Lipopolysaccharide; MT: Moderate training; PAM: Pulmonary alveolar macrophages; PAMP: Pathogen-associated molecular pattern; Poly(I:C): Polyinosine-polycytidadylic acid; PRR: Pathogen recognition receptor; RAO: Recurrent airway obstruction; SET: Standardized exercise test; TLR: Toll-like receptor; UT: Untrained.

Competing interests
The authors declare that they have no competing interests.

Authors' contributions
LF performed all experiments, data analysis and drafted the manuscript. PG and GK participated in preliminary investigations and the first part of the study. PG also advised on study design, participated in data analysis and in drafting the manuscript. AH, CD, DP, FB, PL, TA advised on study design and reviewed the manuscript. DP designed equine primer sets. All authors read and approved the manuscript.

Acknowledgements
The authors thank the University of Liege, the GIGA, the Pasteur Institute in Lille, the ANSES laboratory in Goustranville, Raja Fares, Ilham Sbai and Jean-Clement Bustin for their support during the study. We also acknowledge Frederic Farnir at the University of Liege for his help with the statistical analysis.

Author details
[1]Center of Equine Sports Medicine, University of Liege, Liege, Belgium. [2]CIRALE, École Nationale Vétérinaire de Maisons-Alfort, Goustranville, France. [3]Institut Pasteur de Lille, Centre d'Infection et d'Immunité de Lille, Lille, France. [4]Université Lille Nord de France, Lille, France. [5]Centre National de la Recherche Scientifique, UMR8204 Lille, France. [6]Institut National de la Santé et de la Recherche Médicale, U1019 Lille, France. [7]Institut Fédératif de Recherche 142, Lille, France. [8]Anses – Dozulé, Equine Pathology Laboratory, Virology Unit, Goustranville, France. [9]Laboratory of Cellular and Molecular Immunology, GIGA-Research, University of Liege, Liege, Belgium.

References

1. Traub-Dargatz JL, Salman MD, Voss JL: **Medical problems of adult horses, as ranked by equine practitioners.** *J Am Vet Med Assoc* 1991, **198:**1745–1747.
2. Wilsher S, Allen WR, Wood JL: **Factors associated with failure of thoroughbred horses to train and race.** *Equine Vet J* 2006, **38:**113–118.
3. Rossdale PD, Hopes R, Digby NJ, Offord K: **Epidemiological study of wastage among racehorses 1982 and 1983.** *Vet Rec* 1985, **116:**66–69.
4. Morley PS, Townsend HG, Bogdan JR, Haines DM: **Risk factors for disease associated with influenza virus infections during three epidemics in horses.** *J Am Vet Med Assoc* 2000, **216:**545–550.
5. Folsom RW, Littlefield-Chabaud MA, French DD, Pourciau SS, Mistric L, Horohov DW: **Exercise alters the immune response to equine influenza virus and increases susceptibility to infection.** *Equine Vet J* 2001, **33:**664–669.
6. Cardwell JM, Wood JL, Smith KC, Newton JR: **Descriptive results from a longitudinal study of airway inflammation in British National Hunt racehorses.** *Equine Vet J* 2011, **43:**750–755.
7. Wood JL, Newton JR, Chanter N, Mumford JA: **Inflammatory airway disease, nasal discharge and respiratory infections in young British racehorses.** *Equine Vet J* 2005, **37:**236–242.
8. Allen KJ, Tremaine WH, Franklin SH: **Prevalence of inflammatory airway disease in national hunt horses referred for investigation of poor athletic performance.** *Equine Vet J Suppl* 2006, **36:**529–534.
9. Richard EA, Fortier GD, Pitel PH, Dupuis MC, Valette JP, Art T, Denoix JM, Lekeux PM, Erck EV: **Sub-clinical diseases affecting performance in Standardbred trotters: diagnostic methods and predictive parameters.** *Vet J* 2010, **184:**282–289.
10. Wood JL, Newton JR, Chanter N, Mumford JA: **Association between respiratory disease and bacterial and viral infections in British racehorses.** *J Clin Microbiol* 2005, **43:**120–126.
11. Christley RM, Hodgson DR, Rose RJ, Wood JL, Reids SW, Whitear KG, Hodgson JL: **A case–control study of respiratory disease in Thoroughbred racehorses in Sydney, Australia.** *Equine Vet J* 2001, **33:**256–264.
12. Burrell MH, Wood JL, Whitwell KE, Chanter N, Mackintosh ME, Mumford JA: **Respiratory disease in thoroughbred horses in training: the relationships between disease and viruses, bacteria and environment.** *Vet Rec* 1996, **139:**308–313.
13. Frellstedt L, Waldschmidt I, Gosset P, Desmet C, Pirottin D, Bureau F, Farnir F, Franck T, Dupuis-Tricaud MC, Lekeux P, Art T: **Training modifies innate immune responses in blood monocytes and in pulmonary alveolar macrophages.** *Am J Respir Cell Mol Biol* 2014, **51:**135–142.
14. Parker D, Prince A: **Innate immunity in the respiratory epithelium.** *Am J Respir Cell Mol Biol* 2011, **45:**189–201.
15. Vareille M, Kieninger E, Edwards MR, Regamey N: **The airway epithelium: soldier in the fight against respiratory viruses.** *Clin Microbiol Rev* 2011, **24:**210–229.
16. Proud D, Leigh R: **Epithelial cells and airway diseases.** *Immunol Rev* 2011, **242:**186–204.

17. Diamond G, Legarda D, Ryan LK: **The innate immune response of the respiratory epithelium.** *Immunol Rev* 2000, **173**:27–38.
18. Akira S, Uematsu S, Takeuchi O: **Pathogen recognition and innate immunity.** *Cell* 2006, **124**:783–801.
19. Gleeson M, McFarlin B, Flynn M: **Exercise and Toll-like receptors.** *Exerc Immunol Rev* 2006, **12**:34–53.
20. Pichavant M, Charbonnier AS, Taront S, Brichet A, Wallaert B, Pestel J, Tonnel AB, Gosset P: **Asthmatic bronchial epithelium activated by the proteolytic allergen Der p 1 increases selective dendritic cell recruitment.** *J Allergy Clin Immunol* 2005, **115**:771–778.
21. Ainsworth DM, Matychak M, Reyner CL, Erb HN, Young JC: **Effects of in vitro exposure to hay dust on the gene expression of chemokines and cell-surface receptors in primary bronchial epithelial cell cultures established from horses with chronic recurrent airway obstruction.** *Am J Vet Res* 2009, **70**:365–372.
22. Ainsworth DM, Reyner CL: **Effects of in vitro exposure to autologous blood and serum on expression of interleukin-8, interleukin-1beta, and chemokine (C-X-C motif) ligand 2 in equine primary bronchial epithelial cell cultures.** *Am J Vet Res* 2012, **73**:296–301.
23. Schwab UE, Fulcher ML, Randell SH, Flaminio MJ, Russell DG: **Equine bronchial epithelial cells differentiate into ciliated and mucus producing cells in vitro.** *In Vitro Cell Dev Biol Anim* 2010, **46**:102–106.
24. Abraham G, Shibeshi W, Ungemach FR: **Identification and characterization of beta-adrenergic receptors in isolated primary equine tracheal epithelial cells.** *Pulm Pharmacol Ther* 2011, **24**:174–181.
25. Abraham G, Zizzadoro C, Kacza J, Ellenberger C, Abs V, Franke J, Schoon HA, Seeger J, Tesfaigzi Y, Ungemach FR: **Growth and differentiation of primary and passaged equine bronchial epithelial cells under conventional and air-liquid-interface culture conditions.** *BMC Vet Res* 2011, **7**:26.
26. Quintana AM, Landolt GA, Annis KM, Hussey GS: **Immunological characterization of the equine airway epithelium and of a primary equine airway epithelial cell culture model.** *Vet Immunol Immunopathol* 2011, **140**:226–236.
27. Soboll Hussey G, Ashton LV, Quintana AM, Lunn DP, Goehring LS, Annis K, Landolt G: **Innate immune responses of airway epithelial cells to infection with Equine herpesvirus-1.** *Vet Microbiol* 2014, **170**:28–38.
28. Waldschmidt I, Pirottin D, Art T, Audigie F, Bureau F, Tosi I, El Abbas S, Farnir F, Richard E, Dupuis MC: **Experimental model of equine alveolar macrophage stimulation with TLR ligands.** *Vet Immunol Immunopathol* 2013, **155**:30–37.
29. Zarember KA, Godowski PJ: **Tissue expression of human Toll-like receptors and differential regulation of Toll-like receptor mRNAs in leukocytes in response to microbes, their products, and cytokines.** *J Immunol* 2002, **168**:554–561.
30. Gornik K, Moore P, Figueiredo M, Vandenplas M: **Expression of Toll-like receptors 2, 3, 4, 6, 9, and MD-2 in the normal equine cornea, limbus, and conjunctiva.** *Vet Ophthalmol* 2011, **14**:80–85.
31. Mignot CC, Pirottin D, Farnir F, de Moffarts B, Molitor C, Lekeux P, Art T: **Effect of strenuous exercise and ex vivo TLR3 and TLR4 stimulation on inflammatory gene expression in equine pulmonary leukocytes.** *Vet Immunol Immunopathol* 2012, **147**:127–135.
32. Koff JL, Shao MX, Ueki IF, Nadel JA: **Multiple TLRs activate EGFR via a signaling cascade to produce innate immune responses in airway epithelium.** *Am J Physiol Lung Cell Mol Physiol* 2008, **294**:L1068–L1075.
33. Sha Q, Truong-Tran AQ, Plitt JR, Beck LA, Schleimer RP: **Activation of airway epithelial cells by toll-like receptor agonists.** *Am J Respir Cell Mol Biol* 2004, **31**:358–364.
34. Mayer AK, Muehmer M, Mages J, Gueinzius K, Hess C, Heeg K, Bals R, Lang R, Dalpke AH: **Differential recognition of TLR-dependent microbial ligands in human bronchial epithelial cells.** *J Immunol* 2007, **178**:3134–3142.
35. Wu R, Smith D: **Continuous multiplication of rabbit tracheal epithelial cells in a defined, hormone-supplemented medium.** *In vitro* 1982, **18**:800–812.
36. Lechner JF, McClendon IA, LaVeck MA, Shamsuddin AM, Harris CC: **Differential control by platelet factors of squamous differentiation in normal and malignant human bronchial epithelial cells.** *Cancer Res* 1983, **43**:5915–5921.
37. Wu R, Yankaskas J, Cheng E, Knowles MR, Boucher R: **Growth and differentiation of human nasal epithelial cells in culture. Serum-free, hormone-supplemented medium and proteoglycan synthesis.** *Am Rev Respir Dis* 1985, **132**:311–320.
38. Wu R, Nolan E, Turner C: **Expression of tracheal differentiated functions in serum-free hormone-supplemented medium.** *J Cell Physiol* 1985, **125**:167–181.
39. Gruenert DC, Finkbeiner WE, Widdicombe JH: **Culture and transformation of human airway epithelial cells.** *Am J Physiol* 1995, **268**:L347–L360.
40. Schulz C, Farkas L, Wolf K, Kratzel K, Eissner G, Pfeifer M: **Differences in LPS-induced activation of bronchial epithelial cells (BEAS-2B) and type II-like pneumocytes (A-549).** *Scand J Immunol* 2002, **56**:294–302.
41. Matsukura S, Kokubu F, Kurokawa M, Kawaguchi M, Ieki K, Kuga H, Odaka M, Suzuki S, Watanabe S, Takeuchi H, Kasama T, Adachi M: **Synthetic double-stranded RNA induces multiple genes related to inflammation through Toll-like receptor 3 depending on NF-kappaB and/or IRF-3 in airway epithelial cells.** *Clin Exp Allergy* 2006, **36**:1049–1062.
42. Davis MS, Schofield B, Freed AN: **Repeated peripheral airway hyperpnea causes inflammation and remodeling in dogs.** *Med Sci Sports Exerc* 2003, **35**:608–616.
43. Davis MS, Lockard AJ, Marlin DJ, Freed AN: **Airway cooling and mucosal injury during cold weather exercise.** *Equine Vet J Suppl* 2002, **34**:413–416.
44. Petersen AM, Pedersen BK: **The anti-inflammatory effect of exercise.** *J Appl Physiol* 2005, **98**:1154–1162.
45. Mayer AK, Bartz H, Fey F, Schmidt LM, Dalpke AH: **Airway epithelial cells modify immune responses by inducing an anti-inflammatory microenvironment.** *Eur J Immunol* 2008, **38**:1689–1699.
46. Raz E: **Organ-specific regulation of innate immunity.** *Nat Immunol* 2007, **8**:3–4.

Amino acid substitutions in the neuraminidase protein of an H9N2 avian influenza virus affect its airborne transmission in chickens

Jing Lv[1,2,3†], Liangmeng Wei[1†], Yan Yang[1], Bingxiao Wang[4], Wei Liang[1], Yuwei Gao[5], Xianzhu Xia[5], Lili Gao[1], Yumei Cai[1], Peiqiang Hou[2], Huili Yang[2], Airong Wang[1], Rong Huang[1], Jing Gao[1,6*] and Tongjie Chai[1*]

Abstract

Cases of H9N2 avian influenza virus (AIV) in poultry are increasing throughout many Eurasian countries, and co-infections with other pathogens have resulted in high morbidity and mortality in poultry. Few studies have investigated the genetic factors of virus airborne transmission which determine the scope of this epidemic. In this study, we used specific-pathogen-free chickens housed in isolators to investigate the airborne transmissibility of five recombinant H9N2 AIV rescued by reverse genetic technology. The results show that airborne transmission of A/Chicken/Shandong/01/2008 (SD01) virus was related to the neuraminidase (NA) gene, and four amino acid mutations (D368E, S370L, E313K and G381D) within the head region of the SD01 NA, reduced virus replication in the respiratory tract of chickens, reduced virus NA activity, and resulted in a loss of airborne transmission ability in chickens. Similarly, reverse mutations of these four amino acids in the NA protein of r01/NASS virus, conferred an airborne transmission ability to the recombinant virus. We conclude that these four NA residues may be significant genetic markers for evaluating potential disease outbreak of H9N2 AIV, and propose that immediate attention should be paid to the airborne transmission of this virus.

Introduction

Cases of poultry infected with H9N2 avian influenza virus (AIV) have occurred repeatedly in many countries since its isolation in America in 1966 [1-4]. H9N2 AIV mainly infected feral birds and wild ducks in South America, and were unable to form a stable lineage in poultry [5,6]. H9N2 AIV infection of chickens, turkeys, pheasants, and domestic ducks has been reported throughout Asia, the Middle East, Europe and Africa from 1995 to 1997 [5,7-9]. H9N2 AIV isolated from diseased chickens in Guangdong province in 1994, represented the first documented case of H9N2 AIV in mainland China, and since 1998 the virus has spread widely [10-13]. Although it was considered a low pathogenic AIV, H9N2 caused high morbidity and mortality in poultry when co-infected with other pathogens [3,14]. More importantly, it was reported that H9N2 AIV had crossed the species barrier, infecting humans in Hong Kong and Guangzhou, China [15,16].

The segmented RNA genome of AIV allows genetic reassortment among different subtypes. The major human influenza pandemics have resulted in high mortalities, and genetic analysis of the infecting strains have indicated that the genes are partially derived from AIV [17-21]. These studies highlight the need for greater research into virus gene mutations and recombinations, and their subsequent effects on virus transmission.

H9N2 AIV transmission among chickens occurs by direct contact and aerosols, with the latter responsible for its prevalence beyond 1998 [22,23]. The NA gene of influenza virus has been shown to play an important role in virus transmission, influencing viral enzyme activity and transmissibility [23,24]. Thus, further study of the NA gene is required to help elucidate the mechanism of airborne transmission of H9N2 AIV in poultry.

* Correspondence: gjch306@sina.com; chaitj117@163.com
†Equal contributors
[1]College of Animal Science and Veterinary Medicine, Shandong Agricultural University; Sino-German Cooperative Research Centre for Zoonosis of Animal Origin Shandong Province; Key Laboratory of Animal Biotechnology and Disease Control and Prevention of Shandong Province, Shandong Agricultural University, Daizong Street 61, Taian 271018, China
Full list of author information is available at the end of the article

Our laboratory established an experimental animal model using three groups of specific-pathogen-free (SPF) chickens housed in isolators. The groups were designated inoculated, direct contact and aerosol contact, and were used to study the generation, spread and infection progression of AIV by aerosols. The results showed that the A/Chicken/Shandong/01/2008 (SD01) virus could be transmitted among chickens via aerosols [22]. A/Chicken/Guangdong/SS/94 (SS94) AIV, the earliest H9N2 virus isolated from diseased chickens in mainland China, is not transmitted by aerosol among chickens, while A/Chicken/Shanghai/F/98 (F98) could be transmitted [23]. Interestingly, substituting the NA gene of F98 with that of SS94 completely abolished the airborne transmission of the recombinant virus [23]. There are four identical amino acids in the NA head region of SD01 and F98 viruses, but they were different from the SS94 virus. These differences are at residues 313, 331, 368 & 370 and 381 (N2 number). Amino acids 368 & 370 belong to the 366–373 peptide loop which was one of hemadsorbing (HB) sites affecting neuraminidase activity [25]. However, amino acids 313–381 are on the opposite side of the globular head. To determine whether NA also influences SD01 transmission in chickens, we designed a series of mutations in the NA gene using reverse genetics systems, and evaluated their effects on airborne transmission.

Materials and methods

Virus and cell culture

H9N2 AIV A/Chicken/Shandong/01/2008 (SD01) H9N2 AIV was isolated from diseased chickens as described previously [22]. Viruses were propagated in 9-day-old SPF embryonated chicken eggs and stored at −80 °C. The Reed-Muench method [26] was used to calculate the 50% egg infective doses (EID_{50}).

Madin Darby canine kidney (MDCK) and 293 T cells were maintained in Dulbecco's minimum essential medium (Gibco-BRL, Grand Island, NY, USA) supplemented with 10% fetal bovine serum, penicillin (100 units/mL), and streptomycin (100 mg/mL), and incubated at 37 °C with 5% CO_2.

Site-directed mutagenesis and virus generation

The QuickChange II site-directed mutagenesis kit (Stratagene, La Jolla, CA, USA) was used to create site-specific mutations in the NA genes of H9N2 AIV. The primers used for mutagenesis are listed in Table 1. The eight-plasmid system was used to generate H9N2 reassortant viruses according to published methods [27,28]. Recombinant plasmids were purified using the Genopure Plasmid Midi Kit (Roche, Basel, Switzerland). Recombinant rSD01, r01/NASS, r01/NAHB, r01/NA381 and r01/NASS-381 viruses were rescued according to previously reported protocols with minor modifications [29,30]. Briefly, eight plasmids (0.5 μg each) of influenza virus were transfected into 5:1 mixed 293 T and MDCK cells using Lipofectamine™ 2000 Transfection Reagent (Invitrogen, Carlsbad, CA, USA). OPTI-MEM I (Gibco, USA) was used to substitute the transfection mixture after incubation for 6 h at 37 °C. Twelve hours later, OPTI-MEM I containing 0.5 μg/mL TPCK-trypsin and antibiotics was added. This medium was collected at 48 h post transfection and propagated in 9-day-old embryonated SPF chicken eggs. Rescued viruses were verified by sequencing the complete genes to ensure the induced mutations and the absence of unwanted mutations. The rescued viruses were titrated and stored as described above.

Infection and transmission in chickens

Studies using H9N2 low pathogenic AIV were conducted in a Biosecurity Level 2+ laboratory approved by the China National Accreditation Service for Conformity Assessment. All animal studies were carried out in strict accordance to the guidelines of Laboratory Animal Management by the National Council for Science and Technology.

For virus transmission studies, ten 4-week-old white leghorn SPF chickens (Chinese Academy of Agricultural Sciences) were inoculated intranasally with 10^7 EID_{50} of infectious allantoic fluid and placed in isolator A. A further ten animals, representing direct contact, were introduced into the same isolator 24 h later. Ten animals (aerosol contact) were placed in different cages respectively in isolator B. Isolators A and B were joined by a tube (length: 1 m; diameter: 0.08 m) to allow air flow from A to B. Oropharyngeal and cloacal swab samples, collected at 2-day intervals for all chickens, were immersed in 1 mL sterile PBS. The solutions were filtered through 0.22 μm Millex syringe filters (Millipore Corp., Bedford, MA, USA) and cultivated in 9-day-old embryonated SPF chicken eggs. Sera samples were collected at 7, 14 and 21 days post inoculation (dpi) and seroconversion confirmed by HI assay according to the OIE protocol.

Air samples were collected simultaneously at 2-day intervals from the space of two isolators as previously described [31]. The SPF isolators (Tianjin Jinhang Pure Air Condition Engineering Co., Tianjin, China) were 222 cm (length) × 86 cm (width) × 103 cm (height), and the airflow was 0.1 m/s. The environmental conditions for this study were 20–22 °C and 45–50% relative humidity.

Tropism for the respiratory tract of chickens

The replication ability and tissue tropism of H9N2 AIV, was investigated in five 4-week-old white leghorn SPF chickens inoculated intranasally with 10^7 EID_{50} virus in PBS (0.1 M, pH 7.2). Three chickens were euthanized at 5 dpi and the trachea and lungs were collected for virus titration in SPF embryonated chicken eggs from initial dilutions of 1:10 as previously described [32]. Morbidity

Table 1 Primers used to generate mutations in the NA gene of SD01 virus

Mutation	Primer sequence (5′-3′)	
	Forward	Reverse
D368E&S370L	TGGATGGGACGGACAATCAAAGA**G**GATT**T**ACGCTCAGGTTA	TAACCTGAGCGT**A**AATC**C**TCTTTGATTGTCCGTCCCATCCA
E313K	GTTCTATATATAAATATGGCAGATTATAGTATT**A**AGTCCA GTTATGTGTGC	GCACACATAACTGGACT**T**AATACTATAATCTGCCATATTT ATATAGAAC
G381D	CTTTCAGGGTCGTTG**A**TGGTTGGACCACGGC	GCCGTGGTCCAACCA**T**CAACGACCCTGAAAG

The changed nucleotides are in boldface.

and mortality of all chickens were monitored for 2 weeks for signs of disease and death, and their sera were collected at 14 dpi and were evaluated for seroconversion by an HI assay.

NA activity assays

Virus copy number used for the dose of comparable virus in NA enzymatic assays was calculated by real-time RT-PCR [31]. Virus was incubated with an equal volume (50 μL) of 0–400 μM 4-methylumbelliferyl N-acetylneuraminic acid (4-MUNANA; Sigma-Aldrich, St. Louis, MO, USA) at 37 °C in U-bottomed microtiter plates [33,34]. The fluorescence of liberated 4-methylumbelliferone was measured every 68 s for 45 min on a Spectra MaxM2/Me2 microplate detection system (Molecular Devices, LLC, Sunnyvale, California, USA) with excitation and emission wavelengths of 355 and 460 nm, respectively. Michaelis-Menten constant (*K*m) and maximum velocity of substrate conversion (*V*max) were calculated using the Michaelis-Menten nonlinear regression model (Prism; GraphPad, San Diego, CA, USA).

HA assays were performed on serial two-fold dilutions of viruses in PBS to determine the length of virus elution from agglutinated chicken red blood cells (CRBC) [34]. Microtiter plates with serial 50 μL mixtures were held at 4 °C for 1 h for virus adsorption to CRBC. The plates were transferred to a 37 °C water bath for virus elution. Samples were monitored for a minimum of 48 h, once a decrease in HA titer, coincident with NA-mediated virus elution, was observed.

Results

NA is important for aerosol transmission of H9N2 AIV in chickens

To determine whether NA also influences SD01 transmission in chickens, we first tested two recombinant viruses: recombinant SD01 (rSD01) virus recovered using reverse genetics; and r01/NASS virus, in which the NA of virus SD01 was replaced by that of SS94 (Figure 1A).

As shown in Table 2, virus was detected in the oropharyngeal and cloacal swab samples of all rSD01 and r01/NASS inoculated chickens at 4 dpi. rSD01 and r01/NASS virus were also detected in direct contact chickens at 2–14 dpi or 4–10 dpi. rSD01 virus was detected in the oropharyngeal and cloacal swab samples of six aerosol contact chickens at 4 dpi, and ten chickens at 8 dpi. No virus was detected in aerosol contact chickens for r01/NASS. Seroconversion was observed for all inoculated chickens, with average antibody titers increasing until 21 dpi (Figures 2A and B). Seroconversion was also observed for rSD01 infected direct contact chickens and for aerosol contact chickens (Figure 2A). In contrast, seroconversion was not observed for aerosol contact chickens exposed to r01/NASS (Figure 2B). Virus aerosols were detected in the air of rSD01 isolators from 4–10 dpi, but not for r01/NASS isolators (Figure 3). These results indicate that recombinant virus rSD01 was detected in the air and transmitted by aerosols between chickens, but recombinant virus r01/NASS, in which the NA of virus SD01 was replaced by that of virus SS94, was not detected in the air and was not aerially transmitted. These results suggest that the NA gene is an important determinant in virus transmission by aerosols.

Mutations D368E, S370L, E313K and G381D in NA of SD01 virus abolished airborne transmission in chickens

The NA protein of influenza A virus is not only required for virion release and spread but also impacts on virion infectivity and membrane fusion [24]. Although studies indicated that amino acid deletion in the stalk region contributes to the high virulence and pathogenicity of H5N1 isolates, in our study, there was no difference between airborne transmissible viruses SD01 and F98, and non-transmissible SS94 which all owned 3-amino acid (aa: 61–63, N2 number) deletion in their NA stalk region. So we investigated whether amino acid changes in the head of the NA protein (aa: 78–469) affected the replication and transmission of mutant viruses in chickens. Multiple sequence alignment of the NA proteins of H9N2 AIV isolated in China and submitted to NCBI from 1994 to 2013 revealed that SS94 and A/Chicken/Guangdong/1997 had acidic amino acid K at position 313, whilst almost all other strains had acidic E313 or D313 [35]. SS94 and three Shandong H9N2 AIV had an acidic D381 residue, while all other viruses had neutral G381 or N381 residues (see Additional file 1). The 3D-structure of neuraminidase was generated using PyMOL software (DeLano Scientific LLC, San Carlos, CA, USA). The G381D mutation was in

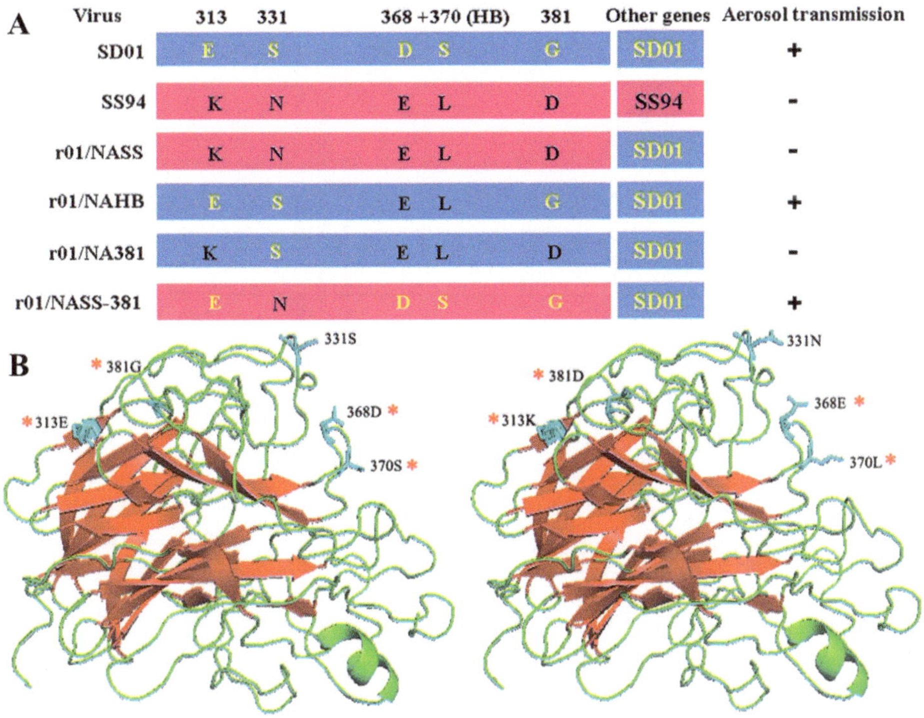

Figure 1 Gene schematic diagrams and 3D-structure of H9N2 neuraminidase used in this study. (A) Gene schematic diagrams of SD01, SS94 and recombinant virus. The blue and red bars indicate the genes originating from SD01 and SS94, respectively. The positions of four amino acid regions in the NA gene are shown at the top of the diagram and differences in the mutants are shown as amino acid abbreviation. Amino acids in NA of SD01 and SS94 are marked up by yellow and black letters respectively. + indicates that the virus could be transmitted among chickens via aerosols, – indicates could not. **(B)** The 3D-structure of H9N2 neuraminidase generated using PyMOL software shows the locations of mutations (PDB access number: 1ivd). The left is the structure before the mutation, and the right is the structure after the mutation. * indicates the positions that will be studied. Amino-acids 368–370 are close to the HB site, while 313–381 are on the opposite side of the globular head.

a random coil region, and the conversion from a non-polar to polar amino acid may result in changes to protein hydrophilicity. When a G381D mutation occurred simultaneously with an E313K mutation in the β-fold region, the protein structure was changed significantly, with the distance between the two reduced amino acids (Figure 1B).

To evaluate whether these amino acid mutations were related to H9N2 virus transmission in chickens, we tested two mutants, r01/NAHB (D368E and S370L) which derives from rSD01 by the two substitutions D368E + S370L in the hemadsorption site, and r01/NA381 (D368E, S370L, E313K and G381D) which derives from r01/NAHB by two further substitutions: E313K + G381D (Figure 1A). r01/NAHB virus shedding was detected in inoculated and direct contact chickens from 2 to 12 dpi, and in aerosol contact chickens, although fewer virus particles were shed compared with rSD01. Virus shedding of r01/NA381 was also detected in inoculated and direct contact chickens, but the number of infected chickens was fewer than those infected by r01/NAHB, and no virus shedding was detected in aerosol contact chickens (Table 2). Seroconversion was observed for all infected chickens (Figures 2C and D), with antibody titers increasing from 7 to 21 dpi. The antibody titers for direct contact or aerosol contact chickens were appreciably lower than for inoculated animals on the same day (Figures 2C and D).

Air samples were collected by an AGI-30 liquid sampler every other day from 2 dpi, and virus titrated in eggs (Figure 3). Virus concentrations were expressed as EID_{50}/L air. Viral aerosols were detected for rSD01 and r01/NAHB at concentrations of 265–13330 EID_{50}/L air. Generally, airborne H9N2 AIV were first detected at 4 or 6 dpi, peaking at 8 dpi and declining at 10 dpi, with no viral aerosols detected at 12 dpi. Airborne virus was not detected for r01/NASS and r01/NA381, which could be associated with the reduced number of virus aerosols produced, and to assay sensitivity.

Recombinant virus r01/NAHB (which derives from rSD01 by the two substitutions D368E + S370L in the HB site) was detected in the air and was aerially transmitted, which demonstrates that the HB site has a modest impact on aerial transmission. Recombinant virus r01/NA381 (which derives from r01/NAHB by two further substitutions: E313K + G381D) was not detected in the air and was not aerially transmitted, which demonstrates the

Table 2 Number of chickens infected by recombinant virus in independent experiments*

Dpi	rSD01			r01/NASS			r01/NAHB			r01/NA381			r01/NASS-381		
	Inoculated	Direct-contact	Aerosol-contact	Inoculated	Direct-contact	Aerosol-contact	Inoculated	Direct-contact	Aerosol-contact	Inoculated	Direct-contact	Aerosol-contact	Inoculated	Direct-contact	Aerosol-contact
2	6/10	2/10	0/10	5/10	0/10	0/10	5/10	2/10	0/10	0/10	0/10	0/10	3/10	0/10	0/10
4	10/10	10/10	6/10	10/10	5/10	0/10	10/10	10/10	3/10	10/10	2/10	0/10	10/10	6/10	2/10
6	10/10	10/10	8/10	10/10	9/10	0/10	10/10	10/10	8/10	10/10	8/10	0/10	10/10	9/10	5/10
8	9/10	9/10	10/10	6/10	6/10	0/10	8/10	7/10	10/10	8/10	4/10	0/10	10/10	10/10	7/10
10	9/10	7/10	9/10	4/10	3/10	0/10	8/10	5/10	7/10	4/10	2/10	0/10	8/10	7/10	6/10
12	7/10	6/10	7/10	2/10	0/10	0/10	4/10	2/10	3/10	1/10	0/10	0/10	6/10	5/10	4/10
14	5/10	3/10	6/10	0/10	0/10	0/10	0/10	0/10	0/10	0/10	0/10	0/10	3/10	2/10	0/10

*In every independent experiment, ten SPF chickens (inoculated) were infected intranasally 10^7 EID_{50} of recombinant virus, then another ten animals (direct contact) were introduced into the same isolator 24 h later, while ten animals (aerosol contact) were placed separately in another isolator B. Oropharyngeal and cloacal swab samples of the chickens were collected at 2 day intervals and inoculated in SPF embryonated chicken eggs for observation virus shedding. The result expressed as infected number/total number of chickens. Repeat transmission experiments of r01/NASS and r01/NA381 which could not transmit by aerosols were performed. The results indicate that there was no virus shedding of all aerosol contact animals.

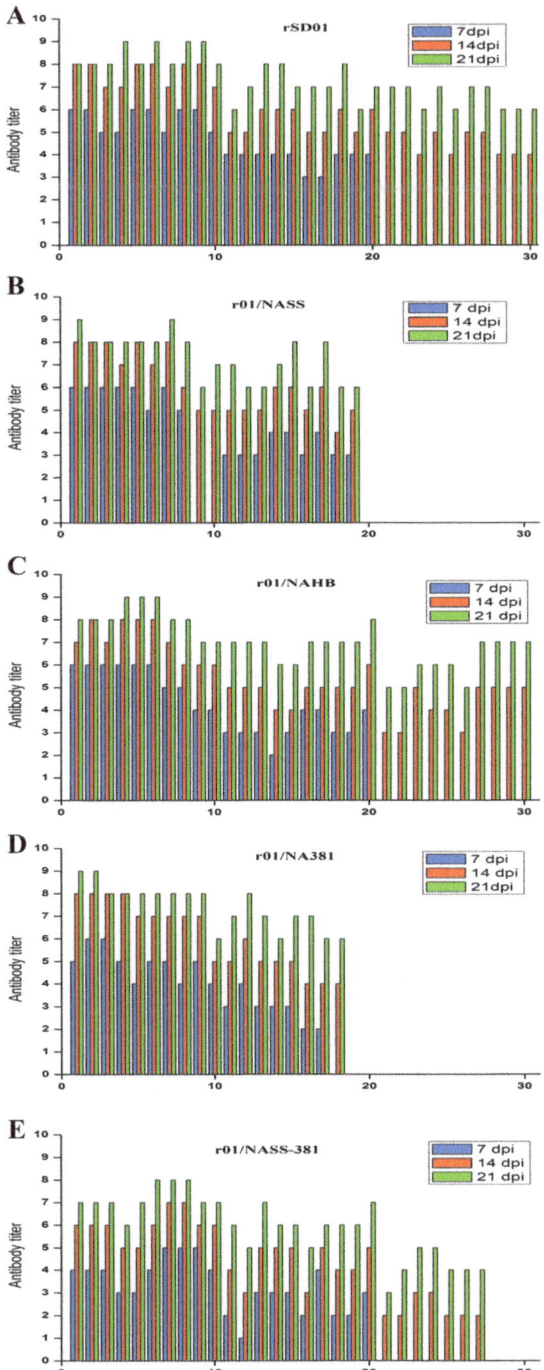

Figure 2 Seroconversion of chickens in the transmission experiments. In every independent experiment, sera of ten chickens in every group were collected at 7 day intervals and seroconversion was confirmed by hemagglutination inhibition (HI) assay. Each color bar represents the antibody titers of every chicken. Repeat seroconversion experiments of r01/NASS and r01/NA381 were performed. The results also indicate that no seroconversion was observed in aerosol contact chickens. 1–10 represents ten inoculated chickens, 11–20 represents ten direct-contact chickens and 21–30 represents ten aerosol-contact chickens. The blue, red and green colors express antibody titers detected on 7, 14 and 21 dpi respectively.

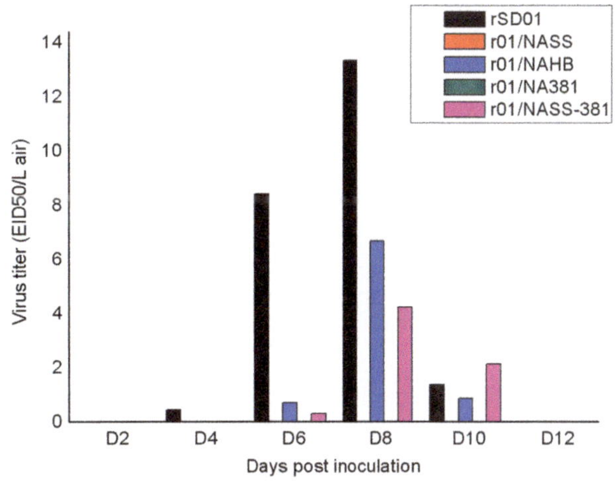

Figure 3 Virus titers of airborne H9N2 AIV in an isolator. Air samples were collected simultaneously from the space of two isolators using an AGI-30 liquid sampler operated continuously for an optimized time of 30 min at an airflow rate of 12.5 L/min. Virus titer in the air was expressed as values of EID_{50}/L air. Each color bar represented the every recombinant virus concentration in the air collected every two days from the beginning of 2 dpi in an independent experiment. No airborne virus was detected in the experiment for r01/NASS and r01/NA381 viruses.

importance of the amino-acid pair 313–381 in aerial transmission. The NA of this virus is close to that of SS94.

Replication of recombinant viruses in the respiratory tract of SPF chickens

Clarified homogenates of tracheas and lungs collected from three chickens at 5 dpi were used for virus titration in SPF embryonated chicken eggs. There were no obvious differences in viral titers between the lungs and tracheas of chickens infected with the same virus (Table 3). However, virus titers for r01/NASS and r01/NA381-infected chickens were lower than for those infected with rSD01 (Table 3). According to the study before, these two viruses also had similar characteristics in transmissibility: the reduced virus shedding of infected chickens and no shedding in aerosol contact chickens, and not being detected in the air. All strains were non-lethal to chickens and did not induce serious clinical symptoms, other than slight inappetence and inactivity, with clinical symptoms generally resolved within 10 days. Seroconversion was observed for all viruses, and HI titers were between 64 and 128 (Table 3).

Substitutions or mutations in the NA gene affected virus NA activity

Replacement or mutations of the NA gene of SD01 were shown to decrease virus airborne transmission efficiency. In the current study, we determined the kinetic parameters, K_M and *V*max, of viral NA using the fluorogenic substrate 4-MUNANA. Differences in K_M values for NA of recombinant viruses were not considered to be statistically

Table 3 Pathogenicity of H9N2 AIV to SPF chickens[a]

Virus	Lethality	Virus titers in trachea ($log_{10}EID_{50}$/gram ± SD)	Virus titers in lung ($log_{10}EID_{50}$/gram ± SD)	Seroconversion (HI titers)
rSD01	None	5.83 ± 0.29	5.33 ± 0.34	64, 128
r01/NASS	None	3.72 ± 0.35*	3.61 ± 0.26*	64, 64
r01/NAHB	None	5.67 ± 0.34	5.21 ± 0.18	128, 64
r01/NA381	None	4.17 ± 0.29*	3.56 ± 0.10*	128, 64

[a]SPF chickens ($n = 5$) were inoculated intranasally 10^7 EID_{50} of each virus. Clarified homogenates of tracheas and lungs from three animals collected on 5 dpi were titrated for virus infectivity in SPF embryonated chicken eggs from initial dilutions of 1:10. Virus titers were expressed as mean $log_{10}EID_{50}$/g wet tissues ± standard deviation (SD). Two chickens were observed for signs of lethality, and seroconversion was confirmed by hemagglutination inhibition (HI) assay on 14 dpi. *$P < 0.05$ compared with rSD01.

significant ($P > 0.05$), suggesting NA enzymatic activity was consistent across all viruses. Enzyme activity was significantly higher (*V*max, $P < 0.05$) for NA of rSD01 compared with NA of r01/NASS, r01/NAHB and r01/NA381 (Table 4). Virus elution times were used to evaluate the effect of NA substitutions or mutations on virus release from CRBC. rSD01 virus was first to be eluted, followed by r01/NAHB, with both r01/NASS and r01/NA381 viruses eluted much later (3.5 and 4 h, respectively). These results indicate that NA gene substitution and mutations at 366–373HB, 313 and 381 played an important role in reducing virus NA activity. What is more, the results also indicate that substitutions at residues 313–381 have more impact than those at the HB site.

Mutations E368D, L370S, K313E and D381G in NA of r01/NASS confer virus airborne transmissibility in chickens

r01/NASS-381 virus with mutations E368D, L370S, K313E and D381G in NA was generated on the backbone of the r01/NASS virus which had lost airborne transmissibility in chickens. We compared the transmissibility of r01/NASS-381 virus with r01/NASS virus in chickens. As shown in Table 2, virus shedding was detected in both r01/NASS-381 and r01/NASS inoculated and direct contact chickens, with a greater number of chickens infected by the former from 4 to 14 dpi. Two aerosol contact chickens were infected with r01/NASS-381 virus at 4 dpi; increasing to seven by 8 dpi. Altogether, fewer chickens were infected with r01/NASS-381 compared with rSD01 and r01/NAHB

Table 4 Neuraminidase activities of H9N2 AIV

virus	K_M(μM)[a]	V_{max}(fluorescence a.u/s)[a]	Relative V_{max} [b]	Elution time(h)
rSD01	54.16 ± 3.12	192.73 ± 6.54	1.00	1.5
r01/NASS	49.167 ± 3.34	118.83 ± 1.43*	0.62	3.5
r01/NAHB	52.43 ± 6.68	123.83 ± 3.40*	0.64	2
r01/NA381	53.84 ± 2.53	92.25 ± 1.69*	0.48	4

[a]The enzyme kinetics data was fit to the Michaelis-Menten equation by nonlinear regression to determine the Michaelis constant (K_M) and maximum velocity (*V*max) of substrate conversion. Results are given as the mean ± standard deviation from three duplicate samples. [b]Relative *V*max: homologous of recombinant virus to SD01. *$P < 0.05$ compared with SD01.

on the same day. Seroconversion occurred in aerosol infected chickens, with average antibody titers of 4–32 recorded at 14 and 21 dpi (Figure 2E). Air samples were collected from the isolators and viruses titrated in SPF embryonated chicken eggs, as described previously. Airborne r01/NASS-381 virus was detected at 6 dpi, at a concentration of 265 EID_{50}/L air, whilst no viral aerosol was detected at 12 dpi (Figure 3). Virus elution times of r01/NASS-381 virus released from CRBC was 2.5 h, which was shorter than that of the r01/NASS virus. These results demonstrate that amino acid mutations E368D, L370S, K313E and D381G in the NA protein of r01/NASS enhanced viral NA activity and viral shedding from chickens, and restored airborne transmissibility in chickens, and the HB site had a minor impact on these characteristics, while the amino-acid pair 313–381 had a major effect.

Discussion

H9N2 AIV was first isolated from dead chickens in the Guangdong Province, China, in 1994, and in the proceeding decades has spread widely throughout other provinces, impacting heavily on the poultry industry and imparting great economic losses [2,10,36]. A number of studies have demonstrated the capability of AIV to cause aerosol infections by the respiratory route, moreover, AIV infections occurred between animals through the airborne route in many experimental models [37,38]. The high prevalence of H9N2 AIV in poultry is also associated with airborne transmission. Aerosol transmission of H9N2 AIV was observed in SPF chicken flocks, and recovered airborne virus particles [22]. Shi et al. demonstrated that the F98 virus could be transmitted through chicken flocks by aerosols, whilst the SS94 virus could not. The authors discovered that the mechanism of airborne transmission was associated with the NA gene [23]. To elucidate the mechanisms underlying airborne transmission mechanisms of H9N2 AIV, reverse genetics technology should be employed to establish the relationship between NA amino acids and transmissibility of AIV.

Influenza virus NA is an important viral surface glycoprotein, possessing exoglycosidase activity, catalyzing the hydrolysis of α-glycosidic bonds between sialic acid residues and adjacent oligosaccharides. NA plays an important role in the virus life cycle, including invading and infecting cells, budding and release, and preventing self-aggregation [24,39-41]. Richard et al. reported that D198N, E119D and I222L mutations in NA of H3N2 influenza virus could alter the biological activity of NA [42]. While a substitution of the NA gene from the 2009 H1N1 influenza virus, the recombinant virus (other genes from H1N1 seasonal influenza virus) failed to increase virus replication in vivo. However, the transmission of droplet infection of the recombinant virus was significantly enhanced among mammals [33]. In a previous study, we demonstrated that the SD01 virus could transmit in chickens by airborne route using the isolator apparatus [22]. To investigate the relationship between the NA gene and virus airborne transmission, a reverse genetics system was employed to rescue recombinant H9N2 AIV. We found that the recombinant virus lost parental airborne transmissibility in chickens when the NA gene of the SD01 virus was substituted with that of the SS94 virus. These results were consistent with the work of Shi et al. [23]. We used DNASTAR software to establish that amino acid residues 313, 331, 366–373 and 381 in the active region of NA differed between airborne transmissible viruses SD01 and F98, and non-transmissible SS94. The aim of our present study was to investigate the role of these amino-acids in conferring the airborne transmission ability.

In the present study, SPF chickens inoculated with r01/NAHB virus, continued to infect aerosol contact chickens, and viral aerosols were recovered from the air of isolators. These results indicate that r01/NAHB virus could still transmit in chickens via the airborne route. The replication capacity of r01/NAHB virus within the trachea and lung tissue of SPF chickens did not differ significantly from rSD01 virus. However, NA activity was lower for the r01/NAHB virus, and time of virus release from CRBC was greater. Therefore, NA activity of H9N2 AIV was affected by amino acid mutations at the HB site, although these did not severely impact the transmission and replication of the virus.

Other studies have also shown that amino acid mutations on NA affect its activity. It was found that the NA activity of A/Moscow/10/99 (H3N2) influenza virus with D198N and E119D mutations in NA was considerably lower than for the parental virus following stable passage in MDCK cells [42]. Some NA amino acids have been shown to play a significant role in airborne transmission of influenza virus. Herlocher et al. reported that substitution of R292K in the NA of A/Sydney/5/97 weakened virus infectivity and abolished parental airborne transmissibility in ferrets. They also demonstrated that substitution H274Y could reduce the transmission ability of H1N1 influenza virus in mammals [43,44]. In the present study, SPF chickens inoculated with a recombinant virus r01/NA381 (containing mutations D368E, S370L, E313K and G381D in SD01 virus NA) failed to infect chickens in the aerosol contact group, and airborne virus was not detected in the isolators. Collectively, these results suggest that r01/NA381 had lost its capacity for airborne infection. The protracted elution of r01/NA381 from CRBC, coupled with a reduction in NA activity, and decreased replication capacity in the respiratory tract of chickens may be important factors in the loss of airborne infection capability of this virus.

r01/NASS (rSD01 containing the SS94 NA gene) and SS94 virus transmission does not proceed via the airborne route in chickens. The introduction of four mutations, E368D, L370S, K313E and D381G, in NA of r01/NASS conferred transmissibility of the recombinant virus by aerosols in chickens, especially, the amino-acid pair 313–381 had a major effect on airborne transmissibility. These amino acid mutations in NA of the SS94 virus, illustrate the potential for conferral of airborne virus transmissibility in poultry, which could lead to rapidly spreading epidemics, and a considerable threat to poultry and the industry it supports.

In recent years, several subtypes of AIV, including H3, H5, H6, H7 and H9, have been circulating and evolving in China [45-47]. In such an environment, AIV can easily recombine with other subtypes to generate new viruses. Recombination of airborne transmissible H9N2 virus with highly pathogenic AIV such as H5 and H7 subtypes, could produce recombinant viruses which are both highly pathogenic and airborne transmissible. Therefore, further research should be directed towards airborne transmission of the H9N2 virus.

In conclusion, we demonstrate that H9N2 AIV NA was important for airborne transmission of virus in poultry. Specifically, residues E368, L370, K313 and D381 of NA contribute to NA activity and replication capacity in the respiratory tract of poultry. More importantly, these amino acids, especially K313 and D381, play a role in preventing virus airborne transmission. During the submission process, Zhong et al. reported the critical roles of HA and PA in the airborne transmission of a couple of H9N2 viruses [48]. These findings can be applied to guide the transmission ability assessment of H9N2 AIV and forecast disease outbreaks in the coming years.

Additional file

Additional file 1: Multiple sequence alignment of the NA proteins of H9N2 AIV. The viruses used for alignment were isolated in China and submitted to NCBI from 1994 to 2013.

Competing interests
The authors declare that they have no competing interests.

Authors' contributions

JL, LMW and TJC participated in the design of the study, performed the experiments, collected and analyzed data, and drafted the manuscript. YY and BXW cloned and sequenced the segments of virus. ARW, RH and WL constructed plasmid and rescued the recombinant viruses. LLG and YMC helped with the animal experiment. YWG, XZX, PQH and HLY participated in preliminary data acquisition and performed the statistical analysis. JG and TJC conceived the study and participated in its design and coordination. All authors read and approved the final manuscript.

Acknowledgments

We thank Dr Robert G. Webster at the St. Jude Children's Research Hospital, Memphis, Tennessee for providing the vector of 8-plasmid-system. This study was supported by the National Science and Technology Support Project (2012BAD39B02); National Natural Science Foundation of China (31270172 and 31470258); the State Key Laboratory of Pathogen and Biosecurity (Academy of Military Medical Science; SKLPBS1449) and China Postdoctoral Science Foundation "Molecular mechanism of H9N2 avian influenza virus airborne transmission" (2013 M531639).

Author details

[1]College of Animal Science and Veterinary Medicine, Shandong Agricultural University; Sino-German Cooperative Research Centre for Zoonosis of Animal Origin Shandong Province; Key Laboratory of Animal Biotechnology and Disease Control and Prevention of Shandong Province, Shandong Agricultural University, Daizong Street 61, Taian 271018, China. [2]Taian Municipal Center for Disease Control and Prevention, Changcheng Street, Taian 271000, China. [3]College of Life Science, Shandong Agricultural University, Taian 271018, China. [4]Qingdao Chia Tai Co., Ltd, Qingwei Street, Qingdao 266109, China. [5]Institute of Military Veterinary PLA, Qinglong Street 1068, Changchun 130000, China. [6]School of dentistry and oral health Taishan Medical University, Tai'an 271000, China.

References

1. Homme PJ, Easterday BC (1970) Avian influenza virus infections. I. Characteristics of influenza A-turkey-Wisconsin-1966 virus. Avian Dis 14:66–74
2. Choi YK, Ozaki H, Webby RJ, Webster RG, Peiris JS, Poon L, Butt C, Leung YH, Guan Y (2004) Continuing evolution of H9N2 influenza viruses in Southeastern China. J Virol 78:8609–8614
3. Nili H, Asasi K (2002) Natural cases and an experimental study of H9N2 avian influenza in commercial broiler chickens of Iran. Avian Pathol 31:247–252
4. Bano S, Naeem K, Malik SA (2003) Evaluation of pathogenic potential of avian influenza virus serotype H9N2 in chickens. Avian Dis 47:817–822
5. Alexander DJ (2000) A review of avian influenza in different bird species. Vet Microbiol 74:3–13
6. Sharp GB, Kawaoka Y, Wright SM, Turner B, Hinshaw V, Webster RG (1993) Wild ducks are the reservoir for only a limited number of influenza A subtypes. Epidemiol Infect 110:161–176
7. Naeem K, Ullah A, Manvell RJ, Alexander DJ (1999) Avian influenza A subtype H9N2 in poultry in Pakistan. Vet Rec 145:560
8. Lee CW, Song CS, Lee YJ, Mo IP, Garcia M, Suarez DL, Kim SJ (2000) Sequence analysis of the hemagglutinin gene of H9N2 Korean avian influenza viruses and assessment of the pathogenic potential of isolate MS96. Avian Dis 44:527–535
9. Perk S, Panshin A, Shihmanter E, Gissin I, Pokamunski S, Pirak M, Lipkind M (2006) Ecology and molecular epidemiology of H9N2 avian influenza viruses isolated in Israel during 2000–2004 epizootic. Dev Biol 124:201–209
10. Guan Y, Shortridge KF, Krauss S, Webster RG (1999) Molecular characterization of H9N2 influenza viruses: were they the donors of the "internal" genes of H5N1 viruses in Hong Kong? Proc Natl Acad Sci U S A 96:9363–9367
11. Xu KM, Li KS, Smith GJ, Li JW, Tai H, Zhang JX, Webster RG, Peiris JS, Chen H, Guan Y (2007) Evolution and molecular epidemiology of H9N2 influenza A viruses from quail in southern China, 2000 to 2005. J Virol 81:2635–2645
12. Guo YJ, Krauss S, Senne DA, Mo IP, Lo KS, Xiong XP, Norwood M, Shortridge KF, Webster RG, Guan Y (2000) Characterization of the pathogenicity of members of the newly established H9N2 influenza virus lineages in Asia. Virology 267:279–288
13. Li C, Yu K, Tian G, Yu D, Liu L, Jing B, Ping J, Chen H (2005) Evolution of H9N2 influenza viruses from domestic poultry in Mainland China. Virology 340:70–83
14. Haghighat-Jahromi M, Asasi K, Nili H, Dadras H, Shooshtari AH (2008) Coinfection of avian influenza virus (H9N2 subtype) with infectious bronchitis live vaccine. Arch Virol 153:651–655
15. Peiris M, Yuen KY, Leung CW, Chan KH, Ip PL, Lai RW, Orr WK, Shortridge KF (1999) Human infection with influenza H9N2. Lancet 354:916–917
16. Butt KM, Smith GJ, Chen H, Zhang LJ, Leung YH, Xu KM, Lim W, Webster RG, Yuen KY, Peiris JS, Guan Y (2005) Human infection with an avian H9N2 influenza A virus in Hong Kong in 2003. J Clin Microbiol 43:5760–5767
17. Kawaoka Y, Krauss S, Webster RG (1989) Avian-to-human transmission of the PB1 gene of influenza A viruses in the 1957 and 1968 pandemics. J Virol 63:4603–4608
18. Webster RG, Bean WJ, Gorman OT, Chambers TM, Kawaoka Y (1992) Evolution and ecology of influenza A viruses. Microbiol Rev 56:152–179
19. Taubenberger JK, Reid AH, Krafft AE, Bijwaard KE, Fanning TG (1997) Initial genetic characterization of the 1918 "Spanish" influenza virus. Science 275:1793–1796
20. Vijaykrishna D, Poon LL, Zhu HC, Ma SK, Li OT, Cheung CL, Smith GJ, Peiris JS, Guan Y (2010) Reassortment of pandemic H1N1/2009 influenza A virus in swine. Science 328:1529
21. Watanabe T, Zhong G, Russell CA, Nakajima N, Hatta M, Hanson A, McBride R, Burke DF, Takahashi K, Fukuyama S, Tomita Y, Maher EA, Watanabe S, Imai M, Neumann G, Hasegawa H, Paulson JC, Smith DJ, Kawaoka Y (2014) Circulating avian influenza viruses closely related to the 1918 virus have pandemic potential. Cell Host Microbe 15:692–705
22. Yao M, Zhang X, Gao J, Chai T, Miao Z, Ma W, Qin M, Li Q, Li X, Liu J, Zhang H (2011) The occurrence and transmission characteristics of airborne H9N2 avian influenza virus. Berl Munch Tierarztl Wochenschr 124:136–141
23. Shi H, Ashraf S, Gao S, Lu J, Liu X (2010) Evaluation of transmission route and replication efficiency of H9N2 avian influenza virus. Avian Dis 54:22–27
24. Su B, Wurtzer S, Rameix-Welti MA, Dwyer D, van der Werf S, Naffakh N, Clavel F, Labrosse B (2009) Enhancement of the influenza A hemagglutinin (HA)-mediated cell-cell fusion and virus entry by the viral neuraminidase (NA). PLoS One 4:e8495
25. Uhlendorff J, Matrosovich T, Klenk HD, Matrosovich M (2009) Functional significance of the hemadsorption activity of influenza virus neuraminidase and its alteration in pandemic viruses. Arch Virol 154:945–957
26. Reed LJ, Muench H (1938) A simple method of estimating fifty per cent endpoints. Am J Hygiene 27:493–497
27. Hoffmann E, Neumann G, Kawaoka Y, Hobom G, Webster RG (2000) A DNA transfection system for generation of influenza A virus from eight plasmids. Proc Natl Acad Sci U S A 97:6108–6113
28. Hoffmann E, Stech J, Guan Y, Webster RG, Perez DR (2001) Universal primer set for the full-length amplification of all influenza A viruses. Arch Virol 146:2275–2289
29. Hoffmann E, Krauss S, Perez D, Webby R, Webster RG (2002) Eight-plasmid system for rapid generation of influenza virus vaccines. Vaccine 20:3165–3170
30. Wan H, Perez DR (2007) Amino acid 226 in the hemagglutinin of H9N2 influenza viruses determines cell tropism and replication in human airway epithelial cells. J Virol 81:5181–5191
31. Lv J, Wei B, Chai T, Xia X, Miao Z, Yao M, Gao Y, Huang R, Yang H, Roesler U (2011) Development of a real-time RT-PCR method for rapid detection of H9 avian influenza virus in the air. Arch Virol 156:1795–1801
32. Lu X, Tumpey TM, Morken T, Zaki SR, Cox NJ, Katz JM (1999) A mouse model for the evaluation of pathogenesis and immunity to influenza A (H5N1) viruses isolated from humans. J Virol 73:5903–5911
33. Yen HL, Liang CH, Wu CY, Forrest HL, Ferguson A, Choy KT, Jones J, Wong DD, Cheung PP, Hsu CH, Li OT, Yuen KM, Chan RW, Poon LL, Chan MC, Nicholls JM, Krauss S, Wong CH, Guan Y, Webster RG, Webby RJ, Peiris M (2011) Hemagglutinin-neuraminidase balance confers respiratory-droplet transmissibility of the pandemic H1N1 influenza virus in ferrets. Proc Natl Acad Sci U S A 108:14264–14269
34. Zhang W, Xue T, Wu X, Zhang P, Zhao G, Peng D, Hu S, Wang X, Liu X, Liu W (2011) Increase in viral yield in eggs and MDCK cells of reassortant H5N1 vaccine candidate viruses caused by insertion of 38 amino acids into the NA stalk. Vaccine 29:8032–8041

35. Multiple Sequence Alignment [http://www.ncbi.nlm.nih.gov/genomes/FLU/FLU.html].
36. Bi J, Deng G, Dong J, Kong F, Li X, Xu Q, Zhang M, Zhao L, Qiao J (2010) Phylogenetic and molecular characterization of H9N2 influenza isolates from chickens in Northern China from 2007–2009. PLoS One 5:e13063
37. Tellier R (2009) Aerosol transmission of influenza A virus: a review of new studies. J R Soc Interface 6(Suppl 6):S783–790
38. Webster RG (1997) Influenza virus: transmission between species and relevance to emergence of the next human pandemic. Arch Virol Suppl 13:105–113
39. Matrosovich MN, Matrosovich TY, Gray T, Roberts NA, Klenk HD (2004) Neuraminidase is important for the initiation of influenza virus infection in human airway epithelium. J Virol 78:12665–12667
40. Colman PM (1994) Influenza virus neuraminidase: structure, antibodies, and inhibitors. Protein Sci 3:1687–1696
41. Yang P, Bansal A, Liu C, Air GM (1997) Hemagglutinin specificity and neuraminidase coding capacity of neuraminidase-deficient influenza viruses. Virology 229:155–165
42. Richard M, Deleage C, Barthelemy M, Lin YP, Hay A, Lina B, Ferraris O (2008) Impact of influenza A virus neuraminidase mutations on the stability, activity, and sensibility of the neuraminidase to neuraminidase inhibitors. J Clin Virol 41:20–24
43. Herlocher ML, Truscon R, Elias S, Yen HL, Roberts NA, Ohmit SE, Monto AS (2004) Influenza viruses resistant to the antiviral drug oseltamivir: transmission studies in ferrets. J Infect Dis 190:1627–1630
44. Herlocher ML, Carr J, Ives J, Elias S, Truscon R, Roberts N, Monto AS (2002) Influenza virus carrying an R292K mutation in the neuraminidase gene is not transmitted in ferrets. Antiviral Res 54:99–111
45. Yang S, Chen Y, Cui D, Yao H, Lou J, Huo Z, Xie G, Yu F, Zheng S, Yang Y, Zhu Y, Lu X, Liu X, Lau SY, Chan JF, To KK, Yuen KY, Chen H, Li L (2014) Avian-origin influenza A(H7N9) infection in influenza A(H7N9)-affected areas of China: a serological study. J Infect Dis 209:265–269
46. Huang K, Bahl J, Fan XH, Vijaykrishna D, Cheung CL, Webby RJ, Webster RG, Chen H, Smith GJ, Peiris JS, Guan Y (2010) Establishment of an H6N2 influenza virus lineage in domestic ducks in southern China. J Virol 84:6978–6986
47. Pepin KM, Wang J, Webb CT, Smith GJ, Poss M, Hudson PJ, Hong W, Zhu H, Riley S, Guan Y (2013) Multiannual patterns of influenza A transmission in Chinese live bird market systems. Influenza Other Resp Viruses 7:97–107
48. Zhong L, Wang X, Li Q, Liu D, Chen H, Zhao M, Gu X, He L, Liu X, Gu M, Peng D (2014) Molecular mechanism of the airborne transmissibility of H9N2 avian influenza A viruses in chickens. J Virol 88:9568–9578

18

Host-specific exposure and fatal neurologic disease in wild raptors from highly pathogenic avian influenza virus H5N1 during the 2006 outbreak in Germany

Judith MA van den Brand[1†], Oliver Krone[2†], Peter U Wolf[3], Marco WG van de Bildt[1], Geert van Amerongen[1], Albert DME Osterhaus[1] and Thijs Kuiken[1*]

Abstract

Raptors may contract highly pathogenic avian influenza virus H5N1 by hunting or scavenging infected prey. However, natural H5N1 infection in raptors is rarely reported. Therefore, we tested raptors found dead during an H5N1 outbreak in wild waterbirds in Mecklenburg-Western Pomerania, Germany, in 2006 for H5N1-associated disease. We tested 624 raptors of nine species—common buzzard (385), Eurasian sparrowhawk (111), common kestrel (38), undetermined species of buzzard (36), white-tailed sea eagle (19), undetermined species of raptor (12), northern goshawk (10), peregrine falcon (6), red kite (3), rough-legged buzzard (3), and western marsh-harrier (1)—for H5N1 infection in tracheal or combined tracheal/cloacal swabs of all birds, and on major tissues of all white-tailed sea eagles. H5N1 infection was detected in two species: common buzzard (12 positive, 3.1%) and peregrine falcon (2 positive, 33.3%). In all necropsied birds (both peregrine falcons and the six freshest common buzzards), H5N1 was found most consistently and at the highest concentration in the brain, and the main H5N1-associated lesion was marked non-suppurative encephalitis. Other H5N1-associated lesions occurred in air sac, lung, oviduct, heart, pancreas, coelomic ganglion, and adrenal gland. Our results show that the main cause of death in H5N1-positive raptors was encephalitis. Our results imply that H5N1 outbreaks in wild waterbirds are more likely to lead to exposure to and mortality from H5N1 in raptors that hunt or scavenge medium-sized birds, such as common buzzards and peregrine falcons, than in raptors that hunt small birds and do not scavenge, such as Eurasian sparrowhawks and common kestrels.

Introduction

Highly pathogenic avian influenza virus causes high mortality in poultry, but is rarely reported to cause clinical disease in wild waterbirds. However, since 2000 there have been several reported outbreaks of highly pathogenic avian influenza virus of the subtype H5N1 causing mortality in wild waterbirds. A major outbreak occurred in 2005 in western China, causing mortality of more than thousand birds, including bar-headed geese (*Anser indicus*), great black-headed gulls (*Larus ichthyaetus*), and brown-headed gulls (*Larus brunnicephalus*) [1,2]. Subsequently, H5N1 spread to Europe in 2005 and 2006, and caused mortality in a variety of wild birds. In Germany, H5N1 infection was detected by real-time reverse transcriptase polymerase chain reaction (RT-PCR) in several wild bird species, not only waterbirds such as whooper (*Cygnus cygnus*) and mute swans (*Cygnus olor*), Canada geese (*Branta canadensis*), tufted ducks (*Aythya fuligula*), greater black-backed gulls (*Larus marinus*), herring gulls (*Larus argentatus*), but also in raptors such as northern goshawks (*Accipiter gentilis*) and common buzzards (*Buteo buteo*) [3,4]. By histology, these birds showed meningitis and encephalitis, characterized by gliosis and inflammation of the grey matter, neuronal degeneration and necrosis, and perivascular cuffing. These brain lesions were associated with influenza virus antigen expression in neurons and cells of the glia, ependyma and choroid plexus

* Correspondence: t.kuiken@erasmusmc.nl
†Equal contributors
[1]Department of Viroscience, Erasmus Medical Center, Dr. Molewaterplein 50, 3015 GE Rotterdam, Netherlands
Full list of author information is available at the end of the article

[3]. Additional lesions outside the brain were necrosis in liver, exocrine pancreas, adrenal glands and spleen, and hemorrhage in lungs and heart [3].

Since several raptor species selectively hunt moribund or otherwise conspicuous prey, including waterbirds, or scavenge on their carcasses, they may be assumed to have a high rate of exposure to H5N1 during outbreaks of this virus. However, there are only rare case reports of natural H5N1 infection in raptors: common buzzard [3,5,6], mountain hawk-eagle (*Spizaetus nipalensis*) [7,8], and saker falcon (*Falco cherrug*) [7], with limited information on virus distribution and associated lesions. Therefore, our goal was to determine whether raptors exposed to H5N1 during an outbreak in wild waterbirds suffered fatal disease, and—if so—how the H5N1-associated lesions compared to those in other avian species. To do so, we tested all raptors that were found dead in the region Mecklenburg-Western Pomerania during the H5N1 outbreak in 2006 for H5N1 by RT-PCR of tracheal and/or cloacal swabs, and performed full necropsies on a selection of these birds for the presence of H5N1-associated lesions.

Material and methods

Birds

Of the total of 9 356 dead wild birds from Mecklenburg-Western Pomerania examined during the 2006 H5N1 outbreak, 624 were raptors (Tables 1 and 2) [9]. Identification to species was not possible for some carcasses due to advanced state of autolysis. Swabs for virology were collected from each carcass, which was subsequently frozen at −20 °C until potential necropsy. According to the instructions of the Federal Research Institute for Animal Health, National Reference Laboratory for Avian Influenza, Isle of Riems, Germany, combined tracheal and cloacal swabs were taken until 3rd of March 2006: the swab was introduced into the oral cavity to reach the lumen of the trachea, or, when the larynx was too narrow, the throat was cut from outside to take the swab; the same swab was used to sample the cloaca. Beginning 4th of March 2006, only tracheal swabs were taken.

Table 1 RT-PCR results in swabs of wild raptor species found dead in Mecklenburg-Western Pomerania in 2006

Species	Number of birds	
	Tested	H5N1-positive (%)
Common buzzard (*Buteo buteo*)	385	12* (3.1)
Eurasian sparrow hawk (*Accipiter nisus*)	111	0
Common kestrel (*Falco tinnunculus*)	38	0
Buzzard, species undetermined (*Buteo sp.*)	36	1** (2.7)
White-tailed sea eagle (*Haliaeetus albicilla*)	19	0
Raptors, species undetermined	12	0
Northern goshawk (*Accipiter gentilis*)	10	0
Peregrine falcon (*Falco peregrinus*)	6	2*** (33.3)
Red kite (*Milvus milvus*)	3	0
Rough-legged buzzard (*Buteo lagopus*)	3	0
Western marsh harrier (*Circus aeruginosus*)	1	0
Total	624	15 (2.4)

*Seven tested by combined tracheal and cloacal swabs, five tested by tracheal swabs only.
**Tested by combined tracheal and cloacal swab.
***Tested by tracheal swabs only.

Table 2 Sex and age of selected raptor species found dead in Mecklenburg-Western Pomerania in 2006

Species	Sex		Age		
	Female	Male	Juvenile	Subadult	Adult
Common buzzard	4	2	2	0	4
Peregrine falcon	2	0	1	0	1
White-tailed sea eagle	12	7	14	2	3

Both selection of carcasses for necropsy and level of sampling of necropsied carcasses differed between white-tailed sea eagles (*Haliaeetus albicilla*) and other raptor species. For white-tailed sea eagles, all 19 individuals underwent necropsy, regardless whether their swabs tested positive or negative for H5N1, and tissue samples of lung, liver, spleen, kidney, pancreas and brain were collected for virology and stored at −70 °C until analysis. Duplicate samples of the same tissues were collected for histopathology and immunohistochemistry and fixed in 10% neutral-buffered formalin until analysis. For other raptor species, only individuals with H5N1-positive swabs and either freshly dead or intact and expected to be in a mild state of autolysis underwent necropsy: six common buzzards (B1 to B6) and two peregrine falcons (*Falco peregrinus*) (F1 and F2). During this necropsy, tissue samples of nasal turbinate, air sac, trachea, bronchus, lung, heart, liver, spleen, kidney, adrenal gland, pancreas, stomach, jejunum, colon, cerebrum, cerebellum, reproductive tract and cloacal bursa (or cloacal area if cloacal bursa was not visible) were collected for virology and stored at −70 °C until analysis. Duplicate samples of the same tissues were collected for histopathology and immunohistochemistry and fixed in 10% neutral-buffered formalin until analysis. In addition, separate pharyngeal and cloacal swabs for virology were placed in Hank's balanced salt solution containing 0.5% lactalbumin, 10% glycerol, 200 U/mL penicillin, 200 μg/mL streptomycin, 100 U/mL polymyxin B sulfate, 250 μg/mL gentamycin, and 50 U/mL nystatin (ICN Pharmaceuticals, Zoetermeer, The Netherlands), and stored at −70 °C until analysis.

Virology

Swabs were examined by testing extracted total RNA for the presence of influenza A virus matrix gene-fragment by

RT-PCR. A positive result was followed by further subtype differentiation using real-time RT-PCR targeting fragments of the H5 and N1 genes [10]. Tissue samples were weighed and subsequently homogenized with a FastPrep-24 (MP Biomedicals, Eindhoven, The Netherlands) in Hank's balanced salt solution and centrifuged briefly before dilution. Quadruplicate 10-fold serial dilutions of tissue samples and swab supernatants (separate pharyngeal and cloacal swabs from common buzzards, B1 to B6, and peregrine falcons, F1 and F2, only) were used to determine the virus titers in confluent layers of Madin-Darby canine kidney cells as described previously [11].

Histopathology and immunohistochemistry

Formalin-fixed tissue samples from common buzzards, B1 to B6, and peregrine falcons, F1 and F2, were embedded in paraffin, sectioned at 4 μm, and stained with hematoxylin and eosin (HE) for histopathological examination by light microscopy. For immunohistochemical detection of influenza virus antigen, duplicate sections of the same tissue samples were stained with a primary antibody against the influenza A nucleoprotein as described previously [12]. Peroxidase activity was revealed using 3-amino-9-ethylcarbazole (AEC) (Sigma, St Louis, MO, USA), resulting in a bright red precipitate. In each staining procedure an isotype control was included as a negative control and a lung section from an H5N1-infected cat was included as a positive control [13].

Results

Virology

Out of 624 individual raptors belonging to 9 different species, H5N1 was detected by RT-PCR in the swabs of only 2 species: common buzzard (12 of 385) and peregrine falcon (2 of 6) (Table 1). All pharyngeal swabs and most cloacal swabs of the necropsied common buzzards and peregrine falcons were H5N1-positive by RT-PCR, with comparable viral RNA levels in pharyngeal and cloacal swabs (Table 3). Multiple tissues in the necropsied common buzzards and peregrine falcons were H5N1-positive by RT-PCR (Table 3) in contrast to tissues of the 19 white-tailed sea eagles, all of which were H5N1-negative. Overall, the viral RNA levels in the brain samples of both common buzzards and peregrine falcons were considerably higher than in any other tissue samples. Interestingly, viral RNA levels were high in pancreas samples of the peregrine falcons but not in those of the common buzzards.

By virus culture, pharyngeal swabs of necropsied common buzzards and peregrine falcons tested positive for H5N1 more frequently than cloacal swabs (Table 3). Far fewer tissue samples tested positive for H5N1 by virus culture than by RT-PCR (Table 3): H5N1 was consistently cultured only from brain and lung samples in both common buzzards and peregrine falcons, always with the highest titers in brain samples.

Gross pathology

The nutritional state of the white-tailed sea eagles ranged from poor to good. All common buzzards and peregrine

Table 3 RT-PCR results and virus titers in swabs and organs of selected H5N1-infected wild raptors

RT-PCR values* (virus titers)**								
Samples	**Common buzzards**						**Peregrine falcons**	
	B1	**B2**	**B3**	**B4**	**B5**	**B6**	**F1**	**F2**
Pharyngeal swab	24.2 (2.2)	26.7 (0.8)	23.9 (0.8)	26.9 (n)	29.0 (1.2)	28.9 (n)	26.8 (2.2)	28.8 (n)
Cloacal swab	25.9 (n***)	np****	n (n)	24.6 (n)	28.2 (n)	31.0 (n)	16.5 (2.5)	28.2 (1.5)
Lung	18.1 (5.1)	19.6 (5.0)	17.6 (2.8)	14.4 (2.0)	22.0 (4.2)	24.5 (3.4)	22.1 (2.8)	34.6 (4.0)
Air sac	17.3 (n)	19.2 (2.6)	21.2 (n)	21.0 (n)	17.5 (2.5)	22.2 (n)	13.2 (n)	25.9 (n)
Liver	n (n)	28.3 (n)	26.1 (n)	21.9 (n)	24.5 (n)	20.7 (n)	20.3 (n)	21.6 (n)
Spleen	21.5 (n)	21.6 (n)	25.5 (n)	27.5 (n)	28.4 (n)	22.1 (n)	26.7 (n)	21.2 (n)
Heart	24.0 (n)	21.9 (2.3)	17.4 (n)	19.6 (n)	15.3 (n)	17.2 (n)	20.1 (n)	19.5 (n)
Kidney	24.5 (1.6)	23.2 (n)	19.7 (n)	15.0 (n)	19.5 (n)	19.9 (n)	18.4 (n)	26.4 (n)
Jejunum	18.9 (1.9)	17.7 (n)	29.7 (n)	29.3 (n)	22.6 (n)	20.7 (n)	21.8 (n)	22.7 (n)
Colon	20.4 (n)	21.4 (n)	29.6 (n)	27.1 (n)	21.4 (n)	19.7 (n)	24.4 (n)	22.4 (n)
Pancreas	26.7 (n)	25.0 (n)	38.0 (n)	34.7 (n)	29.8 (n)	34.3 (n)	9.6 (n)	13.7 (2.5)
Cloaca/Bursa	np	21.4 (n)	29.1 (2.1)	20.8 (n)	np	np	np	20.9 (n)
Brain	15.5 (6.2)	9.5 (6.3)	13.4 (5.5)	11.3 (6.7)	9.1 (6.2)	18.5 (5.2)	8.8 (4.6)	14.1 (6.3)

*Cycle threshold (Ct) value: The cut-off value is 40.
**All titers are given in $TCID_{50}$ log 10.
***n = negative (<0.5 for virus titers).
****np = not present.

falcons were in poor nutritional state, lacking fat in the subcutis or body cavity, and showing mild to advanced atrophy of the breast muscles. Externally, no lesions were found. Internally, there were lesions in several organs: multifocal hemorrhage in the pancreas (B2 and B3); increased redness in the cerebrum (B1, B2, B3, B5, and F2); enlargement of the spleen (B1, B2 and B6) and kidneys (B1, B2, and B5); wet lungs (B4, B5, B6 and F2); many nematodes (most likely *Serratospiculum sp.*) in the abdominal air sac (F1 and F2), and multifocal hemorrhage in thorax or upper respiratory tract, suggestive of trauma (F1 and F2). Freeze-thaw artifacts and autolytic changes often hampered gross examination.

Histopathology

By histopathology, lesions were seen in the brain, air sac, oviduct, coelomic ganglion, heart, pancreas and adrenal gland of common buzzards and peregrine falcons (Figure 1). In the cerebrum and occasionally in the cerebellum, there was multifocal necrosis of neurons with hypereosinophilia of the cytoplasm, nucleomegaly, neuronophagy and mild increase of glial cells. Separately from this neuronal necrosis, there was a multifocal increase of glial cells with mild to moderate diffuse or perivascular infiltration with lymphocytes, plasma cells and macrophages. Furthermore, in the brain of one peregrine falcon (F2), there was multifocal mild to moderate infiltration with mononuclear cells around blood vessels, in meninges and beneath the ependyma, with necrosis of ependymal cells. In the coelomic ganglion (B4 and F2), there was multifocal necrosis of neurons with hypereosinophilia of cytoplasm, nucleomegaly, neuronophagy and mild infiltration with mononuclear cells. In the lamina propria of the air sac of almost all birds (not B4), there was necrosis of epithelial cells and a mild to moderate infiltration with mononuclear cells. In the lamina propria of the oviduct (B1 and F1), there was moderate infiltration with mononuclear cells. In the heart (B1, B2, B4 and B6), there was multifocal necrosis of cardiomyocytes and mild infiltration with mononuclear cells. In the adrenal gland of one common buzzard (B5), there were multiple large areas with central core of necrosis surrounded by a layer of macrophages, heterophils, plasma cells and lymphocytes. In the pancreas (F1 and F2), there was multifocal necrosis of pancreatic acinar cells and marked infiltration with mononuclear cells. In the bronchus (F2) and parabronchus (B1, F1 and F2) in the lungs of few birds there was mild infiltration on predominantly heterophils in the epithelium and interstitium and mild epithelial necrosis. In the parabronchus and air sac of the peregrine falcons (F1 and F2), there were also intralesional helminth eggs in the lumina and in the epithelium (consistent with *Serratospiculum sp.* infection). Freeze-thaw artifacts and mild autolytic changes were present in most tissues, but did not prevent histopathological assessment.

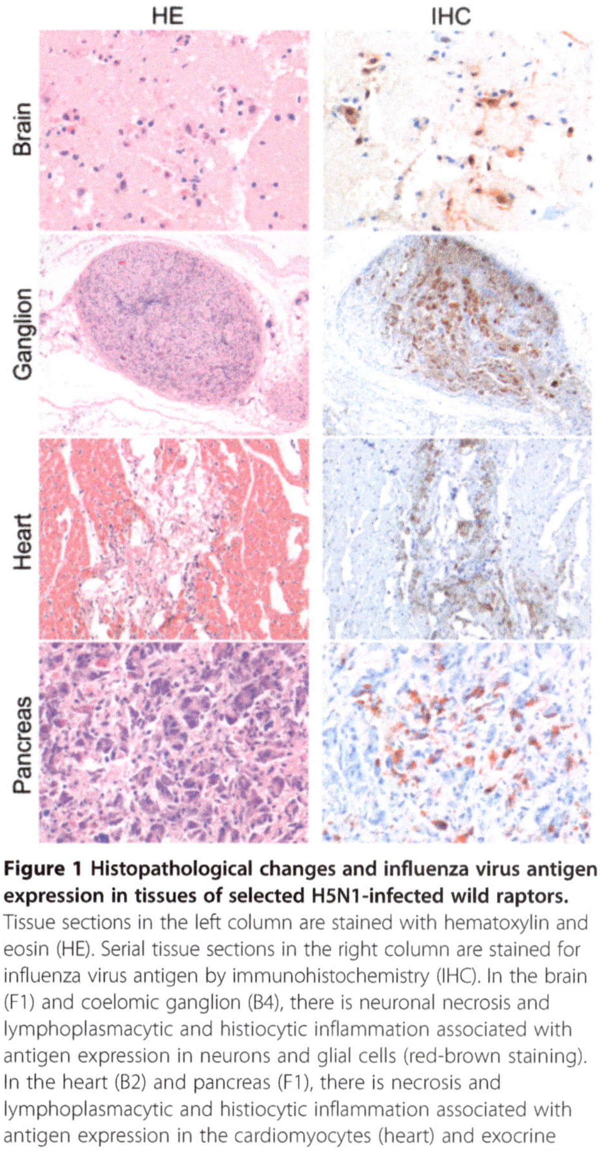

Figure 1 Histopathological changes and influenza virus antigen expression in tissues of selected H5N1-infected wild raptors. Tissue sections in the left column are stained with hematoxylin and eosin (HE). Serial tissue sections in the right column are stained for influenza virus antigen by immunohistochemistry (IHC). In the brain (F1) and coelomic ganglion (B4), there is neuronal necrosis and lymphoplasmacytic and histiocytic inflammation associated with antigen expression in neurons and glial cells (red-brown staining). In the heart (B2) and pancreas (F1), there is necrosis and lymphoplasmacytic and histiocytic inflammation associated with antigen expression in the cardiomyocytes (heart) and exocrine pancreatic cells (pancreas). In all selected tissues freeze-thawn artifacts and mild autolytic changes are visible.

Immunohistochemistry

By immunohistochemistry, influenza virus antigen expression was visible as diffuse red staining mainly in the cytoplasm and occasionally in the nucleus of affected cells. Virus antigen expression was found in multiple tissues (Figure 1) and was associated with histopathological changes. Virus antigen expression was seen most frequently in the brain (all birds) and air sac (B1-3, B5, B6 and F1). In the brain there were multiple foci of positive cells in the cerebrum of all common buzzards and peregrine falcons and in the cerebellum of some birds. In the brain, many neurons and—in one peregrine falcon, F2—ependymal cells, and few glial cells expressed virus antigen. In the coelomic ganglion (B4 and F2), many neurons expressed virus antigen. In the air sac, oviduct (B1, B2 and F1), and bronchus (F2), few epithelial cells expressed virus antigen. In the heart (B2, B4 and B5), few myocardial cells expressed antigen. In multiple granulomas in the adrenal gland of one common buzzard (B5), many macrophages expressed antigen. In the pancreas (F1 and F2), moderate numbers of pancreatic acinar cells expressed antigen.

Discussion

Our study shows that, during the 2006 H5N1 outbreak in wild waterbirds in Mecklenburg- Western Pomerania, Germany, both common buzzards and peregrine falcons were exposed to and suffered fatal disease from H5N1 infection, while seven other raptor species examined showed no evidence of H5N1 infection. In both species, H5N1 showed a distinct neurotropism associated with marked encephalitis, comparable to that observed in most other susceptible wild bird species.

The differences in diet and hunting or scavenging behavior among the nine raptor species was likely an important factor in their exposure to H5N1 in the 2006 outbreak in Germany. This outbreak affected mainly swans, geese, gulls, and diving ducks, all medium-sized birds [14] and the viruses of the waterbirds were closely related to the virus found in a common buzzard that tested positive for H5N1 in the same period and the same area [4]. The Eurasian sparrowhawk and common kestrel do not eat carrion and hunt only small (passerine) birds [15,16] or small mammals [17]; this could explain why H5N1 was not detected in either raptor species, despite the relatively high number of individuals examined. In contrast, the common buzzard and peregrine falcon, both of which were found positive for H5N1, do hunt medium-sized birds—common buzzards up to the size of a pheasant (~1200 g) [15]; peregrine falcons mainly in the range 20 to 300 g for males, and 100–1000 g for females [18,19]—or feed on carrion (common buzzard) [20]. (Interestingly, both H5N1-positive peregrine falcons were females.) The remaining five raptor species (white-tailed sea eagle, northern goshawk, red kite, rough-legged buzzard, and western marsh-harrier) all are known to hunt medium-sized birds and—except for the northern goshawk—to eat carrion, and therefore were at risk of exposure to H5N1 during the outbreak. Remarkably, the white-tailed sea eagles which feed on waterbirds up to the size of swans and also on carrion, were tested negative. The reason why H5N1 was not detected in any individuals of these five species may be due to the small sample size. Alternatively, it may be due to a species-specific resistance to disease from H5N1 infection, similar to that seen in other avian species. For example, in experimental H5N1 infection of six different duck species, tufted ducks (*Aythya fuligula*) and Eurasian pochards (*A. ferina*) showed clinical signs of disease, while the remaining four species, all dabbling ducks belonging to the genus *Anas*, were clinically unaffected [21].

The tissue tropism of H5N1 and the character of the associated lesions in these common buzzards and peregrine falcons correspond with those seen previously in other avian species (reviewed in [22,23], including naturally [3,5,6,24] and experimentally [25,26] H5N1 infected raptors. H5N1 in these common buzzards and peregrine falcons was clearly neurotropic and associated with marked encephalitis, similar to that seen in naturally infected common buzzards from Germany [3] and Sweden [5] and in experimentally infected American kestrels (*Falco sparverius*) [25]. The detection of influenza virus antigen expression and associated lesions in the coelomic ganglion in our birds indicates neurotropism for both the peripheral and central nervous systems. Besides the nervous system, H5N1 in our common buzzards and peregrine falcons also had tropism for other organs, including pancreas, heart, lung, air sac and oviduct. Such pantropism corresponds with that found in other bird species (reviewed in [22,23]. The specific tropism of H5N1 for the pancreas in our peregrine falcons also has been noted in experimental H5N1 infection of American kestrels [25]. In contrast to different swan species, where H5N1 exhibited endotheliotropism [3], no influenza virus antigen expression was seen in endothelial cells of any of these common buzzards or peregrine falcons.

The discrepancy between the results in the immunohistochemistry, RT-PCR and virus titration can most likely be attributed to the extended storage time in the –20 °C freezer and to the difference in sensitivity of the tests. Also, autolysis before storage and freezing artifacts hampered the necropsy and data analyses.

Although it is likely that these common buzzards and peregrine falcons became infected with H5N1 because of feeding on H5N1-contaminated carcasses, as has been shown experimentally in gulls [27], it is not clear by which of three potential portals of entry H5N1 gained entrance. The first possible portal of entry is the intestine, as proven by direct gastric inoculation of H5N1 in different experimental mammals [28-31]. A second possible portal of entry is the olfactory nerve: this was proven by intranasal inoculation of H5N1 in ferrets, in which viral replication in the olfactory mucosa was followed by spread to the olfactory bulb, and from there to the rest of the central nervous system [32]. The third possible portal of entry is the respiratory tract. Because H5N1-contaminated meat in these common buzzards and peregrine falcons would have passed the throat, which is the cross-roads between digestive and respiratory tracts, this latter portal of entry cannot be excluded. More extensive sampling of H5N1-infected raptors at different time points after infection may elucidate the portal of entry and subsequent pathogenesis of H5N1 infection in raptors.

In conclusion, our study implies that the position of raptors at the top of the food pyramid puts them at risk of acquiring infectious pathogens such as H5N1 by eating sick or dead prey. Because of their broad geographic range and migratory nature, they may contribute to long-distance movement of such pathogens; however, this contribution is likely much smaller than that of more numerous species of migratory birds. Our data suggest that some raptor species, such as common buzzards and peregrine falcons, are more likely to eat sick or dead wild waterbirds and subsequently are more exposed to H5N1 infection than other species, such as Eurasian sparrowhawks and common kestrels. Whether there is species-specific resistance to disease from H5N1 infection in some raptor species, such as white-tailed sea eagles, remains to be determined.

Competing interests
The authors declare that they have no competing interests.

Authors' contributions
Conceived and designed the study: JvdB, OK, TK. Performed the necropsies: JvdB, OK, GvA. Analyzed the data: JvdB, PW, MvdB. Drafted the manuscript: JvdB, OK, AO, TK. All authors read and approved the final manuscript.

Acknowledgements
We are grateful for the excellent technical assistance provided by D. de Meulder and P. van Run, and for the figure preparation by F. van der Panne.

Author details
[1]Department of Viroscience, Erasmus Medical Center, Dr. Molewaterplein 50, 3015 GE Rotterdam, Netherlands. [2]Department Wildlife Diseases, Leibniz Institute for Zoo and Wildlife Research, Alfred-Kowalke-Straße 17, 10315 Berlin, Germany. [3]Department for Diagnostic Investigation of Epizootics (LALLF), State Office for Agriculture, Food Safety, and Fishery, Mecklenburg-Western Pomerania, Rostock, Germany.

References
1. Liu J, Xiao H, Lei F, Zhu Q, Qin K, Zhang XW, Zhang XL, Zhao D, Wang G, Feng Y, Ma J, Liu W, Wang J, Gao GF (2005) Highly pathogenic H5N1 influenza virus infection in migratory birds. Science 309:1206
2. Chen H, Smith GJ, Zhang SY, Qin K, Wang J, Li KS, Webster RG, Peiris JS, Guan Y (2005) Avian flu: H5N1 virus outbreak in migratory waterfowl. Nature 436:191–192
3. Teifke JP, Klopfleisch R, Globig A, Starick E, Hoffmann B, Wolf PU, Beer M, Mettenleiter TC, Harder TC (2007) Pathology of natural infections by H5N1 highly pathogenic avian influenza virus in mute (Cygnus olor) and whooper (Cygnus cygnus) swans. Vet Pathol 44:137–143
4. Starick E, Beer M, Hoffmann B, Staubach C, Werner O, Globig A, Strebelow G, Grund C, Durban M, Conraths FJ, Mettenleiter T, Harder T (2008) Phylogenetic analyses of highly pathogenic avian influenza virus isolates from Germany in 2006 and 2007 suggest at least three separate introductions of H5N1 virus. Vet Microbiol 128:243–252
5. Brojer C, Agren EO, Uhlhorn H, Bernodt K, Jansson DS, Gavier-Widen D (2012) Characterization of encephalitis in wild birds naturally infected by highly pathogenic avian influenza H5N1. Avian Dis 56:144–152
6. Marinova-Petkova A, Georgiev G, Seiler P, Darnell D, Franks J, Krauss S, Webby RJ, Webster RG (2012) Spread of influenza virus A (H5N1) clade 2.3.2.1 to Bulgaria in common buzzards. Emerg Infect Dis 18:1596–1602
7. Marjuki H, Wernery U, Yen HL, Franks J, Seiler P, Walker D, Krauss S, Webster RG (2009) Isolation of highly pathogenic avian influenza H5N1 virus from Saker falcons (Falco cherrug) in the Middle East. Adv Virol 2009:1
8. Van Borm S, Thomas I, Hanquet G, Lambrecht B, Boschmans M, Dupont G, Decaestecker M, Snacken R, van den Berg T (2005) Highly pathogenic H5N1 influenza virus in smuggled Thai eagles, Belgium. Emerg Infect Dis 11:702–705
9. Landesamt für Landwirtschaft, Lebensmittelsicherheit und Fischerei Meckelenburg-Vorpommern: Jahrbuch 2006. 1.1 Aviäre influenza (Hausgeflügel, Wildvögel, Säugetiere). 2007, pp. 9–11.
10. Spackman E, Senne DA, Myers TJ, Bulaga LL, Garber LP, Perdue ML, Lohman K, Daum LT, Suarez DL (2002) Development of a real-time reverse transcriptase PCR assay for type A influenza virus and the avian H5 and H7 hemagglutinin subtypes. J Clin Microbiol 40:3256–3260
11. Rimmelzwaan GF, Baars M, Claas EC, Osterhaus AD (1998) Comparison of RNA hybridization, hemagglutination assay, titration of infectious virus and immunofluorescence as methods for monitoring influenza virus replication in vitro. J Virol Methods 74:57–66
12. van den Brand JM, Stittelaar KJ, Leijten LM, van Amerongen G, Simon JH, Osterhaus AD, Kuiken T (2012) Modification of the ferret model for pneumonia from seasonal human influenza A virus infection. Vet Pathol 49:562–568
13. Kuiken T, Rimmelzwaan G, van Riel D, van Amerongen G, Baars M, Fouchier R, Osterhaus A (2004) Avian H5N1 influenza in cats. Science 306:241
14. Globig A, Baumer A, Revilla-Fernandez S, Beer M, Wodak E, Fink M, Greber N, Harder TC, Wilking H, Brunhart I, Matthes D, Kraatz U, Strunk P, Fiedler W, Fereidouni SR, Staubach C, Conraths FJ, Griot C, Mettenleiter TC, Stärk KD (2009) Ducks as sentinels for avian influenza in wild birds. Emerg Infect Dis 15:1633–1636
15. Thiollay JM (1994) Family Accipitridae. In: del Hoyo J, Elliot A, Sargatal J (ed) Handbook of the birds of the world. Volume 2. Barcelona, Spain, Lynx edicions, p 185
16. Newton I (1986) The sparrowhawk. Staffordshire, England, Poyser Monographs
17. Village A (2010) The kestrel. London, England, Poyser Monographs
18. White CM, Olsen PD, Kiff LF (1994) Family Falconidae. In: del Hoyo J, Elliot A, Sargatal J (ed) Handbook of the birds of the world. Volume 2. Lynx Edicions, Barcelona, Spain, p 274
19. Ratcliffe D (1993) The peregrine falcon. London, England, Poyser Monographs
20. Melde M (1983) Der Mäusebussard. Magdenburg, Germany, Neue Brehm Bücherei
21. Keawcharoen J, van Riel D, van Amerongen G, Bestebroer T, Beyer WE, van Lavieren R, Osterhaus AD, Fouchier RA, Kuiken T (2008) Wild ducks as long-distance vectors of highly pathogenic avian influenza virus (H5N1). Emerg Infect Dis 14:600–607
22. Pantin-Jackwood MJ, Swayne DE (2009) Pathogenesis and pathobiology of avian influenza virus infection in birds. Rev Sci Tech 28:113–136
23. Kuiken T, van den Brand J, van Riel D, Pantin-Jackwood M, Swayne DE (2010) Comparative pathology of select agent influenza a virus infections. Vet Pathol 47:893–914
24. Shivakoti S, Ito H, Otsuki K, Ito T (2010) Characterization of H5N1 highly pathogenic avian influenza virus isolated from a mountain hawk eagle in Japan. J Vet Med Sci 72:459–463
25. Hall JS, Ip HS, Franson JC, Meteyer C, Nashold S, TeSlaa JL, French J, Redig P, Brand C (2009) Experimental infection of a North American raptor, American Kestrel (Falco sparverius), with highly pathogenic avian influenza virus (H5N1). PLoS One 4:e7555
26. Bertran K, Busquets N, Abad FX (2012) Garcia de la Fuente J, Solanes D, Cordon I, Costa T, Dolz R, Majo N: Highly (H5N1) and low (H7N2) pathogenic avian influenza virus infection in falcons via nasochoanal route and ingestion of experimentally infected prey. PLoS One 7:e32107
27. Brown JD, Stallknecht DE, Beck JR, Suarez DL, Swayne DE (2006) Susceptibility of North American ducks and gulls to H5N1 highly pathogenic avian influenza viruses. Emerg Infect Dis 12:1663–1670
28. Lipatov AS, Kwon YK, Pantin-Jackwood MJ, Swayne DE (2009) Pathogenesis of H5N1 influenza virus infections in mice and ferret models differs according to respiratory tract or digestive system exposure. J Infect Dis 199:717–725
29. Vahlenkamp TW, Teifke JP, Harder TC, Beer M, Mettenleiter TC (2010) Systemic influenza virus H5N1 infection in cats after gastrointestinal exposure. Influenza Other Respir Viruses 4:379–386

30. Reperant LA, van de Bildt MW, van Amerongen G, Leijten LM, Watson S, Palser A, Kellam P, Eissens AC, Frijlink HW, Osterhaus AD, Kuiken T (2012) Marked endotheliotropism of highly pathogenic avian influenza virus H5N1 following intestinal inoculation in cats. J Virol 86:1158–1165
31. Shinya K, Makino A, Tanaka H, Hatta M, Watanabe T, Le MQ, Imai H, Kawaoka Y (2011) Systemic dissemination of H5N1 influenza A viruses in ferrets and hamsters after direct intragastric inoculation. J Virol 85:4673–4678
32. Schrauwen EJ, Herfst S, Leijten LM, van Run P, Bestebroer TM, Linster M, Bodewes R, Kreijtz JH, Rimmelzwaan GF, Osterhaus AD, Fouchier RA, Kuiken T, van Riel D (2012) The multibasic cleavage site in H5N1 virus is critical for systemic spread along the olfactory and hematogenous routes in ferrets. J Virol 86:3975–3984

Quantification of transmission of foot-and-mouth disease virus caused by an environment contaminated with secretions and excretions from infected calves

Carla Bravo de Rueda[1,2], Mart CM de Jong[2*], Phaedra L Eblé[1] and Aldo Dekker[1]

Abstract

Foot-and-mouth disease virus (FMDV) infected animals can contaminate the environment with their secretions and excretions. To quantify the contribution of a contaminated environment to the transmission of FMDV, this study used calves that were not vaccinated and calves that were vaccinated 1 week prior to inoculation with the virus in direct and indirect contact experiments. In direct contact experiments, contact calves were exposed to inoculated calves in the same room. In indirect contact experiments, contact calves were housed in rooms that previously had held inoculated calves for three days (either from 0 to 3 or from 3 to 6 days post inoculation). Secretions and excretions from all calves were tested for the presence of FMDV by virus isolation; the results were used to quantify FMDV transmission. This was done using a generalized linear model based on a 2 route (2R, i.e. direct contact and environment) SIR model that included information on FMDV survival in the environment. The study shows that roughly 44% of transmission occurs via the environment, as indicated by the reproduction ratio $\hat{R}_0{}^{2R}{}_{environment}$ that equalled 2.0, whereas the sum of $\hat{R}_0{}^{2R}{}_{contact}$ and $\hat{R}_0{}^{2R}{}_{environment}$ equalled 4.6. Because vaccination 1 week prior to inoculation of the calves conferred protective immunity against FMDV infection, no transmission rate parameters could be estimated from the experiments with vaccinated calves. We conclude that a contaminated environment contributes considerably to the transmission of FMDV therefore that hygiene measures can play a crucial role in FMD control.

Introduction

Foot-and-mouth disease virus (FMDV) is the causative agent of foot-and-mouth disease (FMD), a highly contagious disease of livestock. Outbreaks of FMD cause vast sums of money to be spent, to reduce its incidence to low levels [1]. Control measures to restrict the spread of FMDV include movement restrictions, but even when movement restrictions are applied, these do not always prevent new outbreaks (for example in the 2001 FMD epidemic in United Kingdom [2]). Since these restrictions mean that livestock are not allowed to move between farms, direct contact cannot be the (major) cause of transmission, so other, indirect, routes must play a role.

Because most of the secretions and excretions of FMDV infected animals contain virus [3], environmental contamination with secretions and excretions containing FMDV was considered to be one of the causes of FMDV spread [4]. This conclusion was supported by the fact that FMDV remains in the environment, for at least 24 h, after infected animals are killed [5]. Moreover, as studies on survival of FMDV in secretions and excretions have shown, detectable amounts of FMDV persist in the environment (for example, in manure) for up to 14 weeks due to the thermal stability of the virus [6,7]. The suspicion that an environment contaminated with secretions and excretions from FMDV infected animals contributes to the transmission of FMDV has likewise persisted.

SIR (susceptible-infected-recovered) models have been used to model the role of the environment in the transmission of different pathogens [8-12]. Although

* Correspondence: mart.dejong@wur.nl
[2]Department Quantitative Veterinary Epidemiology, Wageningen University, P.O. Box 338, 6700 AH Wageningen, The Netherlands
Full list of author information is available at the end of the article

transmission of FMDV has been quantified in animal experiments [13,14] using a stochastic SIR model [15] and a transient-state algorithm [16], such studies have neither modelled nor quantified the contribution of the environment. In addition, FMDV transmission is known to be reduced through vaccination [17], and that vaccinating 2 weeks before inoculation with the virus reduces the reproduction ratio R_0 to a value below 1 [18]. However, it is unknown whether this could be accomplished through earlier vaccination.

Thus, the aim of the present study is twofold: to utilize a 2 route-SIR model i.e. with both direct contact and indirect (environment) routes, to quantify the contribution of a contaminated environment to the transmission of FMDV, and to examine whether vaccination one week before inoculation with the virus could reduce FMDV transmission through either direct contact or via the environment. As this article shows, a contaminated environment contributes considerably to the transmission of FMDV, and vaccination of cattle 1 week prior to inoculation with the virus does confer protective immunity against FMDV infection.

Materials and methods

Experimental design

We used 46 female calves, aged between 6 and 7 months, born and raised in The Netherlands on conventional dairy farms. Our experiments were performed in rooms approximately 10 m^2 inside the biosecurity facilities of the Central Veterinary Institute (CVI, Lelystad, The Netherlands). The settings for temperature and humidity in the stables were 20 – 24 °C and 40 – 70% relative humidity respectively. The experiments received ethical approval from the animal experiment committee of the CVI in accordance with Dutch law. The experiments with non-vaccinated calves and the experiments with vaccinated calves were performed sequentially. During the experiments, all calves were inspected daily for clinical signs of FMD. In these inspections, rectal temperature above 39.5 °C was considered fever [19] and the calves were checked for the presence of FMD lesions i.e. vesicles. During inspection and/or sampling, animal caretakers changed coveralls and gloves between animal rooms. The animal rooms in which the indirect transmission experiments were performed were not cleaned with water; instead, animal waste was swept daily with a broom to the drainage.

Challenge virus and vaccine

Virus inoculation was performed intranasally using FMDV Asia-1 TUR/11/2000. The inoculum contained $10^{6.1}$ plaque forming units (pfu)/mL (titrated on primary lamb kidney cells). Each inoculated calf received 1.5 mL of inoculum per nostril. The vaccine used was a freshly prepared inactivated FMDV Asia-1 Shamir vaccine, prepared in a double water-in-oil emulsion. The potency of a similarly prepared vaccine was previously determined at > 6 PD_{50} (at 28 days post vaccination).

Direct contact experiments

In both vaccinated and unvaccinated scenarios, 10 calves were randomly assigned to 5 animal rooms in pairs i.e. 2 calves per room. On the day of inoculation i.e. 0 days post inoculation (dpi), 1 calf from each pair was moved to a separate animal room and inoculated with FMDV. Eight hours after inoculation, these calves were reunited with their original roommates. In the experiment in which vaccinated calves were used, all 10 calves were vaccinated intramuscularly with 2 mL of vaccine one week before inoculation (–7 dpi). The direct contact experiments ended at 14 dpi, assuming this duration could allow transmission to occur.

Indirect contact experiments

This experimental design is shown in Figure 1. In both vaccinated and unvaccinated scenarios, 4 calves were inoculated with FMDV at 0 dpi (2 pairs (groups A and B) of inoculated calves, IA and IB). Eight hours after inoculation, they were moved into 2 animal rooms to which they had been randomly assigned, 2 calves per room. At 3 dpi, the inoculated calves were moved to 2 new animal rooms. Subsequently, 1 pair of non-vaccinated contact calves (contacts 1, C1A and C1B) was moved into each of the animal rooms that had been contaminated by the inoculated calves. The inoculated calves stayed in their new rooms from 3 to 6 dpi; at 6 dpi, they were removed from the animal rooms and euthanized. On the same day, each of these now-contaminated rooms was allocated to a pair of non-vaccinated contact calves (contacts 2, C2A and C2B). In the experiment in which vaccinated calves were used, at –7 dpi the 4 inoculated calves were vaccinated intramuscularly with 2 mL of vaccine. The 8 contact calves were not vaccinated. The indirect contact experiments ended at 20 dpi.

Vaccine controls

During the experiment with vaccinated calves, 2 additional calves were vaccinated and used as vaccine control group to evaluate the serological response of the calves in the absence of infection; these controls were housed together in a separate animal room.

Sampling

Oropharyngeal fluid (OPF) swabs, heparinised blood, urine and faeces samples were collected daily from each calf from 0 dpi until the end of the experiment. OPF was collected by inserting a cotton gauze with a 25 cm long forceps into the mouth of the calves and by rubbing

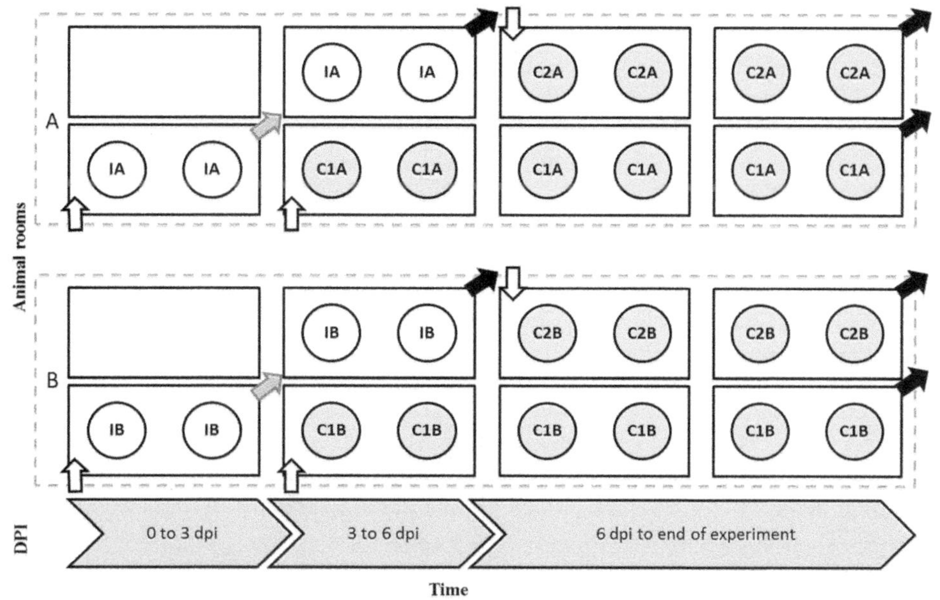

Figure 1 Indirect contact experiment design. Panels **A** and **B** represent groups A and B. IA and IB, calves inoculated at 0 days post infection (dpi); C1A and C1B, contact exposed calves to contaminated environment from 0 to 3 dpi; C2A and C2B, contact exposed calves to contaminated environment from 3 to 6 dpi. Grey arrows indicate movement of animals to an (– other) animal room. Black arrows indicate movement of animals for euthanasia.

the surface of the oropharyngeal cavity. In the laboratory, the pieces of cotton gauze were immersed in 4 mL of Eagle's minimum essential medium (EMEM) containing 2% fetal calf serum (FCS) and 10% antibiotics solution (ABII: 1000 U/mL of penicillin, 1 mg/mL of streptomycin, 20 μg/mL of amphotericin B, 500 μg/mL of polymixin B, and 10 mg/mL of kanamycin). After 20 min of incubation at environmental temperature, the samples were centrifuged (2500 rpm for 15 min). Samples were stored at −70 ℃ until virus isolation and real-time reverse transcriptase polymerase chain reaction (RT-PCR) analysis.

Heparinised blood samples (10 mL per calf) for virus isolation were taken daily, while clotted blood samples (10 mL per calf) for serology were taken twice per week. Blood samples were centrifuged at 2500 rpm for 15 min. Plasma was stored at −70 ℃ until virus isolation analysis and serum was stored at −20 ℃ until serological analysis. Urine samples were collected, as calves were stimulated to urinate spontaneously by rubbing the skin next to the vulva. Urine samples were collected into sterile plastic containers. In the laboratory, 800 μL of urine was mixed with 200 μL of a 50% FCS, 50% ABII solution and stored at −70 ℃ until virus isolation analysis.

Faeces samples were collected from the rectum. In the laboratory, the faeces was suspended 1:10 (w/v) in EMEM containing 10% FCS and 10% ABII solution, and vortexed with glass beads. After 20 min of incubation at environmental temperature, the suspension was vortexed and centrifuged (3000 rpm for 15 min). The supernatants were stored at −70 ℃ until virus isolation analysis.

Virus detection

All OPF, heparinised blood, urine and faeces suspension samples were tested for presence of FMDV by plaque count on monolayers of secondary lamb kidney cells (virus isolation, VI). Samples were tested in 2 wells of a six-well plate using 200 μL per well, as previously described [20]. All OPF samples were also tested for presence of FMDV by RT-PCR. RNA isolation was performed using the Magna Pure LC total Nucleid Acid Isolation kit® (Roche) and the MagNa Pure 96 system® (Roche). Isolated RNA was tested in a LightCycler 480 Real-Time PCR System® (Roche) using a QuantiFast Probe RT-PCR kit® (Qiagen), all in accordance with the manufacturers' instructions. The primers, probes and test protocol used have been previously described [21].

Statistical analysis of virus secretions and excretions

Using data from both the direct and the indirect contact experiments, we calculated, for individual animals, the area under the curve (AUC) of the virus titres. The AUC represents the total amount of FMDV that was secreted and excreted by the infected calves during the experiment. The AUCs were calculated for each calf using the non-logarithm-transformed virus titres observed in its OPF swabs, urine and faeces samples. In the statistical analysis, the logarithm of the AUC was used (log AUC). The maximum FMDV log titres found in OPF swabs, urine and faeces samples from each calf were also calculated. The duration (in days) of FMDV secretion and excretion in OPF swabs, urine and faeces samples was calculated for each calf, counting from the first day until the last day the calf tested positive in the virus isolation assay (in either OPF swabs, urine or faeces samples). A Kruskal Wallis test was used to test whether differences existed between the experimental groups (i.e. inoculated calves, direct contacts, indirect contacts C1 and indirect contacts C2) for either the log AUC, the maximum FMDV log titres or the duration of FMDV secretion and excretion. The log AUC and the maximum FMDV log titres were tested for each type of sample (OPF swabs, urine and faeces). The duration of FMDV secretion and excretion was tested using data from OPF swabs, urine and faeces samples combined.

Antibody detection

A commercially available ELISA (PrioCHECK® FMDV NS, Prionics) was used to detect antibodies against non-structural proteins of FMDV. The test was performed in accordance to the manufacturer's instructions. This test detects antibodies against the non-structural protein 3B of FMDV and differentiates infected from non-infected animals in both non-vaccinated and vaccinated animals. Samples were considered to be positive when the percentage of inhibition was ≥ 50%. The virus neutralization test (VNT) was performed as previously described [22] but using BHK-21 cells instead of porcine kidney cells. Titres were determined against both the vaccine strain (Asia-1 Shamir) and the challenge strain (Asia-1 TUR/11/2000). Samples were considered to be positive when the titres were above 1.2 ^{10}log (cut-off of validated diagnostic test) using the Asia-1 Shamir strain and 0.6 ^{10}log (cut-off based on the score of control samples) using the Asia-1 TUR/11/2000 strain.

Quantification of the FMDV survival rate

The FMDV survival rate (σ day^{-1}), needed for the calculation of the contribution of the environment (E_t) to the transmission of FMDV, was calculated using published data on FMDV thermal inactivation combined with own laboratory data. Because the temperature in the animal rooms was approximately 20 °C during the experiments, the survival rate σ was estimated at 20 °C. The lowest, middle and highest estimates of the time needed for a 10-fold reduction in FMDV titres at 20 °C was used to calculate the FMDV survival rate σ. An additional file shows the calculation of the FMDV survival rate σ in more detail (Additional file 1 with references [7,20,23-27]).

Quantification of FMDV transmission

Transmission rate parameters: β, $\beta_{contact}$ and $\beta_{environment}$

The transmission rate parameter β is defined as the average number of new infections caused by one typical infectious individual per day in a totally "susceptible" (not infected) population [16,28] (Additional file 2: equations 1 and 2, with references [16,28,29]). For the analysis, as described previously [28], it was assumed that the calves were infectious (I) when one of their samples (OPF swabs, urine or faeces) tested positive in the virus isolation assay at the start of the time interval. Contact animals were considered cases (C) when one of their samples (OPF swabs, urine or faeces) tested positive, for the first time, in the virus isolation assay at the end of the time interval. The number of new cases (C) during that time interval is binomially distributed with probability p (which is a function of the transmission rate parameter β, the number of infected animals (I_t) and the total number of animals (N)) and with binomial total S_t, the number of susceptible animals. Thus, the probability of a single susceptible animal becoming infected during a period Δt is, $p = 1 - e^{-e^{C_0} \times \frac{I_t}{N_t} \times \Delta t}$, where e^{C_0} is the transmission rate parameter β. To quantify β, the data from the direct contact experiment were analysed using a generalized linear model (GLM) [30]. The GLM is based on the binomial distribution and the above-mentioned expression for p, using a complementary log-log link function, S as binomial total, a binomial error function and with $\log\left(\frac{I_t}{N_t} \times \Delta t\right)$ as offset [16,28]. This model will be hereinafter referred to as the 1 route-SIR (1R-SIR) model. To quantify the contribution of the environment to the transmission of FMDV, as an extra route to the 1R-SIR model (Figure 2), we included the environment (E). In the new 2 route-SIR model (2R-SIR) we additionally assumed that the amount of FMDV present

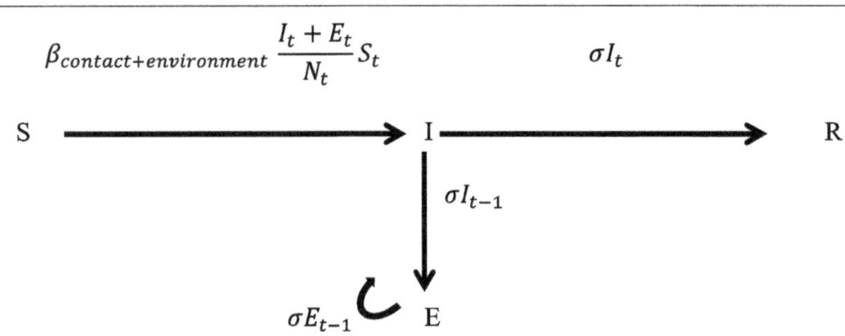

Figure 2 The 2R- SIR model. The combined transmission rate parameter ($\beta_{contact+environment}$) depends on the number of infectious calves (I_t) and/or on the amount of virus in the environment (E_t). E_t depends on FMDV secretion and excretion by the infected calves on previous days (t-1) and on the remaining amount of FMDV in the environment weighted by σ.

in the environment on a specific day (E_t) depends on the secretion and excretion of FMDV by infectious individuals (either I or C) on the previous days, as well as on the remaining FMDV in the environment ($E_{(t-1)}$), both weighted (discounted) by the FMDV survival rate (σ). E_t is represented by the following equation: $E_t = \sigma I_{(t-1)} + \sigma C_{(t-1)\rightarrow t} + \sigma E_{(t-1)}$ with starting condition $E_0 = 0$ (Additional file 2: equation 3). We performed a sensitivity analysis in which we multiplied the new cases (C) in the equation above either by 0 or by 0.5, instead of 1 as it is in the above equation for E_t, to check whether this affected the outcome. Additionally, we performed a sensitivity analysis in which we considered a latent period (counting the inoculated calves as infected but not yet infectious, (1, 2 and 3 days before virus shedding was detected), to check whether the use of an SEIR (susceptible-exposed-infected-recovered) instead of an SIR model would lead to different results for the estimated β and R values (i.e. if β is underestimated) and whether this affected the estimation of the environmental component.

In the 2R-SIR model, there are 2 ways by which the susceptible calves (S_t) can become infected: (1) because they have been in direct contact with an infectious calf (I_t) i.e. being in the same room at the same day as an infectious calf and/or (2) because they have been in contact with a contaminated environment (E_t) i.e. being in an animal room that housed previously one or more infectious individuals (Figure 2). By using the 2R-SIR model, we quantified the transmission rate parameters $\beta_{contact}$ and $\beta_{environment}$. As in the definition of β the transmission rate parameter $\beta_{contact}$ is defined as the average number of new infections per day caused by direct contact to one typical infectious individual in a fully susceptible population. The transmission rate parameter $\beta_{environment}$ is defined as the average number of new infections per day caused by virus in the environment, where the unit of infectivity is equal to the amount of virus secreted and excreted during one day by an infectious animal. An additional file shows the 2R-SIR model in more detail (Additional file 2: equations 4 to 6). In the 2R-SIR model, the number of new cases ($C_{t\rightarrow(t+1)}$), whether caused by I_t and/or E_t, is binomially distributed with parameter p as before (see also below) but now $\beta = e^{C_0 + C_1 \times fe}$ where $f_e = \frac{E_t}{I_t + E_t}$ is the fraction of transmission by the environment and therefore its regression coefficient measures the extra infectivity contributed by the environment. When only direct contact can occur, f_e is 0 and thus $\beta_{contact} = e^{C_0}$. When only environmental exposure can occur, f_e is 1 and $\beta_{environment} = e^{C_0 + C_1}$ (Additional file 2). The latter expression contains $c_0 + c_1$ and thus c_1 is the extra transmission for each unit of infectivity through the environment as compared to one unit through direct contact. Thus the probability of a susceptible animal becoming infected during a period Δt is $p = 1 - e^{-e^{C_0 + f_e \times C_1} \times \frac{I_t + E_t}{N_t} \times \Delta t}$ (Additional file 2: equation 6). To quantify $\beta_{contact}$ and $\beta_{environment}$ we analysed the combined data from both the direct contact experiment and the indirect contact experiment using a GLM. The GLM was based on the binomial distribution and the above mentioned expression for p using a complementary log-log link function, S as binomial total, a binomial error function, f_e as the explanatory variable [28] and with $\log\left(\frac{I_t + E_t}{N_t} \times \Delta t\right)$ as offset (Additional file 2: equations 7 and 8). To test whether $\beta_{contact}$ and $\beta_{environment}$ were significantly different from each other, we used the Wald test on the regression coefficient of f_e. Both analyses (of the 1R-SIR and of the 2R-SIR models) were performed using the statistical program R [31] and the package stats.

Infectious periods: T and τ

The infectious period T was defined as the average infectious period of the inoculated calves that caused transmission from the direct contact experiment. The infectious period of each inoculated calf was defined as the time between the first and the last day on which FMDV was detected (by virus isolation) in OPF swabs, urine, or faeces samples. The 95% confidence intervals (CI) of $\hat{T}$ were calculated using the logarithm of T (log T) and the variance of log T i.e. $e^{logT \pm 1.96\sqrt{var\ (logT)}}$. The infectious period τ represents the infectious period of the contaminated environment. The calculation of τ was based on the amount of infectious material present in the environment (E_t, used in the 2R-SIR model). Considering the loss of infectiousness due to inactivation at environmental temperature, τ was calculated by taking the sum of geometric series: $\tau = \sum_{i=1}^{\infty} \sigma^i \hat{T} = \hat{T}\left(\frac{1}{1-\sigma} - 1\right)$ where σ is the survival rate of FMDV and $\hat{T}$ is the estimated average infectious period of the inoculated calves in the direct contact experiment. The method allowed us to obtain an average period over which one infectious animal contributes to the contamination of the environment, weighted for the amount of infectious material relative to the amount secreted and excreted by an infectious animal on one day. The 95% CI of $\hat{\tau}$ was calculated using the 95% CI of $\hat{T}$.

Reproduction ratio R_0

Using the 1R-SIR model: R_0^{1R}

The reproduction ratio R_0^{1R} is defined as the average number of new infections caused by one typical infectious individual in a population made up entirely of susceptible individuals [32]. R_0^{1R} was estimated by multiplying the transmission rate parameter $\hat{\beta}$ by the infectious period $\hat{T}$. The 95% CI of $\hat{R}_0^{1R}$ was calculated using the variance and the regression constant of the GLM result (log β) and the variance and the logarithm of the average infectious period T, i.e. $e^{log\beta+logT\pm1.96\sqrt{var\ (log\beta)+var\ (logT)}}$.

Using the 2R-SIR model: $R_0{}^{2R}{}_{contact}$, $R_0^{2R}{}_{environment}$ and R_0^{2R}

The reproduction ratio $R_0{}^{2R}$ is defined as the average number of new infections caused by both direct contact to one typical infectious individual in a population made up entirely of susceptible individuals and the virus left in the environment by that one typical infectious individual on the previous days. Both $R_0{}^{2R}{}_{contact}$ and $R_0{}^{2R}{}_{environment}$ were estimated using the results from the 2R-SIR model, i.e. estimated transmission rate parameter $\hat{\beta}_{\ \text{contact}}$ and $\hat{\beta}_{\ \text{environment}}$. The $R_0{}^{2R}{}_{contact}$ was estimated by multiplying $\hat{\beta}_{\text{contact}}$ by the infectious period $\hat{T}$. The $R_0{}^{2R}{}_{environment}$ was estimated by multiplying $\hat{\beta}_{\text{environment}}$ by the infectious period $\hat{\tau}$. Subsequently $R_0{}^{2R}$ was estimated by summing $\hat{R}_0{}^{2R}{}_{contact}$ and $\hat{R}_0{}^{2R}{}_{environment}$. The $\hat{R}_0{}^{2R}{}_{contact}$ is the contribution to $\hat{R}_0{}^{2R}$ by direct contact to virus from an infectious individual (on the day virus secretion and excretion is detected by virus isolation). The $\hat{R}_0{}^{2R}{}_{environment}$ is the contribution to $\hat{R}_0{}^{2R}$ by the virus left in the environment by infectious individuals on previous days. The 95% CI of $\hat{R}_0{}^{2R}{}_{contact,}$ $\hat{R}_0{}^{2R}{}_{environment}$ and of $\hat{R}_0{}^{2R}$ were calculated. For this purpose, we used the variances and the regression constants (see above c_0 and c_1 in equation for p) of the GLM results (log $\beta_{contact}$ or log $\beta_{environment}$) and the variances and the logarithm of the average infectious periods (log T or log τ). Thus, the 95% CI of the $\hat{R}_0{}^{2R}{}_{contact}$ is $e^{log\beta_{contact}+\log T\pm1.96\sqrt{\text{var}\ (log\beta_{contact})+var(logT)}}$ and, the 95% CI of the $\hat{R}_0{}^{2R}{}_{environment}$ is $e^{log\beta_{environment}+\log T+loga\pm1.96\sqrt{\text{var}\ (log\beta_{environment})+var(logT)}}$ where a is $\left(\frac{1}{1-\sigma}-1\right)$. As $\hat{R}_0{}^{2R}$ is the sum of $\hat{R}_0{}^{2R}contact$ and $\hat{R}_0{}^{2R}environment$, its variance is $var\left(e^{\log(\hat{R}_0^{2R})}\right)=var\left(e^{\log(\hat{R}_0^{2R}contact)}\right)+var\left(e^{\log(\hat{R}_0^{2R}environment)}\right)$ and although this is not a linear function we calculated the 95% CI of the $\hat{R}_0{}^{2R}$ using: $var\left(e^{\log(\hat{R}_0^{2R})}\right)=e^{\text{var}(log(\hat{R}_0^{2R}contact))}+e^{var(log(\hat{R}_0^{2R}environment))}$.

Using the final size model: $R_0{}^{FS}$

The transmission parameter R_0 can also be estimated based only on the final outcome (the final size of the experiment, FS) [33]. We estimated the $R_0{}^{FS}$ based on the total number of infected calves at the end of the direct contact experiment under the assumption that the epidemic process ended before the experiment stopped [34]. The animals were considered infected when one or more of their samples tested positive in the virus isolation assay. Because in the direct contact experiment we got all 4 contacts infected in the 4 pairs in which the inoculated calf was considered to be infectious, we used continuity correction, i.e. 3.5 infections in 4 experiments, to avoid an infinite estimate for $R_0{}^{FS}$. The 95% confidence intervals (CI) of $\hat{R}_0{}^{FS}$ were estimated under the FS assumption by using the binomial distribution for the infected fraction [33,35].

Results

Experiments with non-vaccinated calves

Table 1 summarizes the results from the direct and indirect contact experiments with the non-vaccinated calves. FMDV transmission to the contact calves occurred in both experiments.

Direct contact experiment

Inoculated calves

FMD clinical signs were observed in 4 of the 5 inoculated calves. Three of these calves (calves 3643, 3645 and 3649) showed fever and had FMD lesions on the tongue. One of these 3 calves (calf 3643) also had hoof lesions, and another (calf 3651) showed FMD lesions on the nose. Three of the clinically infected calves (calves 3643, 3645 and 3649) shed FMDV in OPF, blood and urine (Table 1). One of these 3 calves (calf 3645) also shed FMDV in faeces. The fourth clinically infected calf (calf 3651) shed FMDV in OPF only. All the inoculated calves were positive in OPF by RT-PCR. Antibodies against non-structural proteins and neutralizing antibodies against FMDV were detected in serum samples from all the inoculated calves. Inoculated calf 3647 became subclinically infected, but shed FMDV in urine, was positive for FMDV in OPF by RT-PCR and developed antibodies against non-structural proteins and neutralizing antibodies against FMDV.

Contact calves

Clinical signs were observed in the 3 contact calves (calves 3644, 3646 and 3650) that were housed together with inoculated calves 3643, 3645 and 3649. The 3 contact calves showed fever and had FMD lesions on the tongue (calf 3646) and hooves (calves 3644 and 3650); they shed FMDV in OPF, blood and urine (Table 1). One of these 3 calves (calf 3650) also shed FMDV in faeces. Another contact calf (calf 3652) became subclinically infected; it shed FMDV in its OPF. Calves 3644, 3646 and 3650 were positive for FMDV in OPF by RT-PCR. All 4 contact calves in which the virus was detected showed antibodies against non-structural proteins and neutralizing antibodies against FMDV. Calf 3648, in contact with inoculated calf 3647, showed no FMD clinical signs and tested negative for FMDV and for antibodies against FMDV. Thus transmission occurred in 4 of the 5 animal

Table 1 Results of virus isolation, RT-PCR (OPF swabs only), antibody detection and detection of FMD clinical signs

Exp[a]	Calf ID	I:C[b]	Group	FMDV detection by virus isolation in OPF swabs (in log10 titres),blood(v), urine(u) and faeces(f) samples and by RT-PCR (OPF swabs only, in bold or as ≡)																				Antibody detection		Clin[c]	Inf[d]
				days post infection of the inoculated calves																				NS-ELISA	VNT		
				1	*2*	*3*	*4*	*5*	*6*	*7*	*8*	*9*	*10*	*11*	*12*	*13*	*14*	*15*	*16*	*17*	*18*	*19*	*20*				
DC	3643	I		≡[e]	**2.2**[f]	≡,v[g]	**2.6**,v,u[h]	**3.8**,v,u	**2.0**,u	-	-	-	-	-	-	-	-							+	+	Yes	Yes
	3644	C		-	-	-	-	**1.5**	-,v,u	**2.1**,v	**1.4**,v	≡	**1.7**,u	-	-	**1.2**	≡							+	+	Yes	Yes
	3645	I		-	-	≡,v	**2.5**,v,f[i]	**2.6**,v	**0.9**,u	**1.2**,u	**0.7**	**0.7**	-	-	-	-	-							+	+	Yes	Yes
	3646	C		-	-	-	-	-	≡	**3.8**	**4.3**,v	**3.0**,v,u	**3.0,u**	-,u	**0.4**	-	-							+	+	Yes	Yes
	3647	I		-	≡	-	-	-	-	-	-	-	-	-	-	-	-,u							+	+	No	No
	3648	C		-	-	-	-	-	-	-	-	-	-	-	-	-	-							-	-	No	No
	3649	I		-	-	**0.7**,v	**2.3**,v,u	**3.4**,v	**0.9**,u	-,u	-,u	-	-	-	-	-	-							+	+	Yes	Yes
	3650	C		-	-	-	-	-	**2.3**,v,u	**1.6**,v,u,f	**0.4**,u,f	≡,u	**0.9**	**0.4**	-,u	-	-							+	+	Yes	Yes
	3651	I		-	-	**1.4**	≡	**4.2**	**1.7**	**0.4**	-	-	-	-	-	-	-							+	+	Yes	Yes
	3652	C		-	-	-	-	-	-	-	0.4	-	-	-	-	-	-							+	+	No	Yes
IC	3653	I	A	-	-	n.t[j]	**1.7**,v,u	**3.4**,v	**2.1**,u															-	-	Yes	Yes
	3654	I	A	-	≡	**6.0**,v	**4.6**,v	**3.7**,v,f	**1.7**															-	-	Yes	Yes
	3657	C1	A			-	-	-	-	-	-	-	-	-	-	-	-	-	-	-	-	-	-	-	-	No	No
	3658	C1	A			-	-	-	-	-	-	-	-	-	-	-	-	-	-	-	-	-	-	-	-	No	No
	3661	C2	A						-	-	-	-	-	**3.7**,v	≡,v,u	≡,v,u	**2.4**	≡,u	≡	≡	-	-	-	+	+	Yes	Yes
	3662	C2	A						-	-	-	-	**2.0**	≡	≡	≡,v	**1.3**,v	**3.8**,v,u	**3.5**,v,u	**3.6**,u	≡	-	≡	+	+	Yes	Yes
	3655	I	B	-	-	**2.1**	**5.2**,v	**4.9**,v,u	**2.6**,u															-	-	No	Yes
	3656	I	B	-	0.4	≡,v	**3.2**,v,u	**5.0**,v,u,f	**3.5**,u															-	-	No	Yes
	3659	C1	B			-	-	**1.9**	**2.0**	**3.6**,v,f	**4.9**,v,u	**4.1**,v,u	**3.4**,u	-	**1.2**	-	-	-	-	-	-	-	-	+	+	Yes	Yes
	3660	C1	B			-	-	-	-	0.9	**1.3**,u	**0.7**	**1.0**	-	-	-	-	-	-	-	-	-	-	-	-	Yes	Yes
	3663	C2	B						-	-	-	-	-	-	-	**2.4**	**0.7**	**1.6**	**3.3**,u	**2.3**,u	≡	-	-	+	+	Yes	Yes
	3664	C2	B						-	**0.4**	**1.0**	1.9	**3.0,v**	**5.2**,v	≡,v	**2.6**	**0.4**	≡	-	-	-	-	-	+	+	Yes	Yes

[a]Exp=experiment: DC=direct contact, IC=indirect contact; [b]I=inoculated, C=contact animal; [c]Clin=clinical signs; [d]Inf=infectious; [e]results of virus isolation (VI) and RT-PCR of oral swab sample: - = VI and RT-PCR negative, ≡ = VI negative and RT-PCR positive; [f]oral swab sample scored positive for FMDV by VI (log10 pfu/mL), RT-PCR positive samples are indicated in **bold**; [g]v=viraemia: blood sample scored positive for FMDV by VI; [h]u=urine sample scored positive for FMDV by VI; [i]f=faeces sample scored positive for FMDV by VI; [j]n.t.=not tested. Table in which the PCR positive samples are indicated (thus either the ≡ or **VI titres in bold**) in an effort to help with the editorial of this table.

rooms in the direct contact experiment. The only moment infectious virus was recovered from inoculated calf 3647 (from urine) was at 14 dpi, at the day of the end of the experiment. Thus, occurrence of transmission was not possible anymore and this pair of calves (calves 3647 and 3648) was excluded from the estimation of the transmission rate parameters and the reproduction ratio.

Indirect contact experiment

Inoculated calves

Clinical signs were observed in 2 out of 4 inoculated calves (number 3653 and 3654; both in pair IA). These 2 inoculated calves showed fever and 1 of them had lesions on the tongue. The other 2 calves (calves 3655 and 3656; pair IB) showed no FMD specific clinical signs. In all 4 inoculated calves, virus was detected in the OPF (IA and IB). All four secreted and excreted FMDV in their blood, urine and/or faeces (Table 1). They all were positive for FMDV in OPF by RT-PCR. Thus, inoculated calves 3655 and 3656 were subclinically infected. Serum samples from all 4 inoculated calves were obtained only at 0 dpi and 3 dpi; in these samples neither antibodies against non-structural proteins nor neutralizing antibodies against FMDV were detected as expected.

Contact calves C1

Contact calves C1 were exposed to the animal rooms that were contaminated by the inoculated calves from 0 to 3 dpi. The contact calves of group C1A (calves 3657 and 3658) did not get infected; no FMD specific clinical signs were seen and both calves tested negative by virus isolation, by RT-PCR and, for antibodies against FMDV. The contact calves of group C1B (calves 3659 and 3660) showed fever and one had FMD lesions on the mouth, tongue, nose and hooves. Both C1B calves had virus detected in their OPF; one of them secreted and excreted virus in blood, urine and faeces, the other one excreted virus in urine. They tested positive for FMDV in OPF by RT-PCR. One C1B calf showed antibodies against non-structural proteins in serum (calf 3660). Both C1B calves showed neutralizing antibodies in serum.

Contact calves C2

Contact calves C2 were exposed to the animal rooms that were contaminated by the inoculated calves from 3 to 6 dpi. All the contact calves of groups C2A and C2B showed clinical signs. Three of them showed fever, and all of them showed FMD lesions on the nose and in the mouth. In all 4 calves, virus was detected in their OPF (Table 1); the calves secreted and/or excreted FMDV in the blood (calves 3661, 3662 and 3664) and in urine (calves 3661, 3662 and 3663). They all were positive for FMDV in OPF by RT-PCR. All developed antibodies against non-structural proteins as well as neutralising antibodies. Thus transmission occurred in the indirect contact experiment in 1 of the 2 animal rooms that were contaminated from 0 to 3 dpi and, in both of the animal rooms that were contaminated from 3 to 6 dpi.

Statistical analysis of virus secretion and excretion

The mean values for the AUC's, peak of virus shedding and duration of virus shedding (and their ranges) for OPF swabs, urine samples, faeces samples and blood samples for the inoculated group, the direct contact group and the indirect contact groups C1 and C2 are shown in Additional file 3.

No significant difference in log AUC could be determined between the different experimental groups i.e. inoculated, direct contacts, indirect contacts C1 and indirect contacts C2, neither for OPF swabs nor for urine nor for faeces ($p > 0.05$). No significant difference in the maximum FMDV log titres was found between the different experimental groups neither for OPF swabs nor for urine nor for faeces ($p > 0.05$). No significant difference in the duration of FMDV secretion and excretion could be determined between the different experimental groups ($p > 0.05$) (Additional file 3).

Experiments with vaccinated calves

At day of challenge (0 dpi, 7 days post vaccination), the average virus neutralisation test (VNT) titre against the vaccine strain FMDV Asia-1 Shamir for all the vaccinated calves (including the vaccine controls) was 2.2 ^{10}log. The average virus neutralisation test (VNT) titre against the challenge strain FMDV Asia-1 TUR/11/2000 was 1.2 ^{10}log.

Direct contact experiment

After challenge, neither the vaccinated inoculated calves nor the vaccinated contact calves showed clinical signs of FMD and all calves tested negative by virus isolation and RT-PCR. Only 2 inoculated calves (calves 3972 and 3976) developed antibodies against non-structural proteins.

Indirect contact experiment

After challenge, neither the vaccinated inoculated calves nor the non-vaccinated contact calves showed clinical signs of FMD. All calves tested negative by virus isolation and RT-PCR. Neither the vaccinated inoculated nor the non-vaccinated contact calves showed detectable antibodies against non-structural protein.

FMDV survival rate (σ)

From the combined published and own experimental data, it was estimated that at 20 °C a 10-fold reduction in FMDV titres occurs in 2.4 days (95% CI: 1.7, 3.3). We calculated the FMDV survival rate (σ) using the lowest (in spiked urine), middle (in spiked faeces) and highest (in spiked buffered solution) estimates obtained at 20 °C. An additional file shows these estimates inside a dashed pointed rectangle (Additional file 4). The estimated time needed for 10-fold reduction in FMDV titres in spiked urine (lowest value) was 0.5 days, indicating an FMDV survival rate (σ) of 0.014 day^{-1}. The estimated time needed for 10-fold reduction in FMDV titres in spiked faecal material (middle value) was 2.8 day indicating an FMDV survival rate (σ) of 0.44 day^{-1}. The estimated time needed for 10-fold reduction in FMDV titres in spiked buffered solution (highest value) was 8.2 days, indicating an FMDV survival rate (σ) of 0.75 day^{-1}. For the quantification of FMDV transmission, we used the middle estimate i.e. $\sigma = 0.44$ day^{-1}.

Quantification of FMDV transmission

Results of the 1R-SIR model

The transmission rate parameter $\hat{\beta}$ was 0.67 per day (95% CI: 0.26, 1.8). The average infectious period from the inoculated calves $\hat{T}$ was 5.5 days (95% CI: 4.5, 6.7). Therefore the estimated reproduction ratio $\hat{R}_0^{1R}$ was 3.7 (95% CI: 1.3, 10.), significantly above 1.

Results of the 2R- SIR model

The regression coefficient of f_e, the extra infectivity contributed by the environment, was not significantly different from 0 which means that $\beta_{contact}$ and $\beta_{environment}$ are not significantly different. Because $\beta_{environment}/\beta_{contact}$ equalled 1.4 (95% CI 0.14, 14), there is contribution of the environment. Using the most parsimonious model $\beta_{contact}$ and $\beta_{environment}$ were estimated both to be 0.45 per day (95% CI: 0.24, 0.85). Because $\hat{T}$ was 5.5 days (95% CI: 4.5, 6.7), $\hat{R}_0{}^{2R}{}_{contact}$ equalled 2.5 (95% CI: 1.3, 5.0). The average infectious period from the contaminated environment $\hat{\tau}$ was 4.3 days (95% CI: 3.6, 5.2), which leads to a $\hat{R}_0{}^{2R}{}_{environment}$ of 1.9 (95% CI: 1.007, 3.8). Combination of the two estimates $\left(\hat{R}_0{}^{2R}{}_{contact} + \hat{R}_0{}^{2R}{}_{environment}\right)$ resulted in $\hat{R}_0^{2R}$ equalled to 4.4 (95% CI: 1.5, 7.4), which is significantly above 1. $\hat{R}^{2R}$ was not significantly different from $\hat{R}_0^{1R}$ as can be seen from their overlapping confidence intervals. The contribution of the environmental transmission to the total transmission of FMDV was 44% $\left(\hat{R}_0{}^{2R}{}_{environment}/\hat{R}_0{}^{2R}.\right)$The sensitivity analysis, i.e. multiplication of the new infections or cases (C) in E_t by either 0 or 0.5, resulted in the same contribution of the environmental transmission (44%). When the lowest and the highest values of σ were used, the contribution of the environmental transmission to the total transmission was estimated to be 31% (when $\sigma = 0.014$ day^{-1}) and 75% (when $\sigma = 0.75$ day^{-1}). The sensitivity analysis in which we included a latent period of 1, 2 or 3 days, resulted in higher estimates for β (Additional file 5) and R_0 (Additional file 6) for the models with a latent period, but the estimated contribution of the environment stayed the same (Additional file 6).

Results of the final size model

The $\hat{R}_0^{FS}$ equalled 14 (95% CI: 1.3, infinite), which is significantly above 1. Based on the comparison of the confidence intervals, $\hat{R}_0^{FS}$ seems to be not significantly different from $\hat{R}_0^{1R}$ nor from $\hat{R}_0^{2R}$.

Experiments with vaccinated calves

After challenge, none of the inoculated or contact calves became infectious; therefore transmission parameters could not be estimated.

Discussion

In this study, we quantified the contribution of a contaminated environment to the transmission of FMDV and analysed whether vaccination one week prior to inoculation of the calves could block FMDV transmission. We show that using a 2R-SIR model allows FMDV transmission to be quantified in two parts: the direct contact component and the indirect i.e. via the environment component. Our results show that roughly 44% of the transmission of FMDV occurs via the environment, in the days after the calves started secreting and excreting the virus. The contribution of the environment to the transmission of FMDV depends on the FMDV survival rate; if the survival rate is high, the contribution of the environment is higher.

An environment that has previously housed infectious animals can contain FMDV if it is not properly disinfected after the removal of the infectious animals [5] and our study shows that this virus accumulation can cause new infections. As we show, environmental transmission of FMDV plays a role in the total transmission of FMDV also in groups of animals that do have direct contact. Transmission of FMDV has been quantified before in several studies by using a 1R-SIR model [14,18,36-41]. We believe that in all of these studies, transmission occurred through both routes: via direct contact to an infected animal and via indirect contact to a contaminated environment. However within the experimental design of those studies, the role of the environment could not be separated from the role of direct contact on the transmission of FMDV. By using both direct and indirect contact experiments we could employ a 2R-SIR model (that included accumulation of FMDV in the environment) to quantify the contribution of the environment $\left(\hat{R}_0{}^{2R}{}_{environment}\right)$ to the total transmission of FMDV. As expected, the estimated $\hat{R}_0^{1R}$, $\hat{R}_0^{2R}$ and $\hat{R}_0^{FS}$ are very similar to each other and moreover, they are similar to the $\hat{R}_0$ (by using a 1R-SIR model) estimated in other direct contact experiments with cattle infected with FMDV O/NET/2001 [18,41]. The consistency of these results indicates that our 2R-SIR model is valid for the estimation of the reproduction ratio and that it is very useful to separate both components i.e. the environment and direct contact transmission, for the quantification of their separate contribution to the transmission of FMDV. Moreover based on the statistical analysis of virus secretion and excretion, the results obtained with the 2R-SIR model are not biased by the route of infection i.e. inoculated and contact infected calves.

In our models, we used an SIR model and we did not incorporate a latent period (then we would have a SEIR i.e. susceptible, exposed, infectious, recovered model), although the data from the virus excretion of the inoculated animals suggest that for this group there is a latent period of approximately 2 days. The main reason why we did not incorporate a latent period in our study is because we did not want to introduce more complexity in the model. Also, incorporation of a latent period affects the estimates for the direct and indirect transmission more or less equally and thus the estimation of the role of the environment (the main interest of this research) was not be affected. Our sensitivity analysis showed that, when a latent period is incorporated in the models, the estimates of the transmission parameters are still "equal" i.e. not significantly different (Additional files 5 and 6). The transmission parameters we provide in Additional files 5 and 6, where a latent period was used, could be useful when the transmission parameters are applied for modelling disease outbreaks and the effect of control measures.

The temporal separation used in our indirect contact experiment allowed us to observe the occurrence of transmission through the environment by taking into consideration virus accumulation in 2 different periods i.e. 0–3 and 3–6 dpi. Temporal separation was also used by Charleston et al. [42] to study FMDV transmission, although they exposed "donor" calves to "recipient" calves by direct contact for 8 hours in separate environments that had been previously disinfected, and thus with no accumulation of virus in the environment. This would, based on our results, reduce transmission of FMDV. They conclude in their study that the occurrence of FMDV transmission is correlated with the presence of clinical signs. However, it has been previously shown that FMDV transmission also can occur before clinical signs are seen [39]. In our study as well, transmission through the environment was caused by one group of calves that contaminated the environment from 0 to 3 dpi but showed no clinical disease. This supports the conclusion that the correlation of FMDV transmission with the presence of clinical signs cannot be generalised to populations, if animals have direct contact to each other for a longer period and/or are present where accumulation of FMDV in the environment is plausible. FMDV transmission may not occur, however, when animals are separated by fences or wooden walls (in pigs [43]; in calves: Charleston et al. (personal communication), [20]), indicating that either exposure to virus secreting and/or excreting animals or exposure to virus contaminated surfaces is important for the occurrence of transmission.

Vaccination can be used as a tool to reduce transmission of FMDV [17]. In our study the calves vaccinated one week prior to inoculation with FMDV did not shed virus. Previously, vaccinating animals 2 weeks prior inoculation with FMDV was reported [18] to reduce FMDV transmission; our results indicate that vaccination reduces FMDV transmission even earlier. As others have demonstrated, vaccination rapidly protects cattle from clinical disease, and reduces virus shedding by infected cattle [44-46]. As our results indicate, vaccination as early as one week before challenge cannot only protect calves against infection but also, can avoid contamination of the environment and so prevent new infections.

In summary, our study shows that the environment is a relevant mechanism in the transmission of FMDV. The quantification of the magnitude of the contribution of transmission via the environment emphasises again that hygiene is an extremely important control measure for FMDV. And that, as already recommended by veterinary authorities, good disinfection of e.g. vehicles, walls and floors previously contaminated by infected animals is necessary to reduce the accumulation of the virus in the environment and therefore FMDV transmission. Also, the data from our experiment give some insight in which secretions and excretions contain FMDV at different times post infection and also this knowledge could be to improve control measures. The accumulation of FMDV in the environment should be taken into account when studying FMDV transmission. Further, the environmental aspect in the transmission of FMDV should be considered during the planning and implementation of measures to control FMD during an outbreak.

Additional files

Additional file 1: On the FMDV survival rate σ. Detailed calculation of the FMDV survival rate σ, which was calculated using published data on FMDV thermal inactivation combined with own laboratory data [7,20,23-27].

Additional file 2: The 2R-SIR model. Detailed information on the quantification of transmission rate parameters. The transmission rate parameters were calculated using a Generalized Linear Model (GLM) based on an stochastic SIR model. In this additional file we describe the SIR model parameters, the inclusion of an extra route i.e. E to the 1 route SIR-model to calculate the contribution of the environment to the transmission of the infection and, the methodology to quantify the transmission parameters using the GLM model [28,29].

Additional file 3: Mean values (plus range) and the Kruskal-Wallis statistics of virus present in secretions, excretions and blood samples, for the inoculated, direct contact and indirect contact groups. For the Kruskal-Wallis statistics, H is the Kruskal-Wallis test statistic and df the degrees of freedom.

Additional file 4: Plotted linear regression estimates of the log time (hours) needed for a 10-fold reduction in FMDV titres. In this additional file we show the obtained times (log hours) that are needed to have a 10-fold reduction in FMDV titres per sample and per temperature. Light blue points correspond to estimates from water; green from buffers; grey from hemal and lymph nodes and bone marrow; black from faeces; red from urine; pink from milk; blue from slurry. Inside the dashed pointed rectangles, only obtained estimates at 20 °C. Red dashed lines, regression lines at 95% CI.

Additional file 5: Sensitivity analysis considering latent periods. In this additional file we show results of the estimation of transmission parameters for latent periods of 0 (as used in the paper), 1, 2 and 3 days.

Additional file 6: Sensitivity analysis considering latent periods. In this additional file we show results of the estimation of R_0's for latent periods of 0 (as used in the paper), 1, 2 and 3 days.

Competing interests
The authors declare that they have no competing interests.

Authors' contributions
CB participated in the design and coordination of the study, participated in the laboratory analysis, carried out the statistical analysis and drafted the manuscript. MJ participated in the design of the study, carried out the statistical analysis and drafted the manuscript. PE participated in the design and coordination of the study and helped to draft the manuscript. AD conceived the study, participated in the design and coordination of the study, carried out the statistical analysis and helped to draft the manuscript. All authors read and approved the final manuscript.

Acknowledgements
The authors would like to thank Mrs. F. van Hemert-Kluitenberg for her assistance with the handling of samples and laboratory assays. The research leading to these results have received funding from the European Community's Seventh Framework Programme (FP7/2007-2013) under grant agreement n° 226556 (FMD-DISCONVAC).

Author details
[1]Central Veterinary Institute (CVI), part of Wageningen UR, P.O. Box 65, 8200 AB Lelystad, The Netherlands. [2]Department Quantitative Veterinary Epidemiology, Wageningen University, P.O. Box 338, 6700 AH Wageningen, The Netherlands.

References
1. Thomson GR (1994) Foot and Mouth Disease. In: Coetzer JAW, Thomson GR, Tustin RC (ed) Infectious diseases of livestock with special reference to Southern Africa. Volume 1. Oxford University Press, Capetown, pp 825–852
2. Woolhouse M, Chase-Topping M, Haydon D, Friar J, Matthews L, Hughes G, Shaw D, Wilesmith J, Donaldson A, Cornell S, Keeling M, Grenfell B (2001) Epidemiology. Foot-and-mouth disease under control in the UK. Nature 411:258–259
3. Bravo de Rueda C, Dekker A, Eblé PL, de Jong MCM (2014) Identification of factors associated with increased excretion of Foot-and-Mouth Disease Virus. Prev Vet Med 113:23–33
4. Parker J (1971) Presence and inactivation of foot-and-mouth disease virus in animal faeces. Vet Rec 88:659–662
5. Sellers RF, Herniman KA, Donaldson AI (1971) The effects of killing or removal of animals affected with foot-and-mouth disease on the amounts of airborne virus present in looseboxes. Br Vet J 127:358–365
6. Botner A, Belsham GJ (2012) Virus survival in slurry: analysis of the stability of foot-and-mouth disease, classical swine fever, bovine viral diarrhoea and swine influenza viruses. Vet Microbiol 157:41–49
7. Turner C, Williams SM, Cumby TR (2000) The inactivation of foot and mouth disease, Aujeszky's disease and classical swine fever viruses in pig slurry. J Appl Microbiol 89:760–767
8. van Bunnik BA, Hagenaars TJ, Bolder NM, Nodelijk G, de Jong MCM (2012) Interaction effects between sender and receiver processes in indirect transmission of Campylobacter jejuni between broilers. BMC Vet Res 8:123
9. van Bunnik BA, Katsma WE, Wagenaar JA, Jacobs-Reitsma WF, de Jong MCM (2012) Acidification of drinking water inhibits indirect transmission, but not direct transmission of Campylobacter between broilers. Prev Vet Med 105:315–319
10. Breban R, Drake JM, Stallknecht DE, Rohani P (2009) The role of environmental transmission in recurrent avian influenza epidemics. PLoS Comput Biol 5:e1000346
11. Rohani P, Breban R, Stallknecht DE, Drake JM (2009) Environmental transmission of low pathogenicity avian influenza viruses and its implications for pathogen invasion. Proc Natl Acad Sci U S A 106:10365–10369
12. Velkers FC, Bouma A, Stegeman JA, de Jong MCM (2012) Oocyst output and transmission rates during successive infections with Eimeria acervulina in experimental broiler flocks. Vet Parasitol 187:63–71
13. Eblé PL, de Koeijer AA, de Jong MCM, Engel B, Dekker A (2008) A meta-analysis quantifying transmission parameters of FMDV strain O Taiwan among non-vaccinated and vaccinated pigs. Prev Vet Med 83:98–106
14. Orsel K, Dekker A, Bouma A, Stegeman JA, de Jong MCM (2007) Quantification of foot and mouth disease virus excretion and transmission within groups of lambs with and without vaccination. Vaccine 25:2673–2679
15. Kermack WO, McKendrick AG (1927) A Contribution to the mathematical theory of epidemics. Proc Roy Soc Lond 115:700–721
16. Velthuis AGJ, de Jong MCM, De Bree J, Nodelijk G, Van Boven M (2002) Quantification of transmission in one-to-one experiments. Epidemiol Infect 128:193–204
17. Cox SJ, Barnett PV (2009) Experimental evaluation of foot-and-mouth disease vaccines for emergency use in ruminants and pigs: a review. Vet Res 40:13
18. Orsel K, Dekker A, Bouma A, Stegeman JA, de Jong MCM (2005) Vaccination against foot and mouth disease reduces virus transmission in groups of calves. Vaccine 23:4887–4894
19. Hajer R, Hendrikse J, Rutgers LJE, van Oldruitenborgh-Oosterbaan MM S, van der Weyden GC (1985) Het klinisch onderzoek bij grote huisdieren. Wetenschappelijke uitgeverij Bunge, Utrecht
20. Bouma A, Dekker A, de Jong MCM (2004) No foot-and-mouth disease virus transmission between individually housed calves. Vet Microbiol 98:29–36
21. Moonen P, Boonstra J, van der Honing RH, Leendertse CB, Jacobs L, Dekker A (2003) Validation of a LightCycler-based reverse transcription polymerase chain reaction for the detection of foot-and-mouth disease virus. J Virol Methods 113:35–41
22. Dekker A, Terpstra C (1996) Prevalence of foot-and-mouth disease antibodies in dairy herds in The Netherlands, four years after vaccination. Res Vet Sci 61:89–91
23. Dekker A (1998) Inactivation of foot-and-mouth disease virus by heat, formaldehyde, ethylene oxide and gamma radiation. Vet Rec 143:168–169
24. Bachrach HL, Breese SS, Callis JJ, Hess WR, Patty RE (1957) Inactivation of foot-and-mouth disease virus by pH and temperature changes and by formaldehyde. Proc Soc Exp Biol Med 95:147–152
25. Blackwell JH, Hyde JL (1976) Effect of heat on foot-and-mouth disease virus (FMDV) in the components of milk from FMDV-infected cows. J Hyg 77:77–83
26. Hyde JL, Blackwell JH, Callis JJ (1975) Effect of pasteurization and evaporation on foot-and-mouth disease virus in whole milk from infected cows. Can J Comp Med 39:305–309
27. Cottral GE (1969) Persistence of foot-and-mouth disease virus in animals, their products and the environment. Bull Off Int Epizoot 70:549–568
28. Velthuis AG, de Jong MCM, Kamp EM, Stockhofe N, Verheijden JH (2003) Design and analysis of an Actinobacillus pleuropneumoniae transmission experiment. Prev Vet Med 60:53–68
29. Bouma A, de Jong MCM, Kimman TG (1995) Transmission of pseudorabies virus within pig-populations is independent of the size of the population. Prev Vet Med 23:163–172
30. McCullagh P, Nelder JA (1989) Generalized Linear Models. Boca Raton, Chapman & Hall/CRC
31. R Development Core Team (2012) R: A Language and Environment for Statistical Computing. The R Foundation for Statistical Computing, Vienna
32. Diekmann O, Heesterbeek JA, Metz JA (1990) On the definition and the computation of the basic reproduction ratio R_0 in models for infectious diseases in heterogeneous populations. J Math Biol 28:365–382
33. de Jong MCM, Kimman TG (1994) Experimental quantification of vaccine-induced reduction in virus transmission. Vaccine 8:761–766
34. Velthuis AG, de Jong MCM, Stockhofe N, Vermeulen TM, Kamp EM (2002) Transmission of Actinobacillus pleuropneumoniae in pigs is characterized by variation in infectivity. Epidemiol Infect 129:203–214
35. Velthuis AG, de Jong MCM, De Bree J (2007) Comparing methods to quantify experimental transmission of infectious agents. Math Biosci 210:157–176

36. Eblé PL, de Koeijer A, Bouma A, Stegeman A, Dekker A (2006) Quantification of within- and between-pen transmission of Foot-and-Mouth disease virus in pigs. Vet Res 37:647–654
37. Eblé PL, Bouma A, de Bruin MG, van Hemert-Kluitenberg F, van Oirschot JT, Dekker A (2004) Vaccination of pigs two weeks before infection significantly reduces transmission of foot-and-mouth disease virus. Vaccine 22:1372–1378
38. Goris NE, Eblé PL, de Jong MCM, De Clercq K (2009) Quantification of foot-and-mouth disease virus transmission rates using published data. Altex 26:52–54
39. Orsel K, Bouma A, Dekker A, Stegeman JA, de Jong MCM (2009) Foot and mouth disease virus transmission during the incubation period of the disease in piglets, lambs, calves, and dairy cows. Prev Vet Med 88:158–163
40. Orsel K, de Jong MCM, Bouma A, Stegeman JA, Dekker A (2007) Foot and mouth disease virus transmission among vaccinated pigs after exposure to virus shedding pigs. Vaccine 25:6381–6391
41. Orsel K, de Jong MCM, Bouma A, Stegeman JA, Dekker A (2007) The effect of vaccination on foot and mouth disease virus transmission among dairy cows. Vaccine 25:327–335
42. Charleston B, Bankowski BM, Gubbins S, Chase-Topping ME, Schley D, Howey R, Barnett PV, Gibson D, Juleff ND, Woolhouse MEJ (2011) Relationship between clinical signs and transmission of an infectious disease and the implications for control. Science 332:726–729
43. van Roermund HJ, Eblé PL, de Jong MCM, Dekker A (2010) No between-pen transmission of foot-and-mouth disease virus in vaccinated pigs. Vaccine 28:4452–4461
44. Golde WT, Pacheco JM, Duque H, Doel T, Penfold B, Ferman GS, Gregg DR, Rodriguez LL (2005) Vaccination against foot-and-mouth disease virus confers complete clinical protection in 7 days and partial protection in 4 days: Use in emergency outbreak response. Vaccine 23:5775–5782
45. Doel TR, Williams L, Barnett PV (1994) Emergency vaccination against foot-and-mouth disease: rate of development of immunity and its implications for the carrier state. Vaccine 12:592–600
46. Cox SJ, Voyce C, Parida S, Reid SM, Hamblin PA, Paton DJ, Barnett PV (2005) Protection against direct-contact challenge following emergency FMD vaccination of cattle and the effect on virus excretion from the oropharynx. Vaccine 23:1106–1113

Experimentally induced lameness in turkeys inoculated with a newly emergent turkey reovirus

Tamer A Sharafeldin[1,3], Sunil K Mor[1], Aschalew Z Bekele[1], Harsha Verma[1], Sally L Noll[2], Sagar M Goyal[1] and Robert E Porter[1*]

Abstract

Newly emergent turkey arthritis reoviruses (TARVs) have been isolated from cases of lameness in male turkeys over 10 weeks of age. In a previous study, experimental inoculation of TARV in one-week-old turkey poults produced lymphocytic tenosynovitis at four weeks post inoculation but without causing clinical lameness. This study was undertaken to determine if TARV infection at an early age can lead to clinical lameness in birds as they age. One-week-old male turkeys were inoculated orally with a TARV (strain TARV-O'Neil) and monitored for the development of gait defects until 16 weeks of age. At 4, 8, 12 and 16 weeks of age, a subset of birds was euthanized followed by the collection of gastrocnemius tendon, digital flexor tendon, and intestines for virus detection by rRT-PCR and for histologic inflammation scoring. Clinical lameness was first displayed in TARV-infected turkeys at 8 weeks of age and ruptured gastrocnemius tendons with progressive lameness were also seen at 12–16 weeks of age. The virus was detected in gastrocnemius tendon of 4- 8- and 12-week-old turkeys but not in 16-week-old turkeys. Histologic inflammation scores of tendons at each of the four time points were significantly higher in the virus-inoculated group than in the control group ($p < 0.01$). Lesions began as lymphocytic tenosynovitis with mild synoviocyte hyperplasia at four weeks of age and progressed to fibrosis as the birds aged. These results demonstrate the potential of TARV to infect young turkeys and to produce subclinical tenosynovitis that becomes clinically demonstrable as the turkeys age.

Introduction

Initially, turkey arthritis reoviruses (TARVs) were detected in tendons of lame, 15-week-old turkeys with swollen intertarsal (hock) joints showing histological lesions of synovial hyperplasia and inflammatory cellular infiltrates in the subsynovium [1,2]. In an effort to reproduce the disease, three different turkey reoviruses were inoculated into the footpad of 1-day-old poults but no clinical disease or histologic lesions were observed [3]. Subsequently, there were no documented reports on reovirus-induced lameness in turkeys until 2013, when we isolated TARVs from lesions of tenosynovitis/arthritis in turkeys [4]. The samples used for TARVs isolation were gastrocnemius and digital flexor tendons of 12- to 15-week-old lame turkeys.

Partial sequence analysis of the avian reovirus S4 gene showed 88.7 to 99.8% nucleotide identity between a panel of TARVs and turkey enteric reoviruses (TERVs); however, the nucleotide identity of TARVs with chicken arthritis reoviruses (CARVs) was only 78% [4]. Experimental inoculation of TARVs through oral, intratracheal, and footpad routes in 1-week-old turkey poults produced histologic lesions of marked lymphocytic tenosynovitis with synovial hyperplasia at 2 and 4 weeks post inoculation (pi). These lesions were absent in poults inoculated with TERV or CARV (5). Although TARV-inoculated birds showed high histologic scores of tenosynovitis and reovirus could be re-isolated from the gastrocnemius and digital flexor tendons, clinical lameness was not observed for up to 4-weeks pi (5 weeks of age) when the study was terminated [5].

The aims of the present work are to determine whether infection in young poults progresses to clinical lameness as they age from 1 to 16 weeks, identify the age at which lameness occurs, and determine if there is a correlation between histological tenosynovitis and clinical lameness. In addition, this work provides a detailed description of lesion progression induced by TARV in turkeys and addresses the potential of the experimental

* Correspondence: porte349@umn.edu
[1]Department of Veterinary Population Medicine and Minnesota Veterinary Diagnostic Laboratory, University of Minnesota, St. Paul, MN 55108, USA
Full list of author information is available at the end of the article

model to study TARV pathogenesis and immune response in turkeys in the future studies.

Materials and methods

Birds

One hundred and sixty 1-day-old male white commercial (Nicholas) turkey poults purchased from a Midwest poultry hatchery were divided into two groups (80/group) and placed in two isolation units. Meconium samples from another ten birds were collected at 1-day of age and examined for reovirus by real time reverse transcription-polymerase chain reaction (rRT-PCR) [6]. Serum samples from an additional 10 birds were tested for anti-reovirus antibodies using a commercial enzyme-linked immune sorbent assay (ELISA; IDEXX, Westbrook, ME). Birds were supplied feed and water *ad libitum*. Turkeys were supplied with a starter ration (≥30% of protein and ≤3% crude fat) until age of 8 weeks then supplied with grower/finisher ration (≥24% of protein and ≤7% of crude fat) from 8–16 weeks of age. The animal use protocol was reviewed and approved by the Institutional Animal Care and Use Committee of University of Minnesota.

Virus

TARV-O'Neil strain of TARV isolated from leg tendons of lame turkeys in Minnesota was kindly supplied by Dr Jack Rosenberger, AviServe LLC, Newark, Delaware. The virus was grown and titrated on Japanese quail fibrosarcoma cell line (QT-35) cells and had a titer of $10^{5.5}TCID_{50}$/mL.

Experimental design

The poults were divided into two groups and housed separately in isolation rooms. One group of poults was orally inoculated at 1 week of age with 0.2 mL of TARV-O'Neil virus. The negative control group was inoculated with virus-free MEM. At 4, 8, 12 and 16 weeks of age, all birds were weighed and their gaits were scored using a newly developed, turkey-specific gait scoring system (Table 1). After weighing and gait scoring at each of the four time points, 10 birds from each group were euthanized by exposure to carbon dioxide gas followed by the collection of tissue samples as described below. Intertarsal (hock) joint, including distal tibiotarsus and proximal tarsometatarsus, was excised and fixed in 10% neutral-buffered formalin for histopathology. Right and left leg tendons (distal part of gastrocnemius and digital flexor tendons) and 2 cm intestinal segments (along with their digesta) were excised and stored at −20 °C for rRT-PCR. At the end of the experiment, the remaining birds (16 weeks of age) were euthanized after recording their body weights and gait scores. At each time point, Dacron swabs were inserted into the sheaths of excised gastrocnemius tendons from the ten turkeys and placed as a pool into 3 mL of brain-heart infusion broth for PCR targeting *Mycoplasma gallisepticum* and *M. synoviae*. Additionally, the gastrocnemius tendon sheaths of five birds from each treatment group were swabbed and cultured for aerobic bacteria and Mycoplasma.

Table 1 Six-point (0–5) gait scoring system

Score	Description
0^N	• Flex and extend legs smoothly and easily
	• No reluctance in movement
	• Walk actively with upright breast
	• Legs are parallel
	• Stand with no shaking in legs or labored breathing
1^N	• Flex and extend legs smoothly and easily
	• Little reluctance in movement
	• Walk actively with upright breast
	• Legs are parallel
	• Legs shake during standing
	• No anatomical changes in legs (swelling, valgus or varus)
2^N	• Flex and extend legs smoothly and easily
	• Little reluctance in movement
	• Walk actively with upright breast
	• Legs are parallel with mild swelling or had mild valgus or varus
	• Legs shake during standing
3^L	• Staggered movement and dropped keelbone
	• Unilateral significant hock joint swelling, varus or valgus
	• Marked bilateral defect, but can walk and stand for more than 30 seconds
4^L	• Staggered movement and dropped keel bone Marked bilateral hock joint swelling, varus or valgus
	• Cannot walk and stand for more than 30 seconds
5^L	• Completely recumbent
	• Stand and walk for seconds if it is pushed to walk
	• Bird then prefers to walk on hocks "creeping"
	• Bird may not be able to stand and creeps when initiated to move

^{N}non-lame.
^{L}lame.

Gait scoring system

A six-point (0–5) scoring system was designed to score the gait of turkeys and to quantify lameness (Table 1). Each bird was observed and scored separately and any recumbent bird was gently prodded to determine if they could stand or walk independently. Turkeys with gait scores of 3 or more were categorized as clinically lame.

Histopathology and histologic inflammation scoring

Bones comprising the intertarsal joint with adjacent gastrocnemius tendon were preserved in 10% neutral-buffered formalin. After decalcification in EDTA solution, the tissues were trimmed, processed, embedded in paraffin, sectioned at 3–4 μm, placed on glass slides, stained with hematoxylin and eosin (H&E), examined under an Olympus BX40 microscope and photomicrographs were taken by Olympus DP71 digital microscope camera. Tenosynovitis was scored histologically using a previously described histologic inflammation scoring system [5].

Virus detection

Samples were homogenized in Hanks' balanced salt solution (HBSS) containing 2% donor horse serum. The homogenates were then centrifuged 1500 × *g* for 20 min and the supernatant stored at −80 °C until subsequent RNA extraction and rRT-PCR. RNA extraction was done by QIAamp Viral RNA Mini Kit (Qiagen, Valencia, CA, USA). Extracted RNA was tested by rRT-PCR for reovirus S4 gene using one step RT-PCR Kit (Qiagen). This rRT-PCR showed high sensitivity and detected as few as 10 viral gene copies [6].

Statistical analysis

The correlation coefficient between tenosynovitis (as determined histologically) and clinical lameness was calculated at 4, 8, 12 and 16 weeks of age. Detection of significant differences between the means of histologic inflammation scores and gait scores of different groups was done using the non-parametric statistical analysis "Mann Whitney U test" (NCSS 8 Statistical Software, NCSS LLC, Keysville, UT, USA). The difference between averages of body weights was tested by two sample t-test.

Results

Gait scoring and lameness

At the age of four-weeks, none of the turkeys in either the inoculated or the control group showed any clinical signs of lameness and their average gait score was 0. However, the gait scores in the inoculated group were significantly higher than those of control group at the ages of 8, 12 and 16 weeks ($p < 0.05$) (Figure 1). Clinical lameness (gait score >3) was observed at 8 weeks of age and progressively increased as the inoculated birds aged; clinical lameness was observed in 26%, 30%, and 48% of inoculated birds at 8, 12, and 16 weeks of age, respectively. There was a minimal increase in gait scores in turkeys of the control group from 4 to 12 weeks of age but 5 of 39 birds (13%) showed lameness at 16 weeks (Figure 2). Virus-inoculated turkeys showed swollen hock joints with breast blisters and breast buttons with a single bird showing ruptured gastrocnemius tendon at 16 weeks (Figure 3).

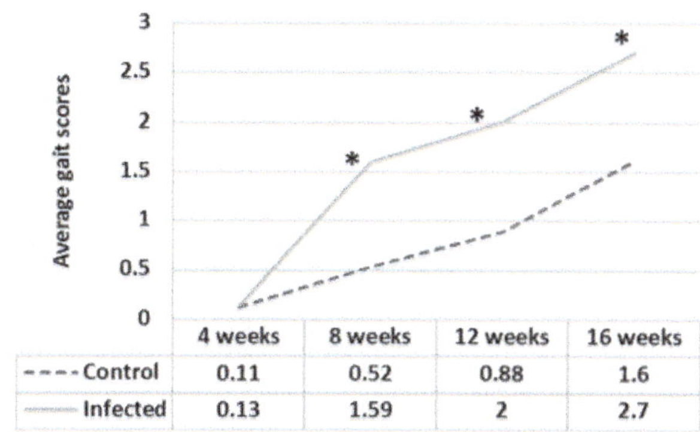

Figure 1 Average gait scoring system at different time points. The average gait scores of infected birds are significantly higher than those of non-infected controls at 8, 12 and 16 weeks of age. *Significant higher gait score at $p < 0.05$.

Histologic inflammation scores

Mean histologic inflammation scores of gastrocnemius tendon sheaths were significantly higher ($p < 0.01$) in the inoculated group as compared to the control group at all ages (4, 8, 12 and 16-weeks) (Figure 4). The lesions consisted of prominent lymphocytic infiltration of the subsynovium and mild synoviocyte hyperplasia at 4 and 8 weeks, along with mild fibroplasia and lymphoid nodule formation at 8 weeks, progressing to decreased lymphocytic infiltration and increasing fibrosis at 12 weeks, and finally a prominent subsynovial fibrosis at 16 weeks (Figure 5).

Correlation between tenosynovitis and gait score

The gait score and histologic inflammation score for each bird were used to calculate correlation coefficient, which was low (0.1) at 4 weeks and progressively increased until a strong positive correlation (0.9) was observed between tenosynovitis and high gait score (lameness) at 16 weeks (Figure 6).

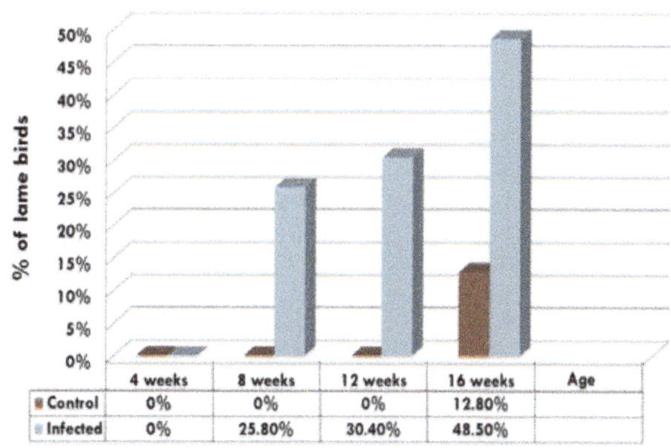

Figure 2 Percentage of lame birds. Lameness, defined as a gait score of 3 or higher, is predominant in infected birds at 8, 12 and 16 weeks of age.

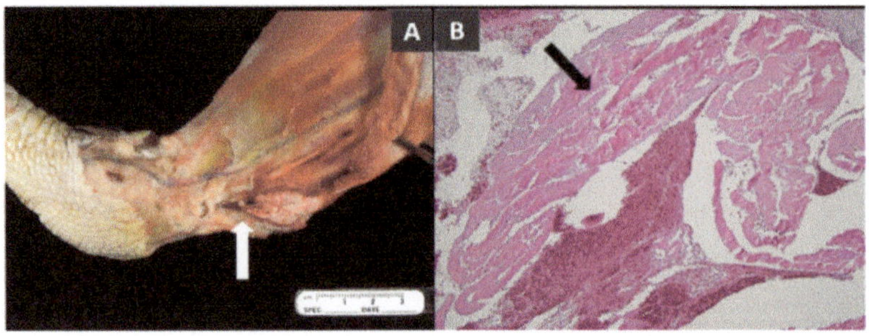

Figure 3 Ruptured tendon with hemorrhage. Tendon rupture was observed in one 16-week-old turkey. **A)** Hemorrhage at the site of ruptured tendon (white arrow). Scale bar, 1 cm. **B)** Microphotograph of shredded tendon fragment (black arrow) surrounded by erythrocytes (hemorrhage). H&E stain (40X magnification).

Body weight

The average body weight of inoculated birds was significantly lower ($p < 0.05$) than that of control birds at 12 and 16 weeks (Figure 7).

Virus detection

Fecal and serum samples taken from 1-day-old poults were negative for reovirus and antireovirus antibodies, respectively. In addition, samples from 1, 4, 8, 12 and 16-week-old turkeys were negative for aerobic bacteria by culture and negative for *Mycoplasma synoviae* and *M. gallisepticum* by culture and PCR. Reovirus was detected by rRT-PCR in 4 of 10 tendon and 3 of 10 intestine samples of 4-week-old turkeys in the virus-inoculated group. In 8-week-old birds, 5 of 10 tendons and 4 of 10 intestines were positive while at 12 weeks, only 2 of 10 tendon and 2 of 10 intestinal samples were positive for reovirus by rRT-PCR. All tissues collected from negative control turkeys at all ages were negative for reovirus by rRT-PCR.

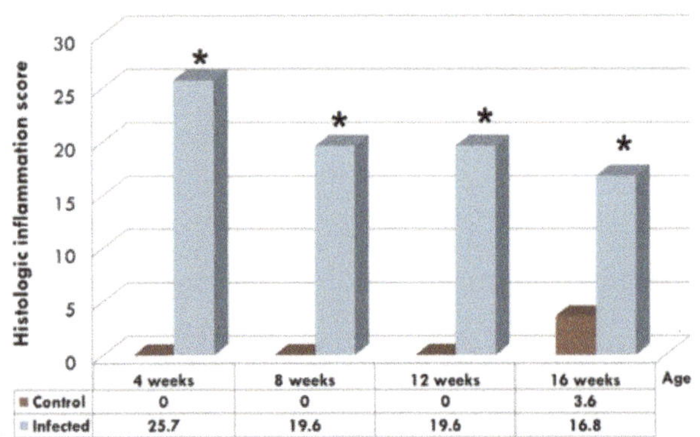

Figure 4 Means of histologic inflammation scores in gastrocnemius tendon sheath. Infected birds had significantly higher averages of histologic inflammation scores at 4, 8, 12 and 16 weeks of age.*Significantly higher score ($p < 0.01$).

Discussion

Previous work in our laboratory showed that poults orally inoculated with TARV at 1-week of age developed lymphocytic tenosynovitis by 4 weeks pi but did not show clinical lameness [5]. Our present study sought to determine if tenosynovitis induced by TARV would progress to clinical lameness as the birds aged, to characterize the lameness through gait scoring, and to determine the relationship between tenosynovitis and gait scores. The study also described the progression of histologic lesions from ages 4 to 16 weeks. The study aimed in general to test the potential of the experimental model for future experimental studies.

Lymphocytic infiltration of the gastrocnemius tendon sheath was prominent in 4-week-old turkeys and progressively decreased by the time the turkeys were 16 weeks of age, while subsynovial fibrosis was initially observed in 8-week-old turkeys and was most prominent in 16-week-old turkeys. These results resemble those shown in a long term study on chicken reoviral arthritis [7], in which oral inoculation of 1-day-old chicks with chicken reovirus led to the development of gastrocnemius lymphocytic tenosynovitis and fibroplasia by 10 weeks of age and predominant fibrosis by 20 weeks of age.

The fibrosis of tendon and tendon sheath might lead to a decrease in the tensile strength of tendons as the birds age and become heavier, especially in domestic turkeys that have a high growth rate. In addition, tendon adhesion with heavy weight as a contributing factor might have led to tendon rupture [8]. Similar results were shown in chickens infected with chicken arthritis reovirus; at 10 weeks pi there was fibrosis and adhesion of the gastrocnemius tendon, which along with the stress of heavier body weight resulted in tendon failure and rupture [9].

Lameness evaluation in this work required a gait scoring system that includes all variations of gait abnormalities. For that reason, a previous 4-point gait scoring system in turkeys [10] did not suit our requirements.

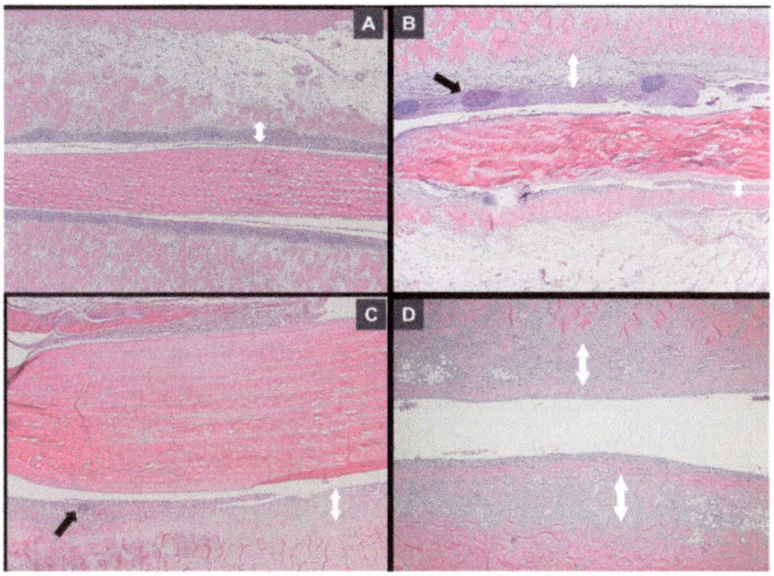

Figure 5 Lesion progression. Microphotographs show the progression of inflammation in gastrocnemius tendon sheath of 4- to 16-week-old infected turkeys. **A)** Prominant lymphocytic infiltration (White up-down arrow) (4-week-old); **B)** Lymphocytic nodules (Black arrow) present and fibroplasia (White up-down arrow) starts (8-week-old); **C)** Fibrosis increases (White up-down arrow) and lymphocytic infiltration (Black arrow) decreases (12-week-old); **D)** Fibrosis (White up-down arrow) is prominent (16-week-old). H&E stain (40X magnification).

The previously designed 6-point (0–5) gait scoring system designed for chickens [11] and its modifications [12] were also not suitable because of behavioral variation between chickens and turkeys. Our newly designed 6-point (0–5) gait scoring system is specific for turkeys in which scores of 3 and above are considered as clinically lame. There was a clear distinction between score 2 and score 3 to avoid confusion and to have a clear cut point that distinguishes between lame and non-lame birds. The average gait score of each infected group was not less than 3, but was significantly higher than the average score of the corresponding control group.

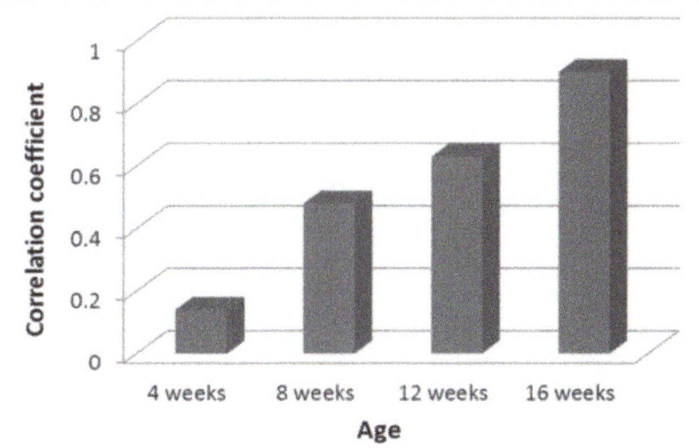

Figure 6 Correlation coefficient between gastrocnemius tendon histologic inflammation score and gait score. The correlation is low at 4 weeks of age as no birds showed clinical lameness though they had high histologic inflammation scores. The correlation gradually increased to 0.9 at 16 weeks of age.

Clinical lameness was first observed in 8-week-old turkeys with 25.8% of inoculated turkeys being lame. The percentage of lame birds in the inoculated group progressively increased at 12 weeks (30.4%) and 16 weeks (48.5%) while negative control turkeys, for the most part, remained clinically normal. The correlation coefficient between tenosynovitis score and degree of lameness was low (0.1) in 4-week-old turkeys; these birds had high tendon inflammation scores (tenosynovitis) but did not show clinical lameness. These findings were in agreement with our previous work that showed no clinical lameness in 5-week-old turkeys that had been orally inoculated with TARV at 1 week of age, despite the presence of high gastrocnemius tendon inflammation scores [5]. In the present study, the correlation between tenosynovitis and gait score increased dramatically from 8 to 16-week-old turkeys with a peak of 0.9 at 16 weeks. This high correlation coefficient was attributed to increased clinical lameness in tenosynovitis birds and this was associated with increased body weight (Figure 6). Studies on reovirus infection in chickens have demonstrated a strong association of lameness with fibrosis of the gastrocnemius tendon and tendon sheath, tendon adhesion and eventual rupture as the chickens increased in body weight [9]. In addition, it has been shown that the greater weight gain in meat producing chickens might

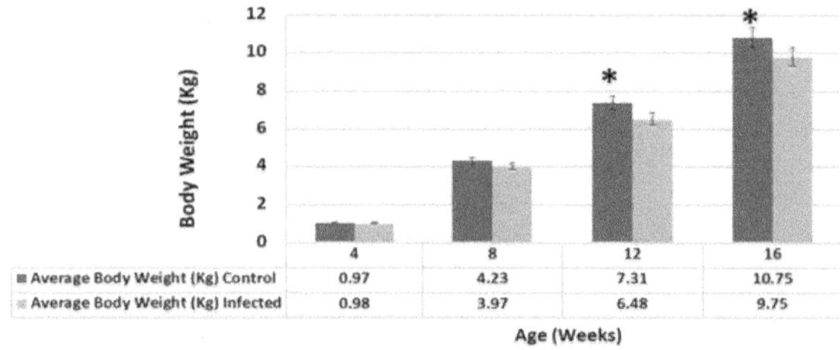

Figure 7 Average body weights at different time points. At 12 and 16 weeks of age, infected birds had a significantly lower average body weight compared with non-infected controls. *Significant higher body weight ($p < 0.05$).

affect the physical consistency of tendons during reovirus infection leading to clinical lameness [13].

In control birds at 16 weeks of age there were 5 lame birds out of 39. These birds were negative for reovirus, bacteria and mycoplasma and they did not show tenosynovitis. A possible noninfectious cause of lameness might be the cause. Tibial dyschondroplasia (TD) which is a genetic disorder in which cartilage at bone epiphysis fails to ossify leading to weak legs and lame birds [14]. When the proximal epiphysis of tibia is cut in necropsy cartilage mass will be seen in epiphysis [15] which we did not do in 16-week-old turkeys. It is possible that it was a valgus–varus deformity which was associated with overgrowth rate and may show gastrocnemius tendon slippage [16]. Perosis and chondrodystrophy may be induced in vitamin B complex and mineral deficiency [16-18] which we think that it was not in our turkeys. We have not found any footpad ulcers and litter was kept dry and clean all the time but this might be a shaky leg lameness which occurs mostly in male turkeys 8–18 weeks of age due to low quality moist litter [19]. TARV-infected turkeys had significantly lower average body weights than control groups at 12 and 16 weeks of age. Because reduced body weights were observed when gait scores started to increase at 8 weeks, we suspect that the discomfort associated with lameness made it more difficult for the affected turkeys to reach the feeders and likely reduced feed consumption.

In a previous study, two-day-old turkeys inoculated with enteric reoviruses showed significantly lower body weight than controls at 2 to 9 days pi [20]. This might be due to the age of inoculation since younger birds have been shown to be most susceptible to reovirus infection. In our study, we inoculated turkeys at 1 week of age. The effect of age of inoculation on TARV infection has not yet been studied in turkeys but this age susceptibility has been demonstrated in chickens challenged with reovirus [21]. TARV not only affects the carcass quality (e.g., hock swelling, breast blisters) of turkeys but, under experimental conditions also results in a significantly lower body weight at market age (Figure 7).

In this study, virus was detected by rRT-PCR in 20%-50% of tendon and intestinal samples in infected turkeys at 4, 8 and 12 weeks of age with the peak of virus detection in 8-week-old turkeys. At 8 and 12 weeks of age, all rRT-PCR positive birds had lameness gait scores (3 or more). In field cases, we originally diagnosed tenosynovitis and successfully isolated reovirus from tendons of 16-week-old turkeys, but under experimental conditions we were not able to detect reovirus in tendons of 16-week-old turkeys by using rRT-PCR, which was previously shown to be of higher sensitivity in TARV detection than virus isolation [6]. Reovirus has been detected in field cases of chickens with tenosynovitis/arthritis at 11 weeks of age and younger [22]. It appears that experimental conditions are different from field conditions, perhaps in terms of overall viral load and viral shedding and cycling in field turkeys. In addition, although we do not know when field turkeys are naturally infected with TARV, our work indicates that surveillance of turkeys for TARV should occur weeks before any anticipated lameness occurs (mostly observed in field cases >12-week-old) in order to increase detection of virus, particularly if field poults are naturally infected vertically through the egg or at a very young age, as has been demonstrated in chickens [23]. In conclusion, infection of poults with TARV causes lymphocytic gastrocnemius tenosynovitis that over time progresses to subsynovial fibroplasia and fibrosis. These changes along with increased body weight lead to clinical lameness and occasional tendon rupture as the birds age. In addition, TARV is most readily detected in infected turkeys prior to or as soon as the lameness is observed. We developed a gait-scoring system that should be useful for veterinarians or production personnel to characterize early alterations in gait, thus identify earlier onset of TARV infection and increase the opportunity for detection of TARV in infected turkeys. These findings augment

the similarity of the experimental model (inoculation of TARV-O'Neil orally at 1-week-old) with the field condition and prove the potentiality of using this model in future immunopathogenesis studies.

Competing interests

The authors declare that they have no competing interests.

Authors' contributions

Conceived and designed the experiment: TAS, SKM, SJN, SMG and REP. Performed the experiment, collected and processed samples: TAS, SKM, AZB, HV, SJN, SMG, and REP. Data analysis: TAS, SKM, HV, SJN, SMG and REP. Wrote the paper TAS, SMG and REP. All authors read and approved the manuscript.

Acknowledgements

This study was funded in part by a grant from the Rapid Agricultural Response Fund, established by the Minnesota legislature and administered by the University of Minnesota Agricultural Experiment Station. We thank Dr Jack Rosenberger for providing TARV-O'Neil for the study.

Author details

[1]Department of Veterinary Population Medicine and Minnesota Veterinary Diagnostic Laboratory, University of Minnesota, St. Paul, MN 55108, USA. [2]Department of Animal Science, University of Minnesota, St. Paul, MN 55108, USA. [3]Pathology Department, Faculty of Veterinary Medicine, Zagazig University, Zagazig 44519, Egypt.

References

1. Levisohn S, Gur-Lavie A, Weisman J (1980) Infectious synovitis in turkeys: isolation of tenosynovitis virus-like agent. Avian Pathol 9:1–4
2. Page RK, Fletcher OJ, Villegas P (1982) Infectious tenosynovitis in young turkeys. Avian Dis 26:924–927
3. Al-Afaleq A, Jones RC (1989) Pathogenicity of three turkey and three chicken reoviruses for poults and chicks with particular reference to arthritis/tenosynovitis. Avian Pathol 18:433–340
4. Mor SK, Sharafeldin TA, Porter RE, Ziegler A, Patnayak DP, Goyal SM (2013) Isolation and characterization of a turkey arthritis reovirus. Avian Dis 57:97–103
5. Sharafeldin TA, Mor SK, Bekele AZ, Verma H, Goyal SM, Porter RE (2014) The role of reoviruses in turkey tenosynovitis/arthritis. Avian Pathol 43:371–378
6. Mor SK, Verma H, Bekele AZ, Sharafeldin TA, Porter RE, Goyal SM (2014) One step real-time RT-PCR for the detection of turkey reoviruses. Avian Dis 58:404–407
7. Hill JE, Rowland GN, Steffens WL, Ard MB (1989) Ultrastructure of the gastrocnemius tendon and sheath from broilers infected with reovirus. Avian Dis 33:79–85
8. Jones RC (2000) Avian reovirus infection. Rev Sci Tech 19:614–625
9. Hill JE, Rowland GN, Glisson JR, Villegas P (1989) Comparative microscopic lesions in reoviral and staphylococcal tenosynovitis. Avian Dis 33:401–410
10. Ferket PR, Oviedo-Rondón EO, Mente PL, Bohórquez DV, Santos AA, Grimes JL, Richards JD, Dibner JJ, Felts V (2009) Organic trace minerals and 25-hydroxycholecalciferol affect performance characteristics, leg abnormalities, and biomechanical properties of leg bones of turkeys. Poult Sci 88:118–131
11. Kestin SC, Knowles TG, Tinch AE, Gregory NG (1992) Prevalence of leg weakness in broiler chickens and its relationship with genotype. Vet Rec 131:190–194
12. Garner JP, Falcone C, Wakenell P, Martin M, Mench JA (2002) Reliability and validity of a modified gait scoring system and its use in assessing tibial dyschondroplasia in broilers. Br Poult Sci 43:355–363
13. Kibenge FSB, Wilcox GE (1983) Tenosynovitis in chickens. Vet Bull 53:431–444
14. Farquharson C, Jefferies D (2000) Chondrocytes and longitudinal bone growth: the development of tibial dyschondroplasia. Poult Sci 79:994–1004
15. Julian RJ (1998) Rapid growth problems: ascites and skeletal deformities in broilers. Poult Sci 77:1773–1780
16. Riddell C (1992) Non-infectious skeletal disorders of poultry: an overview. In: Whitehead CC (ed) Bone biology and skeletal disorders in poultry. Carfax Publishing Co., Abingdon, UK, pp 119–145
17. Ferguson AE, Leeson S, Julian RJ, Summers JD (1978) Leg bone abnormalities and histopathology of cage and floor reared broilers fed diets devoid of selected vitamins and minerals. Poult Sci 57:1559–1562
18. Riddell C (1996) Skeletal system. In: Riddell C (ed) Avian histopathology, 2nd edition. American Association of Avian Pathologists, Kennet Square, PA, pp 45–60
19. Buyse J, Simons PCM, Boshouwers EMG, Decuypere E (1985) Effect of intermittent lighting, light intensity and source on the performance and welfare of broilers. World's Poult Sci J 52:121–130
20. Spackman E, Pantin-Jackwood M, Day JM, Sellers HL (2005) The pathogenesis of turkey origin reoviruses in turkeys and chickens. Avian Pathol 34:291–296
21. Jones RC, Georgiou K (1984) Reovirus-induced tenosynovitis in chickens the influence of age at infection. Avian Pathol 13:441–457
22. Jones RC, Guneratne JR, Georgiou K (1981) Isolation of viruses from outbreaks of suspected tenosynovitis (viral arthritis) in chickens. Res Vet Sci 31:100–103
23. van der Heide L (1977) Viral arthritis/tenosynovitis: a review. Avian Pathol 6:271–284

Mycoplasma iowae: relationships among oxygen, virulence, and protection from oxidative stress

Rachel E Pritchard[1,2] and Mitchell F Balish[1*]

Abstract

The poultry-associated bacterium *Mycoplasma iowae* colonizes multiple sites in embryos, with disease or death resulting. Although *M. iowae* accumulates in the intestinal tract, it does not cause disease at that site, but rather only in tissues that are exposed to atmospheric O_2. The activity of *M. iowae* catalase, encoded by *katE*, is capable of rapid removal of damaging H_2O_2 from solution, and *katE* confers a substantial reduction in the amount of H_2O_2 produced by *Mycoplasma gallisepticum katE* transformants in the presence of glycerol. As catalase-producing bacteria are often beneficial to hosts with inflammatory bowel disease, we explored whether *M. iowae* was exclusively protective against H_2O_2-producing bacteria in a *Caenorhabditis elegans* model, whether its protectiveness changed in response to O_2 levels, and whether expression of genes involved in H_2O_2 metabolism and virulence changed in response to O_2 levels. We observed that *M. iowae* was in fact protective against H_2O_2-producing *Streptococcus pneumoniae*, but not HCN-producing *Pseudomonas aeruginosa*, and that *M. iowae* cells grown in 1% O_2 promoted survival of *C. elegans* to a greater extent than *M. iowae* cells grown in atmospheric O_2. Transcript levels of an *M. iowae* gene encoding a homolog of *Mycoplasma pneumoniae* CARDS toxin were 5-fold lower in cells grown in low O_2. These data suggest that reduced O_2, representing the intestinal environment, triggers *M. iowae* to reduce its virulence capabilities, effecting a change from a pathogenic mode to a potentially beneficial one.

Introduction

H_2O_2 is a dangerous reactive oxygen species (ROS) involved in both pathogenesis and defense against infectious agents. Bacteria may be exposed to multiple sources of H_2O_2 during infection, including macrophages, which produce a variety of ROS that damage and degrade bacteria. A variety of bacterial pathogens can also produce H_2O_2 as a means of causing damage to host tissues [1,2], and some disease states stem from exposure of tissues to ROS including H_2O_2. In particular, in inflammatory bowel disease (IBD), a growing problem in humans in developed countries with a prevalence of 10-20% [3], a direct correlation between increased ROS production and damage to gut epithelial cells has been reported [4-7].

The enzyme catalase catalyzes degradation of H_2O_2 [8]. The production of catalase by microbes can benefit both the microorganisms themselves and a host organism with which they associate. Catalase can protect catalase-producing bacteria from environmental H_2O_2 and prolong infection. As for the host, several reports have examined the ability of catalase-expressing probiotic bacteria to decrease IBD symptoms [9]. In a murine trinitrobenzenesulfonic acid-induced Crohn's disease model, administration of *Lactobacillus casei* engineered to express catalase results in faster recovery from initial weight loss, increased gut enzyme activity, and decreased intestinal inflammation as compared with mice infected with wild-type or no bacteria [10]. Similar bacteria decrease cecal and colonic inflammation in mice treated with dextran sodium sulfate to induce moderate colitis [11].

Mycoplasma iowae is a catalase-positive bacterium that infects poultry animals, primarily turkeys but also occasionally chickens [12,13]. The most common outcome of naturally-occurring *M. iowae* infection in turkeys is late embryo mortality, with a 2-5% reduction in hatchability, and leg abnormalities in offspring [14-16]. Symptoms commonly associated with experimental infection include airsacculitis, stunting, poor feathering, and leg and joint problems [14,16]. The *M. iowae* catalase gene, *katE*, confers both catalase activity and a significant reduction in H_2O_2 production upon *Mycoplasma*

* Correspondence: balishmf@miamioh.edu
[1]Department of Microbiology, Miami University, Oxford, OH 45056, USA
Full list of author information is available at the end of the article

gallisepticum, a robust H_2O_2 producer that elaborates no other known toxins [13,17,18]. It is unclear how *M. iowae* causes disease, but in addition to its attachment organelle-mediated adherence and motility functions [19], its genome encodes potential virulence factors, including two closely linked genes encoding proteins similar to *Mycoplasma pneumoniae* CARDS toxin [13], an ADP-ribosylating toxin that is associated with many of the symptoms of *M. pneumoniae* infection [20-22].

Interestingly, *M. iowae* colonizes a variety of body sites with a range of O_2 concentrations. It has been isolated from the cloacae of healthy poults and mature turkeys [23,24], but also infects the chorioallantoic membrane and a variety of organs in embryos [25], which accounts for the morbidity and mortality associated with *M. iowae*. Significantly, *M. iowae* also has a pronounced tendency to colonize the gut with no ill effects. Following yolk sac inoculation of eight-day-old turkey embryos, *M. iowae* can be detected in the small intestines, with bacteria most often attaching to microvilli [25]. Oral inoculation of day-old poults with *M. iowae* results in bacteria present in both the feces and intestinal wall for at least 21 days post-inoculation, and no differences in fecal appearance or cloaca temperature as compared to control birds [26]. The gut is a very low-O_2 environment [27], whereas *in ovo* embryos, which are commonly damaged by *M. iowae*, are exposed to atmospheric O_2 due to eggshell permeability [28]. It is intriguing that *M. iowae* infection at aerobic sites, but apparently not the gut, causes disease, leading us to suspect that O_2 might play a role in regulating expression of *M. iowae* virulence factors, resulting in different outcomes at different body sites.

Differential gene expression regulation exists in a variety of mycoplasma species despite their reduced genomes. The *M. pneumoniae* promoters for acetate kinase and lactate dehydrogenase are strongly induced in the presence of glucose and glycerol, respectively [29]. *M. pneumoniae* lipoprotein genes are also differentially expressed in response to exposure to host cells, H_2O_2, and low pH [30]. Multiple forms of regulation occur in *Mycoplasma hyopneumoniae* in response to heat shock [31], iron deprivation [32], H_2O_2 treatment [33], and infection of pigs [34]. The means by which most of these regulatory events occur is unknown.

In this study we examined the ability of *M. iowae*, by virtue of its catalase activity, to offer protection to a model host from H_2O_2 stress, and to test whether *M. iowae* experiences differential regulation of catalase as well as possible virulence-associated genes in response to changes in O_2 level. We used *Caenorhabditis elegans* bioassays, developed previously as a model for use with *M. iowae* [13], and reverse transcription-quantitative polymerase chain reaction (RT-qPCR) of selected candidate virulence-associated genes. Our results indicate that catalase contributes to *M. iowae* being protective toward the host against H_2O_2-producing organisms, even though catalase activity is reduced under conditions of low O_2. They also indicate that *M. iowae* grown in low O_2 results in increased survival of *C. elegans* upon co-incubation as compared with *M. iowae* grown in atmospheric conditions, accompanied by a 5-fold decrease in expression of at least one of the CARDS toxin-like protein genes.

Materials and methods

Bacterial strains and growth conditions

Mycoplasma strains used include *M. iowae* serovar K strain DK-CPA, *M. gallisepticum* R_{low}, and *M. gallisepticum* R_{low} transformant 56A. For *M. gallisepticum* and for aerobic growth of *M. iowae*, all strains were grown at 37 °C in 175-cm^2 tissue culture flasks containing 50 mL of SP-4 broth [35] to mid-log phase. Transformant 56A was grown in the presence of 4 μg mL^{-1} tetracycline. SP-4 broth for samples grown in low O_2 was allowed to equilibrate with a 1% O_2/99% N_2 gas mix overnight. Following equilibration, 50 mL of broth was aliquotted into glass bottles that were capped with rubber stoppers in which cultures were grown to mid-log phase at 37 °C.

Escherichia coli DH5α was grown in Luria broth (LB) with 100 μg mL^{-1} ampicillin at 37 °C in a shaking incubator. A *Streptococcus pneumoniae* obtained from the Miami University Department of Microbiology stock collection was grown at 37 °C without shaking in brain heart infusion (BHI) broth. *Pseudomonas aeruginosa* strain PAO1, also from the Miami University Department of Microbiology stock collection, was grown at 37 °C with shaking in LB broth.

Preparation of cell lysates and protein analysis

Fifty- mL cultures of mycoplasma cells were collected by centrifugation at 20 000 × *g* for 20 min and washed three times with cold phosphate-buffered saline (PBS). Cells were resuspended in 1 mL cold PBS containing 1% sodium dodecyl sulfate using a 25-gauge syringe and incubated at 37 °C for 30 min. Cell lysates were stored at −80 °C. Protein concentration in cell lysates was determined using bicinchoninic acid assays (Pierce Biotechnology Inc.).

Catalase enzyme activity

Catalase activity was measured in whole cell lysates of *M. iowae* using the Amplex Red Catalase Assay kit (Invitrogen). Catalase activity was normalized to total protein concentration in cell lysate samples. Statistical significance of results was calculated using unpaired Student's *T*-test. Results represent two biological replicates from each condition with four technical replicates each.

H_2O_2 assays

Methods were adapted from Hames et al. [36]. For *S. pneumoniae* assays, colonies grown on BHI agar plates were picked and grown overnight in 5 mL of BHI broth at 37 °C without shaking. Cultures were diluted 1:100 in pre-warmed BHI broth and grown to mid-log phase at 37 °C without shaking ($OD_{620} = 0.2\text{-}0.3$). Cells were collected by centrifugation at 10 000 × *g* for 6 min and washed three times in cold HNM buffer (67.6 mM HEPES, pH 7.3, 140 mM NaCl, and 7 mM $MgCl_2$. H_2O_2 levels were measured using colorimetric test strips (EM Quant, range 0.5-25 mg L^{-1}). Four biological replicates were examined. Statistical significance was calculated using unpaired Student's *T*-test.

To determine H_2O_2 production by mycoplasmas alone, 50-mL cultures of mycoplasma cells were grown to mid-log phase. Cells were collected by centrifugation at 20 000 × *g* for 20 min and washed three times in cold HNM buffer. Following resuspension in the same buffer to an $OD_{550} = 1.0$, aliquots of 1 mL were added to 24-well plates with 500 μM or 1 mM sucrose and incubated at room temperature for 24 h. H_2O_2 levels were measured and statistical analysis was performed as described above. Two biological replicates, each with 2 technical replicates, were examined.

To determine H_2O_2 production by *S. pneumoniae* when using mycoplasma cells as a source of carbohydrates, both bacteria were grown independently and collected as described above. One-mL aliquots were placed in 24-well plates that contained *S. pneumoniae* at an $OD_{620} = 0.05$ and mycoplasmas at an $OD_{550} = 1.0$ with no sucrose. Samples were incubated at room temperature for 24 h. H_2O_2 levels were measured and statistical analysis was performed as described above. Three biological replicates were examined.

C. elegans growth conditions

All assays were performed with *C. elegans* strain N2 (Bristol). Nematodes were cultured using standard practices [37]. Briefly, worms were cultured on nematode growth media plates seeded with *E. coli* OP50 as a food source at room temperature on the benchtop.

C. elegans survival assays

Plates containing large, gravid nematodes were treated with hypochlorite solution to obtain sterile eggs using standard procedures [37]. Eggs were hatched overnight in 10 mL of M9 buffer with gentle shaking to obtain L1 larvae. L1 larvae were washed with M9 buffer and aliquotted into 24-well plate wells. The number of live larvae per well (indicated by movement) was counted prior to the addition of samples to a final volume of 1 mL. Plates were incubated at room temperature for the designated time, at which time live nematodes were counted again to measure survival. They were considered dead if no movement was observed in response to shaking or tapping the plate. Following the 24-h incubation period, H_2O_2 levels were also recorded with the use of colorimetric test strips as described above. For long-term assays, plates were wrapped in parafilm to prevent evaporation of liquid during the extended incubation time required for the experiment. Long-term assay results represent two biological replicates from each condition with six technical replicates each. Statistical significance of results was calculated using unpaired Student's *T*-test, with $p < 0.05$ being regarded as significant.

For mycoplasma samples, cells were collected and washed as described for H_2O_2 assays. *M. iowae* cells tested alone were resuspended to various OD_{550} values and incubated with *C. elegans* larvae in the presence of the indicated concentrations of H_2O_2. Assays examining protection from abiotic H_2O_2 were performed with mycoplasma cells resuspended to an $OD_{550} = 1.0$ in the presence of 8 mg L^{-1} H_2O_2. Three biological replicates, each with 3–4 technical replicates, were examined.

For assays with *S. pneumoniae*, bacteria were grown and harvested as described for H_2O_2 assays. Samples were added to *C. elegans* larvae with *S. pneumoniae* resuspended to $OD_{620} = 0.05$ (approximately 1.1×10^7 CFUs), mycoplasmas resuspended to $OD_{550} = 1.0$ (approximately 1.2×10^9 CFUs for *M. iowae*), and 500 μM sucrose. Three biological replicates, each with 2 technical replicates, were examined.

For assays with *P. aeruginosa*, colonies grown on LB agar plates were picked and grown overnight in 5 mL of LB broth at 37 °C in a shaking incubator. Cultures were diluted 1:100 in pre-warmed LB broth and grown to mid-log phase at 37 °C and 200 rpm ($OD_{600} = 0.4$). Cells were pelleted by centrifugation at 10 000 × *g* for 10 min and washed three time with cold buffer containing 20 mM L-glutamate, 5 mM K_2HPO_4, 5 mM NaH_2PO_4, 2 mM $MgSO_4 \cdot 7H_2O$, 0.02 mM $FeCl_3$, 12.5 mM glycine, and 50 mM Tris, pH 7.5 [38]. *P. aeruginosa* samples tested alone with worms were resuspended to $OD_{650} = 0.1$, 0.05, and 0.01 in the same buffer. For assays performed in combination with mycoplasmas, *P. aeruginosa* was used at $OD_{650} = 0.1$ (approximately 1.1×10^8 CFUs). Mycoplasmas were washed and resuspended in the same buffer as *P. aeruginosa* and used at an $OD_{550} = 1.0$. Three biological replicates, each with 2–4 technical replicates, were examined.

Sequence analysis

Predicted amino acid sequences for *M. iowae* CARDS1 and CARDS2 [13] and *M. pneumoniae* CARDS toxin [39] were aligned to one another with BLAST.

RNA isolation and quantification
RNA was isolated from *M. iowae* cells using TRI reagent (Sigma). Briefly, cells were collected by centrifugation at 20 000 × *g* for 20 min. Following resuspension of cell pellets in TRI reagent, RNA was extracted with chloroform, pelleted with isopropanol, and washed with 75% ethanol. RNA was resuspended in 100–300 μL DEPC-treated water and stored at −20 °C. To eliminate DNA contamination, samples were treated with DNase I (Invitrogen or QIAGEN) according to the manufacturer's instructions. RNA was then cleaned up using the RNeasy Mini Kit (QIAGEN). Elimination of DNA contamination was confirmed by PCR with *glpF* primers (Table 1). RNA quality was determined by analysis on an RNA Pico Chip (Agilent Technologies) using a Bioanalyzer 2100 (Agilent Technologies).

Reverse transcription (RT)
RT was carried out with the Verso cDNA Synthesis Kit (Thermo Scientific) according to the manufacturer's instructions. One hundred ng of RNA was used as starting material and random hexamers were used as primers in reactions with a final volume of 20 μL. Reactions were incubated at 70 °C for 5 min, 42 °C for 30 min, 95 °C for 2 min, and then chilled on ice. cDNA synthesis was confirmed by PCR with *glpF* primers (Table 1). Controls were performed to exclude the possibility of DNA contamination in which the same reactions were performed with water substituted for Verso Enzyme Mix and RT Enhancer. Control reactions were treated and stored identically to other samples.

Genomic DNA isolation and standard generation
Genomic DNA was isolated from a 50-mL culture using the QIAamp® DNA Mini Kit (QIAGEN). To improve quantification, plasmids were constructed that contained a copy of each gene target. Plasmids were constructed from PCR products amplified from *M. iowae* genomic DNA using gene-specific primers (Table 2) that were ligated into pCR®2.1 (Invitrogen) and transformed into competent *E. coli* DH5α. Plasmids were isolated from clones with the Zyppy™ Plasmid Miniprep Kit (Zymo Research). Insertion was confirmed with digestion by *Eco*RI and sequence was confirmed using vector-specific primers M13F and M13R (Table 2). Gene copy numbers were calculated using the concentration of each plasmid assuming 1.096×10^{-12} g bp^{-1} [40]. Standard curves were generated from ten-fold dilutions of DNA with known copy numbers and were analyzed by qPCR in triplicate.

RT-quantitative PCR (qPCR)
Each RT-qPCR reaction was done in at least triplicate using two biological replicates. Reactions were performed with PerfeCTa® SYBR® Green Supermix (Quanta Biosciences), 1 μL of cDNA or DNA template (5 ng), and 300 nM gene-specific primers (Table 1) in a final volume of 25 μL. Amplification conditions were 5 min at 95 °C for 3 min followed by 40 cycles of 10 s at 95 °C and 45 s at 52 °C. To determine the melting temperature and PCR product specificity, a melting curve was obtained after every run by heating from 50 °C (2 °C below T_a) to 95 °C. Primer specificity was determined by melting curve analysis and agarose gel electrophoresis of PCR products. Controls with no template or reverse transcriptase were included for each sample during each run. Runs were performed using the CFX Connect (Bio-Rad) and analysis was performed using Bio-Rad CFX Manager 3.0 software (Bio-Rad). The 16S rRNA gene was used for normalization. Statistical analysis of results was calculated using unpaired Student's *T*-test. MIQE guidelines were followed for performing and reporting experiments [41].

Results

Catalase confers host protection from peroxigenic bacteria
M. iowae has an active catalase protein, enabling reduction of H_2O_2 by this organism [13]. *C. elegans* is a well-established model for the study of H_2O_2-mediated

Table 1 Primers used for qPCR experiments

Primer Name	Target	Sequence (5'-3')	Tm (°C)
MI16Sleft(qPCR)	16S rRNA gene	CGCAAGACTCACGAGCTTAT	54.6
MI16Sright(qPCR)		GGTACAAACTGTCGCAAACC	54.4
MIcards1left(qPCR)	*cards1 (P271_571)*	TGGGTAGAAGCACAGACGTT	56.1
MIcards1right(qPCR)		ACTCATCTGCATCTGGGTCA	55.8
MIglpFleft(qPCR)	*glpF (P271_673)*	ATCTAGCATGATGGGTGGCG	57.3
MIglpFright(qPCR)		TGTCCAAACATTGCTCCTGT	54.7
MIkatEleft(qPCR)	*katE (P271_534)*	CGTGTAGTTCATCGAAAAGGTG	54.6
MIkatEright(qPCR)		CTTCCAGCTTCACCACCAAC	56.3
MIsodleft(qPCR)	*sodA (P271_491)*	ACACAAAGCATCACCAAGCT	55.2
MIsodright(qPCR)		TGATTGTGATGACCTCCACCA	56.1

Table 2 Primers used for construction and sequencing of qPCR standards

Primer name	Target	Sequence (5′-3′)
Mlcards1up	*cards1*	ATCGTCTGGTGCATATGCAACAGC
Mlcards1down		ATCGGCTCATGCAAGTGTTGCAGC
MlglpFup	*glpF*	ATCGGTAGTGCTTTTGCACTACAC
MlglpFdown		ATCGCTTCCAATGATTCCACCTCC
MlkatEupSalI	*katE*	ATCGGTCGACAAATGCTGCAACAGCTGCAC
MlkatEdownSalI		ATCGGTCGACTAAACACAAAATTTGATTTAATCAAAATTCATG
Mlsodup	*sodA*	ATCGGAACTGGGCCAACAAATGAC
Mlsoddown		ATCGACTTCACATGTCAGTTAGGG
M13Forward	Sequencing	GTTGTAAAACGACGGCCACT
M13Reverse		CAGGAAACAGCTATGACC

bacterial pathogenicity [1,2,42], and has recently been adapted for use with mycoplasma cells [13]. *M. gallisepticum* naturally lacks catalase activity, but *M. gallisepticum katE* transformant 56A, which produces *M. iowae* catalase, produces less H_2O_2 and kills fewer *C. elegans* larvae in the presence of the peroxigenic molecule glycerol than wild-type *M. gallisepticum* R_{low}, suggesting a role for catalase in protection from killing [13]. Incubation with *M. iowae* at $OD_{550} = 0.01$ increased survival of *C. elegans* from 30% in the absence of bacteria to 50% (not shown), a reasonable set of conditions for subsequent assays.

In the vertebrate host, bacteria can come into contact with multiple sources of H_2O_2, including host immune defense mechanisms and other microbial pathogens [1,2,43]. To mimic more closely conditions of H_2O_2 exposure in the host and test whether *M. iowae* was protective under these conditions, *C. elegans* survival assays were performed with the use of H_2O_2 produced continuously by a biotic source. *S. pneumoniae* is a bacterial pathogen that produces H_2O_2 from a variety of substrates including sucrose [44-46], a carbohydrate that *M. iowae* and *M. gallisepticum* are unable to metabolize [17]. When *S. pneumoniae* resuspended to $OD_{620} = 0.05$ was incubated with 500 μM sucrose at room temperature for 24 h, H_2O_2 accumulated rapidly, reaching maximum levels after 8 h of incubation, at which point H_2O_2 levels remained constant for the duration of the 24 h period (Figure 1). *M. iowae* or wild-type *M. gallisepticum* resuspended to $OD_{550} = 1.0$ and incubated under the same conditions produced less than 1 mg L^{-1} H_2O_2, respectively, and the same outcome occurred when mycoplasma cells were co-incubated with *S. pneumoniae* in the absence of sucrose (data not shown; see Figure 2B). Based upon these results, *C. elegans* survival assays were performed with *S. pneumoniae* at $OD_{620} = 0.05$, mycoplasmas at $OD_{550} = 1.0$, and 500 μM sucrose.

When incubated with *S. pneumoniae* alone, approximately 6% of *C. elegans* larvae survived for 24 h in the presence of sucrose (Figure 2A), correlating with an accumulation of 8 mg L^{-1} H_2O_2 (Figure 2B). In the absence of sucrose, very little H_2O_2 accumulated (Figure 2B) and almost all *C. elegans* larvae survived upon incubation with *S. pneumoniae* (Figure 2A), demonstrating that under these conditions the toxicity was associated primarily with H_2O_2. Inclusion of wild-type *M. gallisepticum* with *S. pneumoniae* and sucrose did not significantly alter the amount of *C. elegans* survival as compared to *S. pneumoniae* alone with sucrose (Figure 2A). However, H_2O_2 accumulation decreased to 4.5 mg L^{-1} (Figure 2B), possibly because of loss of H_2O_2 upon reaction with the high number of *M. gallisepticum* cells in suspension. On the other hand, inclusion of catalase-producing *M. iowae* or *M. gallisepticum* transformant 56A resulted in significantly increased amounts of *C. elegans* survival (Figure 2A) and no detectable H_2O_2 (Figure 2B). Taken together, these results suggest that catalase enables *M. iowae* to

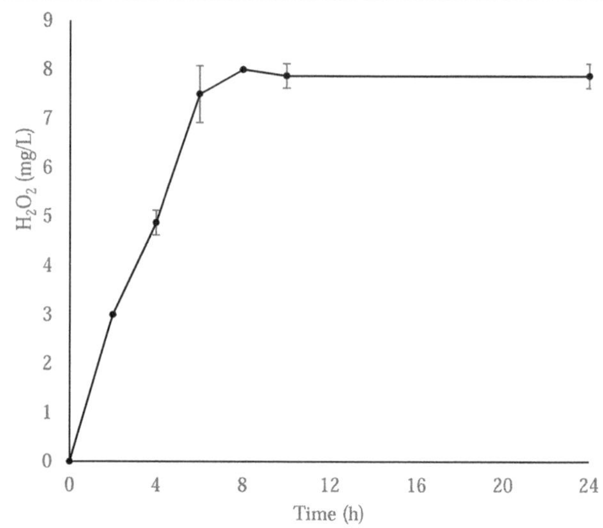

Figure 1 H_2O_2 accumulation by *S. pneumoniae*. Accumulation of H_2O_2 over time by *S. pneumoniae* at an OD_{620} of 0.05 in the presence of 500 μM sucrose. Error bars, SD.

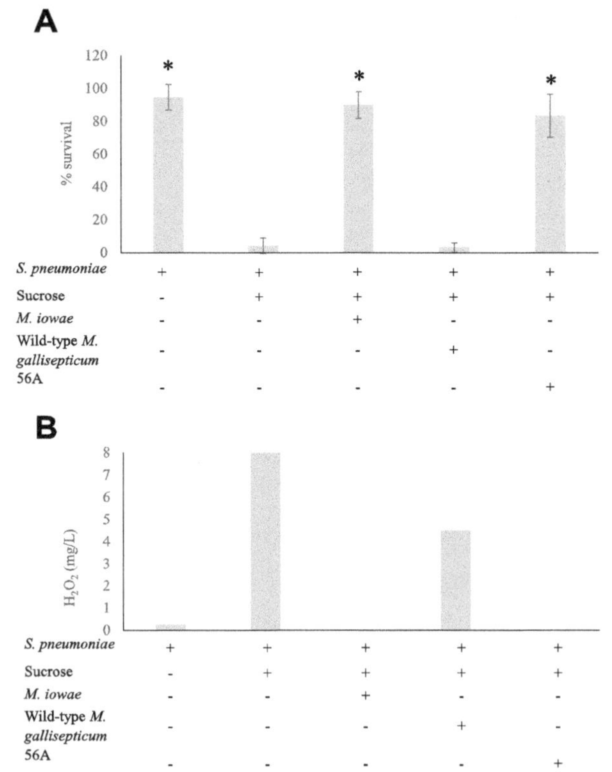

Figure 2 Host protection from *S. pneumoniae*-produced H_2O_2 by catalase-positive mycoplasmas. Survival of *C. elegans* **(A)** and amount of H_2O_2 remaining **(B)** at 24 h upon incubation with *S. pneumoniae* at $OD_{620} = 0.05$ in the presence of 500 μM sucrose. Experiments were performed in triplicate. Results shown are from one representative experiment (B). Error bars, SD. *, statistically significantly different from *S. pneumoniae* alone with 500 μM sucrose ($p < 0.05$).

offer protection from H_2O_2 being continually produced by other organisms.

Reasoning that protection by *M. iowae* is due to catalase and therefore might be specific to H_2O_2-mediated stress, *C. elegans* survival assays were repeated with a non-H_2O_2 producing pathogen. *P. aeruginosa* PAO1 produces the toxic molecule HCN [47], to which *C. elegans* larvae are highly susceptible; incubation with this bacterial strain typically results in complete killing of larvae [48,49]. At $OD_{650} = 0.1$, *P. aeruginosa* caused almost complete killing of larvae at 24 h (data not shown). Under these conditions, co-incubation of *C. elegans* with *P. aeruginosa* and any of the mycoplasma strains resulted in no difference in the survival of larvae at 24 h (Figure 3).

O_2-dependent changes in catalase activity and long-term survival of *C. elegans*

M. iowae lives in both aerobic and reduced-oxygen environments in its natural host, but its pathogenicity appears to be limited or non-existent in the gut, where it accumulates but where O_2 is low. Therefore, we explored whether *M. iowae* grown under low O_2 conditions might be less toxic to host cells. Interestingly, catalase activity of *M. iowae* significantly decreased by 24% ($p < 0.05$) in low O_2 (Figure 4), suggesting that O_2 exposure has an impact on catalase activity in *M. iowae*. *M. gallisepticum* 56A, which offered protection comparable to that of *M. iowae* [13] had 63% less catalase activity ($p < 0.05$) than *M. iowae* under atmospheric conditions (Figure 4). Therefore the decreased catalase activity in *M. iowae* cells grown in 1% O_2 is unlikely to result in a significant decrease in protection.

Whereas diffusible molecules such as H_2O_2 are responsible for damage to *C. elegans* within the first 48 h of incubation, the impact of toxins becomes apparent after 48 h as bacteria are able to establish an infection within the nematode gut [2]. To examine differences in the ability of *M. iowae* to cause damage to its host, long-term *C. elegans* assays were performed with bacterial cells grown under different O_2 concentrations. It is important to consider that the *C. elegans* assay conditions are carried out in a buffer, preventing mycoplasma growth, and at room temperature, which is well below the temperature range at which *M. iowae* can grow. It is therefore very likely that by the end of the incubation with *C. elegans*, *M. iowae* cells have no more catalase or putative toxins than they had at the beginning. A repeated measures ANOVA revealed significant differences between the two groups [$F(1,17) = 27.39$, $p < 0.05$]. Cells grown aerobically caused nematodes to die much more quickly, with 50% survival achieved after approximately 5 days as compared to approximately 9 days with cells grown in the presence of 1% O_2, and death of all larvae by 15 days with aerobically-grown *M. iowae* cells as opposed to 20 days with low O_2-grown mycoplasmas (Figure 5). These data suggest that *M. iowae* cells are less harmful in low-O_2 environments.

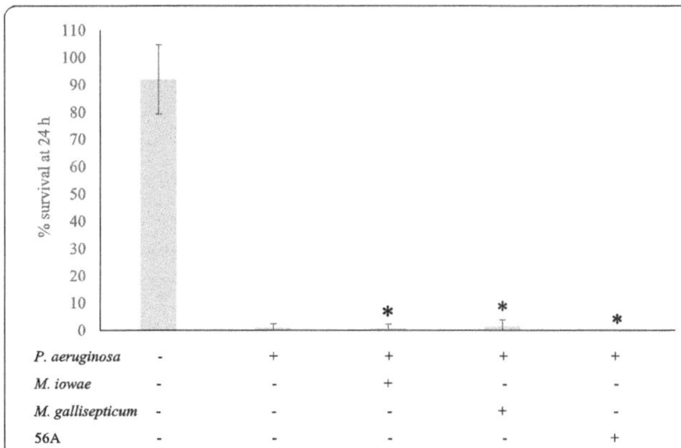

Figure 3 Absence of host protection from *P. aeruginosa* by catalase-positive mycoplasmas. Survival of *C. elegans* at 24 h upon co-incubation with *P. aeruginosa* at $OD_{650} = 0.1$. Experiments were performed in triplicate. Error bars, SD. *, no statistically significant difference from *P. aeruginosa* alone ($p > 0.05$).

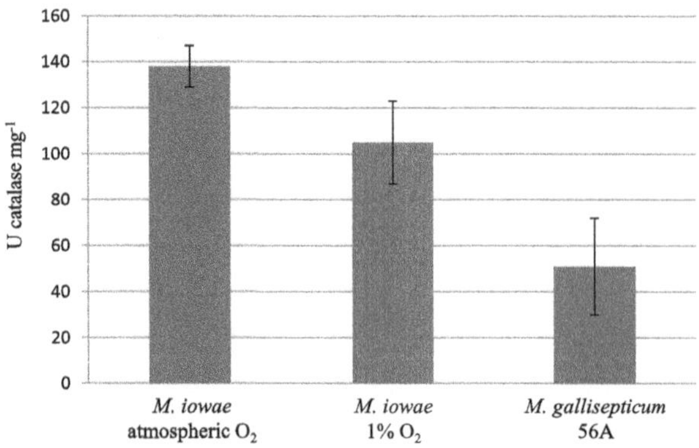

Figure 4 Catalase activity in *M. iowae* and *M. gallisepticum* transformed with *katE*. Extracts from cells grown under atmospheric conditions or in 1% O_2 were assayed for catalase activity as described in Material and methods. Error bars, SD.

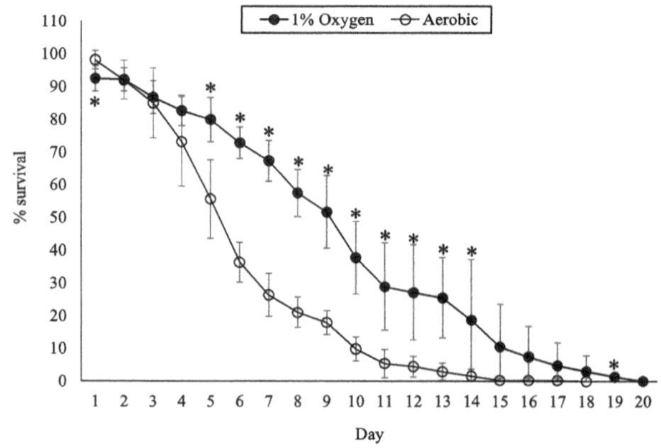

Figure 5 Long-term survival of *C. elegans* when fed *M. iowae* grown aerobically or in the presence of 1% O_2. Error bars, SD. *, statistically significantly different from aerobically-grown *M. iowae* ($p < 0.05$).

O_2 regulation of potential *M. iowae* virulence genes

Because it is unlikely that a relatively small O_2-dependent decrease in *M. iowae* catalase activity was related to increased survival of *C. elegans*, we hypothesized that *M. iowae* genes more directly linked to virulence experienced O_2-dependent regulation. Candidate virulence-associated genes were selected for analysis of regulation of expression by O_2. Transcription of the potential virulence factors *glpF* and *cards1* was examined as well as *katE* and another antioxidant enzyme, *sodA*. *glpF*, which allows uptake of glycerol for production of H_2O_2, was chosen as a representative of the presumptive glycerol catabolism operon that includes *glpK* and *glpO*. Additionally, *M. iowae* serovar K has two copies of genes homologous to *M. pneumoniae* CARDS toxin [13]. We examined the predicted amino acid sequences for the proteins encoded by these genes. There are three common motifs shared by many ADP-ribosylating toxins: a conserved arginine for NAD^+ binding, a serine-threonine-serine motif to maintain structural integrity of the NAD^+ binding site, and a catalytic glutamate [20]. These amino acids are all present in *M. pneumoniae* CARDS toxin, which has ADP-ribosyltransferase activity [20]. When both *M. iowae* CARDS toxin homologs were examined (named CARDS1 and CARDS2), some deviations were observed (Figure 6). CARDS2 has a conservative change of the second serine residue in the STS motif to a threonine. CARDS1 contains multiple changes, with substitutions of like charge at the conserved arginine and glutamate residues and less conservative substitutions for two of the three amino acids in the serine-threonine-serine motif. These *M. iowae* homologues have 28% and 25% identity, respectively, to the *M. pneumoniae* CARDS toxin sequence. Each *M. iowae* gene also has 99% identity to its respective homolog in *M. iowae* serovar I strain 695 [50]. *cards1* was chosen despite the greater degree of disparity from *M. pneumoniae* CARDS toxin since only 20 bases separate *cards1* and *cards2*, likely making both genes transcriptionally linked.

To examine transcript levels in *M. iowae* cells grown under different O_2 concentrations, qPCR was performed (Table 3). Expression of 16S rRNA was used as a control. The putative toxin gene *cards1* and the catalase gene *katE* underwent statistically significant down-regulation in *M. iowae* cells grown in the presence of 1% O_2, with decreases of 4.9- and 5.4-fold, respectively (Table 3). In contrast, *glpF* and *sodA* did not exhibit significant changes in expression in response to O_2 availability. Taken together, these data suggest that *M. iowae* undergoes differential regulation of select genes in response to low O_2 conditions. The reduction in *cards1* expression is consistent with reduced pathogenicity in the gut.

Discussion

Both genome sequences currently available for *M. iowae* [13,50] reveal the presence of a gene for catalase, an H_2O_2-degrading enzyme absent from all other published mycoplasma genomes, which produces an active protein [13]. Bacteria can encounter exposure to H_2O_2 from a variety of different sources, including other bacterial pathogens as well as the host immune response [1,2,43]. Bacteria bearing enzymes that detoxify ROS, including catalase, have been demonstrated to provide benefit to animal hosts in the context of probiotics [9]. Our results support a model wherein protection by *M. iowae* is specific to catalase-mediated reduction of H_2O_2 stress, but other mechanisms are also possible. Catalase is specifically implicated in this protection because *M. gallisepticum*, which does not normally have catalase activity, becomes protective upon transformation with *M. iowae katE* [13], despite 2.7-fold less catalase activity in the *M. gallisepticum* transformant 56A as compared with *M. iowae*.

M. pneumoniae CARDS	^{6}RFVY**R**VDLR	^{44}RSYFI**STS**ET	^{126}SFAYQR**E**WFTD
M. iowae CARDS1	^{21}KYVY**K**IDKR	^{66}RSLLI**SVF**PT	^{145}NFLWQN**D**WFKI
M. iowae CARDS2	^{13}RLVY**R**IDSR	^{58}RSVYV**STT**DS	^{144}DFAYQR**E**WIHV

Figure 6 Alignment of CARDS toxin-like sequences from *M. pneumoniae* and *M. iowae*. Residues generally conserved in other ADP-ribosylating toxins are bolded and enlarged.

Host-associated bacteria live in the presence of a consortium of other microorganisms, some of which may be H_2O_2 producers. We used *S. pneumoniae* as a model pathogen that produces H_2O_2 as an important virulence factor that not only can cause damage to host cells but has also been studied in the context of *C. elegans* [51-53]. Furthermore, *S. pneumoniae* can inhibit the growth of other bacterial competitors by virtue of its H_2O_2 production [54]. The ability of *M. iowae* to protect against H_2O_2-mediated damage caused by *S. pneumoniae*, albeit not against other kinds of damage such as that caused by *P. aeruginosa*, suggests that *M. iowae* could be beneficial to its host provided it is not also producing molecules harmful to its host.

M. iowae causes damage at multiple sites throughout the body of its natural poultry hosts, including legs, joints, air sac, and feathers [14-16]. However, despite many accounts of detection in and isolation from the gut, no clear-cut reports of disease at this site due to *M. iowae* have been documented [23-26]. Because low O_2 concentration is a hallmark of the gut environment that distinguishes it from other sites at which *M. iowae* causes damage and disease [27], we examined the impact of growth in 1% O_2 on *M. iowae* with regard to activities that might be associated with both disease and protection. Our finding that *M. iowae* has an ability to prolong survival when fed to *C. elegans* larvae following growth in 1% O_2 supports the notion that *M. iowae* is not harmful in the gut and might in fact be a beneficial component of the gut microflora. Significantly, at the transcriptional level, this environment causes a significant down-regulation in not only the gene encoding catalase, but also a gene encoding a homolog of CARDS toxin, a causative agent of host damage by *M. pneumoniae* [20,55] and *M. penetrans* [56].

Table 3 Differences in gene expression as determined by qPCR in response to growth in the presence of 1% O_2

Gene	Fold-change of down-regulation in response to 1% O_2^{*}
cards1	4.93 ± 0.78†
glpF	1.67 ± 0.88
katE	5.37 ± 2.60†
sodA	1.35 ± 1.06

*Average ± SD.
†$p < 0.05$ compared to aerobic expression as determined by unpaired Student's *T*-test.

These data suggest that *M. iowae* undergoes differential regulation of select genes in response to growth in low O_2 environments.

The down-regulation of *katE* in 1% O_2 could be a response to a decreased threat of damage from ROS. Despite this reduction, it is important to consider that the catalase activity in low O_2-grown *M. iowae* cells is still 2.1-fold greater than the amount present in *M. gallisepticum* transformant 56A, which itself still confers significant protection of *C. elegans* exposed to H_2O_2 [13]. Therefore, the reduction in *M. iowae* catalase activity in a gut-like environment is not necessarily associated with decreased protection. It is possible that production of catalase facilitates colonization of the gut by *M. iowae*, in parallel with *Campylobacter jejuni*, which expresses an active catalase that is important for colonization of the poultry intestinal tract [57]. The degree of down-regulation of *katE* at the transcription level does not closely match the change in catalase activity in whole cell lysates, with a smaller decrease observed in the latter. The high level of catalase activity might not decrease linearly as the concentration of catalase decreases.

The down-regulation of *cards1*, a homolog of CARDS toxin, which is likely accompanied by similar down-regulation of the very closely linked *cards2*, may be associated with decreased pathogenicity of *M. iowae* in the gastrointestinal tract. The amount of CARDS toxin produced correlates positively with the amount of host damage caused by *M. pneumoniae* [55]. Differential expression of toxins in different environments is well-established in diverse bacteria, including clostridia [58], *Vibrio cholerae* [59], and cyanobacteria [60]. It is conceivable that the environment of the intestine is sufficiently nutritious for *M. iowae* that severe damage to host cells is unwarranted, favoring a strategy in which virulence factors may be used principally in environments in which nutrients are less readily available. In this model, low O_2 provides a cue to *M. iowae* that it is in the gut, where it can conserve energy by down-regulating virulence genes, including those encoding the CARDS toxin-like proteins. The similar down-regulation of both *cards1* and *katE* transcript levels when grown in the presence of 1% O_2, on the order of 5-fold, raises the possibility that a common regulatory mechanism may be acting on both genes, but further work is necessary to elucidate such a mechanism.

Abbreviations
ROS: Reactive oxygen species; IBD: Inflammatory bowel disease; RT-qPCR: Reverse transcription-quantitative polymerase chain reaction; BHI: Brain heart infusion; PBS: Phosphate-buffered saline..

Competing interests
The authors declare that they have no competing interests.

Authors' contributions
REP carried out all the experimentation, participated in the design of the study, participated in the analysis of the results, and drafted the manuscript. MFB conceived of the study, participated in the design of the study, the analysis of the results, and the writing of the manuscript. Both authors read and approved the final manuscript.

Acknowledgments
This work was supported by the National Institutes of Health (Public Health Service grant R15 AI073994) to MFB and by an award from the Sigma Xi foundation to REP. We thank A. Bollmann and members of her research group for assistance with low-O_2 growth of *M. iowae*. We thank A. Kiss of the Miami University Center for Bioinformatics and Functional Genomics for training in RNA quantification. We thank C.N. Bialorucki for assistance with quantification of the relationship among OD_{550} values, colony-forming units, and protein concentrations for mycoplasma species. This work was done in partial fulfillment of REP's doctoral dissertation requirements.

Author details
[1]Department of Microbiology, Miami University, Oxford, OH 45056, USA. [2]Present address: Division of Natural Sciences and Mathematics, Kentucky Wesleyan College, Owensboro, KY 42301, USA.

References
1. Bolm M, Jansen WTM, Schnabel R, Chhatwal G (2004) Hydrogen peroxide-mediated killing of *Caenorhabditis elegans*: a common feature of different streptococcal species. Infect Immun 72:1192–1194
2. Moy TI, Mylonakis E, Calderwood SB, Ausubel FM (2004) Cytotoxicity of hydrogen peroxide produced by *Enterococcus faecium*. Infect Immun 72:4512–4520
3. Whelan K, Quigley EMM (2013) Probiotics in the management of irritable bowel syndrome and inflammatory bowel disease. Curr Opin Gastroenterol 29:184–189
4. Simmonds NJ, Allen RE, Stevens TR, Van Someren RN, Blake DR, Rampton DS (1992) Chemiluminescence assay of musical reactive oxygen metabolites in inflammatory bowel disease. Gastroenterology 103:186–196
5. Sedghi S, Fields JZ, Klamut M, Urban G, Durkin M, Winship D, Fretland D, Olyaee M, Keshavarzian A (1993) Increased production of luminol and chemiluminescence by the inflamed colonic mucosa in patients with ulcerative colitis. Gut 34:1191–1197
6. Lih-Brody L, Powell SR, Collier KP, Reddy GM, Cerchia R, Kahn E, Weissman GS, Katz S, Floyd RA, McKinley MJ, Fisher SE, Mullin GE (1996) Increased oxidative stress and decreased antioxidant defenses in mucosa of inflammatory bowel disease. Dig Dis Sci 41:2078–2086
7. Keshavarzian A, Banan A, Farhadi A, Komanduri S, Mutlu E, Zhang Y, Fields JZ (2003) Increases in free radicals and cytoskeletal protein oxidation and nitration in the colon of patients with inflammatory bowel disease. Gut 52:720–728
8. Switala J, Loewen PC (2002) Diversity of properties among catalases. Arch Biochem Biophys 401:145–154
9. Zhu H, Li YR (2012) Oxidative stress and redox signaling mechanisms of inflammatory bowel disease: updated experimental and clinical evidence. Exp Biol Med 237:474–480
10. LeBlanc JG, del Carmen S, Miyoshi A, Azevedo V, Sesma F, Langella P, Bermúdez-Humarán LG, Watterlot L, Perdigon G, de Moreno de LeBlanc A (2011) Use of superoxide dismutase and catalase producing lactic acid bacteria in TNBS induced Crohn's disease in mice. J Biotechnol 151:287–293
11. Rochat T, Bermúdez-Humarán L, Gratadoux J-J, Fourage C, Hoebler C, Corthier G, Langella P (2007) Anti-inflammatory effects of *Lactobacillus casei* BL23 producing or not a manganese-dependent catalase on DSS-induced colitis in mice. Microb Cell Fact 6:22
12. Al-Ankari AR, Bradbury JM (1996) *Mycoplasma iowae*: a review. Avian Pathol 25:205–229
13. Pritchard RE, Prassinos AJ, Osborne JD, Raviv Z, Balish MF (2014) Reduction of hydrogen peroxide accumulation and toxicity by a catalase from *Mycoplasma iowae*. PLoS One 9:e105188
14. Bradbury JM, Ideris A, Oo TT (1988) *Mycoplasma iowae* infection in young turkeys. Avian Pathol 17:149–171
15. Trampel DW, Goll F, Jr (1994) Outbreak of *Mycoplasma iowae* infection in commercial turkey poults. Avian Dis 38:905–909
16. Ley DH, Marusak RA, Vivas EJ, Barnes HJ, Fletcher OJ (2010) *Mycoplasma iowae* associated with chondrodystrophy in commercial turkeys. Avian Pathol 39:87–93
17. Taylor RR, Mohan K, Miles RJ (1996) Diversity of energy-yielding substrates and metabolism in avian mycoplasmas. Vet Microbiol 51:291–304
18. Papazisi L, Gorton TS, Kutish G, Markham PF, Browning GF, Nguyen DK, Swartzell S, Madan A, Mahairas G, Geary SJ (2003) The complete genome sequence of the avian pathogen *Mycoplasma gallisepticum* strain R_{low}. Microbiology 149:2307–2316
19. Jurkovic DA, Newman JT, Balish MF (2012) Conserved terminal organelle morphology and function in *Mycoplasma penetrans* and *Mycoplasma iowae*. J Bacteriol 194:2877–2883
20. Kannan TR, Baseman JB (2006) ADP-ribosylating and vacuolating cytotoxin of *Mycoplasma pneumoniae* represents unique virulence determinant among bacterial pathogens. Proc Natl Acad Sci U S A 103:6724–6729
21. Hardy RD, Coalson JJ, Peters J, Chaparro A, Techasaensiri C, Cantwell AM, Kannan TR, Baseman JB, Dube PH (2009) Analysis of pulmonary inflammation and function in the mouse and baboon after exposure to *Mycoplasma pneumoniae* CARDS toxin. PLoS One 4:e7562
22. Medina JL, Coalson JJ, Brooks EG, Winter VT, Chaparro A, Principe MF, Kannan TR, Baseman JB, Dube PH (2012) *Mycoplasma pneumoniae* CARDS toxin induces pulmonary eosinophilic and lymphocytic inflammation. Am J Respir Cell Mol Biol 46:815–822
23. Jordan FTW, Amin MM (1980) A survey of mycoplasma infections in domestic poultry. Res Vet Sci 28:96–100
24. Jordan FTW (1983) Recovery and identification of avian mycoplasmas. In: Tully JG, Razin S (ed) Methods in Mycoplasmology. Diagnostic Mycoplasmology, vol II. Academic, New York, pp 69–79
25. Mirsalimi SM, Rosendal S, Julian RJ (1989) Colonization of the intestine of turkey embryos exposed to *Mycoplasma iowae*. Avian Dis 33:310–315
26. Shah-Majid M, Rosendal S (1986) Oral challenge of turkey poults with *Mycoplasma iowae*. Avian Dis 31:365–369
27. He G, Shankar RA, Chzhan M, Samouilov A, Kuppusamy P, Zweier JL (1999) Noninvasive measurement of anatomic structure and intraluminal oxygenation in the gastrointestinal tract of living mice with spatial and spectral ER imaging. Proc Natl Acad Sci U S A 96:4586–4591
28. Wangensteen OD, Rahn H (1970–1971) Respiratory gas exchange by the avian embryo. Respir Physiol 11:31–45
29. Halbedel S, Eiler H, Jonas B, Busse J, Hecker M, Engelmann S, Stülke J (2007) Transcription in *Mycoplasma pneumoniae*: analysis of the promoters of the *ackA* and *ldh* genes. J Mol Biol 371:596–607
30. Hallamaa KM, Tang S-L, Ficorilli N, Browning GF (2008) Differential expression of lipoprotein genes in *Mycoplasma pneumoniae* after contact with human lung epithelial cells, and under oxidative and acidic stress. BMC Microbiol 8:124
31. Madsen ML, Nettleton D, Thacker EL, Edwards R, Minion FC (2006) Transcriptional profiling of *Mycoplasma hyopneumoniae* during heat shock using microarrays. Infect Immun 74:160–166
32. Madsen ML, Nettleton D, Thacker EL, Minion FC (2006) Transcriptional profiling of *Mycoplasma hyopneumoniae* during iron depletion using microarrays. Microbiology 152:937–944
33. Schafer ER, Oneal MJ, Madsen ML, Minion FC (2007) Global transcriptional analysis of *Mycoplasma hyopneumoniae* following exposure to hydrogen peroxide. Microbiology 153:3785–3790
34. Madsen ML, Puttamreddy S, Thacker EL, Carruthers MD, Minion FC (2008) Transcriptome changes in *Mycoplasma hyopneumoniae* during infection. Infect Immun 76:658–663
35. Tully JG, Rose DL, Whitcomb RF, Wenzel RP (1979) Enhanced isolation of *Mycoplasma pneumoniae* from throat washings with a newly-modified culture medium. J Infect Dis 139:478–482
36. Hames C, Halbedel S, Hoppert M, Frey J, Stülke J (2009) Glycerol metabolism is important for cytotoxicity of *Mycoplasma pneumoniae*. J Bacteriol 191:747–753

37. Lewis JA, Fleming JT (1995) Basic culture methods. In: Epstein HF, Shakes DC (ed) Methods in Cell Biology. *Caenorhabditis elegans*: Modern Biological Analysis of an Organism, vol 48. Academic, Boston, pp 3–29
38. Castric PA (1983) Hydrogen cyanide production by *Pseudomonas aeruginosa* at reduced oxygen levels. Can J Microbiol 29:1344–1349
39. Himmelreich R, Hilbert H, Plagens H, Pirkl E, Li B-C, Herrmann R (1996) Complete sequence analysis of the genome of the bacterium *Mycoplasma pneumoniae*. Nucleic Acids Res 24:4420–4449
40. Kong W, Nakatsu CH (2010) Optimization of RNA extraction for PCR quantification of aromatic compound degradation genes. Appl Environ Microbiol 76:1282–1284
41. Bustin SA, Benes V, Garson JA, Hellemans J, Huggett J, Kubist M, Mueller R, Nolan T, Pfaffl MW, Shipley GL, Vandesompele J, Wittwer CT (2009) The MIQE guidelines: *m*inimum *i*nformation for publication of *q*uantitative real-time PCR *e*xperiments. Clin Chem 55:611–622
42. Jansen WTM, Bolm M, Balling R, Chhatwal GS, Schnabel R (2002) Hydrogen peroxide-mediated killing of *Caenorhabditis elegans* by *Streptococcus pyogenes*. Infect Immun 70:5202–5207
43. Slauch JM (2011) How does the oxidative burst of macrophages kill bacteria? Still an open ended question. Mol Microbiol 80:580–583
44. Avery OT, Neill JM (1924) Studies on oxidation and reduction by pneumococcus. II. The production of peroxide by sterile extracts of pneumococcus. J Exp Med 39:357–366
45. Spellerberg B, Cundell DR, Sandros J, Pearce BJ, Idänpään-Heikkilä I, Rosenow C, Masure HR (1996) Pyruvate oxidase, as a determinant of virulence in *Streptococcus pneumoniae*. Mol Microbiol 19:803–813
46. Iyer R, Camilli A (2007) Sucrose metabolism contributes to *in vivo* fitness of *Streptococcus pneumoniae*. Mol Microbiol 66:1–13
47. Castric PA (1974) Hydrogen cyanide, a secondary metabolite of *Pseudomonas aeruginosa*. Can J Microbiol 21:613–618
48. Darby C, Cosma CL, Thomas JH, Manoil C (1999) Lethal paralysis of *Caenorhabditis elegans* by *Pseudomonas aeruginosa*. Proc Natl Acad Sci U S A 96:15202–15207
49. Gallagher LA, Manoil C (2001) *Pseudomonas aeruginosa* PAO1 kills *Caenorhabditis elegans* by cyanide poisoning. J Bacteriol 183:6207–6214
50. Wei S, Guo Z, Li T, Zhang T, Li X, Zhou Z, Li Z, Lui M, Luo R, Bi D, Chen H, Zhou R, Jin H (2012) Genome sequence of *Mycoplasma iowae* strain 695, an unusual pathogen causing deaths in turkeys. J Bacteriol 194:547–548
51. Duane PG, Rubins JB, Weisel HR, Janoff EN (1993) Identification of hydrogen peroxide as a *Streptococcus pneumoniae* toxin for rat alveolar epithelial cells. Infect Immun 61:4392–4397
52. Hirst RA, Sikand KS, Rutman A, Mitchell TJ, Andrew PW, O'Callaghan C (2000) Relative roles of pneumolysin and hydrogen peroxide from *Streptococcus pneumoniae* in inhibition of ependymal ciliary beat frequency. Infect Immun 68:1557–1562
53. Garsin DA, Sifri CD, Mylonakis E, Qin X, Singh KV, Murray BE, Calderwood SB, Ausubel FM (2001) A simple model host for identifying Gram-positive virulence factors. Proc Natl Acad Sci U S A 98:10892–10897
54. Pericone CD, Overweg K, Hermans PW, Weiser JN (2000) Inhibitory and bactericidal effects of hydrogen peroxide production by *Streptococcus pneumoniae* on other inhabitants of the upper respiratory tract. Infect Immun 68:3990–3997
55. Techasaensiri C, Tagliabue C, Cagle M, Iranpour P, Katz K, Kannan TR, Coalson JJ, Baseman JB, Hardy RD (2010) Variation in colonization, ADP-ribosylating and vacuolating cytotoxin, and pulmonary disease severity among *Mycoplasma pneumoniae* strains. Am J Respir Crit Care Med 182:797–804
56. Johnson C, Kannan TR, Baseman JB (2009) Characterization of a unique ADP-ribosyltransferase of *Mycoplasma penetrans*. Infect Immun 77:4362–4370
57. Flint A, Sun Y-Q, Stintzi A (2012) Cj1386 is an ankyrin-containing protein involved in heme trafficking to catalase in *Campylobacter jejuni*. J Bacteriol 194:334–345
58. Carter GP, Cheung JK, Larcombe S, Lyras D (2014) Regulation of toxin production in the pathogenic clostridia. Mol Microbiol 91:221–231
59. Matson JS, Withey JH, DiRita VJ (2007) Regulatory networks controlling *Vibrio cholerae* virulence gene expression. Infect Immun 75:5542–5549
60. Neilan BA, Pearson LA, Muenchhoff J, Moffitt MC, Dittmann E (2013) Environmental conditions that influence toxin biosynthesis in cyanobacteria. Environ Microbiol 15:1239–1253

22

Comparative analysis of cytokine transcript profiles within mediastinal lymph node compartments of pigs after infection with porcine reproductive and respiratory syndrome genotype 1 strains differing in pathogenicity

Obdulio García-Nicolás[1*], Rubén S Rosales[2], Francisco J Pallarés[1], David Risco[3], Juan J Quereda[4], Simon P Graham[5], Jean-Pierre Frossard[5], Sophie B Morgan[5], Falko Steinbach[5,7], Trevor W Drew[5], Tony S Strickland[6] and Francisco J Salguero[6,7]

Abstract

Porcine reproductive and respiratory syndrome virus (PRRSV) induces a weak immune response enabling it to persist in different organs of infected pigs. This has been attributed to the ability of PRRSV to influence the induction of cytokine responses. In this study, we investigated the cytokine transcriptional profiles in different compartments of the mediastinal lymph node of pigs infected with three genotype 1 PRRSV strains of differing pathogenicity: the low virulence prototype Lelystad virus (LV), and UK field strain 215–06 and the highly virulent subtype 3 SU1-Bel isolate from Belarus. We have used a combination of laser capture micro-dissection (LCM) followed by real time quantitative PCR (RT-qPCR) and immunohistochemical (IHC) detection of immune cell markers (CD3, CD79a and MAC387) and RT-qPCR quantification of PRRSV and cytokine transcripts. Compared to mock infected pigs, we found a significant downregulation of TNF-α and IFN-α in follicular and interfollicular areas of the mediastinal lymph node from 3 days post-infection (dpi) in animals infected with all three strains. This was accompanied by a transient B cell depletion and T cell and macrophage infiltration in the follicles together with T cell depletion in the interfollicular areas. A delayed upregulation of IFN-γ and IL-23p19 was observed mainly in the follicles. The PRRSV load was higher in all areas and time-points studied in the animals infected with the SU1-Bel strain. This paper describes the first application of LCM to study the cytokine transcript profiles and virus distribution in different compartments of the lymph node of pigs.

Introduction

Porcine reproductive and respiratory syndrome (PRRS) is characterized by respiratory disease in neonatal and growing pigs and reproductive failure in gilts and sows (increased number of abortions, mummified foetuses, stillbirth and weak-born piglets) [1-3]. PRRS is considered one of the most economically important swine infectious diseases around the world, with estimated losses of up to $664 million annually in the USA alone [4,5].

PRRS virus (PRRSV) is classified into two genotypes, type 1 (European or PRRSV-1) and type 2 (North American or PRRSV-2) [6]. In addition, a high degree of genetic variation in both genotypes has been found, with PRRSV-1 having been divided into 3 subtypes: pan-European subtype 1 and East European subtypes 2 and 3 [7], with the possibility of a fourth subtype being suggested [8]. Significant differences in virulence have also been described between PRRSV-1 subtypes, with the East European subtype 3 seemingly comprising the most virulent strains [9-11].

PRRSV shows a marked tropism for cells of the monocyte-macrophage lineage [12]. The main target of PRRSV are alveolar and other tissue macrophages, and

* Correspondence: ogn14346@um.es
[1]Department of Anatomy and Comparative Pathology, Faculty of Veterinary Medicine, Murcia University, "Mare Nostrum Excellence Campus – 3738", 30100 Murcia, Spain
Full list of author information is available at the end of the article

to a lesser extent, monocytes and dendritic cells [13]. Absent or weak interferon alpha (IFN-α) secretion [14] and a consequent weak and delayed cell-mediated immune response with low levels of IFN-γ has been described following PRRSV infection [15,16]. Pigs infected with PRRSV have also shown a delayed production of neutralizing antibodies [17]. PRRSV replication has been reported in lymphoid organs [18,19] however studies have also shown a lack of homogeneity in proinflammatory cytokine responses [20-22]. This suggests a role for this tissue in the pathogenesis of PRRS but also highlights the need for comparative in vivo studies using PRRSV-1 strains which differ in their virulence. The porcine lymph node (LN) has a dense medulla, where T cells are predominant and which lacks sinuses and cords. The LN cortex is divided into two differentiated areas the follicles (F) and interfollicular (IF) areas. The F is a B cell rich area that also contains follicular dendritic cells (fDC) and $CD4^+$ T helper cells that collaborate in antigen presentation to B cells and subsequent antibody production. The IF area is rich in T cells [21,22]. It has been proposed that the immunopathogenesis of porcine circovirus 2 (PCV2) infection is associated with follicular changes in lymph nodes [23], and it is suggested that this could also be the case for PRRSV infection.

Transcriptional expression profiling studies can aid to the understanding of infection biology and the molecular basis of disease [24]. Several studies have analysed the host transcriptional profiles during PRRSV infection in different organs by taking small pieces of tissue [25-28], but none have addressed transcriptional profiling in defined tissue structures. Laser capture microdissection (LCM) is a powerful tool for the acquisition of homogeneous cell populations or specific tissue structures which can be analyzed by a variety of molecular biology techniques and aid disease pathogenesis investigations [29-31].

The main aim of this study was to compare the cytokine transcriptional profiles in different compartments of lymph nodes from pigs infected with three PRRSV-1 strains of defined virulence. This study included the prototype Lelystad virus (LV) and a field strain from the UK (215–06), both categorized as low virulence subtype 1 viruses, and a divergent and highly pathogenic Eastern European subtype 3 strain from Belarus (SU1-Bel). Using LCM followed by quantitative reverse transcriptase PCR (RT-qPCR), viral RNA and cytokine transcripts were measured in the F and IF areas of mediastinal lymph nodes (Med-LN) collected at selected time-points post-infection. To further contextualize these data, T cells, B cells and macrophages were immunolabelled to characterize these cell populations within the lymph node compartments.

Material and methods

Viruses

Three PRRSV-1 strains were used in this study: the LV-Ter Huurne was selected as the prototype subtype 1 strain (kindly provide by Anne Marie Rebel, CVI Lelystad, The Netherlands) [11]; the subtype 1 215–06 strain was isolated in 2006 from the serum of a post-weaning piglet showing signs of wasting and poor condition on a farm in England and isolated at the Animal and Plant Health Agency (APHA, Addlestone, UK); and the highly pathogenic subtype 3 strain SU1-Bel, isolated at the APHA from lung tissue of a pig from Belarus (kindly provided by Dr Tomasz Stadejek, Warsaw University of Life Sciences, Poland) was also included. Virus propagation was carried out as previously described [10].

Animals and experiment design

Seventy-six specific-pathogen-free five-week-old male piglets from a PRRSV and PCV2 seronegative farm in the Netherlands were used in this study. These animals were matched by weight and randomly allocated to four groups; for the control group 16 animals were allocated, whereas for each infected group 20 animals were used. Each group was housed in separate rooms, which allowed the free airflow from the outside, and were allowed to acclimatise for 14 days prior to the experiment. Measures were taken to prevent cross-contamination between groups, including the change of clothes and equipment between each room. At seven weeks of age, 3 groups of piglets were inoculated intranasally with 1.5 mL of complete Roswell Park Memorial Institute medium supplemented with 10% FBS (cRPMI) containing 10^5 50% tissue-culture infective dose ($TCID_{50}$) of PRRSV-1 strain (LV, 215–06 and SU1-Bel, respectively). The remaining control group was inoculated intranasally with 1.5 mL of uninfected porcine alveolar macrophage cryolysate in cRPMI. Four animals in the control group and five from each virus-inoculated group were euthanized at 3 and at 7 days post-infection (dpi). All remaining animals were euthanized at 35 dpi. This experiment was performed in accordance with the Animals (Scientific Procedures) Act, 1986, UK, following approval of the APHA Ethical Review Committee. A clinical scoring system with predefined humane endpoints was used to prevent undue suffering.

Clinical signs, gross pathology and histopathology

Pigs were monitored daily throughout the study, and clinical signs, including rectal temperatures, were scored and recorded as previously described [10]. The Med-LN is the main draining lymph node for the apical and medial lobes of the lungs. Since PRRSV is most frequently detected in these lung lobes [32], Med-LN was selected for this study and the gross pathology evaluated during post-mortem examination. For the analysis by RT-qPCR, a piece of 10×10×3 mm of Med-LN was embedded and cryopreserved in optimal cutting temperature (OCT) compound (Sakura Finetek Europe B.V., The Nederland) as previously described [33]. For histopathology examination, the remaining Med-LN samples were fixed in 10% buffered formalin, routinely processed, embedded in paraffin-wax, and 4 μm tissue sections stained with haematoxylin and eosin. The histopathological lesions were evaluated in these slides using a light microscope.

Immunohistochemistry (IHC)

The immunolabelling of cell markers was done using the avidin-biotin complex method (ABC Vector Elite, Vector laboratories, USA) as described previously [19,34]. Briefly, 4 μm thick sections were dewaxed and rehydrated, followed by endogenous peroxidase inhibition with 3% H_2O_2 in methanol for 30 min. Depending on the epitope of interest, antigen retrieval in the tissue sections was performed by enzymatic trypsin/alpha-chymotrypsin (for CD3 and MAC-387) or by microwaving the sections in citric acid pH6.0 (for CD79a) or pH6.0 citrate buffer (for PRRSV nucleocapsid N protein). The slides were mounted in a Sequenza Immunostaining Centre (Shandon Scientific, UK) and washed with Tris buffered saline (TBS; pH 7.6, 0.005 M; Sigma–Aldrich, UK) and incubated for 30 min at room temperature with 100 μL per slide of blocking solution. The primary antibodies used were monoclonal anti-human CD3 (1:1000; Dako, UK), monoclonal anti-human CD79a (1:400; Dako, UK), and monoclonal anti-human MAC-387 (1:100; AbDSerotec, UK). Each antibody was applied for 1 h at room temperature. In each case, the corresponding biotinylated secondary antibody (Vector Laboratories, UK) was then incubated for 30 min at room temperature. Slides were then incubated for 30 min with avidin-biotin complex and labelling performed using 3,30-diaminobenzidine tetrahydrochloride (DAB; Sigma-Aldrich, UK). Sections were counterstained with Mayer's haematoxylin, dehydrated and mounted. Positive and negative controls, as well as isotype controls, were included in each IHC run.

The immunolabelled Med-LN sections were examined by light microscopy, and immunolabelling measurements recorded using a score ranking from −3 to 0 (cellular depletion) and from 0 to 3 (cellular increment) compared to the control group. Positive scale: 0 = absence (<1 positive cell/structure); 1 = scarce (1–10 positive cells/structure); 2 mild-moderate (11–30 positive cells/structure); 3 abundant (>31 positive cells/structure). Negative scale: 0 = absence (no different to control group); −1 = scarce (5% less positive cells compares with control group); −2 mild-moderate (6-10% less positive cells compares with control group); −3 abundant (more than 10% less positive cells compares with control group).

Laser capture microdissection (LCM)

Frozen OCT-embedded Med-LNswere cut to 10 μm thick sections using a cryostat. Tissue sections were placed on membrane-coated slides (PEN-Membrane 2.0 μm; Leica Microsystems, Germany). The cryostat was treated with RNAZap Solution (Life Technologies, UK) between each sample in order to avoid cross-contamination of RNA. Sections were air-dried and fixed in 70% ethanol for 5 min and stained with RNase free haematoxylin for 1 min. Two consecutive Med-LN tissue sections were used per animal. All observed F and peripheral IF were dissected and captured separately in RNase-free PCR tubes (Greiner bio-one, UK) using a laser microdissector (Leica LMD6500, Leica, Germany). The samples were immediately frozen and stored at −80 °C until laboratory processing.

RNA extraction and reverse transcription quantitative polymerase chain reaction (RT-qPCR)

For each sample, total RNA was extracted using the RNA queous-Micro Kit (Ambion,Life Technologies, UK) following the manufacturer's instructions for LCM samples, including the DNase I treatment and DNase inactivation steps. The total RNA was quantified using Qubit 2.0 Fluorometer (Life Technologies) and all samples adjusted to an RNA concentration of 2 ng/μL).

PRRSV infection kinetics in the F and IF areas of Med-LN were studied by measuring viral RNA. PRRSV RT-qPCR was performed as previously described [35]. Briefly, 2 μL of sample or standard PRRSV-1 RNA dilutions were added as template to the QuantiTec Probe RT-PCR Kit (Qiagen, UK) following the manufacturer's instructions for a total volume of 25 μL. Data was analysed by changes in the cycle threshold (Ct), and results were calculated as 38 − Ct, which represented the difference between the last cycle of the PRRSV RT-qPCR and the Ct for each sample.

Primers and TaqMan probe sets for porcine cytokines were synthesized by Sigma-Aldrich (Table 1). All cytokines primer pairs produced amplicons smaller than 150 base pairs (bp). All primer and probe sets were optimized for our laboratory conditions.

In order to obtain complementary DNA (cDNA) reverse transcription was carried out using the SuperScript VILO^{TM} cDNA Synthesis Kit (Applied Biosystems, UK) and cDNA was stored at −80 °C until laboratory processing. 2 μL of cDNA diluted 1:100 in RNase free water was used as template for each cytokine qPCR, using the EXPRESS qPCR Supermix (Invitrogen) with ROX reference dye in a total volume of 20 μL. Thermal cycling conditions were 2 min at 95 °C, 45 cycles of denaturation at 95 °C for 15 s and annealing/extension at 60 °C for 1 min. Reverse transcription negative controls and non-template controls were included. PCR plates were centrifuged prior to

Table 1 Primers and probes used for qPCR

Gene	Primer Forward nM	Primer Reverse nM	Probe nM
β-Actin	5′-cactcctaacgctgtggatcag-3′ 300	5′-ccacttaactatcttgggcttatcg-3′ 300	5′-[6FAM]-cacgtgcttcacgcggcagc-[TAM]-3′ 50
TNF-α	5′-tggccccttgagcatca-3′ 900	5′-cgggcttatctgaggtttgaga-3′ 600	5′-[6FAM]-ccctctggcccaaggactcagatca-[TAM]-3′ 50
IFN-α	5′-tcagctgcaatgccatctg-3′ 150	5′-agggagagattctcctcatttgtg-3′ 600	5′-[6FAM]-tgacctgcctcagacccacagcc-[TAM]-3′ 50
IFN-γ	5′-gaaaagctgattaaattccggtag-3′ 300	5′-aggttagatcttggtgacagatc-3′ 900	5′-[6FAM]-tctgcagatccagcgcaaagccatcag-[TAM]-3′ 50
SOCS1	5′-ttcttcgccctcagtgtgaa-3′ 300	5′-ggcctggaagtgcacgc-3′ 300	5′-[6FAM]-ttcgggccccacaagcatcc-[TAM]-3′ 50
IL-10	5′-tgagaacagctgcatccacttc-3′ 300	5′-tctggtccttcgtttgaaagaaa-3′ 300	5′-[6FAM]-caaccagcctgccccacatgc-[TAM]-3′ 150
TGF-β	5′-agggctaccatgccaattt-3′ 600	5′-ccgggttgtgctggttgt-3′ 600	5′-[6FAM]-cactcagtacagcaaggtcctggctctgta-[TAM]-3′ 50
IL-23p19	5′-agaagagggagatgatgagac-3′ 900	5′-agcaggactgactgccgtcc-3′ 300	5′-[6FAM]-ctgaggatcacagccatccccgc-[TAM]-3′ 50

amplification using the Strategene MX3000P qPCR System (Stratagene, UK). Fold-change of cytokine expression was calculated using the $2^{-\Delta\Delta Ct}$ method [36] and β-actin was used as the endogenous calibrator; which was selected due to its stable expression in porcine lymphatic tissue [37]. Relative gene expression results are presented on a base 2 logarithmic scale.

Statistical analysis

Statistical analyses were performed using SPSS 15.0 software (SPSS Inc., USA) and graphs were prepared using SPSS 15.0 software (SPSS Inc., USA) and GraphPad Prism 5 (GraphPad Software, Inc., USA). To determine the non-normal distribution of all data a Kolmogorov-Smirnov test was used. Non-normal distributed data was then analysed using a non-parametric test. The Kruskal-Wallis test was performed to analyse the mean parameters (PRRSV RNA load, immunolabelled cells and cytokine expression) between the animal groups (Control, LV, 2015–06, and SU1-Bel) at three different time-points post inoculation (3 dpi, 7 dpi, and 35 dpi). Thereafter, we performed multiple comparisons using the non-parametric Mann–Whitney-U test with Bonferroni correction as post-hoc to determine significant individual differences. Finally, the presence of differences between results obtained in F and IF tissues were assessed using the non-parametric Wilcoxon signed-rank test. The correlations between PRRSV RNA and cytokine transcripts were determined by Spearman's Rho analysis. A p value of less than 0.05 was considered significant.

Results

Clinical signs, gross pathology and histopathology

Rectal temperatures remained within the physiological range in control as well as infected animals, except for SU1-Bel infected animals that showed hyperthermia at 3, 8–10 dpi (over 40 °C). Only SU1-Bel infected animals developed elevated clinical sign scores (mean score from 5 to 10) compared with the rest of animals in this study (mean clinical score only up to 3) [10]. Macroscopically at post-mortem, a mild to moderate enlargement of Med-LN was observed in infected animals at 3 and 7 dpi, while at 35 dpi no Med-LN damage was observed [10]. The control animals did not show any lesions during the study. The histopathological analysis of Med-LN revealed the presence in the lymphoid follicles of a mild hypertrophy of germinal centres and the presence of apoptotic bodies at 3 and 7 dpi. At 35 dpi virus-infected groups showed no significant histological lesions.

PRRSV RNA quantification

All PRRSV RNA measurements are shown in Figure 1. All PRRSV infected animals showed a higher PRRSV RNA load at 3 and 7 dpi than at 35 dpi ($p < 0.05$). No viral RNA was detected in control animals (data not shown). The LV group showed at 3 dpi higher viral RNA in the IF area of Med-LN (38 - Ct = 18.89 ± 1.27 SD; $p < 0.05$). At 7 dpi the viral RNA amount was similar between Med-LN compartments (38-Ct = 18.89 ± 1.90 SD; 38 - Ct = 19.09 ± 0.58 SD; F and IF areas respectively). At 35 dpi the LV RNA was significantly reduced in Med-LN

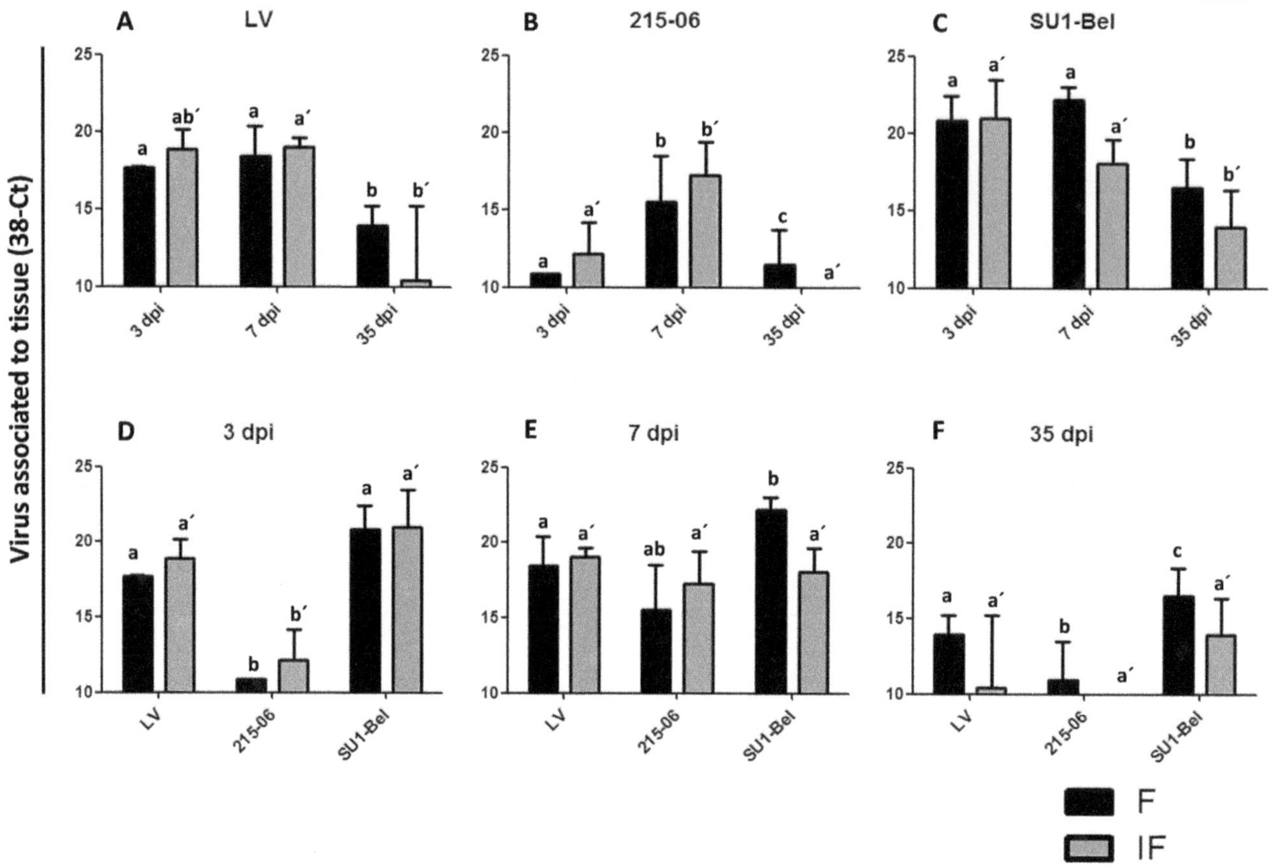

Figure 1 PRRSV viral load in mediastinal lymph node. PRRSV RNA was quantified by RT-qPCR and data represented by changes in the cycle threshold (Ct) in F and IF areas of Med-LN of LV **(A)**, 215–06 **(B)** and SU1-Bel **(C)** infected animals. Differences between distinct PRRSV-1 infected groups are showed for 3 **(D)**, 7 **(E)**, and 35 **(F)** days post-infection. This figure showed the median of each group ± SD. In control animals the viral RNA were not detected (data not shown). Identical superscript letters indicate no significant difference ($p > 0.05$), whereas different superscript letters indicate statistically significant differences ($p < 0.05$) between the same compartment among different groups (a, b, and c for follicle; a´, b´, and c´ for interfollicular area).

compartments (38 - Ct = 13.98 ± 1.23; 38 - Ct = 10.46 ± 4.76; F and IF area respectively; $p < 0.05$) (Figure 1A).

The PRRSV-1 215–06 RNA was detected at 3 dpi mainly in IF area of Med-LN (38 - Ct = 12.16 ± 2.02; $p < 0.05$). At 7 dpi the 215–06 RNA increased to the highest level seen in the study in this group, and was higher in IF area than in F (38 - Ct = 17.27 ± 2.16; 38 – Ct = 15.55 ± 2.96; respectively; $p < 0.05$). Interestingly the 215–06 virus was only detected in F of Med-LN at 35 dpi (38 - Ct = 10.94 ± 2.55; $p < 0.05$) (Figure 1B).

At 3 dpi PRRSV-1 SU1-Bel RNA was mostly detected in IF (38 - Ct = 21.03 ± 2.43; $p < 0.05$), whereas at 7 dpi SU1-Bel RNA was mostly found in F (38 - Ct = 22.20 ± 0.85; $p < 0.05$). At 35 dpi the SU1-Bel RNA decreased but was statistically significant in both Med-LN compartments although predominantly detected in F of Med-LN (38 - Ct = 16.49 ± 1.88; $p < 0.05$) (Figure 1C).

The SU1-Bel group showed the higher load of viral RNA in both Med-LN compartments at each time-point throughout this study (Figures 1D-F; $p < 0.05$). At 3 dpi, PRRSV RNA was mainly detected in IF areas (Figure 1D), where the 215–06 RNA amount was statistically significant lower than in LV and SU1-Bel groups ($p < 0.05$). PRRSV RNA remained higher in IF compartment at 7 dpi for LV and 215–06 groups, but it was higher in F of SU1-Bel-infected pigs ($p < 0.05$; Figure 1E). By 35 dpi, the SU1-Bel RNA in F was statistically significant higher than in LV infected group ($p < 0.05$), and in both groups it was significant higher than in F of Med-LN of 215–06 infected animals ($p < 0.05$; Figure 1F).

Immunohistochemistry (IHC)

CD3 immunolabelling defined the T cell population locations in Med-LN [38,39]. During this study the number of T cells was found to be increased in F of Med-LN at 7 dpi in all infected animals compared with the control animals (2 semi-quantitative immunolabelled cells [s-qic] for LV and 215–06 groups and 3 s-qic for the SU1-Bel group; $p < 0.05$). At 35 dpi this follicular T cell population remained statistically higher in LV infected animals (2 s-qic for LV; $p < 0.05$; Figure 2A). Conversely, the number of T cells decreased in the Med-LN IF from

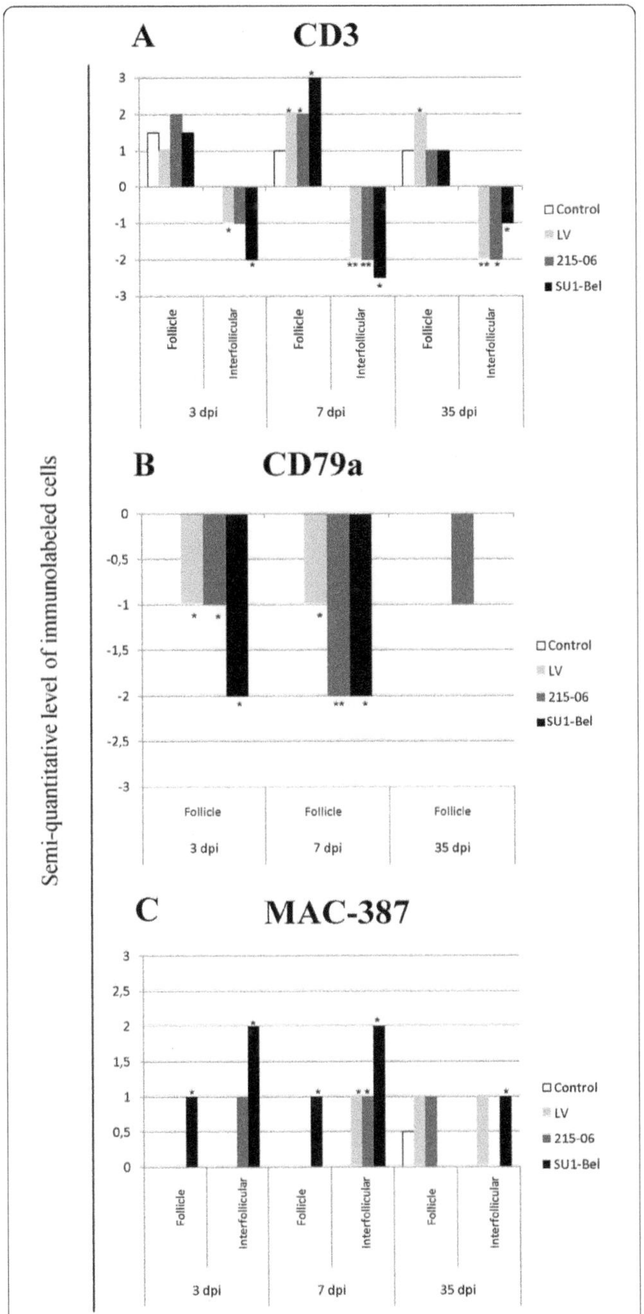

Figure 2 Immunolabelled cell populations in mediastinal lymph node of PRRSV-1 infected pigs. A. CD3 staining for T cells detection; it was observed a general T cell depletion during this study for all PRRSV infected groups, otherwise the T cell immunolabeled cells increased in F at 7 dpi. **B**. CD79a staining for B cell staining in follicle, where was evidence a B cell depletion at 3 and 7 dpi for all PRRSV infected animals. **C**. Macrophage detection with MAC-387 staining, the amount of immunolabeled macrophages increased along this study in SU1-Bel infected pigs. The bars represent s-qic mean values; asterisks indicated the statistically significant differences ($p < 0.05$) against the control group. It is important to note that only a few animals in the control groups showed a higher number of immunolabeled cells in the follicle compared to the rest of animals within this group. For this reason there is a bar in some control groups.

3 dpi in LV (−1 s-qic; $p < 0.05$) and SU1-Bel inoculated animals (−2 s-qic; $p < 0.05$), remaining lower than control animals at 7 and 35 dpi for all infected animals (−2 s-qic for LV and 215–06, and from −2.5 to −1 s-qic for SU1-Bel; $p < 0.05$; Figure 2A).

The immunolabelling of the pan-B cell surface protein CD79a [40,41] showed B cells only in the F of Med-LN. In all infected animals these cells decreased in number compared with control animals at 3 dpi (−1 s-qic for LV and 215–06 and −2 s-qic for SU1-Bel groups; $p < 0.05$) and 7 dpi (−1 s-qic for LVand −2 s-qic for both 215–06 and SU1-Bel groups; $p < 0.05$). At 35 dpi the B cell population did not show a statistically significant change between the infected and control groups (Figure 2B).

Macrophages were identified through MAC-387 imunolabelling of Med-LN sections [21,42]. In the F, macrophage numbers were found to be statistically increased in SU1-Bel infected animals at 3 and 7 dpi (1 s-qic on both days; $p < 0.05$). In the IF areas of SU1-Bel infected animals, the macrophage population was increased at all time-points (from 2 to 1 s-qic; $p < 0.05$). However the animals inoculated with LV and 215–06 PRRSV strains showed a smaller increase in macrophages in the IF area only at 7 dpi (1 s-qic; $p < 0.05$; Figure 2C).

Representative images of CD3, CD79a and MAC387 IHC staining in all the groups are shown in Figure 3.

Cytokine gene expression in Med-LN compartments

To assess immune responses against the selected PRRSV-1 strains within the different Med-LN compartments, IFN-α, TNF-α, IFN-γ, IL-23p19, SOCS1, IL-10 and TGF-β transcript levels were measured by RT-qPCR and compared against control animals (Figure 4). The suitability of the RNA quality was confirmed by testing expression of β-actin in the samples. All cDNA samples produced a positive amplification to each gene by qPCR.

Compared to control animals, in both studied LN compartments the IFN-α was generally downregulated in all infected groups and time-points, which was statistically significant for all PRRSV-1 strains at 7 dpi ($p < 0.05$), when the SU1-Bel group showed the lowest IFN-α transcript levels. The IFN-α remained downregulated at 35 dpi in the Med-LN of 215–06 and Sul-Bel infected pigs ($p < 0.05$; Figure 4A). TNF-α expression was downregulated in IF area of Med-LN of LV infected pigs at 3 dpi ($p < 0.05$) and in Med-LN of 215–06 group at 35 dpi ($p < 0.05$; Figure 4B) compared with the control groups. IFN-γ was significantly upregulated in F of Med-LN of LV ($p < 0.05$) and SU1-Bel infected pigs at 7dpi ($p < 0.05$); on the other hand the IFN-γ was significant downregulated in IF area of Med-LN of 215–06 infected animals at 35 dpi ($p < 0.05$; Figure 4C). At 35 dpi, IL-23p19 was statistically significant upregulated in F of all infected groups ($p < 0.05$; Figure 4D).

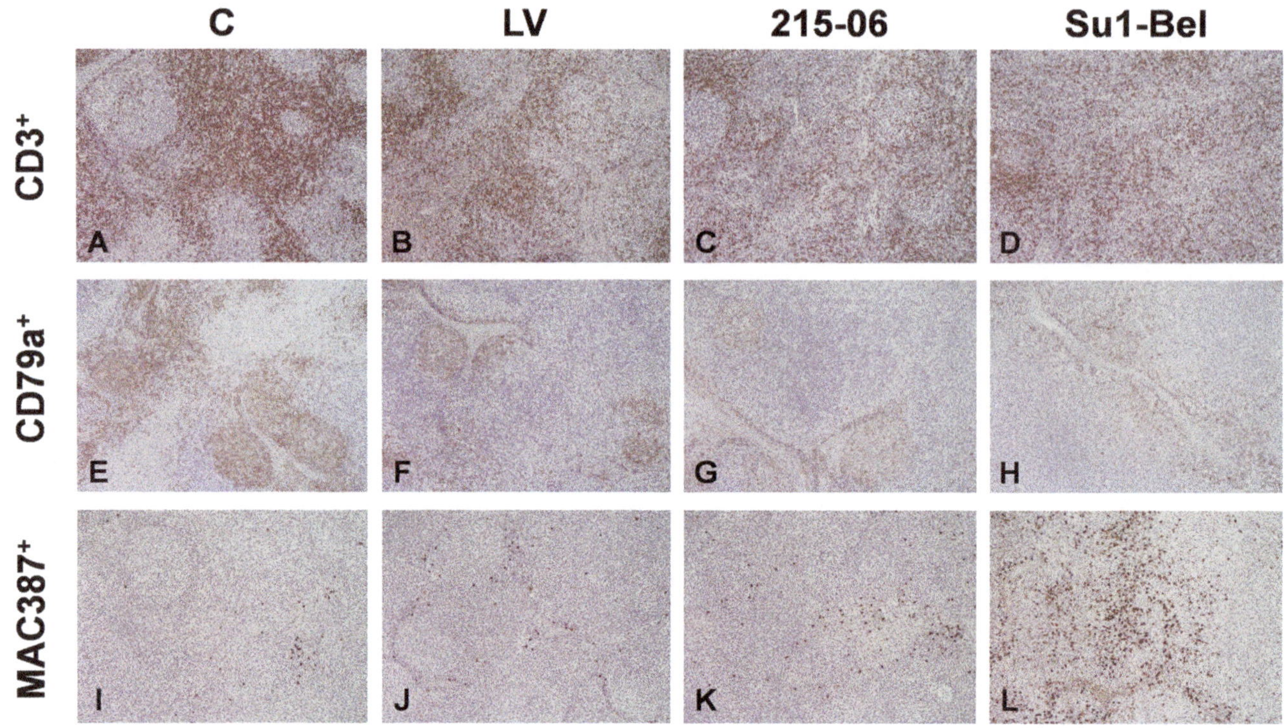

Figure 3 Representative images of CD3, CD79a and MAC387 IHC staining in mediastinal lymph node. CD3 **(A, B, C, D)**, CD79a **(E, F, G, H)** and MAC387 **(I, J, K, L)** in mediastinal lymph nodes of control pigs **(A, E, I)** and infected with LV **(B, F, J)**, 215–06 **(C, G, K)** and SU1-Bel **(D, H, J)** strains, at 7 dpi. An increased in the number of $CD3^+$ cells is observed in the lymphoid follicles from all infected groups together with a depletion of these cells in the interfollicular areas. A decrease in the number of CD79a cells in the follicles is also observed in all the infected groups. A substantial increase in the number of MAC387 is observed in the follicles and interfollicular areas from SU1-Bel infected animals **(L)** together with a mild increase in the LV **(J)** and 215–06 **(K)** groups. Original magnification: 20x.

No significant differences in the expression IL-12 mRNA were detected during the study (data not shown). SOCS1 transcript levels were not statistically significantly regulated for any infected group during the first week of this experiment. However at 35 dpi, SOCS1 transcript levels were increased in the IF area of the Med-LN of animals from the 215–06 group ($p < 0.05$; Figure 4E). At 7 dpi the IL-10 gene expression was significantly downregulated in the F of both 215–06 and SU1-Bel groups ($p < 0.05$) and in the IF area ($p < 0.05$; only 215–06 group). In contrast, IL-10 was significantly upregulated in IF area of Med-LN of the LV infected group ($P < 0.05$; Figure 4F). TGF-β was statistically significantly downregulated at 3 dpi in IF areas of Med-LN of 215–06 and SU1-Bel infected animals ($p < 0.05$), at 7 dpi in Med-LN of SU1-Bel group ($p < 0.05$), and at 35 dpi in IF area of Med-LN of 215–06 infected pigs ($p < 0.05$); contrary, it was statistically upregulated in F of the LV group at 35 dpi ($p < 0.05$; Figure 4G).

The statistically significant correlations between gene expression of immune genes in Med-LN compartments and LV, 215–06 and SU1-Bel PRRSV RNA are respectively represented in the Tables 2, 3 and 4.

Discussion

This study reveals additional data generated from an animal experiment conducted at APHA as part of the EU FP7 PoRRSCon project [10,43]. This study was conceived to directly compare the modulation of immune response transcripts from defined Med-LN compartments of pigs experimentally infected with PRRSV-1 strains of varying virulence.

Pigs infected with the SU1-Bel PRRSV strain have shown greater Med-LN gross pathology compared with the pan-European subtype 1 strains LV and 215–06 [10]. In the present study the highest PRRSV RNA levels were detected in the IF area of Med-LN, which suggest that PRRSV was entering from the apical and medial lung lobes [32] to the Med-LN via draining lymphatics vessels. We have previously shown that for all PRRSV infected groups, the virus load in serum showed a peak at 7 dpi decreasing until 28 dpi, whereas in bronchoalveolar lavage fluid (BALF) the virus persisted until 35 dpi [10]. Interestingly, despite its enhanced virulence the levels of virus in both circulation and BALF were lowest in SU1-Bel infected animals. In contrast, in the present analysis we have detected the higher levels for SU1-Bel in

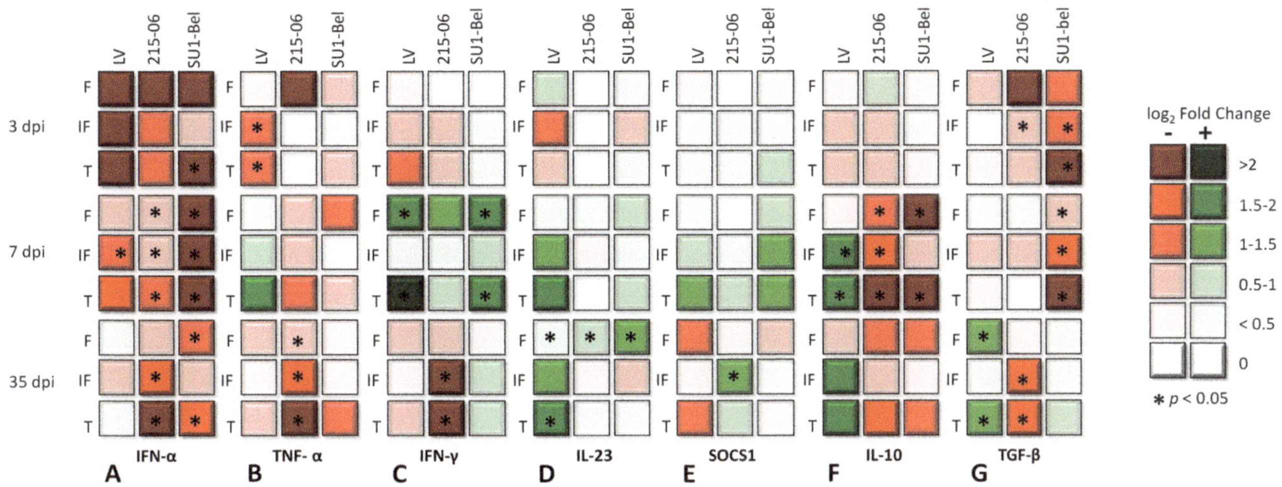

Figure 4 Cytokine gene expression in mediastinal lymph node compartments. Log 2 Fold change in transcript level of IFN-α **(A)**, TNF-α **(B)**, IFN-γ **(C)**, IL-23p19 **(D)**, SOCS1 **(E)**, IL-10 **(F)** and TGF-β **(G)** gene expression relative to the control gene β-Actin; which was calculated by $2^{-\Delta\Delta Ct}$ method. Log_2 fold change of gene expression in follicle **(F)**, interfollicular area (IF) or total Med-LN lymph node (T) values are depicted. Green boxes indicate upregulation and red boxes indicate downregulation as the key showed. The statistically significant differences ($p < 0.05$) with control group are indicated by asterisks on the boxes.

Table 2 Correlations between LV RNA and the gene expression of TNF-α, IFN-α, IFN-γ, SOCS1, IL-23p19, IL-10 and TGF-β

		IFN-α	IFN-γ	IL-23	SOCS1	IL-10	TGF-β	ORF7 PRRSV
TNF-α	F	0.857**	0.094	−0.102	0.064	0.160	0.964**	−0.077
	IF	0.184	0.469	0.643*	0.471	0.687**	0.479	−0.190
	T	0.750**	0.248	0.031	0.091	0.305	0.921**	−0.043
IFN-α	F		−0.255	−0.351	0.009	−0.201	0.901**	−0.110
	IF		0.307	0.276	−0.086	0.094	0.619*	−0.663**
	T		−0.142	−0.156	−0.132	0.167	0.880**	−0.301
IFN-γ	F			0.342	0.607*	0.131	−0.082	0.413
	IF			0.220	0.680**	0.100	0.282	0.144
	T			0.167	0.649**	0.222	0.008	0.438
IL-23	F				0.239	0.112	−0.179	−0.208
	IF				0.109	0.553*	0.183	−0.231
	T				−0.004	0.395	−0.106	−0.154
SOCS1	F					0.809	−0.063	0.527*
	IF					0.310	−0.016	0.303
	T					0.211	−0.139	0.486
IL-10	F						−0308	0.397
	IF						0.116	−0.332
	T						0.144	−0.151
TGF-β	F							−0.206
	IF							−0.557*
	T							−0.245

*$p < 0.05$; **$p < 0.01$. F (follicle of Med-LN), IF (interfollicular area of Med-LN) and T (Total cortical compartments of Med-LN).

Table 3 Correlations between 215–06 RNA and the gene expression of TNF-α, IFN-α, IFN-γ, SOCS1, IL-23p19, IL-10 and TGF-β

		IFN-α	IFN-γ	IL-23	SOCS1	IL-10	TGF-β	ORF7 PRRSV
TNF-α	F	0.66	−0.015	0.679*	0.462	−0.169	0.919**	0.099
	IF	−0.149	0.490*	0.239	0.081	0.204	0.438	0.133
	T	−0.010	0.349	0.380	0.123	0.254	0.386	−0.024
IFN-α	F		−0.316	−0.482	−0.445	−0.666*	0.073	0.129
	IF		0.145	0.091	−0.399	−0.137	0.188	0.252
	T		−0.077	0.070	−0371	−0.476*	0.378	0.205
IFN-γ	F			0.016	0.193	0.257	0.067	0.612*
	IF			0.002	−0.385	−0.123	0.808**	0.661**
	T			−0.068	0.133	0.178	0.436	0.524*
IL-23	F				0.233	0.266	0.526	−0.208
	IF				0.135	0.324	−0.225	0.017
	T				0.395	0.403	0.070	−0.022
SOCS1	F					0.362	0.420	−0.013
	IF					0.374	−0.267	−0.221
	T					0.560*	0.206	−0.201
IL-10	F						−0.173	−0.114
	IF						−0.261	−0.334
	T						0.124	−0.341
TGF-β	F							0.235
	IF							0.582*
	T							0.276

*$p < 0.05$; **$p < 0.01$. F (follicle of Med-LN), IF (interfollicular area of Med-LN) and T (Total cortical compartments of Med-LN).

Med-LN compared with the subtype 1 strains, which suggest that this PRRSV-1 subtype 3 strainmay infect LN resident/transient cell populations more efficiently and this could be linked to the higher pathogenicity of this strain. In support of this data, the PRRSV N protein has been detected by IHC mainly in the cytoplasm of macrophages of the Med-LN of infected pigs from on 3, 7 and 35 dpi, with highest levels of immunolabelled cells found in SU1-Bel infected animals [43].

The use of LMD in the present study, enabled for the first time the measurement of PRRSV-1 RNA within different Med-LN compartments. The results showed the presence of PRRSV in the F of the Med-LN at 35 dpi albeit at low levels, according with a previous report that described the detection of infectious PRRSV in lymphoid tissues for several months [39]. We hypothesize that PRRSV may interact with fDC in secondary lymph organs, such as the Med-LN, and this could impair fDC presentation of PRRSV antigens to B cells, which could contribute to the lack of production of neutralizing antibodies detected in this [10] and other PRRSV infection studies. PRRSV presence in follicles of Med-LN and the non-neutralizing Ab secretion at 35 dpi suggest a role of fDC in the immunopathogenesis of PRRSV.

The B and T cell depletion observed in F and IF areas of Med-LN during this study are in accordance with previous reports that showed B and T cell depletion in cortical areas of secondary lymph organs such as the thymus [44] and lymph nodes [45] of PRRSV infected pigs. The immune cell depletion in lymphoid tissues has recently been associated to apoptotic cell death indirectly induced in bystander cells by PRRSV infected cells [46]. We showed a T cell increase in the F, mostly at 7 dpi, that could be related to the migration of $CD4^+$ helper T cells to the F area to assist the induction of B cell responses. During this study the macrophage population increased in the Med-LN, especially for the SU1-Bel group, which indicates that the SU1-Bel strain induces a higher inflammatory response in the lung than the other PRRSV-1 strains tested, in accordance with previous reports [9,11].

Production of type I IFNs (IFN-α/β) is critical to activation of the innate immune response against viral infection, as well as regulation of the induction of the adaptive immune response [47,48]. We detected either no changes or lower IFN-α transcript levels for all PRRSV inoculated groups, most noticeably at 7 dpi, which likely plays a role in delaying the onset of an effective innate immune

Table 4 Correlations between SU1-Bel RNA and the gene expression of TNF-α, IFN-α, IFN-γ, SOCS1, IL-23p19, IL-10 and TGF-β

		IFN-α	IFN-γ	IL-23	SOCS1	IL-10	TGF-β	ORF7 PRRSV
TNF-α	F	−0.047	−0.146	0.651**	−0.254	0.292	0.471	−0.683**
	IF	−0.419	−0.188	0.107	−0.211	−0.404	0.167	−0.240
	T	−0.138	−0.165	0.436	−0.164	−0.181	0.266	−0.549*
IFN-α	F		−0.401	0.060	−0.449	0.165	0.649**	−.273
	IF		−0.186	−0.557*	−0.258	0.339	0.193	−0.044
	T		−0.402	−0.250	−0.629*	0.373	0.433	−0.265
IFN-γ	F			−0.040	0.432	−0.327	−0.229	0.353
	IF			0.298	0.300	−0.347	−0.079	0.082
	T			0.147	0.476	−0.169	−0.267	−0.74
IL-23	F				−0.037	0.004	0.455	−0.416
	IF				0.594*	−0.318	−0.216	−0.124
	T				0.496*	−0.178	−0.573*	−0.530*
SOCS1	F					−0.406	−0.481	0.515*
	IF					0.002	−0.341	−0.245
	T					−0.121	−0.181	−0.089
IL-10	F						0.088	−0.384
	IF						−0.283	−0.108
	T						−0.246	−0.093
TGF-β	F							−0.541*
	IF							0.052
	T							−0.263

*$p < 0.05$; **$p < 0.01$. F (follicle of Med-LN), IF (interfollicular area of Med-LN) and T (Total cortical compartments of Med-LN).

response [14,49]. We showed that PRRSV can reduce the transcription of TNF-α which would also impair innate immune response and to delay the adaptive immune responses [50,51]. Interestingly, the IFN-α and TNF-α gene expression were positively correlated in LV infected pigs, both LV and SU1-Bel RNA levels were negatively correlated with the IFN-α gene expression, and SU1-Bel RNA levels were negatively correlated with the TNF-α gene expression. These results suggest that PRRSV downregulates these cytokine gene inductions at the site of infection, in agreement with previous studies [52]. These results also support the hypothesis that PRRSV-1 subtype 3 strains have developed the most efficient strategies to avoid the host immune responses among the PRRSV-1 genotype viruses. The upregulation of IFN-γ expression at 7 dpi is evidence of a delayed adaptive immune response in all PRRSV inoculated groups, as it has been previously described [53,54]. During this study a positive correlation between IFN-γ gene expression and PRRSV LV and 215–06 strains suggests that PRRSV-1 subtype 1 induction of IFN-γ expression depends directly on the presence of virus. It has been described that SOCS proteins are a pivotal regulator in both innate and adaptive immune responses [55]. Specifically SOCS1 acts as a negative regulator of IFN-γ signaling, inhibiting the activation of STAT1 and thereby the expression of IFN-γ mediated genes [56]. SOCS1 induction in PRRSV vaccinated/infected pigs has been described [57,58], which suggests SOCS1 expression in infected cells may be a mechanism to evade the host immune response. Nevertheless, the positively correlation of SOCS1 and IFN-γ gene expression in the LV group could be a result of its negative feedback control system. Additional in vitro experiments may be used to elucidate the proposed SOCS1 induction by PRRSV during the initial phase of virus infection.

The IL-23 protein is an IL-12p40-IL-23p19 heterodimer that is secreted by antigen presenting cells such as macrophages and DCs. This cytokine is necessary for the differentiation and survival of Th17 cells, which can induce a pro-inflammatory reaction and the secretion of TGF-β [59]. In this study we did not detect IL-12p40 transcripts; this could be explained by the transcription kinetics of this cytokine being earlier or later compared with the tissue sample collection points. The IL-23p19 is a limiting factor to produce a biologically active IL-23 protein, as IL-23p19 is not secreted in the absence of the IL-12p40 chain [60] and the IL-23p19 induction is typically lower than that of IL-12p40 [61]. In the present study, IL-23p19 was upregulated from 7 dpi, and this was statistically significant at 35 dpi in the F for all PRRSV groups, which suggest that PRRSV may modulate the cytokine environment to drive the differentiation of Th17 as opposed to antiviral Th1 cells.

The IL-10 transcription levels showed considerable variation between PRRSV strains as previously described [62]. Therefore, this study supports the idea that the induction of IL-10 as a mechanism to delay the host immune response is not a common strategy among the PRRSV-1 genotype. The TGF-β gene expression was either unaffected or downregulated in agreement with previous findings [63], and this may explain why a positive correlation between TGF-β and other cytokines were detected in this study.

The standard techniques used to take samples for mRNA extraction cannot select different tissue structures in the way that LMC can. We therefore conclude that LMC in combination with RT-qPCR is a powerful tool to enable the differentiation of transcriptomic profiles between different Med-LN compartments of PRRSV-1 infected pigs. In this study we show several examples that demonstrate how the immunopathogenesis of PRRSV-1 infection is associated with the site of infection; for instance, PRRSV-1 SU1-Bel showed a higher tissue pathogenesis and virulence compared with PRRSV-1 subtype 1 strains. We have also provide further evidence that PRRSV-1 strains avoid the innate immune response in infected pigs through the downregulation of IFN-α and TNF-α in F and IF areas of Med-LN, and inducing a T and B cell depletion in the cortex of Med-LN.

Competing interests

The authors declare that they have no competing interests.

Authors' contributions

SPG, FS, FJS, JPF and TWD conceived the animal experiment and participated in the design and coordination, and helped drafting the manuscript. Experimental work performed by OGN, RSR, DR, FJP and FJS. TSS and SBM participated in the samples collection and processing for histopathology. All authors contributed to the manuscript preparation, revision and provided important intellectual input. All authors read and approved the final manuscript.

Acknowledgements

The authors would like to thank Tomasz Stadejek for provision of material for the isolation of the SU1-Bel strain and Anna Marie Rebel and Eefke Wessendorp for the provision of the Lelystadvirus. This work was supported by the PoRRSCon and NADIR Projects of the European Union Seventh Framework Programme (Grant Agreements #245141 and #228394 respectively), DEFRA project SE0529, EU COST action FA0902 and the British Pig Executive (BPEX). O. García-Nicolás was founded by grant BES-2010-032408 of the Ministry of Economy and Competitiveness, in part by the project AGL2009-12438 from the Government of Spain. F.J. Pallarés was supported by a grant from "Fundación Séneca", Spain. D. Risco has a "Formación de Profesorado Universitario" (FPU) grant from the Ministry of Education (AP2009-0704) from the Government of Spain.

Author details

[1]Department of Anatomy and Comparative Pathology, Faculty of Veterinary Medicine, Murcia University, "Mare Nostrum Excellence Campus – 3738", 30100 Murcia, Spain. [2]Department of Bacteriology, Animal and Plant Health Agency, Addlestone, Surrey KT15 3NB, UK. [3]Red de Grupos de Investigación Recursos Faunísticos, Facultad de Veterinaria, Universidad de Extremadura, 10003 Cáceres, Spain. [4]Spanish National Center of Biotechnology (CSIC), C/Darwin 3, Campus de Cantoblanco, 28049 Madrid, Spain. [5]Department of Virology, Animal and Plant Health Agency, Addlestone, Surrey KT15 3NB, UK. [6]Department of Pathology, Animal and Plant Health Agency, Addlestone KT15 3NB, UK. [7]Department of Pathology and Infectious Diseases, School of Veterinary Medicine, University of Surrey, Guildford GU2 7TE, UK.

References

1. Hopper SA, White ME, Twiddy N (1992) An outbreak of blue-eared pig disease porcine reproductive and respiratory syndrome in four pig herds in Great Britain. Vet Rec 131:140–144
2. Done SH, Paton DJ (1995) Porcine reproductive and respiratory syndrome: clinical disease, pathology and immunosuppression. Vet Rec 136:32–35
3. Rossow KD (1998) Porcine reproductive and respiratory syndrome. Vet Pathol 35:1–20
4. Zimmerman JJ, Benfield DA, Murtaugh MP, Osorio F, Stenvenson GW, Torremorell M (2006) Porcine reproductive and respiratory syndrome virus (porcine arterivirus). InStraw BE, Zimmerman JJ, D'Allaire S, Taylor DJ (eds) Ames, Iowa5. Holtkamp DJ, Kliebenstein JB, Neumann EJ, Zimmerman JJ, Rotto HF, Yoder TK, Wang C, Yeske PE, Mowrer CL, Haley CA (2013) Assessment of the economic impact of porcine reproductive and respiratory syndrome virus on United States pork producers. J Swine Health Prod 21:72–84
5. Holtkamp DJ, Kliebenstein JB, Neumann EJ, Zimmerman JJ, Rotto HF, Yoder TK, Wang C, Yeske PE, Mowrer CL, Haley CA (2013) Assessment of the economic impact of porcine reproductive and respiratory syndrome virus on United States pork producers. J Swine Health Prod 21:72–84
6. Nelsen CJ, Murtaugh MP, Faaberg KS (1999) Porcine reproductive and respiratory syndrome virus comparison: divergent evolution on two continents. J Virol 73:270–280
7. Stadejek T, Oleksiewicz MB, Scherbakov AV, Timina AM, Krabbe JS, Chabros K, Potapchuk D (2008) Definition of subtypes in the European genotype of porcine reproductive and respiratory syndrome virus: nucleocapsid characteristics and geographical distribution in Europe. Arch Virol 153:1479–1488
8. Stadejek T, Stankevicius A, Murtaugh MP, Oleksiewicz MB (2013) Molecular evolution of PRRSV in Europe: current state of play. Vet Microbiol 165:21–28
9. Karniychuk UU, Geldhof M, Vanhee M, Van Doorsselaere J, Saveleva TA, Nauwynck HJ (2010) Pathogenesis and antigenic characterization of a new East European subtype 3 porcine reproductive and respiratory syndrome virus isolate. BMC Vet Res 6:30
10. Morgan SB, Graham SP, Salguero FJ, Sánchez-Cordón PJ, Mokhtar H, Rebel JM, Weesendorp E, Bodman-Smith KB, Steinbach F, Frossard JP (2013) Increased pathogenicity of European porcine reproductive and respiratory syndrome virus is associated with enhanced adaptive responses and viral clearance. Vet Microbiol 163:13–22
11. Weesendorp E, Morgan S, Stockhofe-Zurwieden N, Popma-De Graaf DJ, Graham SP, Rebel JM (2013) Comparative analysis of immune responses following experimental infection of pigs with European porcine reproductive and respiratory syndrome virus strains of differing virulence. Vet Microbiol 163:1–12
12. Lee YJ, Park CK, Nam E, Kim SH, Lee OS, du Lee S, Lee C (2009) Generation of a porcine alveolar macrophage cell line for the growth of porcine reproductive and respiratory syndrome virus. J Virol Methods 163:410–415
13. Van Gorp H, Van Breedam W, Delputte PL, Nauwynck HJ (2008) Sialoadhesin and CD163 join forces during entry of the porcine reproductive and respiratory syndrome virus. J Gen Virol 89:2943–2953
14. Albina E, Carrat C, Charley B (1998) Interferon-alpha response to swine arterivirus (PoAV), the porcine reproductive and respiratory syndrome virus. J Interferon Cytokine Res 18:485–490

15. Meier WA, Galeota J, Osorio FA, Husmann RJ, Schnitzlein WM, Zuckermann FA (2003) Gradual development of the interferon-gamma response of swine to porcine reproductive and respiratory syndrome virus infection or vaccination. Virology 309:18–31
16. Mateu E, Diaz I (2008) The challenge of PRRS immunology. Vet J 177:345–351
17. Lopez OJ, Osorio FA (2004) Role of neutralizing antibodies in PRRSV protective immunity. Vet Immunol Immunopathol 102:155–163
18. Xiao Z, Batista L, Dee S, Halbur P, Murtaugh MP (2004) The level of virus-specific T-cell and macrophage recruitment in porcine reproductive and respiratory syndrome virus infection in pigs is independent of virus load. J Virol 78:5923–5933
19. Barranco I, Gómez-Laguna J, Rodríguez-Gómez IM, Quereda JJ, Salguero FJ, Pallarés FJ, Carrasco L (2012) Immunohistochemical expression of IL-12, IL-10, IFN-α and IFN-γ in lymphoid organs of porcine reproductive and respiratory syndrome virus-infected pigs. Vet Immunol Immunopathol 149:262–271
20. Gómez-Laguna J, Salguero FJ, Barranco I, Pallarés FJ, Rodríguez-Gómez IM, Bernabé A, Carrasco L (2010) Cytokine expression by macrophages in the lung of pigs infected with the porcine reproductive and respiratory syndrome virus. J Comp Pathol 142:51–60
21. Binns RM, Pabst, (1994) Lymphoid tissue structure and lymphocyte trafficking in the pig. Vet Immunol Immunopathol 43:79–87
22. Rezk SA, Nathwani BN, Zhao X, Weiss LM (2013) Follicular dendritic cells: origin, function, and different disease-associated patterns. Hum Pathol 44:937–950
23. Lin CM, Jeng CR, Hsiao SH, Liu JP, Chang CC, Chiou MT, Tsai YC, Chia MY, Pang VF (2011) Immunopathological characterization of porcine circovirus type 2 infection-associated follicular changes in inguinal lymph nodes using high-throughput tissue microarray. Vet Microbiol 149:72–84
24. Mendrick DL (2011) Transcriptional profiling to identify biomarkers of disease and drug response. Pharmacogenomics 12:235–249
25. Lunney JK, Fritz ER, Reecy JM, Kuhar D, Prucnal E, Molina R, Christopher-Hennings J, Zimmerman J, Rowland RR (2010) Interleukin-8, interleukin-1beta, and interferon-gamma levels are linked to PRRS virus clearance. Viral Immunol 23:127–134
26. Miller LC, Fleming D, Arbogast A, Bayles DO, Guo B, Lager KM, Henningson JN, Schlink SN, Yang HC, Faaberg KS, Kehrli ME, Jr (2012) Analysis of the swine tracheobronchial lymphnode transcriptomic response to infection with a Chinese highly pathogenic strain of porcine reproductive and respiratory syndrome virus. BMC Vet Res 8:208
27. Wysocki M, Chen H, Steibel JP, Kuhar D, Petry D, Bates J, Johnson R, Ernst CW, Lunney JK (2012) Identifying putative candidate genes and pathways involved in immune responses to porcine reproductive and respiratory syndrome virus (PRRSV) infection. Anim Genet 43:328–332
28. García-Nicolás O, Quereda JJ, Gómez-Laguna J, Salguero FJ, Carrasco L, Ramis G, Pallarés FJ (2014) Cytokines transcript levels in lung and lymphoid organs during genotype 1 Porcine Reproductive and Respiratory Syndrome Virus (PRRSV) infection. Vet Immunol Immunopathol 160:26–40
29. Okuducu AF, Hahne JC, Von Deimling A, Wernert N (2005) Laser-assisted microdissection, techniques and applications in pathology (review). Int J Mol Med 15:763–769
30. Aranday-Cortes E, Bull NC, Villarreal-Ramos B, Gough J, Hicks D, Ortiz-Peláez A, Vordermeier HM, Salguero FJ (2013) Upregulation of IL-17A, CXCL9 and CXCL10 in early-stage granulomas induced by Mycobacterium bovis in cattle. Transbound Emerg Dis 60:525–537
31. Cheng L, Zhang S, MacLennan GT, Williamson SR, Davidson DD, Wang M, Jones TD, Lopez-Beltran A, Montironi R (2013) Laser-assisted microdissection in translational research: theory, technical considerations, and future applications. Appl Immunohistochem Mol Morphol 21:31–47
32. Halbur PG, Paul PS, Frey ML, Landgraf J, Eernisse K, Meng XJ, Andrews JJ, Lum MA, Rathje JA (1996) Comparison of the antigen distribution of two US porcine reproductive and respiratory syndrome virus isolates with that of the Lelystad virus. Vet Pathol 33:159–170
33. Irving JA, Cain G, Parr A, Howard M, Angus B, Cattan AR (1996) OCT embedded sections of pathological specimens as a source of high quality RNA for reverse transcriptase/polymerase chain reaction. J Clin Pathol 49:258–259
34. Barranco I, Gómez-Laguna J, Rodríguez-Gómez IM, Salguero FJ, Pallarés FJ, Bernabé A, Carrasco L (2011) Immunohistochemical detection of extrinsic and intrinsic mediators of apoptosis in porcine paraffin-embedded tissues. Vet Immunol Immunopathol 139:210–216
35. Frossard JP, Fearnley C, Naidu B, Errington J, Westcott DG, Drew TW (2012) Porcine reproductive and respiratory syndrome virus: antigenic and molecular diversity of British isolates and implications for diagnosis. Vet Microbiol 158:308–315
36. Livak KJ, Schmittgen TD (2001) Analysis of relative gene expression data using real-time quantitative PCR and the 2(–Delta DeltaC(T)). Methods 25:402–408
37. Delgado-Ortega M, Melo S, Meurens F (2011) Expression of SOCS1-7 and CIS mRNA in porcine tissues. Vet Immunol Immunopathol 144:493–498
38. Jones M, Cordell JL, Beyers AD, Tse AG, Mason DY (1993) Detection of T and B cells in many animal species using cross-reactive anti-peptide antibodies. J Immunol 150:5429–5435
39. Batista L, Pijoan C, Dee S, Olin M, Molitor T, Joo HJ, Xiao Z, Murtaugh M (2004) Virological and immunological responses to porcine reproductive and respiratory syndrome virus in a large population of gilts. Can J Vet Res 68:267–273
40. Mason DY, Cordell JL, Brown MH, Borst J, Jones M, Pulford K, Jaffe E, Ralfkiaer E, Dallenbach F, Stein H, Pileri S, Gatter KC (1995) CD79a: a novel marker for B-cell neoplasms in routinely processed tissue samples. Blood 86:1453–1459
41. Marquet F, Bonneau M, Pascale F, Urien C, Kang C, Schwartz-Cornil I, Bertho N (2011) Characterization of dendritic cells subpopulations in skin and afferent lymph in the swine model. PLoS One 6:e16320
42. Soulas C, Conerly C, Kim WK, Burdo TH, Alvarez X, Lackner AA, Williams KC (2011) Recently infiltrating MAC387(+) monocytes/macrophages a third macrophage population involved in SIV and HIV encephalitic lesion formation. Am J Pathol 178:2121–2135
43. Morgan SB, Frossard JP, Pallares FJ, Gough J, Stadejek T, Graham SP, Steinbach F, Drew TW, Salguero FJ Pathology and virus distribution in the lung and lymphoid tissues of pigs experimentally inoculated with three distinct Type 1 PRRS virus isolates of varying pathogenicity. Transbound Emerg Dis, in press
44. He Y, Wang G, Liu Y, Shi W, Han Z, Wu J, Jiang C, Wang S, Hu S, Wen H, Dong J, Liu H, Cai X (2012) Characterization of thymus atrophy in piglets infected with highly pathogenic porcine reproductive and respiratory syndrome virus. Vet Microbiol 160:455–462
45. Gómez-Laguna J, Salguero FJ, Fernández de Marco M, Barranco I, Rodríguez-Gómez IM, Quezada M, Carrasco L (2013) Type 2 Porcine Reproductive and Respiratory Syndrome Virus infection mediated apoptosis in B- and T-cell areas in lymphoid organs of experimentally infected pigs. Transbound Emerg Dis 60:273–278
46. Rodríguez-Gómez IM, Barranco I, Amarilla SP, García-Nicolás O, Salguero FJ, Carrasco L, Gómez-Laguna J (2014) Activation of extrinsic- and Daxx-mediated pathways in lymphoid tissue of PRRSV-infected pigs. Vet Microbiol 172:186–194
47. Overend C, Mitchell R, He D, Rompato G, Grubman MJ, Garmendia AE (2007) Recombinant swine beta interferon protects swine alveolar macrophages and MARC-145 cells from infection with Porcine reproductive and respiratory syndrome virus. J Gen Virol 88:925–931
48. Sadler AJ, Williams BR (2008) Interferon-inducible antiviral effectors. Nat Rev Immunol 8:559–568
49. Labarque GG, Nauwynck HJ, Van Reeth K, Pensaert MB (2000) Effect of cellular changes and onset of humoral immunity on the replication of porcine reproductive and respiratory syndrome virus in the lungs of pigs. J Gen Virol 81:1327–1334
50. Labarque G, Van Gucht S, Nauwynck H, Van Reeth K, Pensaert M (2003) Apoptosis in the lungs of pigs infected with porcine reproductive and respiratory syndrome virus and associations with the production of apoptogenic cytokines. Vet Res 34:249–260
51. Subramaniam S, Kwon B, Beura LK, Kuszynski CA, Pattnaik AK, Osorio FA (2010) Porcine reproductive and respiratory syndrome virus non-structural protein 1 suppresses tumor necrosis factor-alpha promoter activation by inhibiting NF-κB and Sp1. Virology 406:270–279
52. Murtaugh MP, Xiao Z, Zuckermann F (2002) Immunological responses of swine to porcine reproductive and respiratory syndrome virus infection. Viral Immunol 15:533–547
53. Zuckermann FA, Garcia EA, Luque ID, Christopher-Hennings J, Doster A, Brito M, Osorio F (2007) Assessment of the efficacy of commercial porcine reproductive and respiratory syndrome virus (PRRSV) vaccines based on measurement of serologic response, frequency of gamma-IFN-producing cells and virological parameters of protection upon challenge. Vet Microbiol 123:69–85
54. Jung K, Renukaradhya GJ, Alekseev KP, Fang Y, Tang Y, Saif LJ (2009) Porcine reproductive and respiratory syndrome virus modifies innate immunity and alters disease outcome in pigs subsequently infected with porcine respiratory coronavirus: implications for respiratory viral co-infections. J Gen Virol 90:2713–2723

55. Dalpke A, Heeg K, Bartz H, Baetz A (2008) Regulation of innate immunity by suppressor of cytokine signaling (SOCS) proteins. Immunobiology 213:225–235
56. Alexander WS (2002) Suppressors of Cytokine Signalling (SOCS) in the immune system. Nat Rev Immunol 2:410–416
57. Royaee AR, Husmann RJ, Dawson HD, Calzada-Nova G, Schnitzlein WM, Zuckermann FA, Lunney JK (2004) Deciphering the involvement of innate immune factors in the development of the host response to PRRSV vaccination. Vet Immunol Immunopathol 102:199–216
58. Zhou P, Zhai S, Zhou X, Lin P, Jiang T, Hu X, Jiang Y, Wu B, Zhang Q, Xu X, Li JP, Liu B (2007) Molecular characterization of transcriptome-wide interactions between highly pathogenic porcine reproductive and respiratory syndrome virus and porcine alveolar macrophages in vivo. Int J Biol Sci 7:947–959
59. Vignali DA, Kuchroo VK (2012) IL-12 family cytokines: immunological playmakers. Nat Immunol 13:722–728
60. Cooper AM, Khader SA (2007) IL-12p40: an inherently agonistic cytokine. Trends Immunol 28:33–38
61. Shimizu J, Kaneko F, Suzuki N (2013) Skewed helper T-Cell responses to IL-12 ramily cytokines produced by antigen-presenting cells and the genetic background in Behcet's Disease. Genet Res Int 2013:363859
62. Gimeno M, Darwich L, Diaz I, de la Torre E, Pujols J, Martin M, Inumaru S, Cano E, Domingo M, Montoya M, Mateu E (2011) Cytokine profiles and phenotype regulation of antigen presenting cells by genotype-I porcine reproductive and respiratory syndrome virus isolates. Vet Res 42:9
63. Silva-Campa E, Córdoba L, Fraile L, Flores-Mendoza L, Montoya M, Hernández J (2009) European genotype of porcine reproductive and respiratory síndrome (PRRSV) infects monocyte-derived dendritic cells but not induce Treg cells. Virology 396:264–271

Eimeria bovis-triggered neutrophil extracellular trap formation is CD11b-, ERK 1/2-, p38 MAP kinase- and SOCE-dependent

Tamara Muñoz-Caro[1*], Sandra Jaqueline Mena Huertas[2,3], Ivan Conejeros[2], Pablo Alarcón[2], María A Hidalgo[2], Rafael A Burgos[2], Carlos Hermosilla[1] and Anja Taubert[1]

Abstract

Eimeria bovis is an important coccidian parasite that causes high economic losses in the cattle industry. We recently showed that polymorphonuclear neutrophils (PMN) react upon *E. bovis* sporozoite exposure by neutrophil extracellular trap (NET) formation. We focused here on the molecular mechanisms that are involved in this process. The sporozoite encounter led to an enhanced surface expression of neutrophil CD11b suggesting a potential role of this receptor in *E. bovis*-mediated NETosis. Antibody-mediated blockage of CD11b confirmed this assumption and led to a significantly decreased sporozoite-triggered NET. In addition, *E. bovis*-induced NETosis was found to be Ca^{2+}-dependent since the inhibition of store-operated calcium entry (SOCE) significantly diminished NET. Furthermore, NADPH oxidase, neutrophil elastase (NE) and myeloperoxidase (MPO) were confirmed as key molecules in sporozoite-triggered NETosis, as inhibition thereof blocked parasite-triggered NET. PMN degranulation analyses revealed a significant release of matrix metalloprotease-9 containing granules upon sporozoite exposure. We further show a significantly enhanced phosphorylation of ERK1/2 and p38 MAPK in sporozoite-exposed PMN indicating a key role of this signaling pathway in *E. bovis*-mediated NETosis. Accordingly, ERK 1/2 and p38 MAPK inhibition led to a significant decrease in NET formation. Finally, we demonstrate that sporozoite-induced NETosis is neither a stage-, species-, nor host-specific process.

Introduction

Eimeria bovis is an important intracellular apicomplexan parasite of cattle, causing severe haemorrhagic diarrhoea (typhlocolitis) especially in calves leading to high economic losses worldwide [1]. Polymorphonuclear neutrophils (PMN) appear to play a pivotal role in *E. bovis* defense. This leukocyte population was identified in parasitized intestine of *E. bovis*-infected calves [2] and PMN have been shown to interact directly with *E. bovis* stages and antigen, resulting in direct elimination or production of pro-inflammatory cytokines, chemokines and iNOS upon encounter [3]. Additionally, PMN were shown to adhere to *E. bovis*-infected host endothelial cells [4] and their phagocytic and oxidative burst activities were enhanced in response to *E. bovis* sporozoites in vitro or ex vivo during infection [3]. Furthermore, we recently identified sporozoites of *E. bovis* as potent inducers of neutrophil extracellular traps (NET) [5]. Overall, NET formation has been described as a novel form of cell death called ETosis which is distinct from apoptosis, autophagy and necrosis leading to extracellular entrapment and eventually the killing of pathogens [6,7]. NET have been shown to be involved in several infections caused by bacteria, viruses and fungi [8-11]. However, little attention has been paid to the role of NET in the early host innate immune response against protozoan parasites [12,13]. By now, NET formation has been described to be induced by some protozoan parasites, such as *Leishmania* spp. [14], *E. bovis, Toxoplasma gondii, Plasmodium falciparum, E. arloingi*, and *Besnoitia besnoiti* [5,12,15-17].

NETosis is an NADPH oxidase-mediated ROS-dependent mechanism [7-11] which causes the expulsion of a mixture of nuclear and cytoplasmic granule contents leading to the formation of fiber-like structures being decorated with

* Correspondence: Tamara.Munoz-Caro@vetmed.uni-giessen.de
[1]Institute of Parasitology, Justus Liebig University Giessen, Schubertstraße 81, 35392 Giessen, Germany
Full list of author information is available at the end of the article

histones and granular molecules, such as neutrophil elastase (NE) and myeloperoxidase (MPO) amongst others [7,10,11]. On the mechanistic level, parasites are immobilized within these DNA-rich structures and may be killed via high local concentrations of antimicrobial molecules [12,13]. Consequently, some cases of parasite-triggered NETosis have been described as ROS-, NE- or MPO-dependent [5,12,16,17].

So far, few pathogen-derived molecules triggering NETosis have been identified such as bacterial toxins [18], virus [19] or surface lipophosphoglycans of *Leishmania* [14]. In addition, little data are reported on NET-associated PMN-derived ligands and Ca^{2+}-mediated signalling pathways [20]. As such, CD11b and CD18 are described as being involved in *Candida albicans* [21] or *Mannheimia haemolytica*-mediated NETosis [18]. Recently Ca^{2+}-dependent ETosis has been reported [20]. In the case of parasite-triggered NETosis, no data on PMN ligands or Ca^{2+}-dependency are available, so far. This work focuses on molecular mechanisms involved in *E. bovis*-induced NET formation. We here demonstrate that respective NETosis depends on granulocyte NE and MPO activities and on the activation of an ERK1/2- and p38-related signaling pathway. Furthermore store-operated Ca^{2+} entry and CD11b receptor binding is involved in *E. bovis*-triggered NETosis.

Materials and methods

Parasite

The *E. bovis* (strain H) used in the present study was maintained by passages in Holstein–Friesian calves for oocyst production as described by Hermosilla et al. [22]. Calves were infected orally with 5×10^4 sporulated *E. bovis* oocysts. Collection of oocysts, oocyst sporulation and excystation of sporozoites were performed as previously described [22]. Free-released sporozoites were washed three times with sterile PBS ($400 \times g$, 10 min), counted in a Neubauer haemocytometer chamber and thereafter suspended at final concentrations of 2.5×10^5 – 10^6 sporozoites/mL in culture medium (RPMI 1640, 1% penicillin/streptomycin, v/v; Gibco) free of fetal calf serum (FCS) until further experimental use. In addition, sporulated *E. arloingi* oocysts (strain A) [16], *Isospora suis* oocysts (kindly provided by Anja Joachim, University of Veterinary Medicine of Vienna, Austria) and *Toxoplasma gondii* oocysts (kindly provided by Anja Joachim, University of Veterinary Medicine of Vienna, Austria and Peter Deplazes, Faculty of Veterinary Medicine, University of Zurich, Switzerland) were used for comparative analyses on parasite species-specific NET induction. Sporozoite excystation of the latter parasite species was performed according to Pinckney et al. [23] as well as Freyre and Falcon [24].

Isolation of bovine PMN

Adult dairy cows ($n = 3$) were bled by puncture of the jugular vein and blood was collected in 50 mL plastic tubes (Nunc) containing 0.1 mL heparin (Sigma-Aldrich) as anticoagulant. Heparinized blood was diluted in an equal amount of PBS containing 0.02% EDTA (Sigma-Aldrich), layered on Biocoll Separating Solution® (Biochrom AG) and centrifuged at $800 \times g$ for 45 min. After removal of the plasma and PBMC layer, the pellet was suspended in 25 mL distilled water and gently shaken for 40 s to lyse erythrocytes. Osmolarity was immediately re-adjusted by adding 3 mL of Hanks Salt Solution (HBSS 10 x, Biochrom AG). PMN were washed twice, re-suspended in RPMI 1640 medium (Gibco), counted in a Neubauer haemocytometer chamber and subsequently incubated at 37 °C and 5% CO_2 atmosphere for at least 30 min before use.

Flow cytometric analysis of *Eimeria bovis* sporozoites-induced CD11b surface expression on bovine PMN

PMN were incubated with CFSE-stained *E. bovis* sporozoites (1:1 ratio, 30 min, 37 °C) in HBSS containing 0.9 mM $CaCl_2$. For positive controls, PMN were treated with platelet activating factor (PAF 100 nM, 15 min, 37 °C; Calbiochem). For negative controls, non-treated and non-exposed PMN were used. After incubation, cells were pelleted ($300 \times g$, 20 °C, 6 min), resuspended in 200 μL HBSS and incubated with anti-CD11b antibodies coupled to allophycocyanin (APC; clone M1/70; 20 min, in the dark; BD Pharmingen) and washed at $300 \times g$, 20 °C, 6 min. Thereafter, the cells were analyzed using a FACS Canto II cytometer (BD Biosciences, San Diego, CA, USA). The data were displayed as plots of forward versus side light scatter. The mean fluorescence of APC was determined from a minimum of 10^4 cells using BD FACS Diva 6.1 software (BD Biosciences, San Diego, CA, USA).

Inhibition of store-operated calcium entry (SOCE)

Bovine PMN were pre-incubated with the SOCE inhibitor 2-aminoethoxydiphenyl borate (2-APB) for 15 min at concentrations of 50 and 100 μM in HBSS medium prior to exposure to *E. bovis* sporozoites in a 1:2 ratio (2×10^5 PMN: 4×10^5 sporozoites, 60 min, 37 °C).

For NET quantification, 50 μL of micrococcal nuclease buffer containing 0.1 U/μL micrococcal nuclease (both New England Biolabs) were added to each well and incubated (15 min, 37 °C). Afterwards the samples were centrifuged ($300 \times g$, 5 min) and the supernatants were transferred into a 96-well flat-bottom plate (100 μL per well in duplicates). Fifty microliters of Pico Green® (1:200 dilution in 10 mM Tris base buffered with 1 mM EDTA) were added to each sample and the samples were incubated (4 min, in the dark). NET formation was determined by spectrofluorometric analysis at an excitation wavelength of 484 nm and an emission wavelength of 520 nm using an automated plate monochrome reader (Varioskan Flash®; Thermo Scientific). For negative controls,

PMN in plain medium were used. For positive controls, stimulation with zymosan (1 mg/mL) was used.

Immunoblotting for the detection of phosphorylated ERK1/2 and p38 MAPK

PMN (5×10^6 in HBSS containing 0.9 mM $CaCl_2$) were exposed to *E. bovis*-sporozoites (5×10^6) for 15 and 30 min at 37 °C in a final volume of 500 μL. For positive controls, PMN were stimulated with PAF (100 nM). Thereafter, total protein was extracted as described previously by Hidalgo et al. [25] and 40 μg total protein were analyzed by a 10% SDS-PAGE. Immunoblotting was performed according to a protocol previously described by Hidalgo et al. [26]. Antibodies directed against phospho-p38 MAPK and phospho-ERK1/2 (Cell Signalling, Beverly, MA, USA) were used according to the instructions provided by the manufacturer. Anti-mouse HRP-conjugated antisera (Santa Cruz Biotechnology, USA) were used as secondary antibodies (2 h of incubation, RT, in constant agitation). Signals were detected using an enhanced chemiluminescence system (Western Lightning® Plus-ECL; Perkin-Elmer, USA). After signal detection and documentation, the bound antibodies were removed by stripping the membranes (100 mM 2-mercaptoethanol; 2% SDS; 62.5 mM Tris-HCl, pH 6.7, for 2 h at 50 °C with agitation, followed by several washes with TBS-Tween 0.1%) according to Hidalgo et al. [25] and each membrane was re-probed with an antibody recognizing total p38 MAPK (p38 MAPK anti rabbit antibody; Cell signaling technology) and ERK1/2 (rabbit polyclonal IgG; Santa Cruz Biotechnology, USA). The samples were then further processed as described above. The intensities of each band were analyzed using the Software Image J and the signals were normalized to total ERK1/2 for p-ERK1/2 and to total p38 for p-p38.

NET inhibition assays using ERK1/2, p38 MAPK inhibitors and functional CD11b monoclonal antibodies

For the inhibition of ERK 1/2 and p38 MAPK the following inhibitors were used respectively: UO126 (50 μM; Sigma-Aldrich) and SB 203580 (10 μM; Sigma-Aldrich). Therefore, PMN were preincubated with the inhibitors for 30 min at RT in HBSS-buffer without phenol red (Gibco). CD11b was blocked via pre-incubation in mouse anti bovine CD11b monoclonal antibodies (MCA1425, diluted 1:5 in PBS; AbD Serotec). For antibody control, we used an irrelevant antibody at an identical concentration (anti-bovine CD4, AbD Serotec). Then, PMN were exposed to viable *E. bovis*-sporozoites (1:2 ratio: 2×10^5 PMN + 4×10^5 sporozoites) for 60 min at 37 °C. Thereafter extracellular DNA was quantified as described above. All measurements were achieved using an automated monochrome reader (Varioskan Flash; Thermo Scientific). For positive controls, zymosan (Sigma-Aldrich) was used in a final concentration of 0.5 mg/mL.

Visualization of NET and detection of histones (H3), neutrophil elastase (NE) and myeloperoxidase (MPO) in NET structures

Bovine PMN were incubated with *E. bovis* sporozoites (ratio 1:1; 30 min) on poly-L-lysine-treated coverslips and fixed [4% (w/v) paraformaldehyde, Merck, 20 min in the dark]. NET structures were visualized by staining extracellular DNA with 5 mM Sytox Orange dye (Invitrogen) for 10 min at RT according to Martinelli et al. [27]. For the visualization of sporozoites within NET structures, sporozoites were stained with 5(6)-carboxyfluorescein diacetate succinimidyl ester (CFSE, 7.5 μM, 37 °C, 30 min; Invitrogen) according to Hermosilla et al. [28] prior to PMN exposure. After fixation of the cells and three washings in sterile PBS, the samples were mounted in anti-fading buffer (Mowiol®, Sigma-Aldrich) and stored (4 °C, in the dark) until further use. For the detection of histones, MPO and NE within NET structures the following specific antibodies were used: anti-histone monoclonal antibodies [rabbit (E173) anti-bovine histone H3, phospho S10 DyLight® 488, 1:100; ab139848, Abcam], anti-MPO antibodies (rabbit anti-bovine MPO, Alexa Fluor 488, 1:200; ABIN906866) and anti-NE antibodies (rabbit anti-human NE, 1:200; AB68672, Abcam). Therefore, the samples were washed three times with PBS, blocked with BSA [1% (w/v) in PBS, 30 min, RT, Sigma-Aldrich] and reacted with anti-histone, anti-NE or anti-MPO antibodies [1 h, RT, in the dark for bovine anti-histone (H3); 24 h, RT, in the dark for both anti-MPO and anti-NE antibodies]. The samples were then gently washed in PBS and mounted in anti-fading buffer (Mowiol®, Sigma-Aldrich). Visualization was achieved using an inverted Olympus® IX81 fluorescence microscope equipped with a digital camera.

Measurements of NADPH oxidase, NE and MPO enzymatic activities and inhibition of these enzyme activities

For NADPH oxidase-, NE- and MPO-inhibition assays, the following inhibitors were used: the NADPH oxidase inhibitor diphenylene iodonium (DPI, 10 μM, Sigma-Aldrich); the NE inhibitor Suc-Ala-Ala-Pro-Val chloromethyl ketone (CMK; 1 mM, Sigma-Aldrich), according to Scapinello et al. [29] and the MPO inhibitor 4-aminobenzoic acid hydrazide (ABAH; 100 μM, Calbiochem), according to Parker et al. [30]. In brief, PMN and sporozoites (1:1 ratio, $n = 3$) were incubated (30 min, 37 °C) in HBSS-buffer without phenol red (Gibco) for positive controls. In parallel, PMN were pre-incubated with the corresponding inhibitors for 30 min at RT prior to exposure to viable *E. bovis*-sporozoites (1:1 ratio, 30 min, 37 °C). To estimate maximum values of extracellular DNA, PMN were lysed by Triton-X 100 treatment (0.1%; Sigma-Aldrich). To block NET formation, 90 U of DNase I (Roche Diagnostics) were supplemented 15 min before the end of incubation period. NET were quantified via Pico Green®-DNA staining as described above.

NADPH oxidase, NE and MPO enzymatic activities were measured using respective substrates: 10 µg/mL DCFH-DA (Sigma-Aldrich); 3 mg/mL of the NE chromogenic substrate MeoSuc-Ala-Ala-Pro-Val-chloromethyl-ketone (Sigma-Aldrich) and 50 µM Amplex red (Invitrogen), respectively. ROS production was measured by oxidation of DCFH-DA to fluorescent DCF according to Conejeros et al. [31]. The relative fluorescence units (RFU) were recorded at 15 min intervals for a period of 30 min applying 485 nm excitation and 530 nm emission wavelengths. NE activity was measured every 10 min for 30 min at 410 nm wavelength and MPO-peroxidase activity was measured every 10 min for 30 min in 571-585 nm fluorescence ranges. All measurements were achieved using an automated monochrome reader (Varioskan Flash; Thermo Scientific). As positive control, zymosan (Sigma-Aldrich) was used at a final concentration of 0.5 mg/mL.

Determination of matrix metalloproteinase 9 (MMP-9) activities in PMN supernatants

PMN (10^6/500 µL HBSS/0.9 mM $CaCl_2$) were exposed to equal numbers of *E. bovis* sporozoites (15 and 30 min, 37 °C). Stimulation of PMN with PAF (100 nM, 5 min, 37 °C) was used for positive controls. PMN cultivated in plain medium were used for negative controls. After incubation, the cells were centrifuged (600 × *g*, 6 min) and the supernatants were assayed for gelatinase activity by zymography. Therefore, substrate gel electrophoresis was performed using the method described by Conejeros et al. [32]. Briefly, 10 µL of supernatant/slot were loaded on polyacrylamide gels (10%, 0.75 mm thickness) containing 0.28% of gelatin (Sigma-Aldrich). In parallel a recombinant MMP-9 standard (Sigma-Aldrich) and a molecular mass marker (Fermentas International Inc., Canada) were loaded as reference samples. The gels were run at 200 V for 1 h in a Bio-Rad Mini Protean II chamber (Bio-Rad Laboratories, CA, USA). Thereafter, the gels were incubated twice in Triton X-100 (2.5%, under constant shaking, RT, 30 min) and overnight at 37 °C in reaction buffer (100 mM Tris, pH 7.5; 10 mM $CaCl_2$). The gels were stained in Coomassie Brilliant Blue R-250 (Winkler, Santiago, Chile; 0.5% in acetic acid : methanol : water = 1 : 3 : 6). MMP-9 (gelatinase B) enzymatic activity present in the test samples were determined according to the degree of gelatin degradation (visible as clear bands of 82 kDa) relative to the MMP-9-control by means of band intensity measurements (applying ImageJ 1.35 s software).

Host cell infection and production of viable *Eimeria bovis* merozoites I

Primary bovine umbilical vein endothelial cells (BUVEC) were isolated from umbilical cord veins, according to the method of Hermosilla et al. [4]. Confluent BUVEC monolayers ($n = 3$) were infected with 2.5×10^5 freshly excysted *E. bovis*-sporozoites suspended in modified ECGM [ECGM (PromoCell) supplemented with 70% (v/v) M199 (Gibco), 2% FCS (Gibco) and 1% penicillin (Sigma-Aldrich)] per 25 cm^2 flask (Greiner). The cells were fed 24 h after infection and thereafter every third day with modified ECGM. To control for *E. bovis* macromeront development and the release of merozoites I, infected BUVEC cultures were analyzed daily over a period of 22 days using a phase-contrast inverted microscope (IX81 microscope®, Olympus). Free-released merozoites I were harvested from the supernatant of infected BUVEC monolayers (400 × *g*, 5 min) and washed twice in PBS. The merozoites I were counted in a Neubauer chamber haemocytometer.

Scanning electron microscopy (SEM)

Bovine PMN were incubated with *E. bovis* sporozoites, merozoites I or oocysts at a ratio of 1:1 for 90 min on poly-L-lysine (Sigma-Aldrich) pre-coated coverslips. After incubation, the samples were fixed (2.5% glutaraldehyde in 0.1 M cacodylate buffer, 15 min, all Merck) and washed with 0.1 M cacodylate buffer. The samples were post-fixed in 1% osmium tetroxide (Merck) in 0.1 M cacodylate buffer, washed three times in distilled water, dehydrated in ascending ethanol concentrations, critical point dried by CO_2-treatment and sputtered with gold. Specimens were examined using a Philips XL30 scanning electron microscope at the Institute of Anatomy and Cell Biology, Justus Liebig University Giessen, Germany.

Quantification of NET derived from PMN and parasites from different origins

NET formation was quantified using Pico Green® (Invitrogen), a DNA-binding dye. In order to quantify *E. bovis* sporozoite- or merozoite I-induced NET formation, bovine PMN ($n = 3$-5) were re-suspended in serum-free medium RPMI 1640 and incubated (all at 37 °C) with *E. bovis*-sporozoites in a 1:2 ratio (2×10^5 PMN: 4×10^5 sporozoites, 60 min), with *E. bovis*-merozoites I in a 1:1 ratio (1×10^5 PMN: 1×10^5 merozoites, 90 min), with oocysts (5×10^4, 60 min, 1:1) and with sporozoites of *E. arloingi* ($n = 3$; 1×10^5 PMN: 1×10^5 sporozoites, 60 min), *Isospora suis* ($n = 3$; 1×10^5 PMN: 1×10^5 sporozoites; 60 min) and *T. gondii* ($n = 5$; 1×10^5 PMN: 1×10^5 sporozoites; 60 min). In addition, PMN isolated from different host species origin (caprine, horse and dog) were incubated with *E. bovis* sporozoites in a 1:2 ratio (2×10^5 PMN: 4×10^5 sporozoites, 60 min at 37 °C). For positive controls, zymosan was used at a final concentration of 0.5 mg/mL. Plain RPMI 1640 medium served as negative controls. NET-formation was determined based on Pico Green®-DNA staining as described above.

Eimeria bovis sporozoite entrapment assay

For the quantification of sporozoite entrapment within NET structures we followed the method described by Köckritz-Blickwede et al. [8] with slight modifications. Briefly, PMN (2.5×10^5/96-well) were pre-activated by zymosan treatment (30 min, 37 °C). Meanwhile, *E. bovis*-sporozoites were stained with FITC dye (0.2 mg/mL, 30 min, on ice, in the dark, Invitrogen) and washed twice in PBS (3000 × *g*, 10 min). Thereafter, zymosan-stimulated PMN were exposed to FITC-labeled *E. bovis* sporozoites (512 × *g*, 10 min; subsequent incubation for 30 min at 37 °C) in ascendant ratios (0.5:1;1:1 and 1:2). Non-exposed sporozoites were used for controls (1:1; 1:2). The samples were washed twice in RPMI 1640 medium and measured for fluorescence intensity at 485/538 nm wavelength. The percentage of entrapment was calculated as follows: [(A485/538 nm sporozoites exposed to PMN)/(A485/538 nm non-exposed sporozoites)] × 100%.

Ethics statement

All animal procedures were performed according to the Justus Liebig University Animal Care Committee guidelines, approved by the Ethic Commission for Experimental Animal Studies of the State of Hesse (Regierungspräsidium Giessen) and in accordance to the current German Animal Protection Laws. Identification number of animal care and project licence: GI 18/10-Nr.A51/2012 544_AZ952 (*Eimeria bovis*-oocyst production); GI 18/10-Nr.A9/2012 521_AZ877 (Bovine blood samples). European Animal Welfare Legislation: ART13TFEU.

Statistical analysis

Co-culture/stimulation conditions were compared by one- or two-factorial analyses of variance (ANOVA) with repeated measurements in order to compare co-culture/stimulation conditions. All analyses were performed with the GraphPad Prism® 6 software. Differences were regarded as significant at a level of $p \leq 0.05$ (*); $p \leq 0.01$ (**); $p \leq 0.001$ (***).

Results

Exposure to *E. bovis* sporozoites up-regulates neutrophil CD11b surface expression on bovine PMN and triggers NET formation in a CD11b-dependent manner

Since no data are available on PMN-derived receptors being involved in *E. bovis*-mediated NETosis, we here analyzed whether sporozoite exposure would affect CD11b

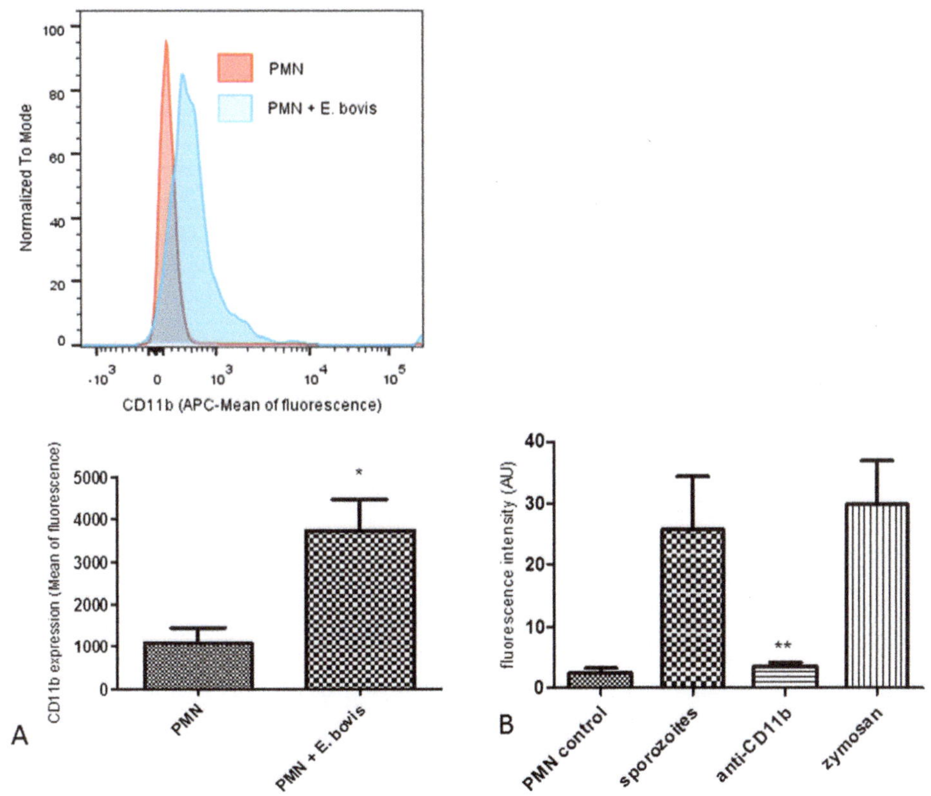

Figure 1 CD11b surface expression and CD11b-dependent-NET formation of bovine *E. bovis* sporozoite-exposed PMN. (A) Bovine PMN were exposed to CFSE-labeled sporozoites (1:1) and subjected to FACS analysis probing with an antibody directed against CD11b. Non-exposed PMN in plain medium served as negative controls. The histograms represent the shift in the mean fluorescence of the PMN population analyzed and are representative of the experiments performed. **(B)** NET formation in the presence of anti-CD11b antibodies. Bovine PMN were pre-treated with anti-CD11b prior to sporozoite exposure. Stimulation with zymosan served as a positive control; PMN in plain medium were used for negative controls.

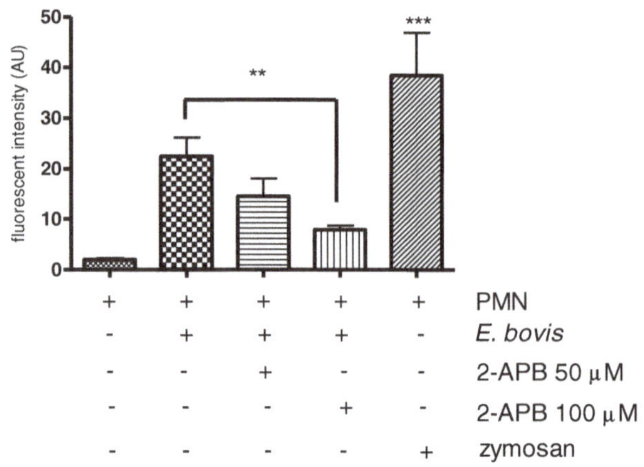

Figure 2 Influence of store-operated calcium entry (SOCE) on *E. bovis* sporozoites-induced NET formation. PMN were treated with the SOCE-inhibitor 2-APB prior to exposure to *E. bovis* sporozoites. For negative controls, non-treated PMN were used. For positive controls, zymosan stimulation was used. NET formation was quantified based on DNA-derived fluorescence intensities using an automate plate reader.

surface expression of bovine PMN. Applying FACS methodology, a significant parasite-triggered increase of CD11b surface expression was shown when compared to non-exposed PMN ($p \leq 0.05$, Figure 1A). In addition, blockage of CD11b via specific antibodies led to a significant reduction in sporozoite-mediated NET formation when compared to antibody-free controls ($p \leq 0.01$; Figure 1B). We also did not observe any significant NET induction using our irrelevant antibody control. Thus, these results suggest CD11b as a potential candidate for neutrophil receptors being involved in NET formation.

Eimeria bovis-induced NET formation is store-operated calcium entry (SOCE)-dependent

As previously shown in the bovine system, ROS production is a Ca^{2+}-dependent process [32]. Since sporozoite-triggered NETosis was recently proven to be ROS-dependent [5], we here analyzed whether the presence of the Ca^{2+} (SOCE) inhibitor 2-APB [31,32] would influence sporozoite-mediated NETosis. The fact that treatment with 100 μM 2-APB resulted in a significant reduction of *E. bovis* sporozoite-induced NET when compared with non-treated but sporozoite-exposed PMN ($p \leq 0.01$, Figure 2), suggests a Ca^{2+}/SOCE-dependent process. Overall, stimulation of PMN with zymosan revealed to be a potent SOCE inducer compared to the negative control ($p \leq 0.001$; Figure 2).

Sporozoite-induced NETosis is a ROS-, NE- MPO-dependent process

Experiments applying specific antibodies against H3, NE and MPO alongside with DNA-staining proved NET structures (estimated via extracellular DNA-positive fibres) as co-localizing with histone H3-, NE- and MPO-positive signals indicated a pivotal role of these molecules in

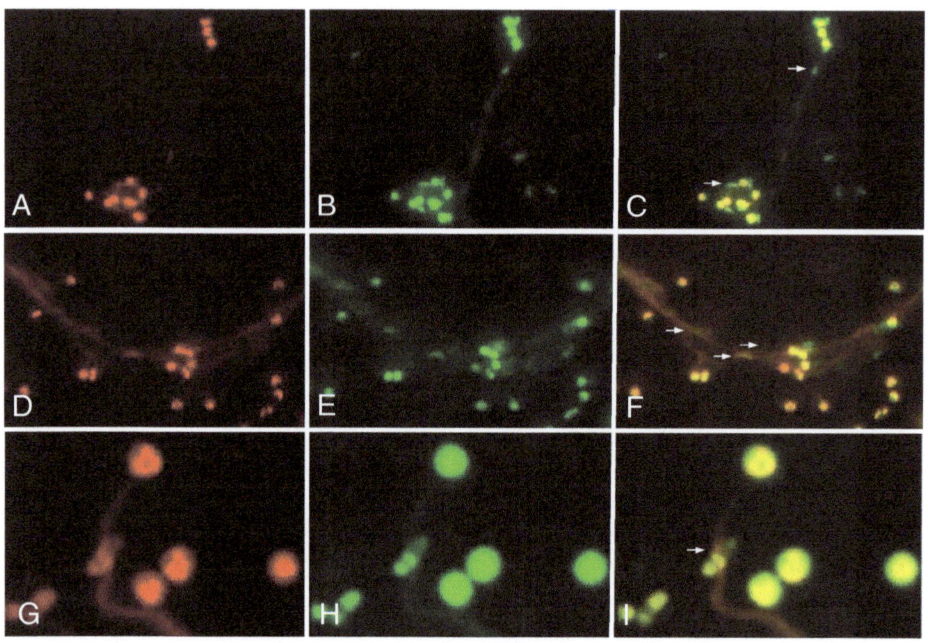

Figure 3 Co-localization of DNA with histones (H3), neutrophil elastase (NE) and myeloperxodase (MPO) in *E. bovis* sporozoite-induced NET structures. Co-cultures of bovine PMN and *E. bovis* sporozoites and oocysts were fixed, permeabilized and stained for DNA using Sytox Orange (red: **A**, **D**, **G**) and probed for histone 3 (H3) (green: **B**), MPO (green: **E**) and NE (green: **H**) using anti-H3, anti-NE and anti-MPO antibodies jointly with adequate conjugate systems. Areas of respective co-localization (merges) are illustrated in **C**, **F**, **I**. Photomicrographs are of representative cells from 3 independent experiments.

sporozoite-triggered NETosis and confirmed classical NET characteristics (Figure 3). In addition, PMN exposure to *E. bovis* sporozoites resulted in a significant up-regulation of NADPH oxidase-, NE- and MPO- enzymatic activities ($p \leq 0.05$ for NADPH oxidase; $p \leq 0.01$ for NE and MPO; Figures 4A-C). Furthermore, we confirmed the key role of these enzymes since inhibition of NADPH oxidase, NE and MPO led to significantly reduced sporozoite-triggered NETosis when compared to non-treated controls (Figure 4D; DPI and ABAH: $p \leq 0.05$; CMK: $p \leq 0.01$). As expected, DNase I treatments led to a significant NET resolution ($p \leq 0.001$, Figure 4D). Total DNA release from PMN was controlled by Triton X treatments revealing a proportion of up to 43% of PMN to be involved in sporozoite-mediated NETosis. Overall, these data confirm the relevance of NADPH oxidase, NE and MPO in *E. bovis* sporozoite-induced NET formation.

E. bovis sporozoite exposure enhances matrix metalloprotease 9 (MMP-9) release of bovine PMN

Given that tertiary granule contents of PMN also contribute to NET formation based on their antimicrobial peptide/protease activities as described by Brinkmann et al. [6], we additionally analyzed PMN supernatants for the enzymatic activity of MMP-9. Co-cultures of PMN with *E. bovis* sporozoites led to a significant increase of MMP-9 release ($p \leq 0.05$; Figure 5) at both time points tested (15 and 30 min) indicating that tertiary granules or MMP-9 may also be involved in sporozoite-triggered NETosis. As expected, stimulation with PAF revealed to be a reliable positive control for MMP-9 release in the bovine system ($p \leq 0.05$).

ERK1/2- and p38 MAPK-signaling pathways are involved in *E. bovis* sporozoite-triggered NET extrusion

We analyzed whether the ERK1/2 and p38 MAPK signaling pathway is involved in sporozoite-triggered NETosis. Exposure of *E. bovis* sporozoites to PMN resulted in a fast and significant phosphorylation of ERK1/2 ($p \leq 0.05$ after 15 and 30 min of incubation, Figure 6A) and p38 ($p \leq 0.05$ at 15 min, Figure 6B) MAPK. Furthermore, experiments applying inhibitors of ERK1/2 and p38 MAPK confirmed the relevance of this signaling pathway since treatments with both inhibitors resulted in a significant reduction of sporozoite-mediated NET formation (UO126: $p \leq 0.01$ and SB 203580: $p \leq 0.05$, Figure 6C).

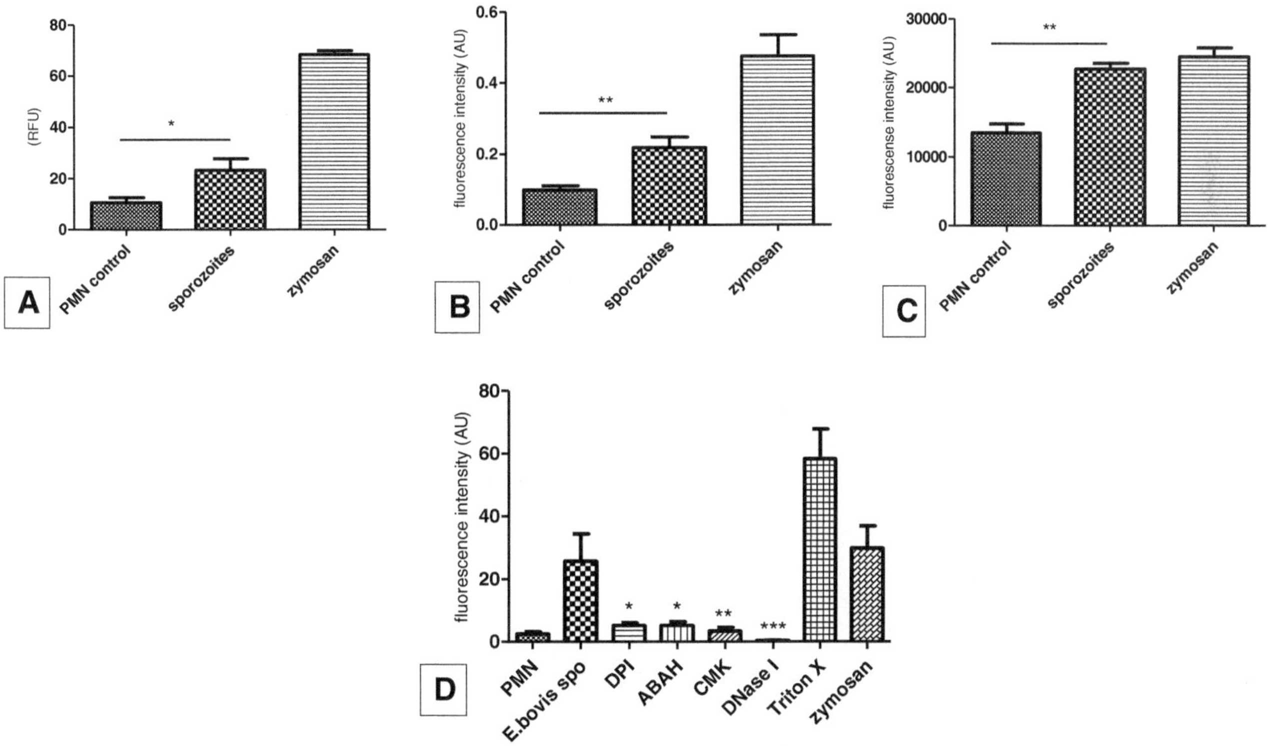

Figure 4 *E. bovis* sporozoite-induced NETosis in bovine PMN is a NADPH oxidase-, NE- MPO-dependent process. (A-C) NADPH oxidase, NE and MPO enzymatic activities in *E. bovis* sporozoite-exposed PMN. PMN were exposed to *E. bovis* sporozoites and enzymatic activities of NADPH oxidase **(A)**, NE **(B)** and MPO **(C)** were measured using via DCFH-DA oxidation, NE-chromogenic substrate analysis and using Amplex red reagent, respectively. **(D)** Sporozoite-triggered NET formation after inhibition of NADPH oxidase (via DPI), NE (via CMK) and MPO (via ABAH). For inhibition and maximum DNA release controls, DNase I and Triton X treatments were used, respectively. Stimulation with zymosan served as a positive control (1 mg/mL) and PMN in plain medium as a negative control.

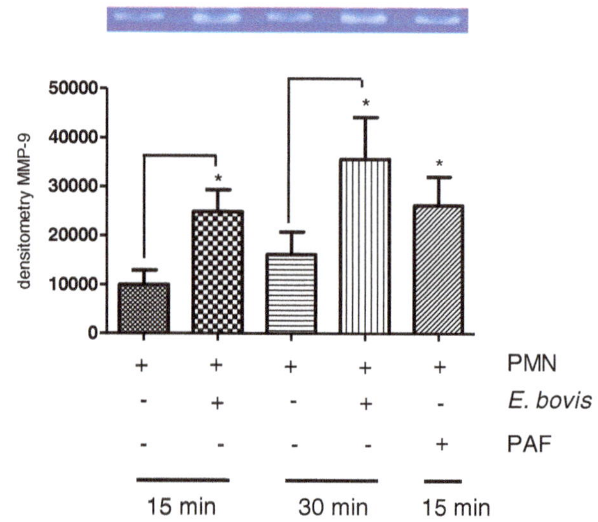

Figure 5 Release of MMP-9 from PMN granule contents after sporozoite-exposure. Bovine PMN were exposed to *E. bovis* sporozoites and the supernatants were analyzed for MMP-9 activities via zymography in gelatin-containing polyacrylamide gels and consecutive densitometric estimations. Recombinant MMP-9 was used as an internal standard. Stimulation of PMN with PAF (100 nM) served as a positive control. Each bar represents arithmetic means ± SEM of x PMN donors.

Sporozoite-triggered NETosis is neither stage- nor parasite species- nor host-specific

To account for stage-specificity we tested *E. bovis* merozoites I for the capability to induce NET. As depicted in Figure 7C, merozoite I stages significantly triggered NET when compared to non-exposed controls ($p \leq 0.01$). These data were confirmed by SEM analyses illustrating the formation of a delicate, NET-like network of thicker and thinner strands of fibres originating from dead PMN and being firmly attached to the merozoites I (Figure 7A). In addition, SEM analyses indicated NET-like structures also to be induced by oocyst stages (Figure 7B). These data clearly argue against a stage-specificity of *E. bovis*-triggered NETosis highlighting the capability of PMN to equally respond to different parasitic stages of this parasite.

In order to analyze whether *E. bovis*-triggered NETosis is a parasite-specific event or rather reflects a general mechanism that commonly accounts for most coccidian parasites, we analyzed NET formation of bovine PMN after exposure to the sporozoite stage of a non-bovine *Eimeria* spp. (the caprine-specific species *E. arloingi*) and of two non-*Eimeria* coccidian species (*T. gondii* and *I. suis*). The data clearly show that the sporozoites of all three parasite species equally induced significant NET formation (*E. arloingi* and *T. gondii*: $p \leq 0.01$, *I. suis*: $p \leq 0.05$, Figure 8B). Overall, these findings rather argue against a parasite-specific mechanism and propose NET formation as a generally valid effector mechanism against the sporozoite stage of different coccidian species.

Given that *E. bovis* is a strict host-specific parasite and, in consequence, exclusively infects bovines, we then analyzed whether *E. bovis*-mediated NET formation is a host-specific event. Therefore, PMN of different host origins (horse, goat, dog and cattle) were controlled for NET formation after exposure to *E. bovis* sporozoites. The data clearly revealed that PMN of all host types reacted by significant NET formation ($p \leq 0.01$, Figure 8A) which argues against a host-specific reaction.

NET structures significantly entrap *Eimeria bovis* sporozoites

In order to analyze the capacity of NET to trap viable *E. bovis* sporozoites, we established a quantitative parasite-entrapment-assay by using FITC-stained parasites and zymosan pre-activated bovine PMN as described elsewhere [17]. The experiments revealed a proportion of 43.4% of sporozoites to be immobilized in NET structures when compared to non-exposed sporozoites (data not shown). These results indicate a rather high efficacy of NET as an effector mechanism considering that almost every second parasite was entrapped and most probably hampered from host cell invasion as reported elsewhere [5].

Discussion

NET formation depends on the assembly/activation of the NADPH oxidase complex and the resulting production of ROS [7]. Since these mechanisms were reported as Ca^{2+}-mediated in the bovine system [31], it appears likely that NETosis is a Ca^{2+}-dependent process, as recently demonstrated by Gupta et al. [20]. The fact that NET formation is induced by thapsigargin [33] which mobilizes Ca^{2+} from intracellular pools, also indicates a key role of Ca^{2+} in NETosis. Since SOCE was proven to play a crucial role in Ca^{2+}-dependent ROS production [34] we here used 2-APB a well-known inhibitor of SOCE for functional assays. The pre-incubation of PMN with 2-APB prior to sporozoite exposure resulted in a significant diminishment of NETosis and therefore confirmed the assumption that parasite-triggered NET formation is a Ca^{2+}-(SOCE)-dependent process.

Besides being SOCE-dependent, ROS production is up-regulated in a CD11b (CR3)-dependent manner in bovine PMN [31]. In turn, up-regulation of CD11b proves as SOCE-dependent since it is inhibited by 2-APB [32] leading us to the assumption that the neutrophil integrin receptor CD11b may also be involved in sporozoite-mediated NETosis. Indeed, we found significantly enhanced levels of surface CD11b expression on parasite-exposed bovine PMN. The fact that antibody-mediated blockage of CD11b additionally resulted in NET diminishment suggests CD11b to be involved in sporozoite-triggered NETosis and to function as a PMN-derived receptor in this effector mechanism. These findings were in accordance

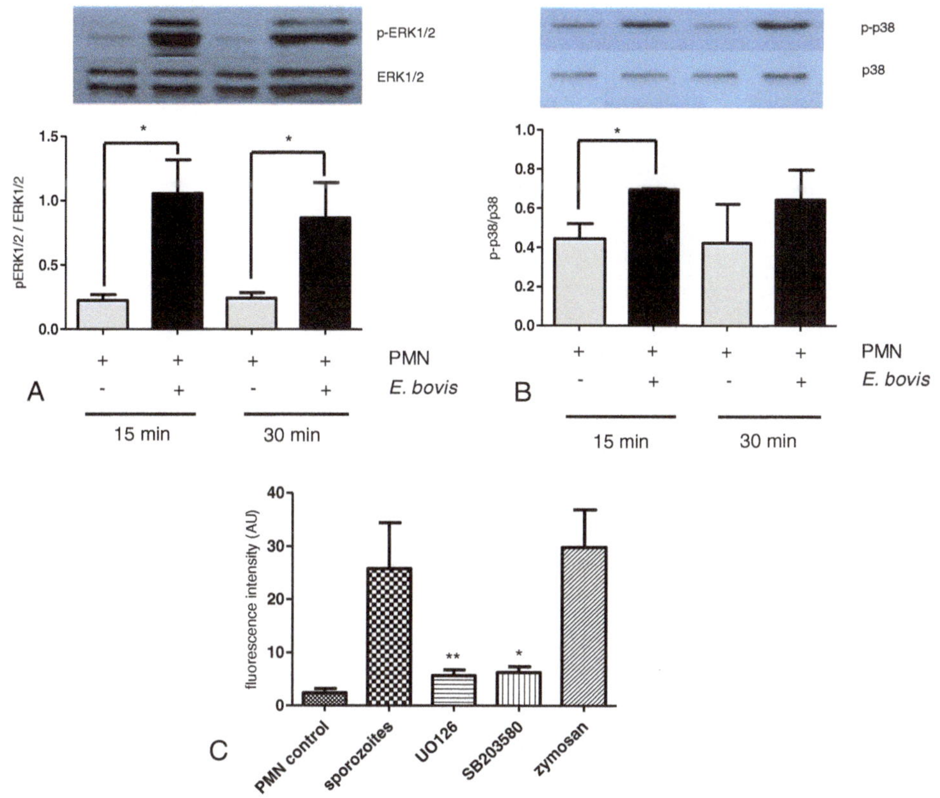

Figure 6 Expression of phosphorylated ERK1/2- and p38 MAPK in sporozoite-exposed PMN and influence of their inhibition on parasite-triggered NETosis. Total proteins of sporozoite-exposed PMN and non-exposed controls were analyzed by SDS/PAGE and immunoblot technique using specific antibodies against non-phosphorylated and phosphorylated ERK1/2 **(A)** and p38 MAPK **(B)**. Respective bands were densitometrically analyzed. Each bar represents the arithmetic means ± SEM of three PMN donors. Differences were regarded as significant at a level of $p \leq 0.05$ compared to negative controls. **(C)** NET formation in presence of ERK 1/2 (UO126) and p38 (SB 203580) MAPK inhibitors. Stimulation with zymosan served as a positive control; PMN in plain medium as a negative control.

with Byrd et al. [21] who reported on CD11b as a potential ligand in NETosis since antibody-mediated blockage of this integrin inhibits fibronectin-dependent NET formation to *C. albicans* hyphae.

Moreover, SOCE is tightly regulated via ERK1/2 MAPK phophorylation, i.e., by a signaling pathway that was recently described to be involved in NETosis [35]. In addition, ROS-dependent activation of ERK and p38 MAPK was demonstrated to mediate PMA-induced NET release from human neutrophils [35]. In accordance to the latter reports and to data on other pathogens [12,21] we here show a sporozoite-triggered up-regulation of ERK1/2 and p38 MAPK phosphorylation in parasite-exposed bovine PMN. The key role of the ERK1/2- and p38 MAPK-dependent signaling pathway in NETosis was confirmed in functional inhibition experiments showing that parasite-triggered NETosis was significantly diminished in the presence of ERK-and p38 inhibitors.

We furthermore focused on the relevance of NE and MPO and confirmed the key role of these two molecules in *E. bovis*-triggered NETosis. As with other bovine pathogens [18], exposure to sporozoites led to an increase of both, NE and MPO enzymatic activities in bovine PMN. Functional inhibition assays confirmed the relevance of these enzymes since parasite-mediated NETosis was significantly blocked when NE and MPO inhibitors were applied. Finally, the co-localization of DNA-rich filaments with NE- or MPO-derived signals in sporozoite-induced NET structures emphasized the classical characteristics of NET. These results were in line with recent findings on other coccidian parasites, such as *E. arloingi* [16] or *B. besnoiti* [17].

Whilst NE and MPO originate from azurophilic PMN granules, other molecules such as metalloproteinases (MMP), are contained in tertiary (gelatinase) granules. We here analyzed whether MMP-9 is released from PMN upon sporozoite exposure. Zymographic analyses of PMN supernatants confirmed a parasite-mediated MMP-9-release into PMN supernatants. So far, the functional role of MMP-9 in NETosis is unclear. However, it is worth noting that the release of MMP-9 is regulated by the ERK 1/2 and p38 MAPK signaling pathway [36]. Interestingly, Carmona Rivera et al. [37] showed an impaired endothelial function induced by NET-externalized

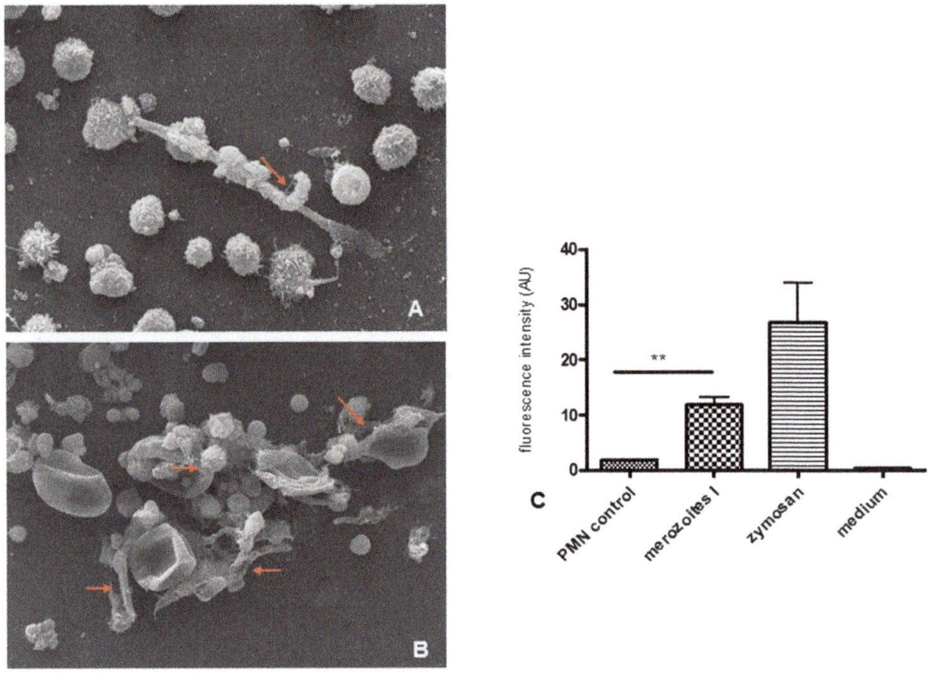

Figure 7 NET formation triggered by *E. bovis* merozoites I and oocyst stages. (A) Scanning electron microscopy (SEM) analysis of *E. bovis* merozoite I-exposed PMN. The arrow indicates a merozoite I being trapped in NET structures. **(B)** SEM analysis of *E. bovis* oocyst-exposed PMN revealing NET-like, delicate PMN-derived filaroid structures being attached to oocysts as indicated by arrows. **(C)** Quantification of *E. bovis* merozoite I-induced NET formation. PMN were exposed to *E. bovis* merozoites I, zymosan (positive control) or plain medium (negative control). NET formation was estimated by Pico Green-derived fluorescence intensities. Arithmetic means of three PMN donors, minimum and maximum.

MMP. Given that *E. bovis* sporozoites infect and mature within endothelial cells, a yet unclear interrelation between NETosis and parasite development within endothelium may exist.

Overall, since the first description of NET as an innate effector mechanism [6], most studies have focused on NETosis driven by bacterial, viral and fungal pathogens and, less frequently, on parasitic pathogens [13]. Nonetheless, there is increasing evidence on the relevance of NET as a defense mechanism against protozoan infections in vitro and in vivo [12,13]. Thus, NET-related data are available on some protozoan pathogens, such as *E. bovis, Toxoplasma gondii, Plasmodium falciparum, E. arloingi,* and *B. besnoiti* [5,12,15-17] and *Leishmania spp.* [14].

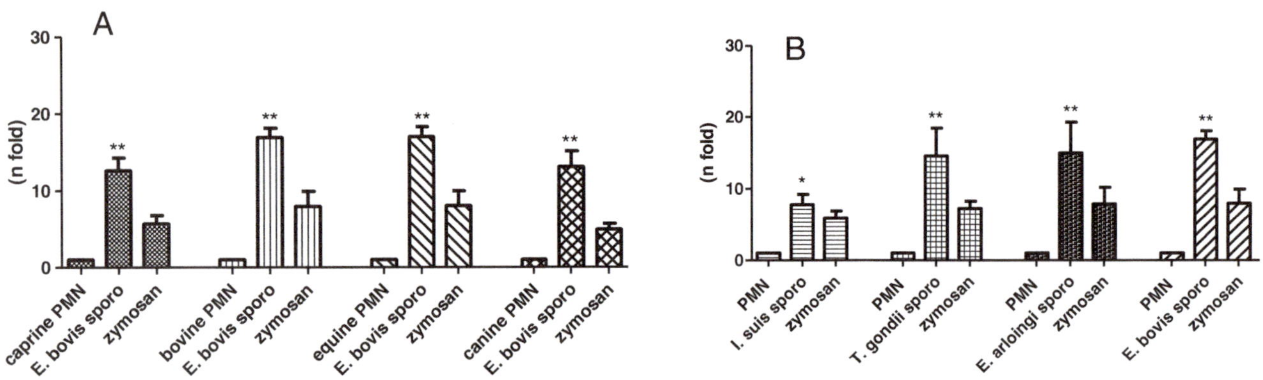

Figure 8 *E. bovis*-sporozoite triggered NETosis of PMN of different host origins and NET formation induced by different coccidian sporozoites. (A) PMN of caprine, bovine, equine and canine origin were exposed to *E. bovis* sporozoites and respective NET formation was measured according to Pico Green-derived fluorescence intensities. **(B)** NET formation of bovine PMN in response to sporozoites of different coccidian species (*I. suis, T. gondii, E. arloingi* and *E. bovis*). In both experiments, stimulation with zymosan served as positive controls and PMN in plain medium were used for negative controls. Arithmetic means of three PMN donors, minimum and maximum.

The current data suggest NETosis as a generally valid effector mechanism against coccidian parasites. Thus, NET release occurred irrespective of the parasite stage (*E. bovis* sporozoites, merozoites I, oocysts), and PMN origin (bovine, caprine, equine, canine). In agreement, data on different *Leishmania* stages [14] also indicated NETosis as a stage-independent defense mechanism. In addition, *T. gondii*-triggered NETosis has been reported for both human and murine PMN [12] indicating host-independent reactions. Overall, it is noteworthy that the degree of entrapment clearly differed amongst different parasite species and stages. Thus, we here report on 43% of *E. bovis* sporozoites to be immobilized within bovine NET structures, whilst in the caprine system even 72% of *E. arloingi* sporozoites were trapped [16] but only 34% of *B. besnoiti* tachyzoites were found ensnared in NET being expelled from bovine PMN [17]. Since all these parasites exhibit an obligatory intracellular replication, extracellular immobilization via NET will have a tremendous implication on the outcome of the disease as previously postulated [16,17].

Furthermore, NETosis was not parasite species-specific since sporozoites of different coccidian parasites (*E. bovis, E. arloingi, I. suis, T. gondii*) equally triggered NET formation. To our best knowledge this is the first report on *T. gondii* and *I. suis* sporozoite-induced NET extrusion whilst tachyzoite stages of *T. gondii* [12] and sporozoites of *E. arloingi* [16] have already been reported before. Especially in the case of *T. gondii*, which exhibits an enormous proliferation at the tachyzoite stage, the intervention of the immune system at a very early time point, i.e. when sporozoites invade the host system and before non-sexual parasite replication occurs, will have a higher impact on the outcome of disease than tachyzoite-triggered reactions. Taking into account that PMN have been demonstrated to actively transmigrate into the intestinal lumen and were found alive in the gut mucus [38], it seems feasible to assume that they may interact with luminal pathogen stages, such as ingested *Eimeria* oocysts, in vivo. Consistently, we here show that oocysts of *E. bovis* are trapped and sometimes almost encaged by NET structures in vitro, thereby most probably preventing proper excystation of sporozoites. This novel anti-excystation mechanism of NET has recently been hypothesized for *E. arloingi* oocysts, in which sporozoites were impeded to escape from NET-covered preformed excystation sites (micropyles) of sporulated oocysts [16]. Thus, in the in vivo situation, luminal occurring NETosis might intervene very early after oral infection with the parasite and abrogate infection even before infectious stages (sporozoites) are able to evade immune reactions via intracellular positioning.

In summary, NET formation seems to be an ancient and highly conserved host effector mechanism of PMN acting against several pathogens as an early host immune reaction. In the present work, we added new data on the molecular mechanisms involved in parasite-triggered NETosis and call for more investigations on receptor-ligand-interactions.

Competing interests
The authors declare that they have no competing interests.

Authors' contributions
Conceived and designed the experiments: TMC, JMH, IC, PA, RAB, MAH, CH, AT. Performed the experiments: TMC, JMH, IC, PA. Analyzed the data: TMC, JMH, IC, PA, RAB, CH, AT. Contributed reagents/materials/analysis tools: TMC, JMH, IC, PA, RAB, MAH, CH, AT. Wrote the paper: TMC, CH, AT. All authors read and approved the final manuscript.

Acknowledgments
We are deeply indebted to Gerd Magdowski (Institute of Anatomy and Cell Biology, JLU Giessen, Germany) for his excellent assistance and kind help on SEM analyses. We further acknowledge Brigitte Hofmann, Christin Ritter and Klaus Becker for their excellent technical assistance in cell culture and blood collection. This work was supported and financed by the German Research Foundation (DFG; grant number: TA 291/4-1).

Author details
[1]Institute of Parasitology, Justus Liebig University Giessen, Schubertstraße 81, 35392 Giessen, Germany. [2]Laboratory of Inflammation Pharmacology, Institute of Pharmacology and Morphophysiology, Faculty of Veterinary Science, Austral University of Chile, Valdivia 5110566, Chile. [3]Department of Biology, University of Nariño, Pasto 520002, Colombia.

References

1. Daugschies A, Najdrowski M (2005) Eimeriosis in cattle: current understanding. J Vet Med B Infect Dis Vet Public Health 52:417–427
2. Friend SC, Stockdale PH (1980) Experimental *Eimeria bovis* infection in calves: a histopathological study. Can J Comp Med 44:129–140
3. Behrendt JH, Hermosilla C, Hardt M, Failing K, Zahner H, Taubert A (2008) PMN-mediated immune reactions against *Eimeria bovis*. Vet Parasitol 151:97–109
4. Hermosilla C, Zahner H, Taubert A (2006) *Eimeria bovis* modulates adhesion molecule gene transcription in and PMN adhesion to infected bovine endothelial cells. Int J Parasitol 36:423–431
5. Behrendt JH, Ruiz A, Zahner H, Taubert A, Hermosilla C (2010) Neutrophil extracellular trap formation as innate immune reactions against the apicomplexan parasite *Eimeria bovis*. Vet Immunol Immunopathol 133:1–8
6. Brinkmann V, Reichard U, Goosmann C, Fauler B, Uhlemann Y, Weiss DS, Weinrauch Y, Zychlinsky A (2004) Neutrophil extracellular traps kill bacteria. Science 303:1532–1535
7. Fuchs TA, Abed U, Goosmann C, Hurwitz R, Schulze I, Wahn V, Weinrauch Y, Brinkmann V, Zychlinsky A (2007) Novel cell death program leads to neutrophil extracellular traps. J Cell Biol 176:231–241
8. Köckritz-Blickwede M, Chow O, Ghochani M, Nizet V (2010) Visualization and functional evaluation of phagocyte extracellular traps. Method Microbiol 37:139–160
9. Guimarães-Costa AB, Nascimento MT, Wardini AB, Pinto-da-Silva LH, Saraiva EM (2012) ETosis: a microbicidal mechanism beyond cell death. J Parasitol Res 2012:929743
10. Brinkmann V, Zychlinsky A (2007) Beneficial suicide: why neutrophils die to make NETs. Nat Rev Microbiol 5:577–582
11. Brinkmann V, Zychlinsky A (2012) Neutrophil extracellular traps: is immunity the second function of chromatin? J Cell Biol 198:773–783
12. Abi Abdallah DS, Lin C, Ball CJ, King MR, Duhamel GE, Denkers EY (2012) *Toxoplasma gondii* triggers release of human and mouse neutrophil extracellular traps. Infect Immun 80:768–777
13. Hermosilla C, Munoz Caro T, Silva LM, Ruiz A, Taubert A (2014) The intriguing host innate immune response: novel anti-parasitic defence by neutrophil extracellular traps. Parasitology 141:1489–1498

14. Guimarães-Costa AB, Nascimento MT, Froment GS, Soares RP, Morgado FN, Conceição-Silva F, Saraiva EM (2009) *Leishmania amazonensis* promastigotes induce and are killed by neutrophil extracellular traps. Proc Natl Acad Sci U S A 106:6748–6753
15. Baker VS, Imade GE, Molta NB, Tawde P, Pam SD, Obadofin MO, Sagay SA, Egah DZ, Iya D, Afolabi BB, Baker M, Ford K, Ford R, Roux KH, Keller TC 3rd (2008) Cytokine-associated neutrophil extracellular traps and antinuclear antibodies in *Plasmodium falciparum* infected children under six years of age. Malar J 7:41
16. Silva LMR, Muñoz Caro T, Rüdiger G, Vila-Viçosa MJM, Cortes HC, Hermosilla T, Taubert A: (2014) The apicomplexan parasite *Eimeria arloingi* induces caprine neutrophil extracellular traps. Parasitol Res 113:2797–2807
17. Muñoz Caro T, Hermosilla C, Silva LMR, Cortes H, Taubert A (2014) Neutrophil extracellular traps as innate immune reaction against the emerging apicomplexan parasite *Besnoitia besnoiti*. PLoS One 9:e91415
18. Aulik NA, Hellenbrand KM, Klos H, Czuprynski CJ (2010) Mannheimia haemolytica and its leukotoxin cause neutrophil extracellular trap formation by bovine neutrophils. Infect Immun 78:4454–4466
19. Juneau RA, Pang B, Weimer KE, Armbruster CE, Swords WE (2011) Nontypeable *Haemophilus influenzae* initiates formation of neutrophil extracellular traps. Infect Immun 79:431–438
20. Gupta AK, Giaglis S, Hasler P, Hahn S (2014) Efficient neutrophil extracellular trap induction requires mobilization of both intracellular and extracellular calcium pools and is modulated by cyclosporine A. PLoS One 9:e97088
21. Byrd AS, O'Brien XM, Johnson CM, Lavigne LM, Reichner JS (2013) An extracellular matrix–based mechanism of rapid neutrophil extracellular trap formation in response to *Candida albicans*. J Immunol 190:4136–4148
22. Hermosilla C, Barbisch B, Heise A, Kowalik S, Zahner H (2002) Development of *Eimeria bovis* in vitro: suitability of several bovine, human and porcine endothelial cell lines, bovine fetal gastrointestinal, Madin-Darby bovine kidney (MDBK) and African green monkey kidney (VERO) cells. Parasitol Res 88:301–307
23. Pinckney RD, Lindsay DS, Toivio-Kinnucan MA, Blagburn BL (1993) Ultrastructure of *Isospora suis* during excystation and attempts to demonstrate extraintestinal stages in mice. Vet Parasitol 47:225–233
24. Freyre A, Falcón J (2004) Massive excystation of *Toxoplasma gondii* sporozoites. Exp Parasitol 107:72–77
25. Hidalgo MA, Ojeda F, Eyre P, LaBranche TP, Smith C, Hancke JL, Burgos RA (2004) Platelet-activating factor increases pH(i) in bovine neutrophils through the PI3K–ERK1/2 pathway. Br J Pharmacol 141:311–321
26. Hidalgo MA, Nahuelpan C, Manosalva C, Jara E, Carretta MD, Conejeros I, Loaiza A, Chihuailaf R, Burgos RA (2011) Oleic acid induces intracellular calcium mobilization MAPK phosphorylation, superoxide production and granule release in bovine neutrophils. Biochem Biophys Res Commun 409:280–286
27. Martinelli S, Urosevic M, Daryadel A, Oberholzer PA, Baumann C, Fey MF, Dummer R, Simon HU, Yousefi S (2004) Induction of genes mediating interferon-dependent extracellular trap formation during neutrophil differentiation. J Biol Chem 279:44123–44132
28. Hermosilla C, Stamm I, Taubert A, Lutz K, Zahner H, Menge C (2008) Fluorescent *Eimeria bovis* sporozoites and meront stages in vitro: a helpful tool to study parasite-host cell interactions. Parasitol Res 102:777–786
29. Scapinello S, Brooks AS, MacInnes JI, Hammermueller J, Clark ME, Caswell JL (2011) Bactericidal activity of porcine neutrophil secretions. Vet Immunol Immunopathol 139:113–118
30. Parker H, Albrett AM, Kettle AJ, Winterbourn CC (2012) Myeloperoxidase associated with neutrophil extracellular traps is active and mediates bacterial killing in the presence of hydrogen peroxide. J Leukoc Biol 91:369–376
31. Conejeros I, Patterson R, Burgos RA, Hermosilla C, Werling D (2011) Induction of reactive oxygen species in bovine neutrophils is CD11b, but not dectin-1-dependent. Vet Immunol Immunopathol 139:308–312
32. Conejeros I, Jara E, Carretta MD, Alarcón P, Hidalgo MA, Burgos RA (2012) 2-Aminoethoxydiphenyl borate (2-APB) reduces respiratory burst, MMP-9 release and CD11b expression, and increases l-selectin shedding in bovine neutrophils. Res Vet Sci 92:103–110
33. Gupta AK, Joshi MB, Philippova M, Erne P, Hasler P, Hahn S, Resink TJ (2010) Activated endothelial cells induce neutrophil extracellular traps and are susceptible to NETosis-mediated cell death. FEBS Lett 584:3193–3197
34. Hallett MB, Davies EV, Campbell AK (1990) Oxidase activation in individual neutrophils is dependent on the onset and magnitude of the Ca2+ signal. Cell Calcium 11:655–663
35. Hakkim A, Fuchs TA, Martinez NE, Hess S, Prinz H (2011) Activation of the Raf-MEK-ERK pathway is required for neutrophil extracellular trap formation. Nat Chem Biol 7:75–77
36. Wang X, Mori T, Jung JC, Fini ME, Lo EH (2002) Secretion of matrix metalloproteinase-2 and -9 after mechanical trauma injury in rat cortical cultures and involvement of MAP kinase. J Neurotrauma 19:615–625
37. Carmona-Rivera C, Zhao W, Yalavarthi S, Kaplan MJ. Neutrophil extracellular traps induce endothelial dysfunction in systemic lupus erythematosus through the activation of matrix metalloproteinase-2. Ann Rheum Dis. in press.
38. Sumagin R, Robin AZ, Nusrat A, Parkos CA (2014) Transmigrated neutrophils in the intestinal lumen engage ICAM-1 to regulate the epithelial barrier and neutrophil recruitment. Mucosal Immunol 7:905–915

Grazing livestock are exposed to terrestrial cyanobacteria

Bruce C McGorum[1*], R Scott Pirie[1], Laura Glendinning[1], Gerry McLachlan[1], James S Metcalf[2], Sandra A Banack[2], Paul A Cox[2] and Geoffrey A Codd[3]

Abstract

While toxins from aquatic cyanobacteria are a well-recognised cause of disease in birds and animals, exposure of grazing livestock to terrestrial cyanobacteria has not been described. This study identified terrestrial cyanobacteria, predominantly *Phormidium* spp., in the biofilm of plants from most livestock fields investigated. Lower numbers of other cyanobacteria, microalgae and fungi were present on many plants. Cyanobacterial 16S rDNA, predominantly from *Phormidium* spp., was detected in all samples tested, including 6 plant washings, 1 soil sample and ileal contents from 2 grazing horses. Further work was performed to test the hypothesis that ingestion of cyanotoxins contributes to the pathogenesis of some currently unexplained diseases of grazing horses, including equine grass sickness (EGS), equine motor neuron disease (EMND) and hepatopathy. *Phormidium* population density was significantly higher on EGS fields than on control fields. The cyanobacterial neurotoxic amino acid 2,4-diaminobutyric acid (DAB) was detected in plant washings from EGS fields, but worst case scenario estimations suggested the dose would be insufficient to cause disease. Neither DAB nor the cyanobacterial neurotoxins β-N-methylamino-L-alanine and N-(2-aminoethyl) glycine were detected in neural tissue from 6 EGS horses, 2 EMND horses and 7 control horses. *Phormidium* was present in low numbers on plants where horses had unexplained hepatopathy. This study did not yield evidence linking known cyanotoxins with disease in grazing horses. However, further study is warranted to identify and quantify toxins produced by cyanobacteria on livestock fields, and determine whether, under appropriate conditions, known or unknown cyanotoxins contribute to currently unexplained diseases in grazing livestock.

Introduction

Cyanobacteria are a diverse group of ubiquitous environmental bacteria which can produce a wide array of toxins (cyanotoxins). While exposure to cyanotoxins from aquatic cyanobacterial blooms, scums and mats is a well-recognised cause of neurologic and hepatic disease in birds and animals [1], exposure of grazing livestock to terrestrial, as opposed to aquatic, cyanobacteria has not been previously described. We hypothesised that grazing livestock are exposed to *Phormidium* spp. since this cyanobacterial genus can grow on turf grasses and golf courses, particularly in favourable weather conditions and following fertiliser application [2-6]. Cyanobacteria including *Phormidium* spp. can produce a wide range of hepato-, neuro- and dermotoxins which cause disease in animals exposed to aquatic cyanobacterial blooms [7-10]. While exposure to anatoxin-a from the benthic cyanobacterium *Phormidium favosum* has been associated with canine neurotoxicosis [9], toxins from terrestrial *Phormidium* spp. have not been previously definitively associated with disease. We hypothesised that cyanotoxins from terrestrial *Phormidium* spp. may trigger or cause currently unexplained diseases of grazing livestock such as equine grass sickness (EGS), a frequently fatal multi-system neuropathy affecting grazing horses, equine motor neuron disease (EMND) and idiopathic hepatopathy. The aims of this study were to: (a) identify and enumerate *Phormidium* filaments in washings of the biofilm on plants collected from livestock-grazing fields; (b) evaluate spatial and temporal variation in the density of *Phormidium* filaments; (c) determine whether *Phormidium* filaments can be detected by microscopy in gastrointestinal contents from grazing horses; and (d) use a genomic approach to identify cyanobacteria in plant washings, equine ileal contents and soil. Additionally, a

* Correspondence: Bruce.mcgorum@ed.ac.uk
[1]Royal (Dick) School of Veterinary Studies and Roslin Institute, University of Edinburgh, Roslin EH25 9RG, Scotland, UK
Full list of author information is available at the end of the article

preliminary investigation of the potential association of cyanotoxins and EGS, EMND and hepatopathy was performed by: (a) comparing the density of *Phormidium* filaments on plants from horse fields immediately after an occurrence of EGS with that of plants from control horse fields; (b) quantifying the cyanobacterial neurotoxins 2,4-diaminobutyric acid [DAB], β-N-methylamino-L-alanine [BMAA] and N-(2-aminoethyl) glycine [AEG] in washings from plants collected from EGS fields; (c) quantifying DAB, BMAA and AEG in archived neural tissue from EGS and EMND horses; and (d) enumerating *Phormidium* spp. in washings of the biofilm on plants collected from fields grazed by horses which had idiopathic hepatopathy.

Materials and methods

Collection of plants

Most plants were collected from livestock-grazing fields ($n = 88$) in Scotland and North England. Most fields were grazed by horses (40 fields; termed horse control fields), cattle (13 fields) or sheep (14 fields) that had no apparent clinical neurological or hepatic disease, although detailed veterinary examinations were not performed. The remaining samples were collected from 21 "EGS" fields as soon as possible (always <96 h) after a horse grazing that field had developed acute EGS. EGS was confirmed by histopathology of autonomic and enteric ganglia [11]. Plants were collected by carefully cutting leaves/petioles with scissors approximately 1 cm above soil level, avoiding sampling of roots and adherent soil. To ensure that plant samples were representative of the entire field, samples comprised a mixture of ≥10 aliquots collected from points situated along an imaginary "W" transect, and comprised plants that were representative of the distribution of species present on the field. The varied mixtures of plants were typical of those growing on livestock grazing fields in Northern Britain. In horse fields, plants were collected only from grazed areas and not from non-grazed "roughs". Samples were analysed within 4 h of collection, or were rapidly frozen within 30 min of collection by mixing with dry ice pellets and then stored in airtight polythene bags at −20 °C or −80 °C pending analysis.

To determine whether there was spatial variation in the density of *Phormidium* filaments within individual fields, samples were collected separately from 10 individual sites along the "W" transect in 2 fields, comprising one EGS field which had high overall *Phormidium* filament population density and one horse control field which had low overall density.

Two experiments were performed to determine whether there was temporal variation in the density of *Phormidium* filaments. To assess short-term variation, *Phormidium* filament population density was determined in samples collected from 9 fields (3 EGS, 6 horse control fields) at both 0700 and 1900 h. To assess longer term variation, *Phormidium* filament density was determined in samples collected from 8 fields at approximately weekly intervals from April to July 2006, including the period of highest incidence of EGS which is typically May in the UK [12]. One of these fields was a control horse field, while 7 were fields where at least one EGS case had occurred in the preceding 2 years; none of the fields had EGS cases during the sampling year. To determine if *Phormidium* filament density was influenced by weather, densities for the 8 individual fields were correlated with average daily air temperature, rainfall and sunshine hours, using data from a Meteorological Office weather station located within 48 km of all fields.

Unfortunately it was not possible to assess the population density of *Phormidium* filaments on fields grazed by EMND horses due to the rarity and sporadic occurrence of this disease [13]. Plants were also collected from 22 fields in France where the grazing horses had idiopathic subclinical hepatopathy, as evidenced by elevated serum activities of gamma glutamyltransferase and glutamate dehydrogenase. Despite extensive investigation, no aetiology had been identified. Samples were collected as described previously, but were kept on ice for 24 h before analysis.

Enumeration of *Phormidium* filaments on plants

To suspend cyanobacteria that were adherent to plants, 20 mL sterile 0.9% saline was added to 10 g wet weight plants in a 50 mL plastic tube which was shaken vigorously by hand for 1 min. As a pilot study indicated that vigorous vortexing (Shaker VX-2500 Multi-Tube Vortexer, VWR International, Lutterworth, UK) of the plant suspension for 0, 1, 2 and 18 h had no significant effect on the yield of free filaments (data not presented), this method was not further employed. A 20 μL aliquot of the suspension was removed immediately after shaking, placed on a microscope slide, a cover-slip added and the total number of *Phormidium* filaments enumerated. The remaining suspension was frozen at −80 °C for future analysis.

Detection of cyanobacterial 16S rDNA in plant washings, soil and equine ileal contents

To confirm identify of cyanobacteria within samples, 16S rDNA amplicons were prepared from plant washings from 6 EGS fields, soil from 1 EGS field and ileal contents from 2 EGS horses and sequenced using an Illumina MiSeq. Ileal contents were harvested within 2 h of death and stored at −80 °C pending analysis. Soil was collected from an EGS field, at a depth of 2–10 cm, and stored at −80 °C pending analysis. The MO-BIO Powersoil DNA Isolation Kit was used to extract total sample DNA following manufacturer's instructions. Before bead beating, samples were heated at 65 °C for 10 min to increase cell lysis. 100 ng DNA was used in a two-round nested PCR protocol to amplify the V2-V3 region of the 16S gene. All PCR steps used the Q5 High-Fidelity 2X Master Mix (New England Biolabs). The first round of PCR consisted of 20 cycles using the primers 28 F (5' GAGTTTGATCNTGGCTCAG 3') and 805R (5' GACTACCAGGGTATCTAATC 3') in a total reaction volume of 50 μL. The reaction ran at 94 °C for 2 min, 20 cycles of 94 °C for 1 min, 55 °C for 45 s, 72 °C for 1.5 min followed by 72 °C for 20 min. After each PCR round, AMPure XP PCR Purification (Agencourt) was used to purify amplified DNA from other components of the reaction mixture. Purified PCR product (20 μL) was added into the second round of PCR along with the mastermix and barcoded primers 104 F (5' GGCGVACGGGTGAGTAA 3') and 519R (5' GTNTTACNGCGGCKGCTG 3') to a total volume of 50 μL. Primers include adapter sequences required for binding to the Illumina flow cell and barcodes for multiplexing. The reaction conditions were 98 °C for 30 s followed by 20 cycles of 98 °C for 10 s, 67 °C for 30 s, 72 °C for 10 s, and 72 °C for 2 min. 250 bp paired-end sequencing was performed using an Illumina Miseq.

Bioinformatic analysis

Primers were removed using CUTADAPT [14] (allowing 1 bp error per 10 bp). MOTHUR [15] was used for quality control and for taxonomic assignment of reads, following a protocol developed for MiSeq by MOTHUR creators [16]. Sequences were removed from analysis if they were of length <350 bp, contained homopolymers of >9 bp or ambiguous base calls, did not align to the SILVA reference alignment [17], were identified as chimeric using UCHIME [18] or were classified as other than bacterial. Taxonomic classification was done using MOTHUR's Bayesian classifier against the Greengenes database [19] trimmed to the V2-V3 16S region [20]. Sequences were assigned taxonomy if there was a >80% chance of correct assignment.

Microscopic examination for cyanobacteria in equine gastrointestinal tract samples

To determine whether cyanobacteria were detectable microscopically in gastrointestinal contents of grazing horses, conventional light and fluorescence microscopy was performed on saline suspensions of freshly collected luminal contents from the stomach ($n = 2$), jejunum ($n = 2$), ileum ($n = 4$), caecum ($n = 2$) and colon ($n = 2$) of horses with acute EGS, and of faeces from 2 horses with chronic EGS and 2 healthy control horses.

Analysis for DAB, BMAA and AEG in plant washings and equine neural tissue

DAB, BMAA and AEG were assayed using UPLC-MS/MS as previously described [21,22] in plant washing pellets from 3 EGS fields after 6 M HCl hydrolysis. The hydrolysate was centrifuge filtered, dried and derivatised with AQC for UPLC-MS/MS analysis, in comparison with synthetic standards [21]. Plant washing pellets were prepared by adding plants (5 g wet mass for sample 1, 6 g for samples 2 and 3) to 10 mL saline, shaking vigorously for 1 min, decanting the fluid, then ultracentrifugation at 13 000 rpm for 10 min before discarding the supernatant. These data were used to calculate the estimated daily DAB intake by a horse grazing for 24 h on each of these EGS fields.

DAB, BMAA and AEG were also assayed in archived formalin-fixed, wax-embedded, neural tissue from EGS and EMND-affected horses and from control horses. Sample 1 (EGS) comprised a pool of cranial cervical (superior) ganglia (CCG) from 6 different EGS-affected horses (mix breed and gender, median age 6 years, range 3–20). EGS was confirmed by histopathology of autonomic and enteric ganglia in all cases [11]. Sample 2 (control) comprised a pool of CCG from 6 different control horses (mix breed and gender; 14, 6–30 years) which were euthanased because of non-neurological disorders. Sample 3 (EMND) comprised pooled neural tissues from a 9 year-old Thoroughbred cross mare that had EMND confirmed at necropsy, including CCG, transverse segments of spinal cord at C1-2, C4-5, C7, C8, T1, T5, L6, S1 and rostral medulla oblongata. Sample 4 (EMND) was a sample of sacrococcygeus dorsalis muscle from a 6 year-old Cob gelding which had EMND. Sample 5 (control) was a wax-embedded formalin-fixed sample of medulla from a 20 year-old Thoroughbred cross mare that had no apparent neurologic disease. Neural samples were excised from formalin-fixed blocks, deparaffinised, washed with xylenes and hydrated using an alcohol series [23]. The subsequent material was hydrolysed with 6 M HCl for 16 h, the supernatant centrifuge filtered and dried in a speedvac. Once dry, the residue was resuspended with 20 mM HCl and derivatised with AQC for UPLC-MS/MS analysis of BMAA and its isomers.

Statistical analysis

Data were not normally distributed. Inter- and within-group comparisons were made using the Mann Whitney and Wilcoxon Rank Sum tests, respectively. Correlations were done using Spearman's Rank correlation. The spatial variability in *Phormidium* filament population density within a field was determined by calculating the coefficient of variance for 10 individual samples collected from that field.

Results

Identification of cyanobacteria in plant samples

During sample collection it was noted that some plants, particularly at the base and branching points, had a slimy coating of mucilage consistent with that produced by cyanobacteria and algae [24]. Light and fluorescence microscopy revealed that these areas had a biofilm containing numerous cyanobacterial filaments. Microscopic examination of plant washings indicated that cyanobacteria were predominantly *Phormidium* spp. (Figure 1), with filaments in washings from many fresh samples exhibiting typical spontaneous oscillatory motion [25]. The numbers of cells per *Phormidium* filament on horse (median 16, range 3–67; $n = 281$), cattle (14, 6–56; $n = 36$) and sheep (18, range 4–76; $n = 85$) fields were not significantly different. Some plant samples also had low numbers of a second, very narrow filamentous cyanobacterium of the *Leptolyngbya* or *Leptothrix* genera, and low numbers of unicellular cyanobacteria of the *Aphanocapsa* genus. Many samples also had filamentous green algae, unicellular green algae, and low numbers of diatoms, motile algal flagellates and desmids (*Closterium* sp.): these were not enumerated.

Density of *Phormidium* filaments in plant samples

Phormidium filaments were present in samples from all EGS ($n = 21$) fields and most horse control (29/40), cattle (11/13) and sheep (13/14) fields. *Phormidium* filament population density was significantly higher in EGS fields (median 2400, range 100–68 900 filaments g wet mass plants^{-1}) than in horse control (250, 0–4200; $p < 0.0001$), cattle (300, 0–1400; $p = 0.0002$) and sheep (700, 0–3300; $p = 0.0012$) fields (Figure 2). There were no significant differences in density among horse

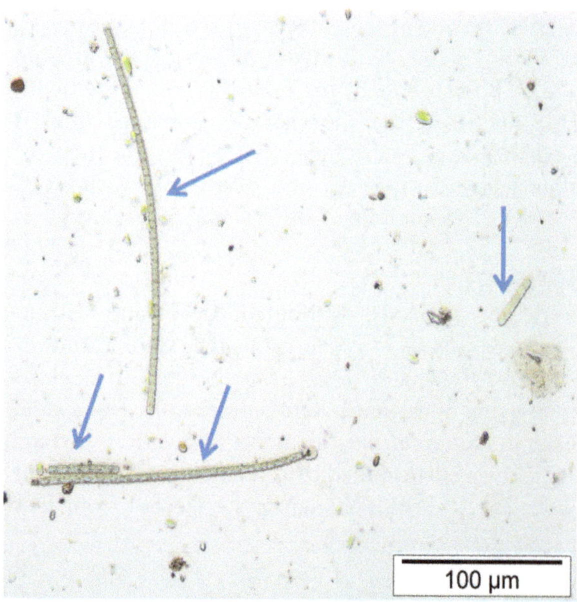

Figure 1 Microscopic appearance of *Phormidium* filaments. Four *Phormidium* filaments (arrows) in plant washings. Unstained specimen.

control, cattle and sheep fields. There was marked spatial variation in *Phormidium* filament population density across transects in an EGS field (coefficient of variance 126%) and a horse control field (143%) (Figure 3). There was marked variation, but no significant difference, in *Phormidium* filament population density in samples collected from 9 horse control fields at 0700 h and 1900 h, with density at 1900 h increased in 5 fields and reduced in 3 fields (Figure 4). There was no apparent consistent pattern to the weekly changes in population density in samples collected from 8 horse fields between April and July (Figure 5), and *Phormidium* filament population density in these samples was not significantly correlated with average air temperature, rainfall or sunshine hours. A low density (50, 50, 100 filaments g wet mass plants^{-1}) of *Phormidium* filaments was present in only 3/22 samples from the French fields.

Genomic identification of cyanobacteria in EGS plant washings, soil and equine ileal contents

Cyanobacterial 16S rDNA sequences were detected in all samples tested (see Additional file 1). Most sequences were attributable to unclassified *Phormidium*. The following sequences were identified; *Anabaena cylindrica* (1 plant washing), 1 unclassified *Nostoc* sp. (2 plant washings), 1 unclassified *Nostocaceae* fam. (2 plant washings), *Phormidium animale* (4 plant washings), 1 unclassified *Phormidium* sp. (6 plant washings, 2 ileal contents), 1 unclassified *Phormidium* sp. (2 plant washings), 1 unclassified *Phormidiaceae* fam. (2 plant washings), 1 unclassified *Oscillatoriales* ord. (1 plant washing), 1 unclassified *Oscillatoriophycideae* class (2 plant washings), *Leptolyngbya frigida* (1 plant washing), 1 unclassified *Leptolyngbya* sp. (1 plant washing), 1 unclassified *Pseudanabaenaceae* fam. (1 plant washing), 1 unclassified *Cyanobacteria* phylum (4 plant washings) and 1 unclassified *Cyanobacteria* phylum (3 plant washings). rDNA from 3 lines of *Melainabacteria* were identified; YS2/4C0d-2 (1 soil sample), mle1-12 (5 plant washings, 1 ileal contents, 1 soil sample) and ML635J-21 (5 plant washings, 1 soil sample). Additionally, rDNA from DAB-producing actinomycetes, including *Clavibacter* spp. and *Rathayibacter* spp., was detected in 6 plant washings and soil.

Examination of cyanobacteria in equine gastrointestinal tract samples

No intact cyanobacteria were apparent. Gastric contents from 2 EGS horses appeared to contain occasional highly degraded and apparently non-viable *Phormidium* filaments.

Analysis for DAB, BMAA and AEG

DAB was detected in all 3 plant washing pellets. Mean free and bound DAB concentrations (pg filament^{-1}),

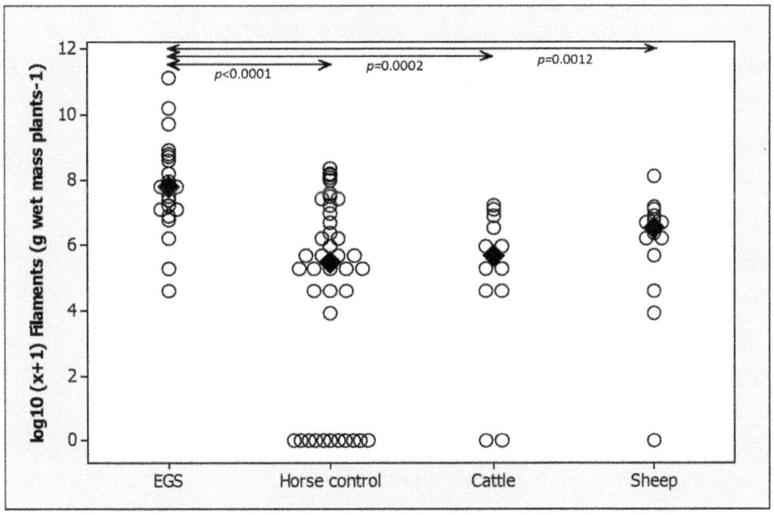

Figure 2 Plants from EGS fields had significantly higher population densities of *Phormidium* filaments than plants from other fields. Population density of *Phormidium* filaments ($\log_{10}$ [x + 1] g wet mass plants^{-1}) on plants from EGS ($n = 21$), horse control ($n = 40$), cattle ($n = 13$) and sheep ($n = 14$) fields. Medians and inter-group significances are marked.

respectively were: pellet 1, 43.5, 355.2; pellet 2, 121.6, 2131.4; pellet 3, 0.4, 8.2. BMAA and AEG were not detected in plant washings. BMAA, AEG and DAB were not detected in neural tissues at minimum detection limits 0.0065 picomoles per injection for L-BMAA and AEG and 0.0013 picomoles per injection for DAB.

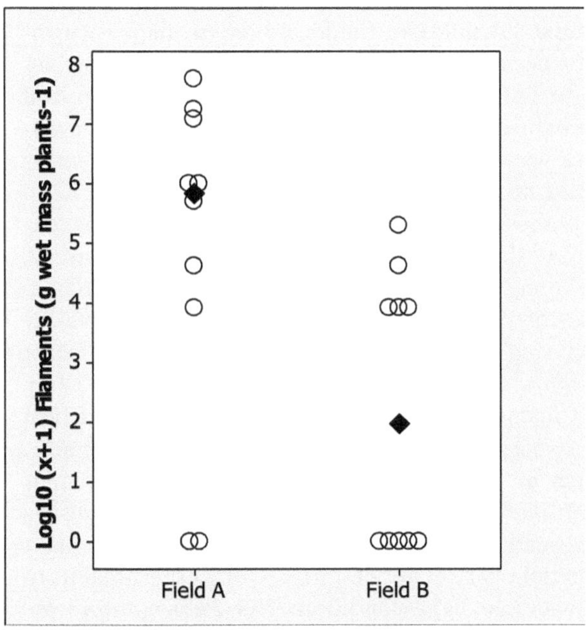

Figure 3 Population densities of *Phormidium* filaments varied considerably, both within and between fields. Spatial variation in density of *Phormidium* filaments ($\log_{10}$ [x + 1] g wet mass plants^{-1}) across transects in an EGS field **(A)** and a horse control field **(B)**. Each datum point represents the density for each of 10 points across the field transect. Medians are marked.

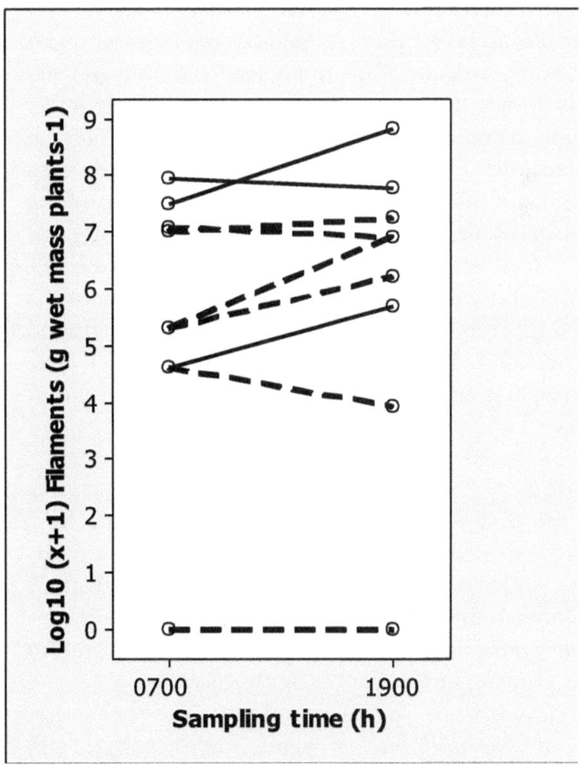

Figure 4 Population densities of *Phormidium* filaments on plants collected at 0700 h and 1900 h did not differ significantly. Comparison of the population density of *Phormidium* filaments ($\log_{10}$ [x + 1] g wet mass plants^{-1}) in 9 fields (3 EGS fields with solid line, 6 horse control fields with broken line) in samples collected at 0700 h and 1900 h (data not significantly different). Medians are marked.

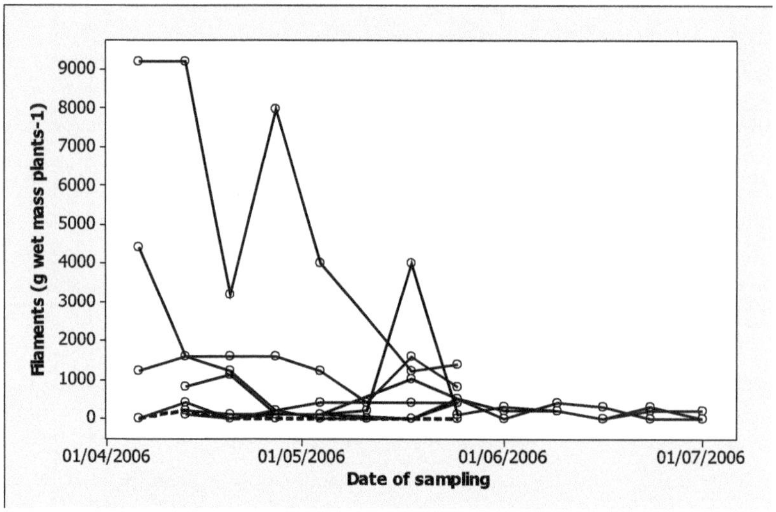

Figure 5 Weekly variation in population density of *Phormidium* filaments on plants. Weekly variation in population density of *Phormidium* filaments (g wet mass plants^{-1}) on plants from one horse control (broken line) field and 7 fields (solid lines) on which there was at least one case of EGS within the preceding 2 years.

Estimation of the worst case scenario daily intake of *Phormidium* filaments and DAB for horses grazing EGS fields

Worst case scenario estimation of daily intake of *Phormidium* filaments for a horse grazing fulltime on the field with the highest *Phormidium* filament population density (68 900 filaments g wet weight plants^{-1}) is 7.6×10^6 filaments kg^{-1}. This estimation assumes that an average 500 kg horse consumes 11.5 kg of herbage dry matter daily, with a typical mean dry matter of 21% [26], equating to 55 kg wet herbage daily. The estimated daily intakes of DAB (mg kg^{-1}) for horses grazing the 3 EGS fields are: Field 1 (free 0.017; bound 0.14; total 0.16); Field 2 (free 0.007; bound 0.12; total 0.12); Field 3 (free 0.004; bound 0.08; total 0.09). Plant-washing pellets 1, 2 and 3 contained, respectively, 2700, 450 and 82 050 *Phormidium* filaments.

Discussion

This is the first study to demonstrate that grazing livestock are exposed to pasture-derived terrestrial cyanobacteria, -microalgae (diatoms, *Closterium*) and their toxins. Indeed, the most commonly identified cyanobacteria, *Phormidium* spp., were identified within the biofilm of plants growing in most of the fields examined.

There was marked spatial variation in the population density of *Phormidium* on plants, both within and between fields, with counts ranging from 0–68 900 filaments g wet plants^{-1}. Repeat sampling at 12 h and weekly intervals suggested there was also apparent marked temporal variation in *Phormidium* population density, although some of this variability could have reflected spatial variation. *Phormidium* density did not appear to follow a consistent diurnal or weekly pattern and was not apparently correlated with average daily air temperature, rainfall or sunshine hours. However these latter findings should be interpreted with caution since these relationships were assessed under limited circumstances and further detailed investigation is required to clarify the influence of weather on *Phormidium* density. Variation in *Phormidium* population density presumably reflects the suitability of the local biofilm microenvironment for cyanobacterial growth and survival. Factors reported to influence cyanobacterial growth and survival include light duration and irradiance, temperature, availability of water, phosphate-, iron- and nitrate concentrations, and numbers of invertebrate prey species [27,28]. We hypothesise that high exposure levels may be encountered when environmental conditions are optimal, as occurs on turf grasses [2-6], a situation akin to the occurrence of cyanobacterial blooms in aquatic environments during eutrophication [29,30]. Indeed the highest *Phormidium* population density recorded in the study (68 900 filaments g wet plants^{-1}) was a clear statistical outlier suggesting that it could be considered to represent such a "bloom" occurrence. Variation in apparent *Phormidium* density also likely reflects the organism's motility, with filaments moving up and down plant leaves/petioles at up to 11 μm s^{-1} [31], presumably to seek favourable light conditions. As *Phormidium* spp. are more likely to be present at the tips of short plants than long plants [5], *Phormidium* population density within plant washings may also reflect plant length and the proportion of lower and upper leaves/petioles sampled. This study may have underestimated *Phormidium* density because an indeterminate number of cyanobacteria may have remained adherent within the plant biofilm despite vigorous shaking. While the *Phormidium* spp. were readily enumerated in plant washings, many of the aforementioned factors which influence *Phormidium* population density will compromise accurate estimation of the number of *Phormidium* filaments ingested by grazing animals. For example, since there was considerable spatial and temporal variation in cyanobacterial density, the number of cyanobacteria ingested may be markedly higher in an animal grazing a cyanobacterium-rich area of grassland. In a worst-case scenario estimation, a 500 kg horse grazing fulltime on the EGS field with the highest *Phormidium* population density (68 900 filaments g wet mass plants^{-1}) and a median number of 16 cells filament^{-1}, would ingest 7.6×10^6 *Phormidium* filaments kg^{-1} day^{-1}or 121×10^6 *Phormidium* cells kg^{-1} day^{-1}.

Ingestion of terrestrial cyanobacteria provides one explanation for the presence of cyanobacterial 16S rDNA in the 2 equine ileal samples in this study. It also provides a more plausible explanation for the previous report of cyanobacterial 16S rDNA in faeces from forage-fed horses than them being homologous sequences from dietary plant chloroplasts [32]. Alternative explanations include ingestion of aquatic cyanobacteria from contaminated water sources and ingestion of foods containing cyanobacterial supplements. Cyanobacterial 16S rDNA sequences detected in ileal contents was attributable to unclassified *Phormidium* spp. (2 horses) and a bacterium of the Order mle1-12 (1 horse). The latter has recently been proposed as a member of a candidate class [33] or sister phylum [34] of non-photosynthetic, filamentous bacteria termed *Melainabacteria*, distinct from extant cyanobacteria, but with ancestral affiliations. The fate of ingested cyanobacteria is currently receiving increasing attention. The ability of ingested cyanobacteria to colonise the gastrointestinal tract has so far received little attention. Indeed cyanobacterial species in aquatic environments do not typically thrive below about pH 6.7 and cell degradation can occur under acid conditions (Codd, personal observations). Intact cyanobacteria were not identified microscopically in the equine gastrointestinal contents, although gastric contents of 2 EGS horses appeared to contain occasional highly degraded and apparently non-viable *Phormidium* filaments. Similarly cyanobacteria in the rumen and abomasum of cattle dying from acute cyanobacterial poisoning are markedly degraded (Codd, personal observations). While spores (akinetes) produced by some cyanobacteria could potentially survive in the gut, akinete production is not widespread among cyanobacteria and does not occur in *Phormidium* which predominated in this study. Further, it is not known whether akinete germination and outgrowth could occur in the aphotic, anaerobic gut. However, it is known that some species of *Phormidium* (*P. uncinatum*) can grow chemoheterotrophically (aphotic growth on glucose, fructose and acetate at a reduced rate) [35]. Furthermore, recent work indicates that the unicellular aquatic cyanobacterium *Microcystis* PCC7806 can survive and potentially produce cyanotoxins for up to 17 days in an in vitro environment mimicking the human gastrointestinal tract [36]. The possibility of gut colonisation by cyanobacteria is further supported by accumulating evidence that *Melainabacteria*, including the mle1-12 present in 1 horse ileum, have differentiated from extant cyanobacteria by niche adaptation, including for symbiosis in the mammalian gut [34,37-39]. Indeed, *Melainabacteria* is considered to have an obligate fermenter role in the gut, and its enrichment in herbivores may reflect a prominent role in plant fibre digestion [34]. Further work, utilising larger numbers of horses, is required to characterise the populations of cyanobacteria within the equine gastrointestinal tract, and to determine whether they are capable of colonisation and in vivo cyanotoxin production. If so, it would add support to the hypothesis that cyanobacteria, while being typically a minor component of the intestinal microflora, may proliferate and produce neurotoxins in vivo, resulting in neurodegenerative diseases [40].

Further study is warranted to identify and quantify the toxins produced by *Phormidium* from livestock fields and to determine whether under appropriate environmental conditions, grazing livestock can ingest sufficient quantities of cyanotoxins from terrestrial cyanobacteria to cause disease. While the range of toxins produced by *Phormidium* is currently unknown, production of BMAA, LPS, microcystins and anatoxin-a is reported [8,9,41-43]. Extrapolation of data from the related cyanobacterial genus *Oscillatoria* suggests that *Phormidium* may also produce, apslysiatoxins, cylindrospermopsin and homoanatoxin-a. These toxins cause hepatotoxicity, neurotoxicity and dermatitis in animals exposed to aquatic cyanobacterial blooms [7-10]. BMAA has been linked with human motor neuron disease, Alzheimer's disease and Parkinson's disease [44-48] and proposed as a potential cause of equine motor neuron disease [40]. The design of this study precluded definitive examination of potential associations between ingested cyanotoxins and disease in grazing animals. Since livestock grazing the horse control-, cattle- and sheep fields had no overt evidence of hepatic or neurological disease (although veterinary examinations were not performed), cyanotoxin exposure in these fields must have been insufficient to cause clinical disease. Additional experiments were performed to test the hypothesis that, under appropriate circumstances, ingestion of cyanobacterial hepato- and neurotoxins contributes to the pathogenesis of some currently unexplained diseases of grazing horses, including EGS, EMND of grazing horses [13] and hepatopathy.

Phormidium population density was significantly higher on EGS fields than on control fields, indicating that horses grazing EGS fields likely ingest higher numbers of *Phormidium* spp. than horses grazing control fields. This brings into question conclusions of a previous study [26] that cyanotoxins can be excluded as a causative factor for EGS. While the present study assessed exposure of horses to terrestrial cyanobacteria, the previous study [26] investigated only exposure to aquatic cyanobacteria, finding no detectable microcystins and no microscopic evidence of cyanobacteria in water samples from 16 premises on which EGS had occurred. While the cause of EGS is unknown, increasing evidence suggests it is a toxico-infectious form of botulism, whereby a dietary trigger induces intestinal overgrowth of *Clostridium botulinum* C and/or D, with resultant in vivo production of botulinum neurotoxins (reviewed in [49]). Potential involvement of cyanotoxins in EGS could therefore reflect their proposed action as triggers for botulism [50-52] or reflect direct neurotoxic effects of cyanotoxins including microcystins, anatoxin-a, DAB and BMAA [1,8,53]. Alternatively the increased *Phormidium* density on EGS fields may be unrelated to EGS pathogenesis, perhaps simply reflecting the elevated total nitrogen and ammonium nitrogen content of soils on EGS fields [26,54], since nitrate promotes growth of some cyanobacteria [55].

Since DAB, BMAA and AEG were not detected in neural tissues from 6 EGS, 2 EMND horses and 7 control horses, a causal role for these neurotoxins in EGS and EMND could not be demonstrated. DAB was however detected in all washing pellets of plants from 3 EGS fields. While DAB is produced by cyanobacteria, additional sources include plant associated actinomycetes and some leguminous plants [56,57]. Indeed the apparent lack of correlation between DAB concentrations and the concentration of *Phormidium* filaments in the 3 plant washing pellets suggests that DAB was derived from a source other than, or in addition to, *Phormidium*. One further potential source of DAB in grass washings is actinomycetes, including the plant pathogenic *Clavibacter* spp. and *Rathayibacter* spp., since 16S rDNA sequences from these bacteria were detected in 6 plant washings and soil. While the effect of ingested DAB on horses is unknown, the estimated worse-case scenario daily intake of DAB (free 0.017; bound 0.14; total 0.16 mg kg^{-1}) is lower than doses used experimentally to induce neurolathyrism in laboratory animals (from 0.7 to approximately 500 mg kg^{-1} [58-60]).

Phormidium was present only in low numbers in plants collected from fields in France where horses had unexplained hepatopathy, indicating that a role in disease aetiology was unlikely.

This is the first study to demonstrate that grazing livestock are exposed to terrestrial cyanobacteria. While it did not yield evidence linking terrestrial cyanotoxins with neurologic or hepatic disease in grazing horses, further study is required to identify and quantify cyanotoxin exposure in grazing livestock, and to determine whether, under appropriate conditions, terrestrial cyanotoxins contribute to currently unexplained diseases. Additional study is also warranted to further identify cyanobacteria within the gastrointestinal tract of herbivores and determine whether some are capable of intestinal colonisation and in vivo toxin production.

Additional file

Additional file 1: Identity of cyanobacterial 16S rDNA sequences detected in EGS plant washings ($n = 6$), equine ileal contents ($n = 2$) and soil ($n = 1$). Numbers in parentheses refer to numbers of plant washings (P), ileal contents (I) and soil (S) which contained each sequence.

Abbreviations

AEG: N-(2-aminoethyl) glycine; BMAA: β-N-methylamino-L-alanine; CCG: Cervical [superior] ganglia; DAB: 2,4-diaminobutyric acid; EGS: Equine grass sickness; EMND: Equine motor neuron disease.

Competing interests

The authors declare that they have no competing interests.

Authors' contributions

BM conceived the study. BM, SP and GC acquired the samples, and identified and quantified cyanobacteria. LG and GM performed genomics. JM, SB and PC performed cyanotoxin assays. All authors contributed to preparation and approval of the manuscript.

Acknowledgements

This project was funded by The Equine Grass Sickness Fund and the Charles Engelhard Foundation. Laura Glendinning was funded by the BBSRC through the EASTBIO program. We thank Bryony Waggett, Karen Wilson, Emily Price and Douglas Callaghan for assistance with sample collection and processing.

Author details

[1]Royal (Dick) School of Veterinary Studies and Roslin Institute, University of Edinburgh, Roslin EH25 9RG, Scotland, UK. [2]The Institute for Ethnomedicine, 240 East Deloney Avenue, Jackson, WY 83001-3464, USA. [3]Biological and Environmental Sciences, School of Natural Sciences, University of Stirling, Stirling FK9 4LA, Scotland, UK.

References

1. Codd GA, Lindsay J, Young FM, Morrison LF, Metcalf JS (2005) Cyanobacterial Toxins. In: Huisman J, Matthijs HCP, Visser PM (ed) Harmful Cyanobacteria. Springer-Verlag, London, pp 1–23
2. Baldwin NA, Whitton BA (1992) Cyanobacteria and eukaryotic algae in sports turf and amenity grasslands: a review. J App Phycol 4:39–47
3. Hodges CF, Campbell DA (1997) Nutrient salts and the toxicity of black-layer induced by cyanobacteria and *Desulfovibrio desulfuricans* to *Agrostis palustris*. Plant Soil 195:53–60
4. Elliott ML (1998) Use of fungicides to control blue-green algae on Bermuda grass putting-green surfaces. Crop Protection 11:631–637
5. Gelernter W, Stowell LJ (2000) Cyanobacteria (A.K.A. blue-green algae): wanted for causing serious damage to turf. PACE Insights 6:1–4
6. Tredway LP, Stowell LJ, Gelertner WD (2006) Yellow spot and the potential role of cyanobacteria as turf grass pathogens. Golf course management. PACE Turfgrass Research Institute, San Diego, pp 83–86
7. Skulberg OM, Carmichael WW, Andersen RA, Matsunaga S, Moore RE, Skulberg R (1992) Investigations of a neurotoxic Oscillatorialean strain

(cyanophyceae) and its toxin. Isolation and characterization of homoanatoxin-a. Environ Toxicol Chem 11:321–329
8. Cox PA, Banack SA, Murch SJ, Rasmussen U, Tien G, Bidigare RR, Metcalf J, Morrison LF, Codd JA, Bergman B (2005) Diverse taxa of cyanobacteria produce-N-methylamino-L-alanine, a neurotoxic amino acid. Proc Natl Acad Sci U S A 102:5074–5078
9. Gugger M, Lenoir S, Berger C, Ledreux A, Druart JC, Humbert JF, Guette C, Bernard C (2005) First report in a river in France of the benthic cyanobacterium *Phormidium favosum* producing anatoxin-a associated with dog neurotoxicosis. Toxicon 45:919–928
10. van Apeldoorn ME, van Egmond HP, Speijers GJA, Bakker GJI (2007) Toxins of cyanobacteria. Mol Nutr Food Res 51:7–60
11. Doxey DL, Pogson DM, Milne EM, Gilmour JS, Chisholm HK (1992) Clinical equine dysautonomia and autonomic neuron damage. Res Vet Sci 53:106–109
12. Doxey DL, Gilmour JS, Milne EM (1991) A comparative study of normal equine populations and those with grass sickness (dysautonomia) in eastern Scotland. Equine Vet J 253:365–369
13. McGorum BC, Mayhew IG, Amory H, Deprez P, Gillies L, Green K, Mair TS, Nollet N, Wijnberg I, Hahn C (2006) Horses on pasture may be affected by equine motor neuron disease. Equine Vet J 38:47–51
14. Martin M (2011) Cutadapt removes adapter sequences from high-throughput sequencing reads. EMBnet J 17:10–12
15. Schloss PD, Westcott SL, Ryabin T, Hall JR, Hartmann M, Hollister EB, Lesniewski RA, Oakley BB, Parks DH, Robinson CJ, Sahl JW, Stres B, Thallinger GG, Van Horn DJ, Weber CF (2009) Introducing mothur: open-source, platform-independent, community-supported software for describing and comparing microbial communities. Appl Environ Microbiol 75:7537–7541
16. Kozich JJ, Westcott SL, Baxter NT, Highlander SK, Schloss PD (2013) Development of a dual-index sequencing strategy and curation pipeline for analyzing amplicon sequence data on the MiSeq illumina sequencing platform. Appl Environ Microbiol 79:5112–5120
17. Pruesse E, Quast C, Knittel K, Fuchs BM, Ludwig W, Peplies J, Glöckner FO (2007) SILVA: a comprehensive online resource for quality checked and aligned ribosomal RNA sequence data compatible with ARB. Nucleic Acids Res 35:188–7196
18. Edgar RC, Haas BJ, Clemente JC, Quince C, Knight R (2011) UCHIME improves sensitivity and speed of chimera detection. Bioinformatics 27:2194–2200
19. DeSantis TZ, Hugenholtz P, Larsen N, Rojas M, Brodie EL, Keller K, Huber T, Dalevi D, Hu P, Andersen GL (2006) Greengenes, a chimera-checked 16S rRNA gene database and workbench compatible with ARB. Appl Environ Microbiol 72:5069–5072
20. Werner JJ, Koren O, Hugenholtz P, DeSantis TZ, Walters WA, Caporaso JG, Angenent LT, Knight R, Ley RE (2012) Impact of training sets on classification of high-throughput bacterial 16 s rRNA gene surveys. ISME J 6:94–103
21. Banack SA, Metcalf JS, Jiang L, Craighead D, Ilag LL, Cox PA (2012) Cyanobacteria produce N-(2-Aminoethyl)Glycine, a backbone for peptide nucleic acids which may have been the first genetic molecules for life on Earth. PLoS One 7:e49043
22. Masseret E, Banack SA, Boumediene F, Abadie E, Brient L, Pernet F, Juntas-Morales R, Pageot N, Metcalf J, Cox P, Camu W (2013) The French network on BMAA/ALS. Detection of BMAA in the marine environment of an ALS cluster in Southern France. PLoS One 8:e83406
23. Scicchitano MM, Dalmas DA, Boyce RW, Thomas HC, Frazier KS (2009) Protein extraction of formalin-fixed, paraffin-embedded tissue enables robust proteomic profiles by mass spectrometry. J Histochem Cytochem 57:849–860
24. Sutherland IW (1996) A natural terrestrial biofilm. J Indust Microbiol 17:281–283
25. Richardson LL, Castenholz RW (1989) Chemokinetic motility responses of the cyanobacterium *Oscillatoria terebriformis*. Appl Environ Microbiol 55:261–263
26. Edwards SE, Martz KE, Rogge A, Heinrich M (2010) Edaphic and phytochemical factors as predictors of equine grass sickness cases in the UK. Front Pharmacol 1:122
27. Mur LR (1983) Some aspects of the ecophysiology of cyanobacteria. Ann Microbiol 134B:61–72
28. Agrawal SC, Singh V (2002) Viability of dried filaments, survivability and reproduction under water stress, and survivability following heat and UV exposure in *Lyngbya martensiana, Oscillatoria agardhii, Nostoc calcicola, Hormidium fluitans, Spirogyra sp.* and *Vaucheria geminate*. Folia Microbiol 47:61–67
29. Fogg GE, Stewart WDP, Fay P, Walsby AE (1972) The Blue-Green Algae. Academic Press, London
30. Sutcliffe DW, Jones JG (1992) *Eutrophication: Research and Application to Water Supply*. Windermere, Freshwater Biological Association
31. Staley JT (1986) Bergey's Manual of Systematic Bacteriology, vol 3. Williams and Wilkins, Baltimore
32. Shepherd ML, Swecker WS, Jensen RV, Ponder MA (2012) Characterization of the fecal bacterial communities of forage-fed horses by pyrosequencing of 16S rRNA V4 gene amplicons. FEMS Microbiol Lett 326:62–68
33. Soo RM, Skennerton CT, Sekiguchi Y, Imelfort M, Paech SJ, Dennis PG, Steen JA, Parks DH, Tyson GW, Hugenholtz P (2014) An expanded genomic representation of the phylum Cyanobacteria. Genome Biol Evol 6:1031–1045
34. Di Rienzi SC, Sharon I, Wrighton KC, Koren O, Hug LA, Thomas BC, Goodrich JK, Bell JT, Spector TD, Banfield JF, Ley RE (2013) The human gut and groundwater harbor nonphotosynthetic bacteria belonging to a new candidate phylum sibling to Cyanobacteria. Elife 2:e01102
35. Bagchi SN, Chauhan VS, Palod A (1990) Heterotrophy and nitrate metabolism in a cyanobacterium *Phormidium uncinatum*. Curr Microbiol 21:53–57
36. Stefanelli M, Vichi S, Stipa G, Funari E, Testai E, Scardala S, Manganelli M (2014) Survival, growth and toxicity of *Microcystis aeruginosa* PCC 7806 in experimental conditions mimicking some features of the human gastro-intestinal environment. Chem Biol Interact 215:54–61
37. Backhed F, Ley RE, Sonnenburg JL, Peterson DA, Gordon JI (2005) Host-bacterial mutualism in the human intestine. Science 307:1915–1920
38. Eckburg PB, Bik EM, Bernstein CN, Purdom E, Dethlefsen L, Sargent M, Gill SR, Nelson KE, Relman DA (2005) Diversity of the human intestinal microflora. Science 308:1635–1638
39. Ley R, Backhed F, Turnbaugh P, Lozupone C, Knight R, Gordon J (2005) Obesity alters gut microbial ecology. Proc Natl Acad Sci U S A 102:11070–11075
40. Brenner SR (2013) Blue-green algae or cyanobacteria in the intestinal micro-flora may produce neurotoxins such as Beta-N-Methylamino-L-Alanine (BMAA) which may be related to development of amyotrophic lateral sclerosis, Alzheimer's disease and Parkinson-Dementia-Complex in humans and Equine Motor Neuron Disease in horses. Med Hypotheses 80:103
41. Mikheyskaya LV, Ovodova RG, Ovodov YS (1977) Isolation and characterization of lipopolysaccharides from cell walls of blue-green algae of the genus *Phormidium*. J Bacteriol 130:1–3
42. Codd GA, Bell SG, Kaya K, Ward CJ, Beattie KA, Metcalf JS (1999) Cyanobacterial toxins, exposure routes and human health. Eur J Phycol 34:405–415
43. Aboal M, Puig MA, Asencio AD (2005) Production of microcystins in calcareous Mediterranean streams: the Alharabe River, Segura River basin in south-east Spain. J Appl Phycol 17:231–243
44. Spencer PS, Nunn PB, Hugon J, Ludolph AC, Ross SM, Roy DN, Robertson RC (1987) Guam amyotrophic lateral sclerosis-Parkinsonism-dementia linked to a plant excitant neurotoxin. Science 237:517–522
45. Cox PA, Banack SA, Murch SJ (2003) Biomagnification of cyanobacterial neurotoxins and neurodegenerative disease among the Chamorro people of Guam. Proc Natl Acad Sci U S A 100:13380–13383
46. Bradley WG, Mash DC (2009) Beyond Guam: The cyanobacteria/BMAA hypothesis of the cause of ALS and other neurodegenerative diseases. Amyotroph Lat Scler 10:7–20
47. Pablo J, Banack SA, Cox PA, Johnson TE, Papapetropoulos S, Bradley WG, Buck A, Mash DC (2009) Cyanobacterial neurotoxin BMAA in ALS and Alzheimer's disease. Acta Neurol Scand 120:216–225
48. Chiu AS, Gehringer MM, Welch JH, Neilan BA (2011) Does α-amino-β-methylaminopropionic acid (BMAA) play a role in neurodegeneration? Int J Environ Res Public Health 8:3728–3746
49. Newton JR, Wylie CE, Proudman CJ, McGorum BC, Poxton IR, Overviews S (2010) Equine grass sickness: are we any nearer to answers on its cause and prevention after a century of research? Equine Vet J 42:477–481
50. Eriksson JE, Lindholm T. Sinilevakukintojen aiheuttamat lintu-ja kalakuolemat. Vesistojen levahaitat. Maakunnallinen vesipaiva. Lahtis Motespublikation. 1998; May 18.
51. Mahakhant A, Klungsugya P, Arunpairojana A, Sano T, Watanabe M, Kaya K, Atthasampunna P (1999) Toxicity of cyanobacterial blooms in Thailand. Thailand Institute of Scientific and Technological Research; Research Project No. 39–02
52. Murphy T, Lawson A, Nalewajko C, Murkin H, Ross L, Oguma K, McIntyre T (2000) Algal toxins - initiators of avian botulism? Inc Environ Toxicol 15:558–567
53. Menga G, Suna Y, Fua W, Guob Z, Lihong X (2011) Microcystin-LR induces cytoskeleton system reorganization through hyperphosphorylation of tau and HSP27 via PP2A inhibition and subsequent activation of the p38 MAPK signaling pathway in neuroendocrine (PC12) cells. Toxicol 290:218–229

54. McCarthy HE, French NP, Edwards GB, Miller K, Proudman CJ (2004) Why are certain premises at increased risk of equine grass sickness? A matched case–control study. Equine Vet J 36:130–134
55. Kumar Saha S, Uma L, Subramanian G (2003) Nitrogen stress induced changes in the marine cyanobacterium *Oscillatoria willei* BDU 130511. FEMS Microbiol Ecol 45:263–272
56. Sasaki J, Chijimatsu M, Suzuki K (1998) Taxonomic significance of 2,4-diaminobutyric acid isomers in the cell wall peptidoglycan of actinomycetes and reclassification of *Clavibacter toxicus* as *Rathayibacter toxicus* comb. nov. Int J Syst Bacteriol 48:403–410
57. Kruger T, Monch B, Oppenhauser S, Luckas B (2010) LC–MS/MS determination of the isomeric neurotoxins BMAA (b-N-methylamino-L-alanine) and DAB (2,4-diaminobutyric acid) in cyanobacteria and seeds of *Cycas revoluta* and *Lathyrus latifolius*. Toxicon 55:547–557
58. Ressler C, Redstone PA, Erenberg RH (1961) Isolation and identification of a neuroactive factor from *Lathyrus latifolius*. Science 134:188–190
59. Mushahwar IS, Koeppe RE (1963) Concerning the metabolism of D- and L-α, γ-diaminobutyric acid-2-C14 in rats. J Biol Chem 238:2460–2463
60. Vivanco F, Ramos F, Jimenez-Diaz C (1966) Determination of γ-aminobutyric acid and other free amino acids in whole brains of rats poisoned with β, β'iminodipropionitrile and α, γ- diaminobutyric acid with, or without, administration of thyroxine. J Neurochem 13:1461–1467

Permissions

All chapters in this book were first published in VR, by BioMed Central; hereby published with permission under the Creative Commons Attribution License or equivalent. Every chapter published in this book has been scrutinized by our experts. Their significance has been extensively debated. The topics covered herein carry significant findings which will fuel the growth of the discipline. They may even be implemented as practical applications or may be referred to as a beginning point for another development.

The contributors of this book come from diverse backgrounds, making this book a truly international effort. This book will bring forth new frontiers with its revolutionizing research information and detailed analysis of the nascent developments around the world.

We would like to thank all the contributing authors for lending their expertise to make the book truly unique. They have played a crucial role in the development of this book. Without their invaluable contributions this book wouldn't have been possible. They have made vital efforts to compile up to date information on the varied aspects of this subject to make this book a valuable addition to the collection of many professionals and students.

This book was conceptualized with the vision of imparting up-to-date information and advanced data in this field. To ensure the same, a matchless editorial board was set up. Every individual on the board went through rigorous rounds of assessment to prove their worth. After which they invested a large part of their time researching and compiling the most relevant data for our readers.

The editorial board has been involved in producing this book since its inception. They have spent rigorous hours researching and exploring the diverse topics which have resulted in the successful publishing of this book. They have passed on their knowledge of decades through this book. To expedite this challenging task, the publisher supported the team at every step. A small team of assistant editors was also appointed to further simplify the editing procedure and attain best results for the readers.

Apart from the editorial board, the designing team has also invested a significant amount of their time in understanding the subject and creating the most relevant covers. They scrutinized every image to scout for the most suitable representation of the subject and create an appropriate cover for the book.

The publishing team has been an ardent support to the editorial, designing and production team. Their endless efforts to recruit the best for this project, has resulted in the accomplishment of this book. They are a veteran in the field of academics and their pool of knowledge is as vast as their experience in printing. Their expertise and guidance has proved useful at every step. Their uncompromising quality standards have made this book an exceptional effort. Their encouragement from time to time has been an inspiration for everyone.

The publisher and the editorial board hope that this book will prove to be a valuable piece of knowledge for researchers, students, practitioners and scholars across the globe.

List of Contributors

David Pérez-Pascual
Área de Microbiología, Departamento de Biología Funcional, Facultad de Medicina, IUBA, Universidad de Oviedo, 33006 Oviedo, Spain
INRA, Institut Micalis, Équipe Peptides et Communication Bactérienne, Domaine de Vilvert, bâtiment 526, 78352 Jouy-en-Josas cedex, France

Esther Gómez
Área de Microbiología, Departamento de Biología Funcional, Facultad de Medicina, IUBA, Universidad de Oviedo, 33006 Oviedo, Spain

José A Guijarro
Área de Microbiología, Departamento de Biología Funcional, Facultad de Medicina, IUBA, Universidad de Oviedo, 33006 Oviedo, Spain

Scott J Weese
Department of Pathobiology, University of Guelph, Guelph, Canada

Jamieson Nichols
Department of Veterinary Clinical Sciences, Purdue University, 625 Harrison St., West Lafayette, IN 47907, USA

Mohammad Jalali
Department of Pathobiology, University of Guelph, Guelph, Canada

Annette Litster
Department of Veterinary Clinical Sciences, Purdue University, 625 Harrison St., West Lafayette, IN 47907, USA

Gry M Grøneng
Norwegian Veterinary Institute, P.O. Box 750 Sentrum, NO-0106 Oslo, Norway

Synnøve Vatn
Animalia - Norwegian Meat and Poultry Research Centre, P.O. Box 396 Løren, NO-0513 Oslo, Norway

Anja Bråthen Kristoffersen
Norwegian Veterinary Institute, P.O. Box 750 Sentrum, NO-0106 Oslo, Norway

Ola Nafstad
Animalia - Norwegian Meat and Poultry Research Centre, P.O. Box 396 Løren, NO-0513 Oslo, Norway

Petter Hopp
Norwegian Veterinary Institute, P.O. Box 750 Sentrum, NO-0106 Oslo, Norway

David Arranz-Solís
SALUVET, Animal Health Department, Faculty of Veterinary Sciences, Complutense University of Madrid, Ciudad Universitaria s/n, 28040 Madrid, Spain

Julio Benavides
Livestock Health and Production Institute (ULE-CSIC), 24346 León, Spain

Javier Regidor-Cerrillo
SALUVET, Animal Health Department, Faculty of Veterinary Sciences, Complutense University of Madrid, Ciudad Universitaria s/n, 28040 Madrid, Spain

Miguel Fuertes
Livestock Health and Production Institute (ULE-CSIC), 24346 León, Spain

Ignacio Ferre
SALUVET, Animal Health Department, Faculty of Veterinary Sciences, Complutense University of Madrid, Ciudad Universitaria s/n, 28040 Madrid, Spain

Maria del Carmen Ferreras
Livestock Health and Production Institute (ULE-CSIC), 24346 León, Spain

Esther Collantes-Fernández
SALUVET, Animal Health Department, Faculty of Veterinary Sciences, Complutense University of Madrid, Ciudad Universitaria s/n, 28040 Madrid, Spain

Andrew Hemphill
Institute of Parasitology, Vetsuisse Faculty, University of Bern, CH-3012 Bern, Switzerland

Valentín Pérez
Livestock Health and Production Institute (ULE-CSIC), 24346 León, Spain

Luis Miguel Ortega-Mora
SALUVET, Animal Health Department, Faculty of Veterinary Sciences, Complutense University of Madrid, Ciudad Universitaria s/n, 28040 Madrid, Spain

Ilias S Frydas
Laboratory of Virology, Department of Virology, Immunology and Parasitology, Faculty of Veterinary Medicine, Ghent University, Salisburylaan 133, B-9820 Merelbeke, Ghent, Belgium

Ivan Trus
Laboratory of Virology, Department of Virology, Immunology and Parasitology, Faculty of Veterinary Medicine, Ghent University, Salisburylaan 133, B-9820 Merelbeke, Ghent, Belgium

Lise K Kvisgaard
National Veterinary Institute, Technical University of Denmark, Frederiksberg C, Denmark

Caroline Bonckaert
Laboratory of Virology, Department of Virology, Immunology and Parasitology, Faculty of Veterinary Medicine, Ghent University, Salisburylaan 133, B-9820 Merelbeke, Ghent, Belgium

Vishwanatha RAP Reddy
Laboratory of Virology, Department of Virology, Immunology and Parasitology, Faculty of Veterinary Medicine, Ghent University, Salisburylaan 133, B-9820 Merelbeke, Ghent, Belgium

Yewei Li
Laboratory of Virology, Department of Virology, Immunology and Parasitology, Faculty of Veterinary Medicine, Ghent University, Salisburylaan 133, B-9820 Merelbeke, Ghent, Belgium

Lars E Larsen
National Veterinary Institute, Technical University of Denmark, Frederiksberg C, Denmark

Hans J Nauwynck
Laboratory of Virology, Department of Virology, Immunology and Parasitology, Faculty of Veterinary Medicine, Ghent University, Salisburylaan 133, B-9820 Merelbeke, Ghent, Belgium

Øystein Wessel
Department of Food Safety and Infection Biology, Norwegian University of Life Sciences, Oslo, Norway

Christel Moræus Olsen
Department of Food Safety and Infection Biology, Norwegian University of Life Sciences, Oslo, Norway

Espen Rimstad
Department of Food Safety and Infection Biology, Norwegian University of Life Sciences, Oslo, Norway

Maria Krudtaa Dahle
Section of Immunology, Norwegian Veterinary Institute, Oslo, Norway

Kristof Moonens
Structural & Molecular Microbiology, Structural Biology Research Center, VIB,

Brussels, Belgium
Structural Biology Brussels, Vrije Universiteit Brussel, Pleinlaan 2, 1050 Brussels, Belgium
College of Veterinary Medicine, Animal Resources and Bio-security, Makerere University, P.O. Box 7062, Kampala, Uganda

Imke Van den Broeck
Structural & Molecular Microbiology, Structural Biology Research Center, VIB,

Brussels, Belgium
Structural Biology Brussels, Vrije Universiteit Brussel, Pleinlaan 2, 1050 Brussels, Belgium

Emmanuel Okello
Structural & Molecular Microbiology, Structural Biology Research Center, VIB,

Brussels, Belgium
Structural Biology Brussels, Vrije Universiteit Brussel, Pleinlaan 2, 1050 Brussels, Belgium
College of Veterinary Medicine, Animal Resources and Bio-security, Makerere University, P.O. Box 7062, Kampala, Uganda

Els Pardon
Structural Biology Brussels, Vrije Universiteit Brussel, Pleinlaan 2, 1050 Brussels, Belgium

Maia De Kerpel
Structural & Molecular Microbiology, Structural Biology Research Center, VIB,

Brussels, Belgium
Structural Biology Brussels, Vrije Universiteit Brussel, Pleinlaan 2, 1050 Brussels, Belgium

Han Remaut
Structural & Molecular Microbiology, Structural Biology Research Center, VIB,

Brussels, Belgium
Structural Biology Brussels, Vrije Universiteit Brussel, Pleinlaan 2, 1050 Brussels, Belgium

Henri De Greve
Structural & Molecular Microbiology, Structural Biology Research Center, VIB,

Brussels, Belgium
Structural Biology Brussels, Vrije Universiteit Brussel, Pleinlaan 2, 1050 Brussels, Belgium

Chaoqun Yao
Department of Biomedical Sciences, Ross University School of Veterinary Medicine, P.O. Box 334, Basseterre, St. Kitts, West Indies

One Health Center for Zoonoses and Tropical Veterinary Medicine, Ross University School of Veterinary Medicine, P.O. Box 334, Basseterre, St. Kitts, West Indies

Liza S Köster
Department of Clinical Sciences, Ross University School of Veterinary Medicine, P.O. Box 334, Basseterre, St. Kitts, West Indies
One Health Center for Zoonoses and Tropical Veterinary Medicine, Ross University School of Veterinary Medicine, P.O. Box 334, Basseterre, St. Kitts, West Indies

Kerstin Wernike
Institute of Diagnostic Virology, Friedrich-Loeffler-Institut (FLI), Suedufer 10, 17493 Greifswald - Insel Riems, Germany

Emiliana Brocchi
Istituto Zooprofilattico Sperimentale della Lombardia e dell'Emilia Romagna, Via Bianchi 7, 25125 Brescia, Italy

Paolo Cordioli
Istituto Zooprofilattico Sperimentale della Lombardia e dell'Emilia Romagna, Via Bianchi 7, 25125 Brescia, Italy

Yann Sénéchal
IDEXX Switzerland AG, Stationsstrasse 12, 3097 Liebefeld-Bern, Switzerland

Christian Schelp
IDEXX Switzerland AG, Stationsstrasse 12, 3097 Liebefeld-Bern, Switzerland

Anne Wegelt
Institute of Diagnostic Virology, Friedrich-Loeffler-Institut (FLI), Suedufer 10, 17493 Greifswald - Insel Riems, Germany

Andrea Aebischer
Institute of Diagnostic Virology, Friedrich-Loeffler-Institut (FLI), Suedufer 10, 17493 Greifswald - Insel Riems, Germany

Gleyder Roman-Sosa
Institute of Diagnostic Virology, Friedrich-Loeffler-Institut (FLI), Suedufer 10, 17493 Greifswald - Insel Riems, Germany

Ilona Reimann
Institute of Diagnostic Virology, Friedrich-Loeffler-Institut (FLI), Suedufer 10, 17493 Greifswald - Insel Riems, Germany

Martin Beer
Institute of Diagnostic Virology, Friedrich-Loeffler-Institut (FLI), Suedufer 10, 17493 Greifswald - Insel Riems, Germany

Antonio Lavazza
IZSLER, Istituto Zooprofilattico Sperimentale della Lombardia e dell'Emilia Romagna "Bruno Ubertini", Via Bianchi 7/9, 25124 Brescia, Italy
OIE Reference Laboratory for Rabbit Haemorrhagic Disease at IZSLER Via Bianchi 7/9, 25124 Brescia, Italy

Patrizia Cavadini
IZSLER, Istituto Zooprofilattico Sperimentale della Lombardia e dell'Emilia Romagna "Bruno Ubertini", Via Bianchi 7/9, 25124 Brescia, Italy
OIE Reference Laboratory for Rabbit Haemorrhagic Disease at IZSLER Via Bianchi 7/9, 25124 Brescia, Italy

Ilaria Barbieri
IZSLER, Istituto Zooprofilattico Sperimentale della Lombardia e dell'Emilia Romagna "Bruno Ubertini", Via Bianchi 7/9, 25124 Brescia, Italy

Paolo Tizzani
Dipartimento di Produzioni Animali, Epidemiologia ed Ecologia, Università degli Studi di Torino, Via Nizza 52, 10126 Torino, Italy

Ana Pinheiro
CIBIO-UP, Centro de Investigação em Biodiversidade e Recursos Genéticos Universidade do Porto, InBio, Laboratório Associado, Campus Agrário de Vairão, Vairão, Portugal
Departamento de Biologia, Faculdade de Ciencias, Universidade do Porto, Porto, Portugal
SaBio - Instituto de Investigacion en Recursos Cinegeticos (CSIC-UCLM-JCCM), Ciudad Real, Spain

Joana Abrantes
CIBIO-UP, Centro de Investigação em Biodiversidade e Recursos Genéticos Universidade do Porto, InBio, Laboratório Associado, Campus Agrário de Vairão, Vairão, Portugal
INSERM, U892, Universite de Nantes, 44007 Nantes, France

Pedro J Esteves
CIBIO-UP, Centro de Investigação em Biodiversidade e Recursos Genéticos Universidade do Porto, InBio, Laboratório Associado, Campus Agrário de Vairão, Vairão, Portugal
CESPU, Instituto de Investigação e Formação Avançada em Ciências e Tecnologias da Saúde, 4585-116 Gandra, Portugal

Guido Grilli
Dipartimento di Scienze Veterinarie e Sanità Pubblica (DIVET), Università degli Studi di Milano, Via Celoria 10, 20133 Milan, Italy

Emanuela Gioia
Veterinary Practitioner, Via Negri 26, 29122 Piacenza, Italy

Mariagrazia Zanoni
IZSLER, Istituto Zooprofilattico Sperimentale della Lombardia e dell'Emilia Romagna "Bruno Ubertini", Via Bianchi 7/9, 25124 Brescia, Italy

Pier Giuseppe Meneguz
Dipartimento di Produzioni Animali, Epidemiologia ed Ecologia, Università degli Studi di Torino, Via Nizza 52, 10126 Torino, Italy

Jean-Sébastien Guitton
ONCFS, National Hunting and Wildlife Agency, Department of Studies and Research, CS 42355, 44323 Nantes, Cedex 3, France

Stéphane Marchandeau
ONCFS, National Hunting and Wildlife Agency, Department of Studies and Research, CS 42355, 44323 Nantes, Cedex 3, France

Mario Chiari
IZSLER, Istituto Zooprofilattico Sperimentale della Lombardia e dell'Emilia Romagna "Bruno Ubertini", Via Bianchi 7/9, 25124 Brescia, Italy

Lorenzo Capucci
IZSLER, Istituto Zooprofilattico Sperimentale della Lombardia e dell'Emilia Romagna "Bruno Ubertini", Via Bianchi 7/9, 25124 Brescia, Italy
7OIE Reference Laboratory for Rabbit Haemorrhagic Disease at IZSLER Via Bianchi 7/9, 25124 Brescia, Italy

Aurora Romero Tejeda
Istituto Zooprofilattico Sperimentale delle Venezie (IZSVe), OIE/FAO and National Reference Laboratory for Newcastle Disease and Avian Influenza, OIE Collaborating Centre for Infectious Diseases at the Human-Animal Interface, Viale dell'Università 10, Legnaro, 35020 Padova, Italy

Roberta Aiello
Istituto Zooprofilattico Sperimentale delle Venezie (IZSVe), OIE/FAO and National Reference Laboratory for Newcastle Disease and Avian Influenza, OIE Collaborating Centre for Infectious Diseases at the Human-Animal Interface, Viale dell'Università 10, Legnaro, 35020 Padova, Italy

Angela Salomoni
Istituto Zooprofilattico Sperimentale delle Venezie (IZSVe), OIE/FAO and National Reference Laboratory for Newcastle Disease and Avian Influenza, OIE Collaborating Centre for Infectious Diseases at the Human-Animal Interface, Viale dell'Università 10, Legnaro, 35020 Padova, Italy

Valeria Berton
Istituto Zooprofilattico Sperimentale delle Venezie (IZSVe), OIE/FAO and National Reference Laboratory for Newcastle Disease and Avian Influenza, OIE Collaborating Centre for Infectious Diseases at the Human-Animal Interface, Viale dell'Università 10, Legnaro, 35020 Padova, Italy

Marta Vascellari
Histopathology Laboratory, IZSVe, Viale dell'Università 10, Legnaro, 35020 Padova, Italy

Giovanni Cattoli
Istituto Zooprofilattico Sperimentale delle Venezie (IZSVe), OIE/FAO and National Reference Laboratory for Newcastle Disease and Avian Influenza, OIE Collaborating Centre for Infectious Diseases at the Human-Animal Interface, Viale dell'Università 10, Legnaro, 35020 Padova, Italy

Fernando Núñez-Hernández
Centre de Recerca en Sanitat Animal (CReSA), UAB-IRTA, Campus de la Universitat Autònoma de Barcelona, Bellaterra, Cerdanyola del Vallès, Spain

Lester J Pérez
Centro Nacional de Sanidad Agropecuaria (CENSA), La Habana, Cuba

Gonzalo Vera
Departament de Genètica Animal, Centre de Recerca en AgriGenòmica (CRAG), CSIC-IRTA-UAB-UB, Universitat Autònoma de Barcelona, Barcelona, Bellaterra, Spain

Sarai Córdoba
Departament de Genètica Animal, Centre de Recerca en AgriGenòmica (CRAG), CSIC-IRTA-UAB-UB, Universitat Autònoma de Barcelona, Barcelona, Bellaterra, Spain

Joaquim Segalés
Departament de Sanitat i Anatomia Animals, Universitat Autònoma de Barcelona, Barcelona, Bellaterra, Spain

Armand Sánchez
Departament de Genètica Animal, Centre de Recerca en AgriGenòmica (CRAG), CSIC-IRTA-UAB-UB, Universitat Autònoma de Barcelona, Barcelona, Bellaterra, Spain
Departament de Ciència Animal i dels Aliments, Universitat Autònoma de Barcelona (UAB), Barcelona, Bellaterra, Spain

José I Núñez
Centre de Recerca en Sanitat Animal (CReSA), UAB-IRTA, Campus de la Universitat Autònoma de Barcelona, Bellaterra, Cerdanyola del Vallès, Spain

Kimberly Crawford
National Animal Disease Center, United States Department of Agriculture-Agricultural Research Services, Ames, IA, USA

Kelly Lager
National Animal Disease Center, United States Department of Agriculture-Agricultural Research Services, Ames, IA, USA

Laura Miller
National Animal Disease Center, United States Department of Agriculture-Agricultural Research Services, Ames, IA, USA

Tanja Opriessnig
Veterinary Diagnostic and Production Animal Medicine, Iowa State University College of Veterinary Medicine, Ames, IA, USA
The Roslin Institute, University of Edinburgh, Midlothian, UK

Priscilla Gerber
Veterinary Diagnostic and Production Animal Medicine, Iowa State University College of Veterinary Medicine, Ames, IA, USA
The Roslin Institute, University of Edinburgh, Midlothian, UK

Richard Hesse
Diagnostic Medicine/Pathobiology, College of Veterinary Medicine, Kansas State University, Manhattan, KS, USA

Stephanie C Talker
Institute of Immunology, Department of Pathobiology, University of Veterinary Medicine, Vienna, Austria

Hanna C Koinig
Institute of Immunology, Department of Pathobiology, University of Veterinary Medicine, Vienna, Austria
University Clinic for Swine, Department for Farm Animals and Veterinary Public Health, University of Veterinary Medicine, Vienna, Austria

Maria Stadler
Institute of Immunology, Department of Pathobiology, University of Veterinary Medicine, Vienna, Austria

Robert Graage
University Clinic for Swine, Department for Farm Animals and Veterinary Public Health, University of Veterinary Medicine, Vienna, Austria
Institute of Veterinary Pathology, Vetsuisse-Faculty, University of Zurich, Zurich, Switzerland

Eva Klingler
University Clinic for Swine, Department for Farm Animals and Veterinary Public Health, University of Veterinary Medicine, Vienna, Austria

Andrea Ladinig
University Clinic for Swine, Department for Farm Animals and Veterinary Public Health, University of Veterinary Medicine, Vienna, Austria

Kerstin H Mair
Institute of Immunology, Department of Pathobiology, University of Veterinary Medicine, Vienna, Austria

Sabine E Hammer
Institute of Immunology, Department of Pathobiology, University of Veterinary Medicine, Vienna, Austria

Herbert Weissenböck
Institute of Pathology and Forensic Veterinary Medicine, Department of Pathobiology, University of Veterinary Medicine, Vienna, Austria

Ralf Dürrwald
Viral Vaccines, Business Unit Animal Health, IDT Biologika GmbH, Dessau-Rosslau, Germany

Mathias Ritzmann
University Clinic for Swine, Department for Farm Animals and Veterinary Public Health, University of Veterinary Medicine, Vienna, Austria
Clinic for Swine, Ludwig-Maximilians-University, Munich, Germany

Armin Saalmüller
Institute of Immunology, Department of Pathobiology, University of Veterinary Medicine, Vienna, Austria

Wilhelm Gerner
Institute of Immunology, Department of Pathobiology, University of Veterinary Medicine, Vienna, Austria

Linda Frellstedt
Center of Equine Sports Medicine, University of Liege, Liege, Belgium
CIRALE, École Nationale Vétérinaire de Maisons-Alfort, Goustranville, France

Philippe Gosset
Institut Pasteur de Lille, Centre d'Infection et d'Immunité de Lille, Lille, France
Université Lille Nord de France, Lille, France
Centre National de la Recherche Scientifique, UMR8204 Lille, France
Institut National de la Santé et de la Recherche Médicale, U1019 Lille, France
Institut Fédératif de Recherche 142, Lille, France

Gwenola Kervoaze
Institut Pasteur de Lille, Centre d'Infection et d'Immunité de Lille, Lille, France
Université Lille Nord de France, Lille, France
Centre National de la Recherche Scientifique, UMR8204 Lille, France

Institut National de la Santé et de la Recherche Médicale, U1019 Lille, France
Institut Fédératif de Recherche 142, Lille, France

Aymeric Hans
Anses - Dozulé, Equine Pathology Laboratory, Virology Unit, Goustranville, France

Christophe Desmet
Laboratory of Cellular and Molecular Immunology, GIGA-Research, University of Liege, Liege, Belgium

Dimitri Pirottin
Laboratory of Cellular and Molecular Immunology, GIGA-Research, University of Liege, Liege, Belgium

Fabrice Bureau
Laboratory of Cellular and Molecular Immunology, GIGA-Research, University of Liege, Liege, Belgium

Pierre Lekeux
Center of Equine Sports Medicine, University of Liege, Liege, Belgium

Tatiana Art
Center of Equine Sports Medicine, University of Liege, Liege, Belgium

Jing Lv
College of Animal Science and Veterinary Medicine, Shandong Agricultural University; Sino-German Cooperative Research Centre for Zoonosis of Animal Origin Shandong Province; Key Laboratory of Animal Biotechnology and Disease Control and Prevention of Shandong Province, Shandong Agricultural University, Daizong Street 61, Taian 271018, China
Taian Municipal Center for Disease Control and Prevention, Changcheng Street, Taian 271000, China
College of Life Science, Shandong Agricultural University, Taian 271018, China

Liangmeng Wei
College of Animal Science and Veterinary Medicine, Shandong Agricultural University; Sino-German Cooperative Research Centre for Zoonosis of Animal Origin Shandong Province; Key Laboratory of Animal Biotechnology and Disease Control and Prevention of Shandong Province, Shandong Agricultural University, Daizong Street 61, Taian 271018, China

Yan Yang
College of Animal Science and Veterinary Medicine, Shandong Agricultural University; Sino-German Cooperative Research Centre for Zoonosis of Animal Origin Shandong Province; Key Laboratory of Animal Biotechnology and Disease Control and Prevention of Shandong Province, Shandong Agricultural University, Daizong Street 61, Taian 271018, China

Bingxiao Wang
Qingdao Chia Tai Co., Ltd, Qingwei Street, Qingdao 266109, China

Wei Liang
College of Animal Science and Veterinary Medicine, Shandong Agricultural University; Sino-German Cooperative Research Centre for Zoonosis of Animal Origin Shandong Province; Key Laboratory of Animal Biotechnology and Disease Control and Prevention of Shandong Province, Shandong Agricultural University, Daizong Street 61, Taian 271018, China

Yuwei Gao
Institute of Military Veterinary PLA, Qinglong Street 1068, Changchun 130000, China

Xianzhu Xia
Institute of Military Veterinary PLA, Qinglong Street 1068, Changchun 130000, China

Lili Gao
College of Animal Science and Veterinary Medicine, Shandong Agricultural University; Sino-German Cooperative Research Centre for Zoonosis of Animal Origin Shandong Province; Key Laboratory of Animal Biotechnology and Disease Control and Prevention of Shandong Province, Shandong Agricultural University, Daizong Street 61, Taian 271018, China

Yumei Cai
College of Animal Science and Veterinary Medicine, Shandong Agricultural University; Sino-German Cooperative Research Centre for Zoonosis of Animal Origin Shandong Province; Key Laboratory of Animal Biotechnology and Disease Control and Prevention of Shandong Province, Shandong Agricultural University, Daizong Street 61, Taian 271018, China

Peiqiang Hou
Taian Municipal Center for Disease Control and Prevention, Changcheng Street, Taian 271000, China

Huili Yang
Taian Municipal Center for Disease Control and Prevention, Changcheng Street, Taian 271000, China

Airong Wang
College of Animal Science and Veterinary Medicine, Shandong Agricultural University; Sino-German Cooperative Research Centre for Zoonosis of Animal Origin Shandong Province; Key Laboratory of Animal Biotechnology and Disease Control and Prevention of Shandong Province, Shandong Agricultural University, Daizong Street 61, Taian 271018, China

Rong Huang
College of Animal Science and Veterinary Medicine, Shandong Agricultural University; Sino-German Cooperative Research Centre for Zoonosis of Animal Origin Shandong Province; Key Laboratory of Animal Biotechnology and Disease Control and Prevention of Shandong Province, Shandong Agricultural University, Daizong Street 61, Taian 271018, China

Jing Gao
College of Animal Science and Veterinary Medicine, Shandong Agricultural University; Sino-German Cooperative Research Centre for Zoonosis of Animal Origin Shandong Province; Key Laboratory of Animal Biotechnology and Disease Control and Prevention of Shandong Province, Shandong Agricultural University, Daizong Street 61, Taian 271018, China
School of dentistry and oral health Taishan Medical University, Tai'an 271000, China

Tongjie Chai
College of Animal Science and Veterinary Medicine, Shandong Agricultural University; Sino-German Cooperative Research Centre for Zoonosis of Animal Origin Shandong Province; Key Laboratory of Animal Biotechnology and Disease Control and Prevention of Shandong Province, Shandong Agricultural University, Daizong Street 61, Taian 271018, China

Judith MA van den Brand
Department of Viroscience, Erasmus Medical Center, Dr. Molewaterplein 50, 3015 GE Rotterdam, Netherlands

Oliver Krone
Department Wildlife Diseases, Leibniz Institute for Zoo and Wildlife Research, Alfred-Kowalke-Straße 17, 10315 Berlin, Germany

Peter U Wolf
Department for Diagnostic Investigation of Epizootics (LALLF), State Office for Agriculture, Food Safety, and Fishery, Mecklenburg-Western Pomerania, Rostock, Germany

Marco WG van de Bildt
Department of Viroscience, Erasmus Medical Center, Dr. Molewaterplein 50, 3015 GE Rotterdam, Netherlands

Geert van Amerongen
Department of Viroscience, Erasmus Medical Center, Dr. Molewaterplein 50, 3015 GE Rotterdam, Netherlands

Albert DME Osterhaus
Department of Viroscience, Erasmus Medical Center, Dr. Molewaterplein 50, 3015 GE Rotterdam, Netherlands

Thijs Kuiken
Department of Viroscience, Erasmus Medical Center, Dr. Molewaterplein 50, 3015 GE Rotterdam, Netherlands

Carla Bravo de Rueda
Central Veterinary Institute (CVI), part of Wageningen UR, P.O. Box 65, 8200 AB Lelystad, The Netherlands

Mart CM de Jong
Department Quantitative Veterinary Epidemiology, Wageningen University, P.O. Box 338, 6700 AH Wageningen, The Netherlands

Phaedra L Eblé
Central Veterinary Institute (CVI), part of Wageningen UR, P.O. Box 65, 8200 AB Lelystad, The Netherlands

Aldo Dekker
Central Veterinary Institute (CVI), part of Wageningen UR, P.O. Box 65, 8200 AB Lelystad, The Netherlands

Tamer A Sharafeldin
Department of Veterinary Population Medicine and Minnesota Veterinary Diagnostic Laboratory, University of Minnesota, St. Paul, MN 55108, USA
Pathology Department, Faculty of Veterinary Medicine, Zagazig University, Zagazig 44519, Egypt

Sunil K Mor
Department of Veterinary Population Medicine and Minnesota Veterinary Diagnostic Laboratory, University of Minnesota, St. Paul, MN 55108, USA

Aschalew Z Bekele
Department of Veterinary Population Medicine and Minnesota Veterinary Diagnostic Laboratory, University of Minnesota, St. Paul, MN 55108, USA

Harsha Verma
Department of Veterinary Population Medicine and Minnesota Veterinary Diagnostic Laboratory, University of Minnesota, St. Paul, MN 55108, USA

Sally L Noll
Department of Animal Science, University of Minnesota, St. Paul, MN 55108, USA

Sagar M Goyal
Department of Veterinary Population Medicine and Minnesota Veterinary Diagnostic Laboratory, University of Minnesota, St. Paul, MN 55108, USA

Robert E Porter
Department of Veterinary Population Medicine and Minnesota Veterinary Diagnostic Laboratory, University of Minnesota, St. Paul, MN 55108, USA

Rachel E Pritchard
Department of Microbiology, Miami University, Oxford, OH 45056, USA
Present address: Division of Natural Sciences and Mathematics, Kentucky Wesleyan College, Owensboro, KY 42301, USA

Mitchell F Balish
Department of Microbiology, Miami University, Oxford, OH 45056, USA

Obdulio García-Nicolás
Department of Anatomy and Comparative Pathology, Faculty of Veterinary
Medicine, Murcia University, "Mare Nostrum Excellence Campus - 3738",30100 Murcia, Spain

Rubén S Rosales
Department of Bacteriology, Animal and Plant Health Agency, Addlestone, Surrey KT15 3NB, UK

Francisco J Pallarés
Department of Anatomy and Comparative Pathology, Faculty of Veterinary
Medicine, Murcia University, "Mare Nostrum Excellence Campus - 3738",30100 Murcia, Spain

David Risco
Red de Grupos de Investigación Recursos Faunísticos, Facultad de Veterinaria, Universidad de Extremadura, 10003 Cáceres, Spain

Juan J Quereda
Spanish National Center of Biotechnology (CSIC), C/ Darwin 3, Campus de Cantoblanco, 28049 Madrid, Spain

Simon P Graham
Department of Virology, Animal and Plant Health Agency, Addlestone, Surrey KT15 3NB, UK

Jean-Pierre Frossard
Department of Virology, Animal and Plant Health Agency, Addlestone, Surrey KT15 3NB, UK

Sophie B Morgan
Department of Virology, Animal and Plant Health Agency, Addlestone, Surrey KT15 3NB, UK

Falko Steinbach
Department of Virology, Animal and Plant Health Agency, Addlestone, Surrey KT15 3NB, UK

Trevor W Drew
Department of Virology, Animal and Plant Health Agency, Addlestone, Surrey KT15 3NB, UK

Tony S Strickland
Department of Pathology, Animal and Plant Health Agency, Addlestone KT15 3NB, UK

Francisco J Salguero
Department of Pathology, Animal and Plant Health Agency, Addlestone KT15 3NB, UK
Department of Pathology and Infectious Diseases, School of Veterinary Medicine, University of Surrey, Guildford GU2 7TE, UK

Tamara Muñoz-Caro
Institute of Parasitology, Justus Liebig University Giessen, Schubertstraße 81,35392 Giessen, Germany

Sandra Jaqueline Mena Huertas
Laboratory of Inflammation Pharmacology, Institute of Pharmacology and Morphophysiology, Faculty of Veterinary Science, Austral University of Chile, Valdivia 5110566, Chile
Department of Biology, University of Nariño, Pasto 520002, Colombia

Ivan Conejeros
Laboratory of Inflammation Pharmacology, Institute of Pharmacology and Morphophysiology, Faculty of Veterinary Science, Austral University of Chile, Valdivia 5110566, Chile

Pablo Alarcón
Laboratory of Inflammation Pharmacology, Institute of Pharmacology and Morphophysiology, Faculty of Veterinary Science, Austral University of Chile, Valdivia 5110566, Chile

María A Hidalgo
Laboratory of Inflammation Pharmacology, Institute of Pharmacology and Morphophysiology, Faculty of Veterinary Science, Austral University of Chile, Valdivia 5110566, Chile

Rafael A Burgos
Laboratory of Inflammation Pharmacology, Institute of Pharmacology and Morphophysiology, Faculty of Veterinary Science, Austral University of Chile, Valdivia 5110566, Chile

Carlos Hermosilla
Institute of Parasitology, Justus Liebig University Giessen, Schubertstraße 81,35392 Giessen, Germany

Anja Taubert
Institute of Parasitology, Justus Liebig University Giessen, Schubertstraße 81,35392 Giessen, Germany

Bruce C McGorum
Royal (Dick) School of Veterinary Studies and Roslin Institute, University of Edinburgh, Roslin EH25 9RG, Scotland, UK

R Scott Pirie
Royal (Dick) School of Veterinary Studies and Roslin Institute, University of Edinburgh, Roslin EH25 9RG, Scotland, UK

Laura Glendinning
Royal (Dick) School of Veterinary Studies and Roslin Institute, University of Edinburgh, Roslin EH25 9RG, Scotland, UK

Gerry McLachlan
Royal (Dick) School of Veterinary Studies and Roslin Institute, University of Edinburgh, Roslin EH25 9RG, Scotland, UK

James S Metcalf
The Institute for Ethnomedicine, 240 East Deloney Avenue, Jackson, WY 83001-3464, USA

Sandra A Banack
The Institute for Ethnomedicine, 240 East Deloney Avenue, Jackson, WY 83001-3464, USA

Paul A Cox
The Institute for Ethnomedicine, 240 East Deloney Avenue, Jackson, WY 83001-3464, USA

Geoffrey A Codd
Biological and Environmental Sciences, School of Natural Sciences, University of Stirling, Stirling FK9 4LA, Scotland, UK